LOCAL INVASION AND SPREAD OF CANCER

Cancer Growth and Progression

SERIES EDITOR: HANS E. KAISER
Department of Pathology, University of Maryland, Baltimore, Md, U.S.A.

Scientific Advisors:
Kenneth W. Brunson / Harvey A. Gilbert / Ronald H. Goldfarb / Alfred L. Goldson / Elizier Gorelik / Anton Gregl / Ronald B. Herberman / James F. Holland / Ernst H. Krokowski[†] / Arthur S. Levine / Annabel G. Liebelt / Lance A. Liotta / Seoras D. Morrison / Takao Ohnuma / Richard L. Schilsky / Harold L. Stewart / Jerome A. Urban / Elizabeth K. Weisburger / Paul V. Woolley

Volume 1: Fundamental Aspects of Cancer
Volume Editor: Ronald H. Goldfarb
ISBN 0-89838-990-9

Volume 2: Mechanisms of Carcinogenesis
Volume Editor: Elizabeth K. Weisburger
ISBN 0-89838-991-7

Volume 3: Influence of Tumor Development on the Host
Volume Editor: Lance A. Liotta
ISBN 0-89838-992-5

Volume 4: Influence of the Host on Tumor Development
Volume Editor: Ronald B. Herberman
ISBN 0-89838-993-3

Volume 5: Comparative Aspects of Tumor Development
Volume Editor: Hans E. Kaiser
ISBN 0-89838-994-1

Volume 6: Etiology of Cancer in Man
Volume Editor: Arthur S. Levine
ISBN 0-89838-995-X

Volume 7: Local Invasion and Spread of Cancer
Volume Editor: Kenneth W. Brunson
ISBN 0-89838-996-8

Volume 8: Metastasis / Dissemination
Volume Editor: Elizier L. Gorelik
ISBN 0-89838-997-6

Volume 9: Cancer Management in Man: Detection, Diagnosis, Surgery, Radiology, Chronobiology, Endocrine Therapy
Volume Editor: Alfred L. Goldson
ISBN 0-89838-998-4

Volume 10: Cancer Management in Man: Biological Response Modifiers, Chemotherapy, Antibiotics, Hyperthermia, Supporting Measures
Volume Editor: Paul V. Woolley
ISBN 0-89838-999-2

Complete set: ISBN 0-89838-989-5

Local Invasion
and
Spread of Cancer

Edited by

KENNETH W. BRUNSON

Department of Immunology and Infectious Diseases
Pfizer Central Research, Groton, Conn., U.S.A.

Kluwer Academic Publishers

DORDRECHT / BOSTON / LONDON

Library of Congress Cataloging in Publication Data
Local invasion and spead of cancer / edited by Kenneth W. Brunson.
        p.   cm. -- (Cancer growth and progression ; v. 7)
    Includes index.
    ISBN-13:978-94-010-6982-3   e-ISBN-13:978-94-009-1093-5
    DOI:10.1007/978-94-009-1093-5

    1. Cancer invasiveness.   I. Brunson, Kenneth W.   II. Series.
    [DNLM: 1. Neoplasm Invasiveness. 2. Neoplasm Metastasis.   QZ 200
C2151518 v. 7]
RC268.5.L63 1988
616.99'407--dc19
DNLM/DLC
for Library of Congress   88-8822
ISBN-13:978-94-010-6982-3   CIP

Published by Kluwer Academic Publishers,
P.O. Box 17, 3300 AA Dordrecht, The Netherlands.

Kluwer Academic Publishers incorporates
the publishing programmes of
Martinus Nijhoff, Dr W. Junk, D. Reidel, and MTP Press.

Sold and distributed in the U.S.A. and Canada
by Kluwer Academic Publishers,
101 Philip Drive, Norwell, MA 02061, U.S.A.

In all other countries, sold and distributed
by Kluwer Academic Publishers Group,
P.O. Box 322, 3300 AH Dordrecht, The Netherlands.

Cover design by Jos Vrolijk.

TABLE OF CONTENTS

Introduction vii

List of Contributors ix

1. Characteristics and pattern of direct tumor spreading
   H.E. KAISER 1

2. Comparison of the progression of selected, topographically particular, tumors in the head and neck region
   G. BROICH 17

3. Spreading on the coelomic (peritoneal, pleural and pericardial) surface
   H.E. KAISER 30

4. Spreading by implantation on epithelial surfaces and iatrogenic spreading by implantation
   H.E. KAISER 38

5. Progression of embryonal and mixed neoplasms
   H.E. KAISER 42

6. Multicentric paragangliomas and associated neuroendocrine tumors
   P.M. GRIMLEY 49

7. Rare types of neoplastic progression
   H.E. KAISER 62

8. The occult primary malignancy: Concepts of spread and scheme for evaluation
   J.A. ARCADI and H.A. GILBERT 111

9. Neoplasms of the immune system with involvement of lymphoreticular structures
   H.E. KAISER and J. SUTHERLAND 115

10. Progression of lymphoproliferative disorders and hematologic malignancies
    E.S. GROVES and D.L. LONGO 122

11. Neoplastic progression of the myeloid leukemias
    H.D. PREISLER and A. RAZA 148

12. Systemic mastocytosis
    W.R. HENDERSON and E.Y. CHI 154

13. Histiocytic tumors: Immunologic classification
    S. WATANABE 162

14. Eosinophilic granuloma
    W.R. HENDERSON and E.Y. CHI 172

15. Malignant lymphomas: Immunologic aspects
    S. WATANABE 178

16. Dormancy and local recurrence of neoplasms
    F.E. WHEELOCK and T. OKAYASU 186

17. Local recurrence
    H.E. KAISER 187

18. Effusions
    R.C. ULIRSCH and D.M. GOMEZ 195

19. Infection in the patient with cancer
    S.C. SCHIMPFF 214

20. Effects of cancer chemotherapy on gonadal function
    R.L. SCHILSKY 219

Index of subjects 227

INTRODUCTION

In this volume the process of local invasion and the spread is emphasized. Volumes I–VI have already provided knowledge pertaining to the importance of tumor invasion and metastasis in the morbidity and mortality of human neoplasms.

The characteristics of local, direct tumor spreading at various sites, including head and neck, the coelomic surface, and neuroendocrine tumors are presented. Emphasis is placed on the spreading of neoplasm by implantation on epithelial surfaces, the spread of occult primary malignancies, and rare types of neoplastic progression, as well as neoplasms of the immune system, the progression of lymphoproliferative disorders and hematologic malignancies, myeloid leukemias, histiocytic tumors, eosinophilic granulomas, and systemic mastocytosis.

The exploration of local recurrence of neoplasms, and the relationship of recurrence to tumor dormancy, is reviewed as it relates to local tumor invasion and progression to metastasis. The elucidation of the mechanisms underlying local tumor invasion and tumor recurrence, as well as those maintaining tumor dormancy of local neoplasms or disseminated micrometastases, will not only lead to advances in the early detection and treatment of primary neoplasms but also detection and eradication of disseminated metastatic foci.

Series Editor   Volume Editor
Hans E. Kaiser   Kenneth W. Brunson

ACKNOWLEDGEMENT

Inspiration and encouragement for this wide ranging project on cancer distribution and dissemination from a comparative biological and clinical point of view, was given by my late friend E. H. Krokowski.

Those engaged on the project included 252 scientists, listed as contributors, volume editors and scientific advisors, and a dedicated staff. Special assistance was furnished by J. P. Dickson, J. A. Feulner, and I. Theloe.

I. Bauer, D. L. Fisher, S. Fleishman, K. Joshi, A. M. Lewis, J. Taylor and K. E. Yinug have provided additional assistance.

The firm support of the publisher, especially B. F. Commandeur, is deeply appreciated. The support of the University of Maryland throughout the preparation of the series is acknowledged.

To the completion of this undertaking my wife, Charlotte Kaiser, has devoted her unslagging energy and invaluable support.

CONTRIBUTORS

John A. ARCADI, M.D.
Department of Radiation Oncology
Whittier Presbyterian Hospital
12401 East Washington Boulevard
Whittier, California 90602, USA

Guido BROICH, M.D.
Divisione di Otorinolaringoiatria
Istituti Ospitalieri di Cremona
USSL N. 51, Cremona, Italy

Kenneth W. BRUNSON, Ph.D.
Department of Immunology and Infectious Diseases
Pfizer Central Research
Eastern Point Road
Groton, Connecticut 06340, USA

Emil Y. CHI, M.D.
Department of Pathology
University of Washington
Seattle, Washington 98105, USA

Harvey A. GILBERT, M.D.
Department of Radiation Oncology
Whittier Presbyterian Hospital
12401 East Washington Boulevard
Whittier, California 90602, USA

Dena M. GOMEZ, M.D.
Department of Pathology
University of California, San Francisco,
San Francisco, California 94143, USA

Philip M. GRIMLEY, M.D.
Department of Pathology
Uniformed Services University of the Health Sciences
4301 Jones Bridge Road
Bethesda, Maryland 20814, USA

Eric S. GROVES, Ph.D.
Medicine Branch, National Cancer Institute/NIH
Bethesda, Maryland 20892, USA
Present mailing address: Cetus Corporation
1400 53rd Street
Emeryville, California 94608, USA

William R. HENDERSON, M.D.
Department of Medicine
University of Washington
Seattle, Washington 98905, USA

Hans E. KAISER, D.Sc.
Department of Pathology
School of Medicine
University of Maryland
10 S. Pine Street
Baltimore, Maryland 21201, USA

Dan L. LONGO, M.D.
Biological Response Modifiers Program
National Cancer Institute/NIH
Frederick Cancer Research Facility
Building 567, Room 135
Frederick, Maryland 21701, USA

Takeshi OKAYASU, Ph.D.
Department of Pathology and Laboratory Medicine
Hahnemann University
Philadelphia, Pennsylvania 19102, USA

Harvey D. PREISLER, M.D.
Department of Hematologic Oncology
Roswell Park Memorial Institute
666 Elm Street
Buffalo, New York 14263, USA

Azra RAZA, M.D.
Department of Hematologic Oncology
Roswell Park Memorial Institute
666 Elm Street
Buffalo, New York, 14263, USA

Richard L. SCHILSKY, M.D.
Section of Hematology and Medical Oncology
Blood Center Michael Reese Hospital & Medical Center
Lakeshore Drive at 31st Street,
Chicago, Illinois 60616, USA

Stephen C. SCHIMPFF, M.D.
University of Maryland Medical System
22 S. Greene Street
Baltimore, Maryland 21201, USA

John SUTHERLAND, M.D.
Department of Surgery
University of Arizona
Tuscon, Arizona 85724, USA

Rudolf C. ULIRSCH, M.D.
Hematology Section
Department of Pathology
Loyola University of Chicago Medical Center
Maywood, Illinois 60153, USA
and
Hematology Section
Laboratory Service
Hines Veterans Administration Medical Center
Hines, Illinois
and
Department of Pathology
Uniformed Services University of the Health Sciences
Bethesda, Maryland

Shaw WATANABE, M.D.
National Cancer Center Research Institute
5-1-1, Tsukiji
Chuo-ku, Tokyo 104, Japan

Frederick E. WHEELOCK, M.D., Ph.D.
Department of Pathology
Hahnemann University
Philadelphia, Pennsylvania 19102, USA

CHARACTERISTICS AND PATTERN OF DIRECT TUMOR SPREADING

H.E. KAISER

Malignant neoplastic spread can occur in form of infiltration into the surrounding tissues, even before metastasis appears; the malignant spread may appear in form of metastasis; or malignant neoplastic spread may be by direct extension. In reality, these three modes of tumor progression are in most cases interwoven into each other. Direct spread of neoplasms has been determined as a mode of distribution from malignant tumors. But also venous deposits, as of leiomyoma, can grow independently in veins after the original connections with the primary uterine tumor have been severed. The literature contains approximately 50 cases, three of which extended from the pelvic veins into the right atrium (81). Direct extension is one of the mechanisms of cancer dissemination, either spontaneous or iatrogenic (10). Early stages, and those after settlement in the soil tissue during direct extension, follow along lines of least tissue resistance (11). Our challenge lies in the opportunity to obtain better insight into the mechanisms of direct tumor spreading and metastatic neoplastic spreading, to use this knowledge to curtail tumor spreading (17). Direct tumor spread is also a malignant process, more localized, and strongly influenced by the topography of structures surrounding the primary neoplasm. The direct tumor spread can be considered as tumor-specific, following a specific topographic path. This pattern depends much more on the topographic location of the primary tumor than is the case in distant, metastatic spread. Again, in contrast to metastasis, the potency of direct spreading diminishes as the distance from the primary tumor increases. Direct spreading is more vigorous around the primary tumor, as opposed to metastasis, where distant dissemination exhibits strong aggressiveness. A continued connection with the primary tumor and diminishing aggressiveness in proportion to increasing distance from the primary tumor may be viewed as typical characteristic of direct tumor spreading. Such direct infiltration of neoplasms may take place via (1) tissue spaces; (2) lymph vessels; (3) blood vessels, veins and arteries; (4) nerve pathways; (5) the coelomic cavity; (6) spaces associated with the distribution of fasciae and aponeuroses; (7) cerebrospinal spaces; and (8) epithelial cavities.

The cascade spread of metastases is more common than direct tumor spread in many neoplasms but there are, however, some exceptions, such as in rectal adenocarcinoma (85), or in basal cell cancer of the skin.

RETROGRADE DIRECT SPREAD

Retrograde functional extension of direct spreading occurs if the tumor, as in the case here described, grows from the primary prostatic carcinoma upward along the ureter, with strong involvement of the renal pelvis (68). Retrograde growth is a typical characteristic of direct spreading. A direct-spreading tumor may grow in the nonfunctional direction- as in the above-mentioned case of growth of the prostatic carcinoma to the renal pelvis via the ureter. In a vein, the ureter, or comparable organs, metastatic cells may move only with the bloodstream, lymph stream or flow of urine etc. but not vice versa.

Neoplastic invasion of tissue spaces

Invading neoplastic cells tend to follow the path of least resistance, exploiting spaces between cells, and areas lying between different tissues exhibiting less resistance. The malignant cells intrude first, but not only, in spaces between cells; they also invade the cells themselves (see Chapter 11/Volume I) and later may expand within the primary spaces of intrusion. In this manner such cells may sometimes surround nerves, arteries or veins, appearing as cuff-like bands around the loose connective tissues or spaces associated with these structures. Other anatomical structures constitute natural barriers against tumor spread, such as organ capsules, like those associated with liver and kidney, periosteum around bones, ligaments, tendons, aponeurosis fasciae, and the dermis; a metastatic deposit in the liver may be prevented from continuing its spread outside the liver by the barrier of the organ capsule. Similarly, a tumor developing outside the liver may be prevented from entering the liver by direct growth, again, by virtue of the barrier of the organ capsule. In some instances, regional recurrences of neoplasms may be considered as a delayed direct tumor spreading, occurring along the perineural spaces, as observed in cases of adenoid cystic carcinoma of the minor salivary glands (40). Direct invasion is also seen in noncontiguous primary carcinomas along the fasciae and mesenteric attachments, as evidenced in metastases to the digestive tract (7).

Direct neoplastic expansion (invasion) via the lymphatic system

Direct growth of neoplasms in the lymph vessels was recognized approximately 130 years ago (Klinger, 1857 (33); Waldeyer, 1867 (87); Hoggan, 1878 (26); von Recklinghausen,

---

*References of historically older cases are given in the right hand column of the tables.

K.W. Brunson (ed) Local invasion and spread of cancer.
© 1989, Kluwer Academic Publishers, Dordrecht.

Table 1. Selected cases of tumors with direct spread into or along veins (Historically older cases).

Body region	Primary neoplasm	Vein with tributaries	Case No	Growth		Metastasis	Comments	References
				Intravascular	Extravascular			
Face, oral cavity	Pharyngeal carcinoma	Internal jugular vein and tributaries	1	+		Cervical	Intravascular growth started from metastases	Sick, P. (1864) Virchows Arch. 31, 265
Pharynx	Squamous cell carcinoma of tongue	Jugular and innominate veins	1	+		Cervical, visceral	Growth started from cervical metastasis	Cited after Willis (89) (1973)
	Squamous cell carcinoma of tongue	Both jugular veins	1	+		Visceral		Poland, J. (1885) Trans. Path Soc. Lond. 36, 411
	Cancer of head and neck	Main veins	30	+		25 Cases		Willis, R. (1973) (89)
	Nasopharyngeal carcinoma	Internal jugular vein	11	+		Remote		Teoh, T.B. (1957) J. Path. Bact. 73, 451
Esophagus	Carcinoma	Acygos vein, superior vena cava, right ventricle	1	+				Leichtenstern, O. (1891) Dtsch. med. Wschr. 17, 535
	Carcinoma	Portal vein	1	+		Hepatic	The intravascular spread started from the metastasis	Willis, R. (1973) (89)
	Squamous cell carcinoma	Atrium	1	+				Kajita, M. et al. (1983) Kyobu Geka 36(2):122-6
Stomach	Gastric carcinoma	Gastric, splenic, mesenteric and portal vein	1	+				Späth, E. (1866) Virchows Arch. 35, 432
	Carcinoma	Vena cava, innominate, jugular, subclavian, axillary and cephalic	1	+		Lymph node metastasis in mediastinum	The intravenous spread started from the metastasis	Schlagenhaufer, A. (1909) Verh. dtsch. path. Ges. 13, 219
	Carcinoma	Portal vein	1	+				Worringen, K. (1921) Zbl. allg. Path. u. path. Anat. 32, 366
	Anaplastic adeno-carcinoma of pilorus	Portal branch veins	1	+		Regional lymph glands, bile duct, duodenum, liver, lungs, kidneys, adrenals		Willis, R. (1973) (89)
	Adenocarcinoma	Anterior branch of right main branch of portal vein	1	+		Lymph glands and liver		Willis, R. (1973) (89)
Intestine	Adenocarcinoma	Mesenteric vein	1	+			Colon	Kettle, E.H. (1925) The Pathology of Tumours, London: Lewis
	Rectal carcinoma	Veins	17%/1000 cases	+				Dukes, C.E. (1944) Proc. R. Soc. Med. 37, 131
	Mucoid adenoca. of cecum	Inferior vena cava, right atrium and to left atrium	1	+		No	Tumor emboli in pulmonary arterioles	Attwood, H.D. and Giles, P.F. (1966) J. Path. Bact. 91, 267

Organ	Tumor	No.	+	Vessel	Metastasis	Notes	Reference
Small intestine	Carcinoid tumors	x	+	Small veins		Frequent presence of tumor thrombi	Marangos, G.N. (1931) Beitr. path. Anat. 86, 48
Duodenum	Adenocarcinoma	1	+	Inferior vena cava			Rutishauser E, (1932) Zbl. allg. Path. u. path Anat. 53, 305
Gallbladder	Cancer	1	+	Superior vena cava	Thoracic	Direct spread started from thoracic metastases	West, S. (1986) Trans. path. Soc. Lond. 37, 141
Pancreas	Cancers	x	+	Mesenteric, portal, hepatic and splenic veins		Main veins are often penetrated by pancreatic cancers	Willis, R. (1973) (89)
Liver	Hepatic carcinoma	x	+	Portal and efferent hepatic veins	Intrahepatic and pulmonary	Frequent occurrence	Willis, R. (1973) (89)
	Hepatic carcinoma	1	+	Vena cava inferior into right atrium			Counseller, V.S. and McIndoe, A.H. (1926) Arch. intern. Med. 37, 363
	Hepatic carcinoma	1	+	Vena cava, atrium, azygos vein, superior vena cava, mammary veins, subcutaneous vessels of chest			Lochlein, W. (1907) Beitr. path. Anat. 42, 531
	Hepatoblastoma	2	+	inferior vena cava up to right atrium		Sometimes	Pang, L.S.C. (1961) J. Path. Bact. 82, 273
Breast	Carcinoma	1	+	Subclavian vein, main pulmonary vein	Pulmonary metastases	Invasion of pulmonary vein started from metastasis	Kantorowicz L (1893) Zbl. allg. Path. u. path. Anat. 4, 817
	Carcinoma	x	+	Small veins			Scheel, O. (1906) Beitr. path. Anat., 39, 187
	Carcinoma	1	+	Axillary vein			Newcomb W.D. (1924) Lancet 1, 1056
	Carcinoma	24	+	Blood vessels			van Raamsdonk, W. (1921) Ned. Tijdschr. Geneesk 1, 3355
	Carcinoma	x	+	Small veins		Tumor occlusion	Fraser J. (1927) Surg. Gynec. Obstet. 45, 266
	Carcinoma	x	+	Many small veins		Vessel permeation	Dawson E.K. and Shaw J.J.M. (1937) Br. J. Surg. 25, 100; Willis, R. (1973) p. 10 (89)
Breast	Carcinoma	2	+	Large pulmonary veins	Pulmonary metastases		Seelig, A. (1895) Virchows Arch. 140, 80
	Uterine carcinoma	1	+	Inferior vena cava		Extension into large veins of female genitals; carcinoma is rare	Willis, R. (1973) p. 10 (89)
Uterine carcinoma		11	+	Vessel			Friedell, G.H. & Parsons, L. (1962). Cancer 15, 1269

Table 1. Continued.

Body region	Primary neoplasm	Vein with tributaries	Case No	Growth — Intravascular	Extravascular	Metastasis	Comments	References
	Ovarian carcinoma						Ovarian growth into the bloodstream occurs only occasionally	Beneke, R. (1890) Beitr. path. Anat. 7, 95
	Ovarian carcinoma	Veins of the broad ligament	1	+				
	Ovarian papillary carcinoma	Subclavian vein, superior vena cava, and right atrium	1	+		Direct growth started from metastasis in the neck region		Gibson, H.J.C. & Findlay, G.M. (1923). J. Obstet. Gynaec. Brit. Emp. 30, 204
	Chorionepithelioma						Invasion of blood vessels is common	
Lung	Bronchial carcinoma	Pulmonary veins and main tributaries	x	+			Frequent occurrence	
		Along the lumen of pulmonary veins into left atrium	x	+				Andre (1865). Trans. path. Soc. Lond. 16, 51 Willis, R. (1973) p. 10 (89)
		Innominate veins or superior vena cava into right atrium	x	+				Dana, H.W. & McIntosh, R. (1922) Am. J. Med. Sci. 163, 411
	Lung carcinoma	Main blood vessels	14	+				Willis, R. (1973) p. 10 (89)
Thymus	Tumor	Superior vena cava or innominate veins	x	+				Brannan, D. (1926) Arch. Path. 1, 569; Foot, N.C. (1926) Am. J. Path. 2, 33; Danisch, F. & Nedelmann, E. (1928) Virchows Arch. 268, 492
Thyroid	Carcinoma	Jugular and innominate veins	x	+			The anaplastic thyroid carcinoma grows frequently and extensively into these blood vessels	Scheiber, S.H. (1872) Virchows Arch. 54, 285; Carrington, R.E. (1886) Trans. path. Soc. Lond. 37, 508; Pitt, G.N. (1887). Trans. path. Soc. Lond. 38, 151, 398; Zenker, K. (1890) Virchows Arch. 120, 68 and others
		Superior vena cava to right atrium	1	+				Wylegschanin, N.J. (1930) Frankfurt. Z. Path. 40, 51
	Well differentiated papillary and cystic carcinoma with benign appearance	Small veins	x	+			This invasion of small veins is the first assured indication of malignancy	Cohnheim, J. (1876) Virchows Arch. 68, 547

Organ	Tumor	Vessels involved	No.	+	Notes	Reference
Kidney	Carcinoma	Renal veins and inferior vena cava	x	+	Intravascular invasion over long distances is notorious for these tumors, of which several extended into the right chambers of the heart*	Wallmann, H. (1858) Virchows Arch. 13, 550; Tuner, F.C. (1885). Trans. path. Soc. Lond. 36, 275, 464; Sudeck, P. (1893). Virchows Arch. 133, 405 and 558; *Polayes, S.H. & Taft, H. (1931). Am. J. Path. 7, 63
	Embryonic and mixed tumors	Main veins even into heart	x	+		Merkel, H. (1898). Beitr. path. Anat. 24, 475 and others
	Wilms' tumor	Spermatic vein into cord and testis	1	+		Dew, H.R. (1928). Surg-Gynec. Obstet. 46, 447
	Transitional cell carcinoma	Renal vein and inferior vena cava	8/2	+		Hartman, D.S., Pyatt, R.S.; Dailey, E. (1983) Urol. Radiol. 5(2):83-7
Adrenal gland:	Carcinoma	Veins	x	+	Extensive invasion	Dreschfeld, J. (1904). J. Path. Bact. 10, 71
Cortex	Neuroblastoma	Small veins, inferior vena cava	1	+		Tileston, W., and Wolbach, S.B. (1908) Am. J. Med. Sci. 135, 871
Bladder	Bilharzial carcinoma	Vesical veins	x	+	Extensive invasion	Ferguson, A.R. (1911) J. Path. Bact. 16, 76
Prostate	Carcinoma	Veins	1	+	Invasion of veins from widespread metastases	Armstrong, E. & Oertel, H. (1919) Am. J. Med. Sci. 158, 359
	Carcinoma	Large veins	2	+		Willis, R. (1973)
Testis	Teratoma	Spermatic veins, vena cava, sometimes into right heart chamber	x	+	These tumors grow frequently in the veins cited, in contrast to seminomas.	Billroth, S. (1855) Virchows Arch. 8, 268; Waldeyer, W. (1868) Virchows Arch. 44, 83; a.o. Dew, H.R. (1925) Malignant Disease of the Testicle. London
		Renal veins, vena cava, right heart chambers, pulmonary arteries to peripheral branches	1	+	Metastasis in the neck invaded jugular and innominate veins	Herzog G. (1917), Beitr. path. Anat. 63, 755
Skin and special locations	Melanoma	Saphenous vein	1	+	Frequently invades the bloodstream but only the small veins, rarely large ones.	See Ch. 16, Vol. VIII
General	Sarcomas	Large or small	x	+	Common in rapidly growing, especially anaplastic sarcomas	Hertzler, A.E. and Gibson E.T. (1914). Ann. Surg. 60, 88

Table 1. Continued.

Body region	Primary neoplasm	Vein with tributaries	Case No	Growth Intravascular	Growth Extravascular	Metastasis	Comments	References
	Sarcoma of pelvic soft tissues	Along iliac, hypogastric, gluteal and vesical veins	1		+			André, C. (1874) Virchows Arch. 61, 383
	Sarcoma of forearm	Large cubital vein	1	+				Eve F.S. and Targett, J.H. (1889) Trans. path. Soc. Lond. 40, 297
	Sarcoma of thigh	Femoral and iliac veins	1	+	+	Lung metastases invaded large pulmonary veins		Zenker, K. (1890) Virchows Arch. 120, 68
	liposarcoma of groin	Extension in femoral and iliac veins	1	+		Invasions of pulmonary veins from lung metastases		Jaffé, R.H. (1926) Arch. Path. 1, 381
	Osteosarcoma of femur	Femoral and iliac veins	1	+				Von Albertini, A. (1928) Virchows Arch., 268, 295
	Rhabdomyosarcoma of leg	Inferior vena cava	1	+		Invasion took place from lumbar lymph node involvement		Hirsch E.F. (1929) Arch. Path. 8, 9; Am. J. Path, 5, 303
	Neurogenic sarcoma	Veins	1	+				Quick, D. and Cutler, M. (1927) Surg. Gynec. Obstet., 45, 320
	Retroperitoneal fibrosarcoma	Inferior vena cava	1	+				Kaufman, E. (1929) Pathology. Transl. by Reimann, S.P. of the Lehrbuch d. Patholog. Anat., Philadelphia, Saunders.
Thigh	Round cell sarcoma of soft tissue	Iliac vein, inferior vena cava, ovarian, uterine and vesical veins				Lungs and myocardia	In branch arteries of lungs: tumor emboli	Willis, R. (1973) (89)
	Chondrosarcoma		x	+				Weber, O. (1866) Virchows Arch. 35, 501.
	Chondrosarcoma	x	+				Benign-appearing, well-differentiated cartilaginous tumor cells	Fry, H. & Shattock, C.E. (1926). Br. J. Surg. 14, 337.
	Meningioma	Dural sinuses, jugular veins innominate, and superior vena cava	2	+				Towne, E.B. (1926). Ann. Surg. 83, 321.

x = multiple or frequent

1885 (86); among others). In 1905, Handley (21) introduced the scientific term "permeation" to characterize the spread of cancer cells within the lymph vessels in continuous columns. In reality, the columns of cancer cells in the case of permeation are not absolutely continuous, but may reveal intervals of discontinuity ((54); see also (15)).

In areas such as the visceral pleura such growths can be macroscopically observed as white lines. Microscopic investigations show coverage extending widely and for long distances. Willis (1973) notes a parotid carcinoma with direct extension to the lower half of the thighs. Similarly, according to Willis a breast cancer may spread by direct extension to thoracic, abdominal, and lumbar lymph nodes. Small and large vessels, even the thoracic duct, may be involved. As first noted by Fitzwilliams (1924) (16), lymphatic vessels undergo increasing destruction and replacement by neoplastic cells, with the greatest magnitude of neoplastic growth (cancerous infestation) occurring in the closest vicinity of the tumor. On the other hand, direct growth should not be considered as involved in only one type of spread, affecting such structural elements as tissue spaces, the circulatory system, or others. Generally speaking, tumor spread takes advantage of every available, and where possible, even a different, avenue. Certain neoplasms prefer to spread via the circulatory system, as in renal cancer; others, via the lymphatics, as in breast cancer. The majority of neoplasms, however, spread via a combination of routes.

Direct neoplastic spread via the circulatory system

Direct spread via the veins (Table 1)
The work of Folkman and his co-workers pointed out the importance of angiogenesis for the progression of tumors (see Chapter 11, Volume I). If neoplastic cells of a carcinoma *in situ* are enzymatically unable to promote capillary growth to the neoplasm, a cancer *in situ* could not invade the tissues beneath the basement membrane. But not only in the begin-

ning of tumor growth do the vessels, as part of the stroma, play an important role, but they are also actively involved in later stages of secondary tumor development as well.

Invasion of the wall of the vein proceeds from the adventitia to the intima. It may not come immediately to full obliteration; a minute channel may remain in the center of an expanding tumor. The lumen can also remain uninvaded and an intact endothelium may be present, but, terminally, the vessel may be completely obliterated. In any event, the elastic tissue of the vessel resists destruction. Indeed, it may be the remaining trace of a vein that has otherwise disappeared in the bulk of the tumor. In other cases, beginning with an endothelial destruction, a thrombus may be formed with malignant infiltration until the lumen of the vein is totally obliterated. The connection between metastatic and direct spreading is documented in the case of a 37-year-old man with a chondrosarcoma metastatic to the lung and from there, exhibiting direct spread to the left atrium via the pulmonary veins (16). Leiomyosarcoma of the inferior vena cava, of which some 67 cases have been described, spreads by extension into adjacent tissues. Direct extension into the heart, but not into the kidneys, adrenals or viscera, has also been observed (18).

Direct tumor spread via arteries (Table 2)
The walls of arteries, due especially to their elastic fiber components in contrast to those of veins, are nearly completely resistant to invasion by, and the spread of, neoplastic cells. Intact, uninvaded arteries have been seen to pass through dense neoplasms. The walls of arteries, however, are susceptible to some types of infection which may precede neoplastic invasion. High blood pressure in arteries may perhaps be linked to the rarity of neoplastic invasion, but this almost certainly cannot be the full explanation. Rarely, arteries have been invaded by direct spread from contiguous neoplastic growth. Table 2 cites a number of historic cases. Hebert (1918) (23) and others observed intact aorta and arteries remaining intact even when invaded by neoplastic

Table 2. Direct neoplastic invasion of the arterial wall. (Historically older cases).

Region	Primary neoplasm	Artery	Metastasis	Comment	Reference
Thorax	Carcinoma of lung	Aorta	–	The tumor tissue had invaded the wall of aorta to the media; started from med. deposits	Geipel P. (1899) Zbl. allg. Path. path. Anat. 10, 846
Abdomen	Chorionepithelioma	Artery		Invasion of media	Bostroem (1927) see Willis, 1973, p. 15 (89)
Abdomen	Squamous cell cancer of the kidney	Renal artery and its branches	–	Caused nearly total infarction of kidney and tumor	Rabinovitch, J. (1932) Arch. Surg. 24, 581
		Invasion of small artery			Ewing, J. (1940) Neoplastic Diseases 4th ed., Philadelphia and London p. 910.
Pelvis	Carcinoma of uterine cervix	Invasion of the iliac artery		Invasion started from pelvic tumor deposits	Willis, R. (1973) (89)

growth. Beneke (1890) (4) and others noted the resistance of small arteries and arterioles to invasion.

Direct spread via nerves

The most common involvement of the nervous system in malignant disease is by direct invasion or metastasis (62).

Direct spread of neoplasms has been found to be inside or along the nerve pathways. A 63-year-old woman with a choroidal melanoma exhibited extension of the tumor outside the sclera, filling the orbit and invading the optic nerve intracranially to the chiasm. Treatment consisted of orbital exenteration and neurosurgical resection of the intracranial remnant of the optic nerve. The patient is alive without metastases, almost four years after surgery (72).

Direct spread of neoplasms in the coelomic cavity

Primary as well as secondary growth may be the agent of direct spreading into the coelomic cavities. Tumors of the heart, as well as those of the mediastinum, may extend through the pericardium. Likewise, tumors of the pleura, the lungs, esophagus and trachea may extend to adjacent structures and viscera. In the peritoneal cavity, the main source of such growth may be the gastrointestinal organs exhibiting large glands, including the female urogenital system (with partial exception of the kidneys).

Direct spread of neoplasms influenced by spaces due to the distribution of fasciae and aponeuroses

Tense connective tissue in form of fasciae or aponeuroses acts as a barrier against the direct spreading of neoplasms composed of less compact (taut) tissue structures. In the case of metastatic spreading, these barriers can be breached by travelling metastatic cells, which is not the case in growth by direct spreading. The situation can be compared to the easier penetration of venous or lymphatic walls in contrast to the arterial wall attacked by spreading neoplastic cells. That a tumor variation may occur with regard to this behavior becomes evident if it is pointed out that aponeuroses may bar the distribution of certain rhabdomyosarcomas located within the aponeuroses to the exterior of the enclosed muscle, or, vice versa, other exterior tumors may not penetrate from the outside.

Direct spread of neoplasms in cerebrospinal spaces and epithelial cavities

In contradistinction to the conditions described under the previous heading, direct tumor growth in cerebrospinal spaces and epithelial cavities is able to proceed without restrictions within the framework of those localities.

Direct spreading of smaller neoplasms may result in sizeable, fungating masses formed in the oral cavity, the nasal cavity, pharynx, larynx, esophagus, trachea, stomach, intestine, uterus, renal pelvis, bladder, bronchus, and other areas. Such neoplasms have also been observed, however, in tube-like organs, such as the Fallopian tubes.

Peritoneal folds of the abdominal aorta, the coeliac axis and superior mesentery artery form the spaces in which

neuroblastomas and other abdominal tumors extend by direct spreading, which is clearly indicated by computed tomography (52, 53).

Direct tumor spread involved in combined types of tumor distribution, including metastasis

As stated earlier in this chapter, the possibility exists that a spreading tumor may take its course, combining different types of direct and distant tumor spreading simultaneously. Such a spread may begin with invasion of a tissue, then spread, and further on, proceed via the components of the lymphatic system; finally, continue its course in the veins and heart, and from there, in the arteries. Such a course would reflect the normal path of the body fluids; from the tissue spaces, to distribution by the arteries. Rare cases of this all-embracing type of spreading may exist.

More often, however, there may be a very highly mixed combination of distribution types. Thus, primary neoplasms or, frequently, propagating metastatic growth and primary tumor may spread directly and simultaneously. One of the metastases involved may also spread directly, whereas, on the other hand, another metastasis may be the origin of secondary growth and the resulting metastasis may be the source of metastatic growth (Chapter 15/ Volume I). Table 3 presents older examples of the direct spreading of tumors into selected organs.

REGIONAL DIRECT SPREAD OF TUMORS: SELECTED EXAMPLES

Stratified squamous epithelium

The most common kind of spread to the skin by carcinomas is by direct extension (35). In the case of Hodgkin's disease, direct extension may develop from an underlying nodal focus (88).

Simple cuboidal/columnar epithelium

Tumor spread in the perineural space suggests spreading by direct extension around the prostatic nerves and not within vascular channels (22).

Simple columnar epithelium

In three patients, direct metastatic spread occurred from the right colon to the duodenum (13). Rectal cancer spreads by direct extension or by lymphatic, hematogenous, transperitoneal, and iatrogenic extension (24).

Transitional epithelium

Penile secondary neoplasms occur by direct extension, retrograde lymphatic or venous spread, direct arterial extension, embolism, iatrogenic action, or in some still unknown manner (2).

Table 3. Nonmetastatic, direct spreading of tumors into selected organs. (Historically older cases).

Organ	Direct spreading from contiguity	Direct spreading via lymphatics	Direct invasions via blood vessels	Comments	References
Lung	Primary growth of thymus, esophagus, thyroid. Invasion through diaphragm, from thoracic duct, by abdominal neoplasms. Mammary gland neoplasms via chest wall. Pleural carcinomatosis.	Hilar and tracheobronchial lymph nodes from the following primary neoplasms: gastric carcinoma (1, 2); carcinoma of breast (3); lung carcinoma (4); carcinoma of stomach, of gallbladder (5); of tongue, of cervix uteri (6).	Rarely via veins to heart and pulmonary arteries from primary renal cancer (7); teratoma of testis (8); intravascular chondroma (9); tumors of left auricle via pulmonary vein to lung (10).		(1) Bristowe J.S. (1860), Trans. path. Soc. Lond. 11, 25; (1860), Trans. path Soc. Lond. 19, 228, 415; (2) Waldeyer, W. (1867), Virchows Arch. 41, 470, (3) Bennett J.R. (1871) Trans. path. Soc. Lond. 22, 76 (4), Ebstein, W. (1890), Dtsch. med. Wschr p. 921, (5) Dürbeck K. (1926), Klin. Wschr 5, 99, (6) R. Willis, (1973) (case 440), (7) Oberndorfer, (1907). Verh. dtsch. Path. Ges. 11, 263, (8) Herzog, G. (1917), Beitr. path. anat. 63, 755; (9) Kos, M. (1929), Virchows Arch. 272, 166; (10) Sternberg C. (1901), Zbl. allg. Path. path. Anat. 12, 625
Liver	Frequent: neoplasms of stomach and gallbladder. Less frequent: neoplasms of esophagus, pancreas, bile ducts, kidney, adrenals, colon; carcinoma of the oviduct (1)	Portal lymph gland invasion of retrograde permeation (2). Most common primary tumor is the gastric carcinoma followed by pancreatic carcinoma, small cell carcinoma of ovary, squamous cell carcinoma of cervix uteri (3, 4). The last cases are unusual, lymphatic permeation is less common, then important in the lung.	Portal vein invasion by uterine carcinoma (5), piloric carcinoma, pancreatic carcinoma. Retrograde growth along inferior vena cava into hepatic vein (6).		(1) Willis, R. (1973), case 131; (2) Vogel, L. (1891), Virchows Arch. 125, 495, (3) (4) Willis, R. (1973); (5) Virchow, R. (1849), Virchows Arch. 2, 587; (6) Weber F.P. (1914), Proc. R. Soc. Med. 8, Sec. Med. 6;
Kidneys	Primary neoplasms: carcinoma of pancreas, stomach, intestines, malignancies of adrenals and of retroperitoneal space. Secondary neoplasms: lumbar lymph node metastases, as of ovarian carcinoma and carcinoma of bladder (1)	Carcinoma of stomach (2); carcinoma of pancreas (3); carcinoma of gallbladder (4); carcinoma of renal pelvis (5)	Veins, carcinoma of other kidney (6); malignant ovarian teratoma via vena cava and renal vein (7)		(1) Willis, R. (1973), case 58, 214; (2) Schierge, M. (1922), Virchows Arch. 237, 129; (3/4) Vogel, L. (1891), Virchows Arch. 125, 495; (5) Frank, P. & Gruber, G.B. (1923), Z. urol. Chir. 13, 116; (6) Weber, F.P. (1914), Proc. R. Soc. Med. 8, Sec. Med. 6; (7) Kaufmann, E. (1929), Pathology, Philadelphia, Saunders
Adrenals	Renal tumors, carcinomas of pancreas, stomach, and esophagus and from metastatic deposits in retroperitoneal lymph nodes (gastric, ovarian and pancreatic carcinoma (1))	Cirrhous tumors of stomach (2)	Teratoma of testis (3)	Direct invasion to the adrenals occurs infrequently	(1) Willis, R. (1973), cases 305, 41, 58 and 459; (2) Schierge, M. (1922), Virchows Arch. 237, 129; (3) Dew, H.R. (1925), Malignant Disease of the Testicle, London, case 7
Spleen	Primary neoplasms of stomach, pancreas, colon, left kidney; secondary tumors of splenic hilar lymph glands and peritoneal growth. Primary tumors of these deposits were carcinoma of the pancreas around the capsule (1); metastatic splenic lymph glands from adenocarcinoma of rectum; anaplastic carcinoma of renal pelvis peritoneal carcinomatosis from carcinoma of lung; from	Tumors in the hilar region of the spleen may develop retrograde permeation (3); carcinoma of stomach (4)	Retrograde invasion from portal venous system (5)		(1) Willis, R. (1973), cases 244, 459; (2) Willis, R. (1973), cases 217, 383, 131; (3) Schmücker, K. (1928). Virchows Arch. 267, 339; (4) Findlay, G.M. (1921), J. Path. Bact. 34, 362; (5) Virchow, R. (1849), Virchows Arch. 2, 587

Table 3. Continued.

Organ	Direct spreading from contiguity	Direct spreading via lymphatics	Direct invasions via blood vessels	Comments	References
	metastasis of carcinoma of the bladder and primary carcinoma of the Fallopian tube (2)				
Intestines	Gastric carcinoma (1); carcinoma of gallbladder, pancreatic carcinoma (2), cystic ovarian carcinoma (3), adenocarcinoma of colon (4). Direct spreading of tumors in the intestines occurs generally via metastatic deposits, or if invasion by contiguous adherent neoplasms is known from tumors of the testis (5), carcinoma of stomach (6), carcinoma of ovary, prostate, colon and cervix uteri (7).	Frequently from gastric carcinoma (8)			(1) Toyosumi, H. (1908), Virchows Arch. 191, 70; (2) Willis, R. (1974), (cases 212, 244), (3) Ley, G. (1919) Proc. R. Soc. Med. 13, Obst. Sec. 95 (case 12); (4) Norbury, L.E.C. (1929), Proc. R. Soc. Med. 23, 712; (5) Borrmann, R. (1907), Verh. dtsch path. Ges. 11, 108; (6) Willis, R. (1974), p. 77; (7) Willis, R. (1974); (8) Seemann, G. & Krasnopolski, A. (1926), Virchows Arch. 262, 697.
Stomach	Liver, pancreas, kidneys or adrenals penetrate the wall of the stomach, extremely rarely.	Neoplasms extending along lymphatic channel may extensively invade the stomach, as primary carcinoma of the esophagus (2) or a primary carcinoma from the stomach itself (2)	This type of distribution is rare. The primary growth shows the following frequency: melanoma, mammary ca, lung ca, kidney ca, thyroid ca, tumors of testis, chorionepithelioma, pharynx, others (3)		(1) Zahn, F.W. (1889), Virchows Arch. 11 71; 117, 30, 37? (2) Fleiner, W. (1905). Beitr. path. Anat. Suppl. 7, 388; (3) Willis, R. (1974), p. 216
Heart	From primary tumors: lung (1), esophagus (2), from hepatic carcinoma through diaphragm into right atrium (3). From secondary tumors: mediastinal lymph glands (4), metastatic sarcoma in lung (5). Atria are invaded more often than the ventricles (rare).	Bronchial carcinoma, esophageal carcinoma (6), gastric carcinoma (7)	Via vena cava inferior: cancer of kidney (8), embryonic renal tumors (9), adrenal tumors (10), teratoma of testis (11), chondroma and chondrosarcoma (12), liver (13) Via vena cava superior: carcinoma of thyroid (14), carcinoma of lung (15), carcinoma of esophagus (16). Invasion via pulmonary vein is rare: carcinoma of the lung (17)	Growth in the ventricles from the atria is rare.	(1) Wilks (1855), Trans. path. Soc. Lond. 6, 112; (2) Handford, H. (1888), Tran. path. Soc. Lond. 39, 48; (3) Strong, G.F. & Pitts, H.H. (1930), Arch. intern. Med. 46, 105; (4) Moxon, W. (1867), Trans. path. Soc. Lond. 18, 38; (5) Powell, R.D. (1873), Trans. path. Soc. Lond. 24, 28; (6) Kaufmann, E. (1929), Pathology. Transl. by Reimann, S.P. of the Lehrbuch d. Pathologischen Anatomie, Philadelphia: Saunders, p. 18; (7) Schierge, M. (1922), Virchows Arch. 237, 129; (8) Oberndorfer (1907), Verh. dtsch. Path. Ges. 11, 263; (9) Merkel, H. (1898), Beitr. path. Anat. 24, 475; (10) Fox, T.C. (1885), Trans. path. Soc. Lond. 36,460; (11) Breuss, C. (1878), Wien. med. Wschr. 767; (12) Ernst, P. (1900), Beitr. path. Anat. 28, 255; (13) Loehlein, W. (1907), Beitr. path. Anat. 42, 531; (14) Wylegschanin, N.J. (1930). Frankfurt Z. Path. 40, 51; (15) Dana, H.W. & McIntosh, R. (1922), Am. J Med. Sci. 163, 411; (16) Leichtenstern, O. (1891), Dtsch. med. Wschr. 17, 535; (17) Andrew (1865), Trans. path. Soc. Lond. 16, 51.
Pancreas	The pancreas is frequently invaded from contiguous neoplasms, such as carcinoma of the	Occasionally from the carcinoma of the stomach (1)			(1) Seemann, G. & Krasnopolski, A. (1926), Virchows Arch. 262, 697

	stomach and transverse colon as primary sources; and secondary ones of all kinds of the surrounding area		
Gallbladder	Direct invasion occurs rarely: from porta of liver and gastric and pancreatic neoplasms.	Lymphatic penetration from viscera of upper abdomen may be extensive	(1) Wechsler, H.F. (1926), Arch. Path. 2, 161
Ovaries	Primary intestinal or uterine tumors or secondary peritoneal growth may be the source of tumor invasion. Carcinoma of the Fallopian tube may continue onto the ovary (1):		(1) Cleland, J.B. (1903), Br. med. J. 2, 1584; (2) Willis, R. (1973), case 296; (3) Geschickter, C.F. (1932), Arch. Surg. 24, 231?
Bones	Cutaneous, oral or pharyngeal carcinomas invade the facial skeleton, skull base, neck and shoulder girdle. The submaxillary gland carcinoma may invade the mandible (1); meningiomas invade the skull. The thoracic skeleton is penetrated from mammary, pulmonary or esophageal carcinoma. Chordoma permeates vertebrae, sacrum and base of skull (2); sarcoma of soft tissues, adjacent bones (3).		
Brain	Infiltrative invasion of the brain is rare, but occurred from nasopharyngeal carcinoma (1), meningioma (2), sarcoma of skull or ear (3), retinoblastoma (4), nasal olfactory tumor (5), adenocystic carcinoma of parotid, suprapituitary adamantinoma	Lymphatic permeation from extracerebral tumors is impossible due to the lack of lymphatics in the brain.	(1) Woltmann, H.W. (1922), Arch. Neurol. Psychiat. 8, 412; (2) Bernstein, S.A. (1933), Virchows Arch. 290, 501; (3) Russell, D.S. & Rubinstein, L.J. (1971), Pathology of Tumours of the Nervous System, 3rd ed., London: Arnold, pp. 262–263; (4) Hu, C.H. (1930), Am. J. Path. 6, 27; (5) Mendeloff, J. (1957), Cancer 10, 944; (26) Willis, R. (1973), case 19
Spinal cord	Occasionally, gross invasion from metastatic carcinoma (1); medulloblastoma (2); and meningeal melanoma (3)		(1) von Scanzoni, C. (1897), Z. Heilk. 18, 381; (2) Wanke, R. (1933), Arch. klin. Chir. 177, 528; (3) Forbes, W. & Maloney, A.F.J. (1950), J. Path. Bact. 62, 403
Leptomeninges	Intracranial and intrathecal tumors: most common, medulloblastoma, astrocytoma, glioblastoma, ependymoma, oligodendroglioma, pinealoma, carcinoma of choroid plexus (1); rarely, pituitary neoplasms (2). Spinal cord; meningeal gliomatosis (3); teratomas and dermoid cysts (4). Extracranial and extrathecal tumors; retinoblastoma (best known), rarely, other tumors of eye, rhabdomyosarcoma of ear region or orbit (5); adenocystic carcinoma (6)	Neoplasms of the leptomeninges spread frequently in perivascular manner as microscopic invasion	(1) Kono, N. (1924), Frankfurt. Z. Path. 30, 92; (2) Cagnetto, G. (1904). Virchows Arch. 176, 115; (3) Pels-Leusden (1898). Beitr. path. Anat. 23, 69; (4) Rossknecht, E. (1913). Frankfurt. Z. Path. 13, 300; (5) Constance, T.J. (1955), J. Path. Bact. 70, 365; (6) Dagnelie, J. (1956), Rev. Belge. Path. 25, 198

Table 3. Continued.

Organ	Direct spreading from contiguity	Direct spreading via lymphatics	Direct invasions via blood vessels	Comments	References
Thyroid gland	Primary neoplasms of pharynx, larynx, esophagus. Metastatic deposits in cervical lymph glands and metastases from small lingual carcinoma (1). Thyroid invasions are generally macroscopic.	Very rare (2)	Invasion via veins unknown (3)		(1) Willis, R. (1973) p. 269; (2) Schierge, M. Willis, R. (1973), p. 269
Skin	Mammary carcinoma	Lymphatic permeation, nodules from permeated deep fascial plexus, cancer en cuirasse. Interchanges occur.			

Exocrine pancreas

Cancer spreading from the pancreas does so by direct invasion into the retropancreatic tissue (49). Primary retroperitoneal sarcomas spread by direct invasion (46). In 7/13 patients, metastases into the duodenum took place by direct invasion, retro- or intraperitoneally (36).

Desmal epithelium

Neoplastic spread within the peritoneal cavity occurs by direct invasion; seeding; and embolic metastases (43). In the case of cancerous pleurisy, direct cancer invasion via the diaphragm was found in some of the intra-abdominal tumor patients with peritonitis (28). Gastric, ovarian, bladder, cervical and endometrial malignancies may spread directly via the greater omentum to the transverse colon (65).

Reticular connective tissue

One mode of spreading of malignant lymphoma to the heart from other intrathoracic tumors is by direct spread (42). Extraskeletal spread by direct extension into paraosseous tissue has been observed in multiple myeloma (30). In the case of malignant non-Hodgkin's lymphomas, direct spread from the bone marrow may not be so important as hematogenous dissemination (29).

Bone

Direct bone invasion by squamous cancers of head and neck is particularly well known from tumors of the oral cavity. The responsible osteoclasts appear to be stimulated by compounds released in the areas of the tumor (8). Direct extension of non-intracranial neoplasms may involve the temporal bone (5).

Cardiac musculature

Cardiac impairment by secondary tumor extension occurs by direct invasion, implantation, hematogenic and lymphatic spread. Malignant melanomas, lung and breast cancers are in the forefront, whereas acute leukemias can account only for implantation and hematogenous or lymphatic spread (57).

Meninges

Cancers of the head and neck region are known to invade locally, also into the meninges. This occurrence of direct spread is more pronounced than is the case with distant metastases, but malignant cells in the cerebrospinal fluid have also been observed (61). Extraneural spread of metastasizing gliomas is ascribable to the direct access of the tumor to extrameningeal tissues (39). A small number of cases of cancerous invasion of the pia-arachnoid from neighboring primary tumors take place by direct spread (34).

Direct spread into the surrounding area

A number of interesting cases derived from clinical practice are provided in the following: It is reported that a recurrent oncocytoma arose from the lateral nasal wall and posterior ethmoid sinus and invaded the orbit (9). During direct invasion of the brain parenchyma, B16 melanoma cells were seen directly attached to the basolateral site of the blood vessel basal lamina, establishing their location by dislodging the perivascular astrocytes (32). Eight brain tumors, namely, two sphenoidal meningiomas, one CP angle meningioma, one CP angle neurofibroma, two pituitary adenomas and two jugular foramen chemodectomas were investigated by Hanakita (19). Plain films showed only expansion of the pituitary adenomas into the paranasal sinuses and the pharynx. CT scans served as a valuable aid, demonstrating extracranial extension resulting in the destruction of the skull. According to the investigator, hyperostosis of the skull with enlargement of the skull foramina could be observed. CT scans proved to be a useful method for analysis (20). Laryngeal cancers below the apex of the arytenoid exhibit a very marked association with cartilage invasion. Predilection for neoplastic invasion of thyroid, crycoid and arytenoid cartilages is pronounced. At these sites, collagen fibers have been observed by Archer (1) to pass through the perichondrium and attach directly to cartilage. These same fibers may serve as a pathway to direct growth of tumor cells.

Unusual, but well documented is the direct invasion of the trachea by an aggressive primary tumor in the thyroid. The vice versa situation is rare. An adenoid cystic carcinoma arising in the trachea has been reported as invading the thyroid gland and recurrent laryngeal nerve, causing vocal cord paralysis (93). Furthermore, direct spread of a primary cancer in proximity to the CNS accounts for a small proportion of cases of cancerous invasion of the pia-arachnoid (34). Finally, in 16 cases, direct invasion of the mediastinum from primary bronchial cancer was described by Pelle and co-worker (56). Of 32 patients with known gastric cancer, 9 exhibited direct spread to structures surrounding the tumor (12). Carcinoma of the pancreatic head has shown the following characteristics: continuous spreading along the caudal pancreatic duct wall; dysplastic lesion; multicentric cancer lesion; lymphatic infiltration; lymph node metastasis and direct invasion of the retroperitoneal space (27). Patients with carcinomas of the rectum established by contiguous spread have a poor prognosis (14). An undifferentiated small cell carcinoma of the renal pelvis exhibited a massive invasion of the kidney (61). Cells from the Nara bladder tumor line (NBT-II), an invasive tumor in the rat, invaded and progressively occupied the cardiac muscle, which degenerated. Cells from a dog kidney line (MOCK), which are of low tumorigenicity in nude mice, failed to accomplish invasion of the cardiac muscle, *in vitro* (69). Sixteen of 51 patients with primary and metastatic cancer of the spine displayed paravertebral tumors involving the spine by direct extension; 28 were suffering from blood-borne metastases to the spine (79). A patient was kept alive for four years by radical nephrectomy and partial resection of the liver for a primary renal carcinoma with direct invasion to the liver; bronchial arterial infusions; and irradiation for the two pulmonary metastases (91). Parenchymal lymphatic vessel invasion alone provides grounds for a poor prognosis (73).

DIRECT SPREAD OF TUMORS FROM SPECIFIC TISSUES-SELECTED EXAMPLES

Stratified squamous epithelium

In 95% of cases, basal cell carcinomas with a diameter below 2 cm extend beyond their visible borders into a distance of 4 mm. This finding is important in evaluating the start of direct spread from surgical remnants (90). This tumor is one of the neoplasms which rarely metastasizes, but patients with AIDS may be at greater risk for metastasis of basal cell carcinoma (75). The primary mode of spread of basal cell carcinoma is the direct extension (66), but the direct spread into the bones of the skull takes a long period of time (44).

Simple cuboidal/columnar epithelium

Direct invasion of the caval wall by very large kidney carcinomas was seen in 2 patients. Treatment consisting of mitomycin C microcapsule therapy led to a tumor-free condition two and eight years after treatment, respectively (31).

Simple columnar epithelium

A 51-year-old woman exhibited an adenocarcinoma of the esophagogastric junction to the cervical esophagus. This situation was at first thought to be the result of direct spreading, but later seemed to be a lymphogenous metastasis (79). Carcinoma of the Fallopian tubes spread directly to the peritoneum (70) and adjacent organs, also with following transcoelomic dissemination (92). Locally advanced carcinoma of the large bowel showed direct spread to neighboring organs in 33% of cases (58). Of 195 cases of colon cancer, 56 cases with macroscopic invasion into surrounding organs revealed 26 cases with direct spread to the abdominal wall – 7 to the bladder and 6 to the stomach (41). Tumor extension in a patient with adenocarcinoma of the prostate, and spreading to prepuce and glans of the penis may have resulted from direct spread, or implantation (55).

Pseudostratified columnar epithelium

Adenocystic carcinomas of the bronchus spread mainly directly to the neighboring trachea (76).

Transitional epithelium

Muscular invasion by recurrent bladder carcinomas depends on the size of the neoplasm and upon cellular anaplasia (51). If the connective stalk in transitional cell papillary tumors of the bladder is invaded, the prognosis is poor (82).

Salivary glands

To prevent microscopic direct spread adenoid cystic carcinomas in minor salivary glands should be irradiated in accordance with the width of the margin of the tumors (63).

Thyroid gland

Direct, lymphatic, and hematogenic spread has been determined in thyroid tumors (80).

Testis

Hoeltl and coworkers (25) reported vascular invasion in 27% of patients with seminomas and in 53% with nonseminomatous germ cell testis tumors. Visceral metastases appeared in 9 and 32%, respectively. Vascular invasion is important for staging and treatment.

A presumed pineal germinoma spread from known spinal metastases by direct extension via the lumbar foramina (64).

Ovary

Ovarian carcinomas spread via the retroperitoneal route, either by direct spreading to contiguous tissues or by different paths of lymphatic extension (48).

Desmal epithelium

Epithelial mesotheliomas may show characteristics of carcinomas, such as direct spreading (37). A 9-year-old Siamese cat exhibited an abdominal mesothelioma which probably arose in the abdominal cavity and spread to the thorax, including the lung, by direct spread through the diaphragm, or by hematogenous or lymphatic extension (60).

Reticular connective tissue

At autopsy, the unusual case of extensive direct spread with infiltration of the chest wall, but without metastases, was seen in a male patient with pulmonary lymphosarcoma (84). In another case, leukemic cells seen in the central nervous system may have arisen (1) by direct derivation from the bone marrow passing the dura by hematogenous spread, or (2) by metastasis from extracranial bone marrow moving through lymphatic channels, or (3) *de novo* from the choroid plexus or the walls of the arachnoid veins (59). Local tumor invasion may be promoted in C57 BL/6 mice due to inhibition of the desmoplastic response (3). In 4 of 6 patients, computed tomography suggested direct invasion by gastric leiomyosarcomas. The most frequent sites were spleen and pancreas (67).

Smooth musculature

A 46-year-old woman suffered from a leiomyoma which invaded the uterine veins, obstructed the inferior vena cava, extending into the right atrium and partially obstructing the tricuspid valve and the coronary sinus. Excision was performed but a residual tumor extended from the inferior vena cava to a point approximately 5 cm below the right atrium. Approximately 50 cases are known including three reports of direct extension of a leiomyoma from the pelvic veins into the right atrium (81).

Transverse striated musculature

Rhabdomyosarcomas with direct and progressive extension to the CNS were seen in 50.6% of neoplasms at autopsy (74).

Neurons of the central nervous system

Twenty-seven patients exhibited spreading of a neuroblastoma into the lung either by direct spread or via hematogenic or lymphatic pathways (83). In contrast to medulloblastoma, ependymoma and glioblastoma, retinoblastoma spreads by direct extension into the optic nerve, originating from the retina and continuing into the meningeal spaces by extension from the choroid, or along the central retinal vessels to the subarachnoid space (38).

Summary

Direct neoplastic spreading has been compared with metastatic spreading; the various modalities of direct neoplastic spreading have been outlined. An extensive case material reveals the diversity of direct spread of neoplasms deriving from selected types of tissues, and intruding into various organs. The historically older cases have been set forth in tabular form.

REFERENCES

1. Archer CR, Yeager VL, Herbold DR: Computed tomography vs. histology of laryngeal cancer: their value in predicting laryngeal cartilage invasion. *Laryngoscope* 93(2):140, 1983
2. Bachrach P, Dahlen CP: Metastatic tumors to the penis. *Urology* 1(4):359, 1973
3. Barsky SH, Goaplakrishna R: Increased invasion and spontaneous metastasis of BL6 melanoma with inhibition of the desmoplastic response in C57 BL/6 mice. *Cancer Res* 47(6):1663, 1987
4. Beneke R: *Beitr path Anat* 7:95, 1890
5. Berlinger N, Koutroupes S: Patterns of involvement of the temporal bone in metastatic and systemic malignancy (meeting abstract). *Amer Laryngological, Rhinological and Otological Soc*, Broomall, PA 48 pp, 1979
6. Boland TW, Winga ER, Kalfayan B: Chondrosarcoma. A case report with left atrial involvement and systemic embolization. *J. Thorac Cardiovasc Surg* 74(2):268, 1977
7. Caramella E, Bruneton JN, Roux P et al.: Metastases of the digestive tract. Report of 77 cases and review of the literature. *Eur J Radiol* 3(4):331, 1983
8. Carter RL, Pittem MR: Squamous carcinomas of the head and neck: some patterns of spread. *J R Soc Med* 73(6):420, 1980
9. Chui RT, Liao SY, Bosworth H: Recurrent oncocytoma of the ethmoid sinus with orbital invasion. *Otolaryngol Head Neck Surg* 93(2):267, 1985
10. Cole WH: Dissemination of cancer: the need for stimulation of the immune process during the immunosuppression produced by major operations. *South Med J* 75(12):1479, 1982
11. Deeley TJ: The spread of malignant disease. *Radiography* 41(482):29, 1975
12. Derchi LE et al.: Sonographic staging of gastric cancer. *AJR* 140(2):273, 1983
13. Diamond RT, Greenberg HM, Boult IF: Direct metastatic spread of right colonic adenocarcinoma to duodenum – bartum and computed tomographic findings. *Gastrointest Radiol* 6(4):339, 1981
14. Durdey P, Williams NS: The effect of malignant and inflammatory fixation of rectal carcinoma on prognosis after rectal excision. *Br J Surg* 71(10):767, 1984
15. Fidler IJ, Gersten DM, Hart IR: The biology of cancer invasion and metastasis. *Adv Cancer Res* 28:149, 1978
16. Fitzwilliams DCL: Carcinoma of the breast and its method of spread embolism or permeation. *Br J Surg* 12: 650, 1924
17. Greig RG, Trainer DL: Shaping future strategies for the pharmacological control of tumor cell metastases. *Cancer Metastasis Rev* 5(1):3, 1986
18. Griffin AS, Starchi JM: Primary leiomyosarcoma of the inferior vena cava: a case report and review of the literature. *J. Surg Oncol* 34(1):53, 1987
19. Hanakita J, Handa H: Neuroradiological examinations of extracranial extension of brain tumors. *No Shinkei Geka* 12(4):445, 1984
20. Hanakita J, Kondo A, Yamamoto Y et al.: Cervical dural ectasia in von Recklinghausen's disease. *No Shinkei Geka* 13(7):785, 1985
21. Handley WS. *Arch Middx Hosp* 7:52, 1906.
22. Hassan MO, Maksem J: The prostatic perineural space and its relation to tumor spread. An ultrastructural study. *Am J Surg Pathol* 4(2):143, 1980
23. Hebert GT: *Quart J Med* 11:165, 1918
24. Hickey RC, Romsdahl MM, Johnson DE et al.: Recurrent cancer and metastases. *World J Surg* 6(5):595, 1982
25. Hoeltl W, Kosak D, Pont J et al.: Testicular cancer: prognostic implications of vascular invasion. *J Urol* 137(4):683, 1987
26. Hoggan G: *Trans path Soc Lond* 29:384, 1878
27. Ishikawa O et al.: Clinico-pathological study on the appropriate range of pancreatic resection to obtain operative curability of pancreatic head cancer. *Nippon Geka Gakkai Zasshi* 85(4):363, 1984
28. Iwai K, Yoshikawa H, Koyama A: Clinico-pathological study on cancerous pleurisy, with emphasis on extra-pulmonary malignancy (meeting abstract). Internat'l Assoc for the Study of Lung Cancer, 2nd World Confer on Lung Cancer, Copenhagen, Denmark, 1980
29. Jellinger K, Radaszkiewicz T: Involvement of the central nervous system in malignant lymphomas. *Virchow Arch Pathol Anat Histol* 370(4):345, 1976
30. Kapadia SB: Multiple myeloma: a clinicopathologic study of 62 consecutively autopsied cases. *Medicine (Baltimore)* 59(5):380, 1980
31. Kato T, Abe R, Sato K et al.: Treatment of renal cell carcinoma invading the inferior vena cava; role of preoperative targeting chemotherapy. *Gan To Kagaku Pyoho* 14(3 Pt 2):956, 1987
32. Kawaguchi T et al.: Cellular behaviour of metastatic B16 melanoma in experimental blood-borne implantation and cerebral invasion. An electron microscopic study. *Invasion Metastasis* 5(1):16, 1985
33. Klinger C: *Virchow Arch* 12:538, 1857
34. Kokkoris CP: Leptomeningeal carcinomatosis: how does cancer reach the PIA-arachnoid? *Cancer* 51(1):154, 1983
35. Krumerman MS, Garret R: Carcinomas metastatic to skin. *NY State J Med* 77(12):1900, 1977
36. Lammli J, Buhler H, Bosseckert H et al.: Metastases to the duodenum. *Schweiz Rundsch Med Prax* 71(25):1054, 1982
37. Law MR, Hodson ME, Heard BE: Malignant mesothelioma of the pleura: relation between histological type and clinical behaviour. *Thorax* 37(11):810, 1982
38. Lipper MH, Kishore PR: Intraspinal metastases from retinoblastoma. *Radiology* 131(1):161, 1979
39. Liwnicz BH, Rubinstein LJ: The pathways of extraneural

spread in metastasizing gliomas. *Hum Pathol* 10(4):453, 1979

40. Man D, McInnes G: Adenoid cystic carcinoma of minor salivary glands. *Del Med J* 52(8):423, 1980

41. Matsumura KJ, Tanaka S, Ito T et al.: Colon cancer with macroscopic invasion into surrounding organs. *Gan No Rinsho* 33(1):49, 1987

42. McDonnell PJ, Mann RB, Bulkley BH: Involvement of the heart by malignant lymphoma. *Cancer* 49(5):944, 1982

43. Meyers MA: Intraperitoneal spread of malignancies and its effect on the bowel. *Clin Radiol* 32(2):129, 1981

44. Mikhail GR, Boulos RS, Knighton RS et al.: Cranial invasion by basal cell carcinoma. *J Dermatol Surg Oncol* 12(5):459, 1986

45. Minami K, Kumada K, Mori K: Echocardiographic findings of renal cell carcinoma extending into the right atrium via the inferior vena cava. *Nippon Geka Hokan* 54(4):281, 1985

46. Moore SV, Aldrete JS: Primary retroperitoneal sarcomas: the role of surgical treatment. *Am J Surg* 142(3):358, 1981

47. Muraguchi T, Sakai K, Yamada T et al.: Surgical management of renal cell carcinoma with inferior vena caval and right atrial involvement. *Jpn J Surg* 15(5):399, 1985

48. Musumeci R: Study of the metastatic spread via the retroperitoneal route by means of lymphography. *Radiol Diagn (Berl)* 22(4):521, 1981

49. Naitro A, Suzuki T, Tobe T: Degree of cancer spread of the pancreas seen in computerized tomograms. Proc 12th Annual Meeting of Japan Pancreatic Disease Res Soc, Tokyo, 1981

50. Nakamura Y, Tamura A, Fijimoto H et al.: A case of hepatocellular carcinoma with growth into the right atrium, pulmonary tumor embolism and cerebral metastasis. *Nippon Shokakibyo Gakkai Zasshi* 82(2):319, 1985

51. Novak R: Course of superficial carcinoma of bladder (Ta-T1). Apropos of 171 cases. *J. Urol (Paris)* 93(1):21, 1987

52. Oliphant M, Berne AS: Computed tomography of the subperitoneal space: demonstration of direct spread of intraabdominal disease. *J Comput Assist Tomogr* 6(6):1127, 1982

53. Oliphant M, Berne AS: Mechanism of direct spread of abdominal neuroblastoma: CT demonstration and clinical implications. *Gastrointest Radiol* 12(1):59, 1987

54. Onuigho WI: Cancer permeation: processes, problems and prospects. *Cancer Res* 33(4):633, 1973

55. Patel NP, Ward JN: Carcinoma of prostate metastatic to prepuce and glans penis. *Urology* 11(3):269, 1978

56. Pelle C et al.: Comparison between the findings of X-ray computed tomography and thoracotomy in the evaluation of locoregional extensions of primary bronchial cancer. Apropos of 45 cases. *Rev Mal Respir* 19(5):295, 1984

57. Perry MC: Cardiac metastasis. In: *Cancer and the Heart*, edited by Kapoor AS, New York: Springer Verlag, pp. 76–81, 1986

58. Pittam MR, Thornton H, Ellis H: Survival after extended resection for locally advanced carcinomas of the colon and rectum. *Ann R Coll Surg Engl* 66(2):81, 1984

59. Pochedly C: How does leukemia invade the CNS? In: *Leukemia and Lymphoma in the Nervous System*, edited by Pochedly C, Springfield, IL: Charles C Thomas

60. Raflo CP, Nuernberger SP: Abdominal mesothelioma in a cat. *Vet Pathol* 15(6):781, 1978

61. Redman BG, Tapazoglou E, Al-Sarraf M: Meningeal carcinomatosis in head and neck cancer. Report of six cases and review of the literature. *Cancer* 58(12):2656, 1986

62. Riddoth D: Neurological manifestations of cancer. *Practitioner* 225(1356):819, 822, 826, 1981

63. Rounthwaite FJ, Wallace AC, Watson TA: The effect of radiotherapy in the treatment of adenoid cystic carcinoma of the head and neck arising in minor salivary glands. *J Otolaryngol Jpn* 6(4):297, 1977

64. Rubery ED, Wheeler TK: Metastases outside the central nervous system from a presumed pineal germinoma. *J. Neurosurg* 53(4):562, 1980

65. Rubesin SE, Levine MS: Omental cakes: colonic involvement by omental metastases. *Radiology* 154(3):593, 1985

66. Scanlon EF, Volkmer DD, Ovledo MA et al.: Metastatic basal cell carcinoma. *J Surg Oncol* 15(2):171, 1980

67. Scaterige JC, Fishman EK, Jones B et al.: Gastric leiomyosarøcoma: CT observations. *J Comput Assist Tomogr* 9(2):320, 1985

68. Schmidt SS: Prostatic carcinoma with direct extension to renal pelvis. *Urology* 3(6):775, 1974

69. Schroyens W et al.: Comparison of invasiveness and non-invasiveness of two epithelial cell lines *in vitro*. *Invasion Metastasis* 4(3):160, 1984

70. Sedlis A: Carcinoma of the Fallopian tube. *Surg Clin North Am* 58(1):121, 1978

71. Senecal L: Undifferentiated small cell carcinoma of the renal pelvis with massive invasion of the kidney. *Union Med Can* 114(2):147, 1985

72. Shields CL, Shields JA, Yarian DL et al.: Intracranial extension of choroidal melanoma via the optic nerve. *Br J Ophthalmol* 71(3):172, 1987

73. Shields TW: Prognostic significance of parenchymal lymphatic vessel and blood vessel invasion in carcinoma of the lung. *Surg Gynecol Obstet* 157(2):185, 1983

74. Shimada H, Newton WA Jr, Soule EH et al.: Pathology of fatal rhabdomyosarcomas. *Proc Annu Meet Am Soc Clin Oncol* 4:245, 1985

75. Sitz KV, Keppen M, Johnson DF: Metastatic basal cell carcinoma in acquired immunodeficiency syndrome-related complex. *JAMA* 257(3):340, 1987

76. Spencer H: Bronchial mucous gland tumours. *Virchows Arch (Pathol Anat)* 383(1):101, 1979

77. Sundaresan N et al.: Vertebral body resection in the treatment of cancer involving the spine. *Cancer* 53(6):1393, 1984

78. Takeda T, Ishikawa N, Sakakibara Y et al.: A giant tumor thrombus in the right atrium clearly detected by 111n-oxine labeled platelet scintigraphy. *Eur J Nucl Med* 11(1):49, 1985

79. Taniki T, Nishimura T, Hatakeyama S et al.: Carcinoma of the esophagogastric junction with extension to the cervical esophagus. *Gan No Rinsho* 33(1):97, 1987

80. Taylor S: Clinical features of thyroid tumours. *Clin Endocrinol Metabol* 8(1):209, 1979

81. Timmis AD, Smallpiece C, Davies AC et al.: Intracardiac spread of intravenous leiomyomatosis with successful surgical excision. *N Engl J Med* 303(18):1043, 1980

82. Tomasini-Degna A, Negri R: Neoplastic invasion of the connective stalks in transitional cell papillary tumors (TCPT) of the bladder. *Urol Res* 15(1):31, 1987

83. Towbin R, Gruppo RA: Pulmonary metastases in neuroblastoma. *AJR* 138(1):75, 1982

84. Veliath AJ, Khanna KK, Subhas BS et al.: Primary lymphosarcoma of the lung with unusual features. *Thorax* 32(5):632, 1977

85. Viadana E, Bross ID, Pickren JW: The metastatic spread of cancers of the digestive system in man. *Oncology* 35(3):114, 1978

86. Von Recklinghausen F: Über die venöse Embolie und die retrograden Transporte in den Venen und in den Lymphgefässen. *Virch Arch* 100:503, 1885

87. Waldeyer W: Die Entwicklung der Carcinome. *Virch Arch* 41:470, 1867

88. White RM, Patterson JW: Cutaneous involvement in Hodgkin's disease. *Cancer* 55(5):1136, 1985

89. Willis RA: *The Spread of Tumors in the Human Body* (3d ed). London: Butterworth, 1973

90. Wolf DJ, Zitelli JA: Surgical margins for basal cell carcinoma. *Arch Dermatol* 123(3):340, 1987

91. Yamasaki Y et al.: A case of the coexistence of renal cysts and renal cell carcinoma associated with direct invasion of the liver (stage IV). *Hinyokika Kiyo* 30(6):817, 1984

92. Yeung HH, Bannatyne P, Russell P: Adenocarcinoma of the Fallopian tubes: a clinicopathological study of eight cases. *Pathology* 15(3):279, 1983

93. Zirkin HJ, Tovi F: Tracheal carcinoma presenting as a thyroid tumor. *J Surg Oncol* 26(4):268, 1984

COMPARISON OF THE PROGRESSION OF SELECTED, TOPOGRAPHICALLY PARTICULAR, TUMORS IN THE HEAD AND NECK REGION
Laryngeal pseudosarcoma, primary cholesteatoma, paraganglioma and schwannoma of the VIIIth cranial nerve

G. BROICH

The head and neck region can be host to a great variety of tumors. In fact with the exception of those arising from the reproductive system, every type of neoplastic growth has its representative in this area. Carcinomas can arise from skin and mucosal surfaces, contained in the cephalic region. The sarcoma family is represented by tumors from all mesenchymal cell types (17), including connective tissue and its derivatives, endothelial tissue, lymphoid and both striated and smooth muscular tissue. Tumors from glial and nervous cells are present as well. Adipose tissue is less abundant and lipomas are less frequent in the oropharyngeal region than in the extremities and the retroperitoneum (42, 43, 62, 107, 113, 115, 124, 204), but Fu and Perzin (63) described a nasopharyngeal liposarcoma and recently a myxoid liposarcoma has been seen by Gaia and Coll. (143) confirming the presence of tumors of all tissue types in the cephalic region. The cephalic region harbors also several peculiar types of tissue. The teeth are formed by both an epithelial element, the ameloblasts, and mesenchymal elements, such as the odontoblasts, cementoblasts and fibroblasts. The former are only transient cells in the odontogenesis of the human, different from the rodents, where the continuously growing incisor teeth are maintained by a vital ameloblastic population. Neoplastic growth from both the ameloblast and the odontoblast has been described, sometimes as mixed odontogenic tumors (217). Ameloblastic growth is thought to derive from islets of less differentiated cells in the periodontal spaces, that are embryonic remnants of the epithelial sheet of the enamel organ, while the odontoblastic component may derive from fibroblasts exposed to cells of the early amelogenic epithelium of the dental lamina. Neoplasms can also arise from cell remnants of another transient organ present in the rhinopharynx, the chorda, and are called chordomas.

The main interest for a separate look on some forms of abnormal growth in the area rises not so much from special histologic features, but from the sometimes peculiar behavior expressed by these tumors. This can be due to special growing patterns or based on the conditions imposed by the unique anatomical relationship between the tumor and a multitude of close lying organ systems in the cephalic extremity. The presence of spaces limited by rigid, bony, structures together with anatomic entities of vital importance, as are the parts of the nervous system harbored in the cephalic extremity, introduces us to a special concept of tumoral behavior. The neoplastic growth, whose degree of malignancy is generally measured in terms of local histologic invasiveness and ability to metastasize, shows here a new feature of potentially life threatening behavior, that can be called topographical and functional malignancy. The neoplasm, growing in a fixed space, will extend first to occupy that area, displacing the other anatomical structures present in the space and limited by it. Encountering the borders of said area, the tumor will continue its growth by eroding and displacing them. The erosion of the generally bony borders happens not in an invasive, and so frankly malignant, process, but through compression induced resorption of bone. It is so a secondary phenomenon, well different from the invasion of bone by truly malignant cells. The result, perhaps, is in both cases the destruction of bone and the impairment of the structural integrity of the surrounding anatomical structures. Therefore the term topographical malignancy, since the neoplasm would behave in an unthreatening way if growing in other areas of the body, where expansion can be easily accomplished without immediate negative effects on the surrounding anatomical structures. Perhaps not only histologically benign tumors can express topographical malignancy. A malignant tumor may arise in areas where its growth becomes a danger for the life of the host not only by its invasiveness or metastasizing ability, but also by local factors. So a laryngeal carcinoma, certainly a malignant tumor, can cause death by obstruction of the airways much earlier than by general dissemination, if untreated. Local recurrences in the neck after surgery may produce exitus due to the erosion of the major local vessels, mainly the carotic artery and jugular vein, with a fatal catastrophic blood loss. The head and neck region with its abundance of vital structures and rigid anatomical spaces offers prime examples for topographical malignancy.

The concept of malignancy as distinct from histological features can be found in other living tissues as well. A reverse behavior is known in plants, where malignant growing cells may not threaten the survival of the plant as a unit, due to the lack of a proper dissemination medium (given in animals by the vascular circulation). Moreover, in a reverse condition that could be called topographical benignity, the local destruction of tissues in a plant, if peripheral to the roots, may not interfere with the general survival of the plant.

Four tumors which in this way can acquire a special interest under both clinical and pathological viewpoints will be brought here as brief examples for this concept. The selection is aimed to comprise a specimen of each major tissue system. It is not supposed to give a comprehensive look on the head and neck oncology, but to introduce the concept of the malignant progression of tumors due to their topography as distinct from their histology. Three histologically benign lesions will be described in conjunction with a malignant one.

K.W. Brunson (ed) Local invasion and spread of cancer.
© 1989, Kluwer Academic Publishers, Dordrecht.

LARYNGEAL PSEUDOSARCOMA

The Laryngeal Pseudosarcoma, described for the first time by Szmurlo (215) and Kahler (112) and delimited as a histopathologic entity of the larynx by Lane (125) and Goellner (79), consists of the association of a laryngeal epidermoid carcinoma, generally of small dimensions, contained in a polypoid mass of great dimensions of proliferating tissue which at the microscopic examination shows cytoplasmatic and nuclear cellular abnormalities peculiar of a sarcoma. The gross appearance is generally that of a polypoid or pedunculated mass without areas of necrosis or ulcerations.

At the microscopic examination there is a great prevalence of sarcomatoid stroma with cellular anomalies and frequent mitosis. At certain times the intercellular edema allows the proliferating cells to assume a stellate and myxomatoid appearance and giant cells with clear nuclear anomalies are abundant. More frequently the cells maintain a fusiform shape embedded in a great amount of collagen and precollagen fibers and assume a disposition in parallel streaks. In rare areas of reduced cellular anomalies the tissue may resemble a granulomatous reaction, but more generally the overall appearance is more like a fibrosarcoma or leiomyosarcoma (79, 114). At certain times the anomalies are so expressed to resemble a liposarcoma or a xantofibrosarcoma (for the classification and review of these soft tissue tumors see (3)).

With exhaustive enough microscopic examination of the tumor, in a restricted area there can always be found a zone of clearly epithelial origin and with an aspect of a generally well-differentiated epidermoid carcinoma. This zone arises from the mucous covering of the polypoid tumor and remains or delimitated to the superficial area, or shows a droplet like ingrowth into the stroma.

Clinically the pseudosarcoma shows a rapid enlargement of the polypoid mass which brings the laryngeal lesions to be rapidly obstructive. It may request an emergency tracheotomy to maintain the airways patent. The further clinical behavior of the tumor is perhaps much less dramatic than could be expected by a sarcoma of that dimensions. It behaves generally much more according to the carcinomatous part embedded in it (7, 184). The incidence of the disease is referred to as rare, but it seems much less exceptional than generally stated. In 1965, Appelman and Oberman (5) could find 54 descriptions present in the literature and add 11 of their own. Additional cases have been reported (68, 69, 186). The overall presence of this type of lesion may well be greater than previously suspected (18).

The fact that the tumor behaves more according to the small carcinoma embedded in it than to the large sarcomatoid mass accompanying it, is of great importance for the treatment, since also large lesions which would have been considered only for palliative radiotherapy, can largely benefit from surgical treatment with a good survival prognosis.

The histogenesis of the tumor has long been debated. The problem lies clearly with the interpretation of the sarcomatoid component. In 1865, Virchow created the term 'carcinosarcoma' for such associated tumors with the definition of the epithelial part as true epidermoid carcinoma. Laryngeal carcinosarcomas have been described by Szmurlo (215), Kahler (112), Uhlman (222), Ricci (174) and Lang and Krainz (126). In a first general survey Saphir and Vass (183)

consider the stroma as purely reactive. Carcinosarcomas can arise also in other oropharyngeal areas, in the esophagus about 50 cases have been described (21, 100, 176, 193, 205). Other areas of pseudosarcomatous growth in the cephalic region are among others the maxillary sinus (220) and the tongue (190). Several authors after 1938 have described carcinomas associated with a fusocellular atypic component (19, 29, 39, 45, 53, 90, 148, 149, 152), but it is with Lane (125) that this form is defined for the first time as a special entity, called pseudosarcoma, excluding other types of apparently mixed growth as for example the nodular fascitis (140). The tumor needs to be held distinct from other forms of atypic growth arising from mesodermal tissue, since, also if rarely, each tissue type present in the larynx may give origin to a neoplastic growth, from fibrous xanthomas (177) to synovial sarcomas (17, 187).

Several major opinions have been expressed regarding the histogenesis of the tumor. Some authors consider the stroma as a true sarcomatoid malignant tissue. Legier (135) and Minchler (141) report three cases with a highly malignant discourse, the presence of sarcomatoid lymphonodal metastasis, and without carcinomatous cells. They sustain the malignancy of the nonepithelial component. This view is held up also by Invernizzi (108), Kupper and Blessing (120) and Szimivasan and Tavalkar (214). A second group, with Lane, considers the tissue as an excessive stromal reaction to the carcinoma. The stroma is considered as exclusively reactive, an opinion expressed also by Baker (10) and Kratz and Ritterhoff (118). Goellner in 1973 (79) expresses the same theory presenting 25 cases of his own. It is supposed to be a special characteristic of these epithelial malignant cells to induce a mesenchymal reaction, for this is found also in the lymphonodal metastases (140, 197). A third group, with Aubry and Leroux-Robert (9) and Kleinsasser and Glanz (114) consider the stroma as of atypic epitheliomatous origin. They explain the whole tumor as of epithelial origin with the pseudosarcomatous component constituted by peculiarly differentiated epithelial cells. This theory has found many followers especially in Europe with Pietrantoni (165), Pizzetti and Leonardelli (166), de Vido (38), Fini-Storchi (46), Rucco and Zerneri (180), Himalstein and Humphrey (96). Rucco and Zerneri (180) and Minnigerode (142) suppose an inducing effect of the radiotherapy of the carcinoma on the pseudosarcomatous component. This theory has been further developed by Randall et al. (171) and especially Kleinsasser and Glanz (114) who describe the fusiform cells as carcinomatous epithelial cells which have lost unspecified surface characteristics becoming able to grow individually.

Finally it may be mentioned a further opinion by Haubrich (89), in which the tumor is seen as a primary benign mesenchymal reaction with the secondary insurgence of a carcinoma.

Also if the origin of the spindle cell component is still unsettled, recent new findings add new biochemical data to its assessment. A protein, called keratin, has been found to be specifically associated with almost all cells of epithelial origin (54, 55, 207, 208, 210). These proteins belong to the intermediate filament family as do vimentin in the mesenchyme, desmin in the muscle, neurofilaments in the nerves and glial filaments in the astrocytes. The keratin has up to now been found in all epithelial cells tested, but is absent in cells of nonepithelial origin (8, 54–57, 207, 208, 210) and can so be considered a marker for cells of epithelial origin, both normal and pathologic. The keratoproteins have been shown to be formed by distinct keratin molecules and more than 17 proteins have been isolated (145, 212). Specific keratin types have been found according to epithelial cell type (40, 58, 221), cellular growth environment (64, 66, 208, 209), stage of cell differentiation (41, 65, 216), stage of development (233) and disease (146, 151, 227). The keratins have been catalogued and their expression in the different epithelial types has been followed (145, 211). Attempts to sequentiate the keratins have been done (59, 198–200) and cDNA sequences have been obtained (86, 87), showing that each keratin type is formed by the expression of a specific gene and not through modification of a primordial common protein. These findings have prompted the research of keratin in cells of uncertain origin, since its presence can be taken as an excellent evidence for their epithelial origin. Specific antibodies to the keratins have been developed (60) with a special effort for standardization by the group directed by Sun (41, 212, 227). The use of antikeratin antibodies on carcinosarcomas or other tumors with an uncertain cell component has given mixed results for different tissues (191). Its application on pseudosarcomatous tumors arising from the larynx has not shown any keratin-like reactivity in the sarcomatoid component (234). It has to be said perhaps, that only Woods tested specifically the pseudosarcoma, excluded in the more recent work of Shi *et al.* (190). Each used different monoclonal antikeratin antibodies, in no series Sun's AE1, AE2 and AE3 antibodies were used. Furthermore, the nonreactivity cannot exclude the presence of keratoproteins definitively. Nonetheless these results generate certainly more evidence for a mesenchymal, and so reactive, origin of the sarcomatoid stroma.

It can be concluded that the pseudosarcoma is certainly determined in its behavior by the carcinomatous component imbedded in it. Besides rare cases in which a true association of sarcoma and carcinoma may be present (141, 205, 214) the pseudosarcomatous part behaves as benign growth. The therapy has so to be focussed on the dimensions, site and extension of the original carcinoma, which generally permits a radical surgical cure, a surgery which may have been renounced of if the whole polypoid mass would have been considered as a sarcoma (18). The tumor will progress as a laryngeal carcinoma, regardless of its sarcomatoid component.

PRIMARY CHOLESTEATOMA

A cholesteatoma is a whitish mass, arising in the middle ear and petrous bone. It consists of lamellar or 'onion-skin-like' disposed layers of keratinizing epidermal cells around an amorphous center, constituted by the desquamated keratinocytes, forming an epidermal cyst. The continuous growth of the keratinocytes with desquamation in a closed cavity is the base of the clinical destructiveness of the tumor, which works its way through the petrous bone without invading it. Cholesteatomas are generally present as a complication of chronic middle ear inflammation. In this case the ingrowth of epidermis through a tympanic perforation is thought to

give origin to the lesion. The tissue forms first a pocket in the middle ear cavity and autonomizes finally itself closing its internal cavity by losing the connection with the external ear canal. Sometimes identical tumors can be found in the petrous bone without any history of middle ear disease and with an intact eardrum. These tumors have generally been considered very rare if not exceptional, but a review of the literature shows easily a large amount of isolated case reports and the impression is that the overall incidence may be greater than originally assumed. They may arise at the cerebellopontine angle, at the jugular foramen, in the petrous pyramid or in the middle ear and mastoid (102). Described as 'tumeur perlée de l'oreille' by Cruveilhier in 1849 (30), Cushing in 1922 (32) expressed the hypothesis that the primary cholesteatomas showed a different pathogenesis than the usual growth found in chronic middle ear disease and were perhaps epidermoid cysts arising from epidermal cell inclusions formed during ontogenesis. This theory is sustained also by Cawthorne *et al.* (23) and Cawthorne (24, 25). The tendency to ascribe cholesteatoma-like lesions to embryonic cell remnant proliferation went so far as to try to describe some middle ear diseases with inflammations and eardrum lesions, principally middle ear cholesteatomas, as secondary to epidermal growth from embryonic cell nests. This point of view is today only of historical significance in middle ear lesions with a perforated eardrum. The majority of authors tend to ascribe only the origin of primary cholesteatomas to the proliferation of cells arising from ectodermal remnants included in the temporal bone during embryogenesis (136). For the diagnosis of primary cholesteatoma an intact eardrum should be present. Obviously the possibility of an unrelated coexistence of a primary cholesteatoma and a chronic middle ear inflammation exists, in which case the diagnosis should be given only if there is clear anatomical distinction and lack of continuity between the lesions. It is rather difficult in these cases to come to a clear diagnosis of origin. Tumors arising in or near to the middle ear cavity are considered to originate from remnants of the first branchial arch, where the cholesteatomas of the petrous bone apex arise from Sessel's pouch (26, 223). This theory has encountered some opposition lately, especially regarding the tumors of the middle ear and those of attical location. Ruedi (181) and Friedman (61) in extended histological studies could not find any epidermal cell remnants in normal temporal bones. Wullstein (235) describes as a frequent finding the presence of small perlaceous tumors right behind an intact attical membrane. The theory of Ruedi, which ascribes these attical cholesteatomas behind intact tympanic membranes to an ingrowth of the basal layer of the epidermis of the membrane of Shrapnell, gains to renewed interest (26, 236), leaving the disontogenetic theory to true apical primary cholesteatomas. Classifications have followed these interpretative difficulties (37) and a definitive viewpoint has still to be agreed upon.

The clinical onset is generally subtle with headaches and Eustachian tube compression as frequent signs, as well as a deficit of the trigeminal nerve, especially in its third branch (67, 156). The nerves of the extrinsic ocular muscles (III, IV, VI) and the acoustico-facial bundle are involved at a second time due to the mostly apical position of the tumor in the petrous bone, i.e. anteriorly to the internal ear canal. Finally the foramen jugulare nerves and the hypoglossus may become involved. The differential diagnosis includes other expansive growth of the petrous bone apex, such as neuromas and meningiomas. The diagnosis relies mainly on radiographic exploration and especially the computerized tomography, which shows a lipidic hypodensity with geographic map like borders (20). A 'truncated' aspect of the apex and asymmetries are of special importance in the radiologic findings.

Due to its continuous expansion in a closed cavity and compression damage to the cranial nerves and the central nervous system these epidermal cysts may acquire a fatal decourse if untreated. The surgery is difficult because of the deep position of the tumor and only few ways of approach are possible (194). One way, reserved for small lesions on the upper side of the bone, is the extradural middle fossa approach (47, 48), the second is a translabyrinthine and transcochlear surgery (101, 106, 169, 170). For a short discussion of these approaches see the Schwannoma of the VIIIth nerve in this chapter. Complete removal is advocated by most surgeons, but it has to be kept in mind that this is not always possible, due to brainstem adherences and deep location. In this case it is of main importance to maintain the cyst's cavity open to the outside through the mastoidectomy opening for draining of the desquamating cells (permanent fistolization) and further medical cure (67). Since the expansion of the cholesteatoma is accomplished through the accumulation of centrally desquamating cells, the presence of a permanent fistula will relieve the internal pressure and arrest the expansive growth of the neoformation.

Comparing finally the local aggressiveness of the lesion with that of the basal cell carcinoma, several important differences have to be noted. The cells of the cholesteatoma remain always typical and with a mitotic count within the normal range. An organization in cell layers, closely resembling normal skin, can be observed. There are visible a basal proliferative layer, a spinous layer and a squamous layer, proceeding from the outside to the inside. There is no visible differentiation toward skin annexes like hairs or sebaceous glands. The local aggressiveness relies only on the expansive pressure created by continuous central desquamation. In the basal cell carcinoma cellular atypias are perhaps present and the dermal/epidermal junction is abnormal and at histologic sections isolated cell nests can be seen, distant from the primary tumor. Perhaps the cell differentiation in the cholesteatoma shows little deviation from the normal. The basal cell carcinoma is surprisingly similar in this, since the evaluation of at least one molecular marker of epithelial cell differentiation, the expression of keratoproteins, has shown no abnormalities or differences from normal skin (119). Keratoproteins as cell differentiation markers have been briefly referenced in the section of the laryngeal pseudosarcoma in this chapter.

The progression of the primary cholesteatoma is that of a topographical, functional malignancy, there is no known tendency of the cells to become histologically malignant. Carcinoma cells may exceptionally be coexistent, but there is no significant relationship of incidence. Three histologically distinct lesions can arise from epidermal tissue, which progress from the topographical malignancy with cellular benignity of the cholesteatoma, to the locally invasiveness of the basal cell carcinoma and finally to the frankly malignant cells of the squamous cell carcinoma.

PARAGANGLIOMA

Paragangliomas or glomus tumors arise from the paraganglia, small cell groups of close association to blood vessels and high vascularization (2), that originate from the neural crest according to the thesis of Masson (160). In the paraganglionic system the adrenal medulla is comprised as well as the carotic body (Luschka's gland, paraganglion of Kohn) and the vagal glomus. Extraadrenal paraganglia are nonchromaffin but are today supposed to possess neuroamine producing capacity (44, 132) and, according to certain authors, may produce neurotransmitting polypeptides. The carotic body and the aortic paraganglionic tissue have a well-established chemoreceptive role in the homeostasis of the blood O_2, CO_2 and pH (71, 74, 75). Specific O_2 partial pressure values in different areas in the glomus tissue have been described by Acker (1). A sensory innervation of the carotic body has been demonstrated in 1928 by De Castro (33) and is established through the nerve of Hering (IX). The aortic paraganglia are innervated by fibers from the vagus (157), which form a distinct nerve only in the rabbit. Sympathetic fibers reach the intraglomic vessels. Microscopically the tissue is characterized by an extremely high vascularization (the carotic glomus has a unit blood flow of 2000 ml/ 100 g/min versus a renal flow of 420 ml/100 g/min!). Two main cell types are found in the glomus, around which some terminologic confusion has arisen and which we will continue to call type I and II cells (17). Type I cells contain a catecholamin, probably dopamin, and show reciprocal synapsis' with intraglomal nerve endings. These cells have been included by Pearse (159, 161) in his Amine Precursor Uptake and Decarboxylase system (APUD) due to cytochemical and ultrastructural characteristics.

Besides the first recognition of the paraganglia by Haller (cited by Rosenwasser (179)) two centuries ago and the studies of the carotic body by Kohn (116), as well as the description of the aortic glomera, paraganglionic tissue has been described in relation to the nodose ganglion of the vagus (229) and in various sites in the temporal bone (rediscovered by Guild (82, 83)), which are now known as a group, as glomus jugulare. Laryngeal paraganglia have been described in the larynx (131) and recently also in the recurrent laryngeal nerve (22). Normal paraganglionic tissue is also present in the trachea, thyroid capsule, orbita, mandible and in various extracephalic regions, not all of which have been clearly proven in humans. The first carotic body tumor has been described by Marchand (139) and the first aortic tumor by Monro (147). Perhaps the detection of tumors from paraganglionic tissue has sometimes preceded the histologic determination of normal tissue in that site, as happened with the laryngeal glomus, where tumors had been described as early as 1955 (4). Today more than 30 laryngeal paragangliomas have been described (99, 122, 225). So tumors in regions where up to now normal tissue has not been demonstrated, as in the nasopharynx (105), may herald the presence of paraganglia in that sites too (14).

Hyperplasia of carotic bodies has been described as a normal adaptation reaction in high altitude dwellers, in which a higher incidence of chemodectomata is also reported (6, 91, 121).

Tumors arising from glomus tissue, called also chemodectomata, are generally well delimitated and firm. Focal hemorrhage and trabecular fibrosis may be present. The 'Zellballen' (cell clusters) of the type I cells are generally somewhat larger than in the normal glomera and are separated by an extensive capillary network. The type I cells have a pale eosinophilic cytoplasm and its granules stain brown and black with Grimelius stain (80, 195, 224). A capsule is generally present also if it can be very thin or even absent in certain areas (123). There is evidence of an increase in connective stromal tissue and hemosiderin deposition with the formation of fibrosiderotic Gamna-Gandy nodules. Small nerve bundles are sometimes visible, also if large nerves are seen exclusively in vagal tumors. The vessels have a thickened wall due to sclerosis, myxoid degeneration and hyperplasia of the smooth muscle tissue.

Malignant degeneration is relatively rare in extramedullary locations, in the head and neck region the most frequent site seems to be the laryngeal glomus (70). The transformation is heralded by the presence of necrosis in the 'Zellballen', invasion of the vascular spaces and presence of mitotic figures. Pluricentricity is present in 10–20% of the cases (133), also if the percentages vary widely in the literature. In certain cases a familial incidence has been observed and these cases account for the greatest part of the pluricentricity seen. The genetic transmission follows an autosomal dominant pattern (206, 232). The most widely accepted classification of these tumors has been established by Grimley et al. (81) and Glenner and Grimley (78), dividing intramedullary and extramedullary tumors.

The clinical symptoms are linked to the site of the tumor. Most forms show no endocrine activity (167), also if neoplasms secerning catecholamines have been described (137). The carotid body tumor appears as a growing tumefaction in the upper carotid region with well-defined margins, horizontal mobility, vertical fixity and transmitted or intrinsic pulsatility. Pain and dysphagia may be present in later stages, symptoms of carotic sinus hypperreflexia are rather rare if present at all. Carotic artery compression finally can give symptoms of reduced blood flow in its internal branch with cephalalgia and vertigo. The tumor can extend up to the skull base and in the parapharyngeal spaces. For surgical purposes three classes have been defined: 1. localized tumor not attached to the vessel wall, 2. tumor attached to the vessel and partially surrounding it, 3. tumor completely surrounding the vessel. Since in the last type the preservation of the carotid is impossible, some authors (134) have advocated surgical treatment only in the first two classes, due to the otherwise high mortality. Better techniques in vascular surgery have perhaps lately widened the surgical indications in these cases (34, 109). The surgeon has always to be prepared to perform vascular reconstruction in paraganglioma removals (189).

Glomus jugulare and tympanicum tumors, known since their description by Rosenwasser (178), arise from the IX and X cranial nerves. The jugularis tumor, laying lower in the tympanic cavity, can produce large bone defects with only few clinical symptoms. When it enters the tympanic cavity tinnitus and hearing loss become evident, a paresis of the VII cranial nerve is rare at this stage. Tympanic glomera tumors arise from the paraganglia along the nerve of Jacobson and give a much earlier symptomatology with pulsatile tinnitus, hearing impairment and visibility of the tumor through the tympanic membrane (94). To establish the diagnosis a radiologic assessment is always necessary and different techniques are used (138, 164, 218, 219) also if arteriography and CT scan remain the most useful ones. A retrograde jugular venography is generally necessary to assess sigmoid sinus invasion and complete the identification of the feeding blood vessels. The tumors have to be differentiated from vascular anomalies present in the middle ear (95). Nonsurgical ways of treatment have been attempted but have been disappointing. Radiotherapy can have only palliative effect (77) and embolization is useful only as a preoperatory attempt to reduce intraoperatory blood loss. The surgery of these tumors is difficult and different techniques have been described (76, 84, 196), but the determination of the surgical treatment is largely the merit of Fisch, who laid the basis of the modern surgical treatment of paragangliomas. Surgery remains the only way of treatment that carries a favorable longterm prognosis (213). Since a clear classification is the first major step for a successful clinical assessment and treatment, Oldring and Fisch (154) and Fisch (52) divided the glomus jugulare and tympanicus tumors in four categories with subdivisions in types C and D, the classification is here reported due to its importance (from Fisch (52)):

A – tumor limited to the middle ear cleft
B – tumor limited to the tympanomastoid area without destruction of bone in the infralabyrinthine compartment
C – tumors extending and destroying bone of the infratemporal and apical compartment of the temporal bone
    C1: tumors destroying the jugular foramen and jugular bulb and with limited involvement of the vertical portion of the carotic canal
    C2: tumors destroying the infralabyrinthine compartment of the temporal bone and invading the vertical portion of the carotic canal
    C3: tumors involving the infralabryinthine and apical compartments with invasion of the horizontal portion of the carotic canal
D – tumors with intracranial extension
    D1: tumors with intracranial extension of less than 2 cm in diameter
    D2: tumors with intracranial extension greater than 2 cm in diameter
    D3: tumors with inoperable intracranial extension

Types A and B are generally removable through a conventional tympanoplasty, while types C1–3 and D1 require the infratemporal fossa approach described by Fisch (51, 110). D2 tumors require a combined otoneurosurgical two-stage approach and D3 tumors need a similar technique for the removal of the extracranial portion of the tumor when indicated. The prognosis of the involved cranial nerves depends on the extension of the tumor. A lack of proper presurgical assessment leads invariably to long-term recurrences of the tumor, which bring to death the patient, like the untreated primary growth, through intracranial invasion and irrefrenable hemorrhage. The high vascularity of the tumor poses in fact certain special problems. A very precise assessment of the feeding vessels of the neoplasm is necessary, large vessels may be in direct contact with the vascular spaces of the tumor. The natural decourse of the tumor ends in fact mostly with a rupture of these vascular spaces and catastrophic blood loss as the terminal event. In this case expansion itself contributes less to the functional malignancy of the tumor than does a special feature of the growth itself, its vascularity.

SCHWANNOMA

The Schwannoma of the VIIIth nerve has been described for the first time by Sandifort in his 'Observationes anatomicopathologicaes' in 1777 (182), reporting a small nodule arisen from the right acoustic nerve. In 1810 Levesque-Lasource recognizes the correlation between the autoptic finding of such growth and the clinical signs of vertigo, deafness, tinnitus, headache and deviation of the tongue. Ballance (11, 12) is supposed to have for the first time successfully excised an acoustic neuroma and with Olivecrona (155) starts the time of serious attempts to preserve the facial nerve in this surgery. Early comprehensive discussions of the tumor can be found in Henschen (31, 92, 93) and Cushing (1917).

Schwannomas can arise from cranial or proximal spinal nerves. They form round or oval, well defined and encapsulated masses with a smooth surface and are generally solitary and monolateral outside v. Recklinghausen's neurofibromatosis. In the latter disease a certain incidence of histologically malignant tumors have been described, but otherwise the neoplasm is mostly benign. The tumor arises from the Schwann cell of the nerve, generally at the transition from the oligodendroglia to the Schwann cell. This latter cell is known to be able to produce collagen and other stromal fibers and especially to give origin to the myelinic sheet of the peripheral nerves. The cell has also phagocyte abilities and originates from the neural crest epithelium. The tumor has an excentric location in the nerve, dislocating and compressing the fibers more than penetrating in between them. Nerve fibers are typically absent in the Schwannoma, a difference with the neurofibroma, where the tumor appears intimately mixed with the nervous fibers. The neoplastic cells are disposed in bundles and the nuclei may show a pseudopalisading pattern around the blood vessels. Fibroreticular tissue as well as hemorrhages and myxoid or xanthomatous degeneration may be present. Areas of high and low cellularity, called Antoni A and B tissue, are also found in Schwannomas, but not in neurofibromas (150, 173, 175).

Also if the solitary Schwannoma of the skull base can arise from virtually every cranial nerve, the more frequent sites are the superior vestibular nerve, the facial nerve and the nerve group of the foramen jugulare. The tumor retains in the majority of cases its benign histologic characteristics and slow growth, but its position in the cranial cavity makes it a life-threatening disease. The acoustic neuroma originates inside the internal auditory canal and in its growth it will then finally extend outside the porus acusticus internus and towards the pontocerebellar angle. The neoplasm will so compress the trigeminus and facial nerves, besides the nervus acusticus, and finally press against the bulbus and pons. This will block the normal liquoral deflux and cause an obstructive hydrocephalus. Besides growing towards the encephalon the neuroma may extend itself inside the temporal bone due to pressure induced bone resorption. In this way it may finally invade the inner ear labyrinth (85, 188, 230). Few cases of isolated primarily intralabyrinthine neuromas, without connection with the internal auditory canal, have been described (36, 231).

The Schwannoma constitutes 8–9% of the intracranial tumors and the incidence, after data from the Swedish Cancer Research Institute, is 0.7 clinically evident cases in 100,000 persons. The real incidence may even be higher, Moberg (144) found one Schwannoma every 100 autopsies done for reasons other than brain tumors.

To understand better the clinical and surgical implications of this neoplasm, a brief discussion of the surgical anatomy of the region of the internal ear canal may be appropriate. Excellent and comprehensive studies by Lang (127–130) have been published; they comprise the topography of the complete canal system of the os temporale, including the facial canal, semicircular canals, vestibule, internal acoustic meatus, sigmoid sinus, superior bulb of the jugular vein, carotic canal, eustachian tube, perilymphatic and endolymphatic ducts and sac, glossopharyngeal nerve and mastoid cell; these studies may be consulted for more information. The internal ear canal presents itself as an invagination of the posterosuperior face of the petrous bone. The porus acusticus internus is situated at about 30 mm from the temporal squama at the union between the medial third with the two lateral thirds of the petrous bone. The canal penetrates in the bone obliquely in a medio-lateral and postero-anterior fashion, forming an angle of about 45° with the major axis of the temporal bone. A posteriorly open angle of 91.7°–92.7° is formed with the mediosagittal line (129). Four internal faces of unequal length of the canal can be described, with the posterior longer than the anterior wall. The median length of the canal is 8.1 mm (129). The diameter of the canal is between 4 and 5 cm with a median value of 3.8 mm. The porus acusticus internus is cut obliquely by the surface of the petrous bone and has so an oval form, with the major diameter in the horizontal plane. The internal end of the canal is formed by an osseous lamina which is divided horizontally by the falciform crest in two parts. The superior fossa is divided again by a small crest, called "Bill's Bar" in otologic surgery. The cranial opening of the fallopian canal (VIIth nerve) is located in the anterior subfossa and in the posterior subfossa the superior vestibular nerve enters the bony labyrinth structures. The inferior fossa is formed anteriorly by the tractus spiralis foraminosus, exit of the cochlear nerve and base of the modiolus, and posteriorly by two foramina for the inferior vestibular nerve and, called foramen singularis Morgagni, for the nerve of the posterior semicircular canal.

The canal contains the VIIth and VIIIth cranial nerves, organized according to the described bony entrance sites. The fibers in the facial nerve are, from front to back: motor fibers, nasolacrimal parasympathetic fibers (from the nucleus Yagitae), gustatory fibers and fibers from the superior salivary nucleus of Kohnstamm. The so-called acoustico-facial anastomotic fibers are present between the facial nerve and the superior vestibular nerve and transport parasympathetic cochlear fibers or, according to other opinions, the efferent regulatory fibers of Rasmussen. Outside the canal the nervous bundle travels in the lateral pontocerebellar cysterna for about 29 mm while performing a rotation that positions the vestibular nerves on top of the cochlear nerve.

The vessels that enter the internal ear canal have been described for the first time by Siebenmann (1982) and subsequently by Konaschko (117). Two major distribution patterns have been seen by these authors. In the first type (of Siebenmann) the internal auditory artery forms one trunk, which then divides into the anterior vestibular artery and the common cochlear artery. This latter vessel then divides into the arteria cochlearis proper and the arteria cochleovestibularis. In the second version (of Konaschko) two distinct arteries enter the canal, called anterior vestibulo-cochlear artery and posterior vestibulo-cochlear artery. The first will then divide into the anterior vestibular artery and the arteria cochlearis proper. Clinically a certain variability of the vascular pattern can be observed, but the labyrinthic arteries enter the canal always through the antero-inferior area, penetrating the area between the facial and the cochlear nerve (228). The antero-inferior cerebellar artery can form a loop inside the canal by itself, with consequent surgical dangers. Lymphatics have not been clearly demonstrated in the canal, but recently a case of facial hemispasm due to a lymph node inside the internal ear canal has been described (153).

The anterior canal wall is in direct relationship with the carotic artery canal, from which it sometimes is divided by a few air cells, and with the basal part of the cochlea. The inferior wall faces the bulbus of the jugular vein. The posterior wall corresponds initially to the postero-superior face of the rocca and more laterally to the vestibular cavity. Its lateral end is in direct continuity of an imaginary plane passing parallel to the anterior wall of the ampulla of the lateral semicircular canal. The superior wall is separated from the middle cranial fossa by a thin bony lamina. Some air cells may be present also in this site, but they are exceptional. On the supero-anterior face of the petrous bone, in the middle fossa, from medial to lateral, the foramen spinosum of the middle meningeal artery, the Fallopian hiatus of the greater superficial petrous nerve, several small foramina for the lesser superficial petrous nerve and the deep petrous nerve and finally the eminentia arcuata can be seen. It should be stressed that the eminentia arcuata cannot be taken as a point of reference for the topographic site of the superior semicircular canal (13).

The treatment of the acoustic neuroma can basically be accomplished through three surgical approaches ((16, 97, 98, 103, 104, 162, 170) among others). The first is given by the suboccipital approach, done for the first time by Ballance and developed further by Dandy and Olivecrona. It consists of the opening of the posterior cranial fossa through the squama occipitalis posteriorly to the sigmoid sinus. The necessary dislocation of the cerebellar hemisphere was originally often followed by brain stem compression. Olivecrona was able to reduce the mortality of this surgery significantly through an hemicerebellectomy with conservation of the tectal and dentate nuclei, allowing so for a better postoperative functional recovery. The access is oriented towards the postero-superior face of the pyramid, reaching the porus acusticus internus through the pontocerebellar angle. It is rather large and permits the excision of tumors of greater dimensions, but generally it does not carry a good prognosis as far as the functionality of the facial nerve is concerned. A combination of neurologic and otologic techniques to approach the posterior wall of the internal ear

canal and to open it has been proposed. So the complete tumor, which originates deep inside the canal, can be removed and the prognosis for the facial nerve will be decisively better, also if the incidence of postoperative functional indemnity remains rather low. The use of microsurgical techniques for the approach of the intracanalicular part of the neuroma is today definitively warranted.

The second way of access is given by the translabyrinthine approach. This technique has been used for the first time by Panse in 1904 (158) and, after a certain time of virtual oblivion, been reproposed mainly by House (104) and Garcia-Ibanez (72). Initially an as wide as possible mastoidectomy is done with wide exposure of the triangle of Trautman between the facial nerve and the sigmoid sinus. Posteriorly the opening should extend to the dura medially of the sinus and superiorly arrive at the dura of the fossa media and the tegmen tympani. Anteriorly the cavity will be delimitated by the geniculate ganglion, as well as the second and the third part of the facial nerve. Through the atticus the hammer and incus become visible and are extirpated. Medially the cavity is closed by the bony labyrinth block. Drilling on this bone block now, the lateral semicircular canal is encountered first. The posterior canal, which forms with the lateral canal a 90° angle, is found at a slightly deeper level. Sometimes a few air cells divide the canal from the dura of the posterior fossa, at other times the canal is in direct contact with the cortical layer of the petrous bone. At a significantly deeper level in the area superior to these canals the superior semicircular canal can be found, both following the posterior canal to the crus commune and the lateral canal to the ampulla. The bony vestibulum is now exposed with attention on preserving the anterior wall of the ampulla of the lateral semicircular canal, which lies in one plane with the lateral extremity of the internal auditory canal. The anterior wall of the lateral semicircular canal forms the anterosuperior limit of the dissection. The internal auditory canal is now opened and the nervous bundle exposed, encountering the two vestibular nerves at a primary level. This facilitates the enucleation of the neuroma. The superior and the facial nerves are divided by a small bony ridge, useful for the surgical separation of the nerves, especially if widely dislocated and compressed by the expanding tumor. The dissection of the facial nerve along the capsule of the tumor and the excision of the neuroma with special care for the possibly present major vessels follow. Finally the closure of the mastoidectomy and labyrinthectomy cavities concludes the operation. If the operating space should result insufficient due to an expansion of the tumor greater than originally assumed, it can be easily extended posteriorly by sectioning the sigmoid sinus and including a part of the occipital squama in the craniotomy.

The third access is given by the transtemporal operation. This more recent type of surgery has been developed and refined mainly by Fisch in Zurich (49, 50). A trapezoidal craniotomy of 4 × 3 cm with the minor basis at the level of the zigomatic radix of the temporal bone is done. The dura is detached from the anterosuperior face of the rocca petrosa up to the foramen spinosum medially and the superior petrous sinus posteriorly. The eminentia arcuata is so exposed and on a line between it and the foramen spinosum, at about 15 mm from the latter, the greater superficial petrosal nerve can be seen. To identify the location of the lateral, deep, extremity of the internal auditory canal several procedures have been proposed. The most interesting are: 1. House (103) – identify the greater petrosal nerve and follow it to the genicolate ganglion first, by drilling the covering bone. The facial nerve can then be followed into the internal auditory canal. The extensive exposure of the facial nerve can result in damage of the nerve itself or of its vascularization. 2. Portmann et al. (168) – a line parallel to the superior ridge of the petrous bone passing through the superior extremity of the eminentia arcuata, should encounter the lateral extremity of the internal auditory canal at about 10 mm medially. The anatomical variances of the eminentia arcuata and the non direct visibility of the reference points constitute a major drawback of this method. 3. Fisch (48) – the angle between the superior semicircular canal and the internal auditory canal is supposed to be at a fixed angle of 60°. After drilling the bone until exposing the 'blue line' of the semicircular canal, the internal auditory canal should lay at 10 mm medial from it. An accidental opening of the semicircular canal with resulting deafness is the major danger. The drill may also contribute to an acoustic trauma to the ear. As said, the eminentia arcuata cannot be taken as a reference point for the semicircular canal due to a certain degree of anatomical variation. 4. Sterkers et al. (201–203) and Chouard (27) – the binaural axis is thought to cross the internal auditory canal, which should be found at 28–30 mm distance medially from the squama of the temporal bone. A major difficulty arises from having the reference points lying outside the surgical field. 5. Garcia-Ibanez (72) – the eminentia arcuata and the greater superficial petrosal nerve are taken as reference points. Two lines are drawn, the first along the course of the petrosal nerve and corresponding to the ampulla of the superior semicircular canal, the second along the eminentia arcuata. The two lines form an angle whose bisecting line should encounter the internal auditory canal the nervous bundle is visualized. Sectioning the dura longitudinally with a Wullstein scalpell the superior vestibular nerve posteriorly and the facial nerve anteriorly, united by the acoustico-facial anastomosis', will be in the primary plane. The neuroma is separated from the facial nerve and excised. The cochlear nerve lies deep in the field and can be preserved in a certain amount of cases, due to the dimensions of the tumor.

The anatomical topography of the vestibular nerves in the inner ear canal can explain most of the early signs of the neuroma of the acousticus. This tumor has a peak incidence at 45 years with a greater prevalence in the female. The clinical onset is mostly subtle, if compression of the labyrinthine arteries does not result in an inner ear infarct. In 1917 Cushing (31) described the sequence of symptoms as follows: 1. auditory and vestibular dysfunctions, 2. headache, 3. cerebellar signs, 4. cranial nerve deficits, 5. intracranial hypertension, 6. dysarthria and dysphagia, 7. respiratory dysfunction. It can be seen that besides point 1, all other signs are expressions of major tumors which expand widely into the pontocerebellar angle. Basically tumors larger than 20 mm can given origin to headaches that have no specific time pattern in their insorgence, equilibrium disorders of cerebellar origin with dysmetry, adiadochocinesis, asynergy and atony and finally compression signs from basically all cranial nerves in a very multiform pattern. The olfactory and optic nerves can be damaged through the endocranial

hypertension, the other nerves may be compressed directly. Finally pyramidal signs may be present due to bulbar compression. This compression is then also the final cause of death with respiratory arrest. The tumor never invades the bulbus histologically. The dysfunctions of the nerves VII and VIII are the only useful signs for an early diagnosis. A generally slowly progressive hypoacusia centered on the higher frequencies is often the first and only sign. Tinnitus is frequently present, the damage is monolateral. Newer audiologic techniques are most helpful in detecting also very small tumors, under the 1.5 cm limit of the computerized tomography. A test battery including tonal audiometry, speech audiometry, tympanic reflex studies (28, 111) and especially electric potential audiometry (15) is generally able to detect small-sized intracanalicular tumors. The slow growth of the tumor allows the vestibular system to reach a good clinical compensation and the vestibular tests are of less use than originally thought, showing an aspecific hyporeflexia, which may confirm but not establish a diagnosis. The motor fibers of the facial nerve are more resistant to compression than the afferent fibers and so electrogeusimetry may monitor facial nerve damage before a paresis becomes visible. Radiological tests used are principally the computerized tomography (185), which generally can show tumors that sprout from the inner ear canal, but is of less use for the detection of intracanalicular tumors due to its separation limit at around 1.5 cm, pneumoencephalography and contrast cisternography. The use of air enhancement in computer tomography has been proven valuable for the assessment of intracanalicular tumors (172). The angiographic study of the pontocerebellar angle is important, especially to detect the presence of an intracanalicular loop of the antero-inferior cerebellar artery and the tumors' vascularization.

The main significance of this tumor is the striking importance of an early detection, which may not only allow its radical removal but also to preserve the function of the facial nerve in the inner ear canal. Every unilateral neurosensorial hearing loss has to be evaluated in this sense. An early detection leads to a good functional prognosis for the facial nerve, while big tumors show a rapidly worsening outlook and when the tumor extends towards the brain stem it may request a suboccipital approach with extensive manipulation of the cerebellum and consequent functional damage. Small tumors can benefit from transtemporal or translabyrinthine surgery which allow in a high percentage of cases the preservation of the facial nerve. The selection of the surgical approach is in fact mainly based on the size of the tumor. Neuromas may be classified in small (< 8 mm), medium (8–35 mm) and large (> 35 mm). For small neuromas the transtemporal approach may be used. It is the least traumatic, does not destroy the labyrinth and opens the dura only in a small area in the internal ear canal. Only minimal bony removal is necessary. Major dangers are a non-exact localization of the end of the internal ear canal with damage to the nearby cochlea and to the facial nerve after opening the geniculatum. The chief disadvantage is the small exposure. The major advantage is the possibility to preserve hearing, which may be as high as 25% (49). For tumors of median size the translabyrinthic approach is favored. This technique produces a complete destruction of the posterior labyrinth and consequent deafness. The dural opening is wider than in the transtemporal approach and large part of the pontocerebellar angle can be explored. The facial nerve can be preserved in 80–90% of the cases. The access is limited by the sigmoid sinus posteriorly and the plane of the fallopian canal anteriorly. It can be widened by sectioning the sigmoid sinus towards the occipital side. An anterior extension of the surgical field is more cumbersome and would include the execution of a so-called transcochlear approach (35, 73, 106, 169). In this the facial nerve is freed in its whole length and rerouted posteriorly. The cochlea is then drilled out and the bone is removed up to the carotic artery and the apex of the petrous bone. This allows a large vision of the middle and posterior fossa's skull base. This technique is generally used for clivus or petrous apex tumors and not for neuromas which grow principally in the posterior fossa. Large tumors still warrant the suboccipital approach which permits an ample approach to the pontocerebellar angle, but carries a bad functional prognosis for the facial nerve and a significantly higher postoperative morbidity and mortality.

Concluding, the acoustic Schwannoma is a prime example for a histologically benign tumor with clear topographical malignancy. The lesion, due to its expansive growth, produces a sequence of functional failures of the cranial nerves first and the cerebellum later. Functional malignancy is expressed here through multiple impairments in the nervous system. Finally, if untreated, the neoplasm, while still histologically benign, will bring the patient to death due to brain stem compression with obstructive hydrocephalus and respiratory arrest. Early diagnosis is essential to eradicate the tumor before it reaches large dimensions. The diagnosis and cure of the tumor warrants a close collaboration between several medical specialties, especially neurosurgery and otorhinolaryngology.

REFERENCES

1. Acker: Local oxygen tension field in the glomus caroticum of the cat and its change at changing arterial pO2. *Pflügers Archiv ges Physiol* 329:136, 1971
2. Adams WE: The comparative morphology of the carotid body and carotid sinus, Springfield, Illinois, C.C. Thomas, 1958
3. Anderson WAD. Pathology, 7th edition, Saunders, 1978
4. Andrews AH: Glomus tumor (non chromaffin paraganglioma) of the larynx. Case Report; Ann Otol 64:1034, 1955
5. Appelman HD, Oberman HA: Squamous cell carcinoma of the larynx with spindle cell carcinoma and 'Pseudosarcoma': *Am J Clin Path* 44:135, 1965
6. Arias-Stella J, Valcarel J: Chief cell hyperplasia in the human carotid body at high altitudes. *Hum Path* 7:361, 1976
7. Ascenzi A, Scalori G: Sul problema del cosiddetto carcinosarcoma della laringe. *Bol Mal Orecchio, Gola, Naso* 83:140, 1965
8. Asch BB, Burstein NA, Vidrich A, Sun TT: Identification of mouse mammary epithelial cells by immunofluorescence with rabbit and guinea pig antikeratin sera. *Proc Natl Acad Sci USA* 78:5643, 1981
9. Aubry M, Leroux-Robert J: Deux cas de tumeurs pediculees de l'endolarynx. Discussion histologique: Fibro-granulome? Sarcome fibroblastique? Epitelioma atipique a cellules fusiformes? *Ann Otolaryng* 3:207, 1937
10. Baker DC Jr: Pseudosarcoma of the pharynx and larynx. *Ann Otol Rhinol Laryng* 68:471, 1959
11. Ballance CA: Some points in the surgery of the brain and its membranes. London, Macmillan, 1907
12. Beevor CE, Ballance CA: A case of subcortical cerebral tumor treated by operation. *Brit Med J* 5:9, 1895
13. Bellocq P: L'os temporale chez l'homme adulte. Iconographie et description de l'os et de sous caverns. Paris, Masson Cie, 1924
14. Bertogalli D, Calearo C, Pignataro O: Les paragangliomas non chromatophiles a siege rare. *Ann Otol (Paris)* 76:688, 1959
15. Brackman DE: Electric response audiometry in a clinical practice. *Laryngoscope* 87:Suppl 5, 1977
16. Brackmann DE: Acoustic neuroma surgery: Otologic Medical Group Results. In *Neurological Surgery of the Ear*, Aesculapius Publ Co, Birmingham Ala, Vol 2, 1979
17. Broich G: Anatomia e clinica delle tumefazioni croniche cervicali. Thesis, Clinica Otorinolaringoiatrica dell'Università di Pavia, Pavia, 1980
18. Broich G: Lo pseudosarcoma laringeo. Le ipotesi istogenetiche correlate al trattamento curativo. *Otorinolaringologia* 31:21, 1981
19. Brooks SM: Carcinoma which simulates sarcoma. A study of 110 specimens from various sites. *Arch Pathol* 36:144, 1943
20. Calabro A, Horn YE, Kulesza E, Gardeur D, Haddad K, Dakar A, Metzger J: Tumeurs Primitives de l'angle pontocerebelleux. Aspect tomodensimetrique (TDM). *Revue de Laryngol* 100:69, 1979
21. Calhoun T, Ali SD, Muna D, Kurz L, Simmons L, Nash E: Carcinosarcoma of the oesophagus. Case report and review of literature. *J Thorac Cardiovasc Surg* 66:315, 1973
22. Carlson B, Dahlquist A, Domeij S: Carotid body like tissue within the recurrent laryngeal nerve: An endoneural chemosensitive micro-organ? *Am J Otolaryngol* 4:334, 1983
23. Cawthorne T, Griffith A: Primary cholesteatoma of the temporal bone. *Arch Otolaryngol* 73:252, 1961
24. Cawthorne T: Congenital cholesteatoma. *Acta Otolaryngol* 78:248, 1963
25. Cawthorne T: Cholesteatome congenital. *Acta Otorhinolaryng Belg* 25:833, 1971
26. Charachon R: Les tumeurs due rocher. *Revue de Laryng* 100:119, 1979
27. Chouard CH: Le traitement chirurgical des vertiges par la neurectomie vestibulaire. Principle et technique. *Rev Laryngol Otol Rhinol (Bord)* 94:51, 1973
28. Clemis JD, Sarno CN: The acoustic reflex latency test: Clinical application. *Laryngoscope* 90:601, 1980
29. Clerf LH: Sarcoma of the larynx. Report of eight cases. *Arch ORL* 44:517, 1946
30. Cruveilhier J: Traité d'anatomie pathologique generale. Paris, JB Bailliere, 1849–1864
31. Cushing H: Tumors of the nervus acousticus. Saunder Co, Philadelphia, 1917
32. Cushing H: A large epidermal cholesteatoma of parietotemporal region deforming left hemisphere without cerebral symptoms. *Surg Gynec Obst* 34:557, 1922
33. De Castro F: Sur la structure et l'innervation du sinus carotidien de l'homme et des mammiferes. Noveaux faits sur l'innervation et la fonction du glomus caroticum. Etudes anatomiques et physiologiques. *Trab Inst Cajal Invest Biol* 25:331, 1928
34. Dent TL, Thomson NW, Fry WJ: Carotid body tumors. *Surgery* 80:365, 1976
35. De la Cruz A: Transcochlear approach to lesions of the cerebellopontine angle and clivus. *Rev Laryng* 102:33, 1981
36. DeLozier HL, Gacek RR, Dana ST: Intralabyrinthine Schwannomas. *Ann Otol Rhinol Laryngol* 88:187, 1979
37. Derlacki EL, Clemis JD: Congenital cholesteatoma of the middle ear and mastoid. *Ann Otol Rhinol Laryngol* 74:706, 1965

38. de Vido G: Tumore misto laringo-faringeo a singolare evoluzione. *Valsalva* 29:187, 1953
39. Diehl KL: Sarcoma of the larynx. Report of two cases. *Arch ORL* 57:40, 1953
40. Doran TL, Vidrich A, Sun TT: Intrinsic and extrinsic regulation of the differentiation of skin, corneal and esophageal epithelial cells. *Cell* 22:17, 1980
41. Eichner R, Bonitz P, Sun TT: Classification of epidermal keratins according to their immunoreactivity, isoelectric point, and mode of expression. *J Cell Biol* 98:1388, 1984
42. Enterline H, Culberson JD, Rochlin DB, Luther WB: Liposarcoma. A clinical and patholgical study of 53 cases. *Cancer* 13:932, 1960
43. Enzinger FM, Weiss SW: Soft tissue tumors. The CV Mosby Co, St Louis, 1983
44. Farrior JB, Hyams VJ, Benke RH, Brown-Farrior J: Glomus carcinoid apudoma. *Laryngoscope* 90:110, 1980
45. Figi FA: Sarcoma of the larynx. *Arch Otolaryng* 21:21, 1933
46. Fini-Storchi C: Carcinomi della laringe simulanti carcinosarcomi e sarcomi. *Boll Mal Orecchio, Gola, Naso* 78:234, 1960
47. Fisch U: Die transtemporale, extralabyrinthare Chirurgie des inneren Gehörganges. *Arch Klin Exp Ohr Nas Kehlk* 194:232, 1969
48. Fisch U: Transtemporal surgery of the internal auditory canal. Report of 92 cases, technique, indications and results. *Adv Otorhinolaryng* 17:203, 1970
49. Fisch U: The middle fossa approach to the internal auditory meatus. In *Ballantyne: Ear-Operative Surgery*, Butterworth, London, 179–192, 1976
50. Fisch U: Facial nerve surgery. Birmingham Ala, Aesculapius Publishing Co, 1977
51. Fisch U: Infratemporal fossa approach for extensive tumors of the temporal bone and base of the skull. In: *Neurological Surgery of the Ear*, edited by Silverstein H, Norell H, Birmingham, Alabama, Aesculapius, 1977
52. Fisch U: Infratemporal fossa approach for glomus tumors of the temporal bone. *Ann Otol Rhinol Laryngol* 91:474, 1982
53. Frank I, Lev M: Carcinosarcoma of the larynx. *Ann Otol Laryng* 49:113, 1940
54. Franke WW, Weber K, Osborne M, Schmid E, Freudenstein C: Antibody to prekeratin: Decoration of tonofilament-like arrays in various cells of epithelial character. *Exp Cell Res* 116:429, 1978
55. Franke WW, Schmid E, Osborn M, Weber K: Different intermediate sized filaments distinguished by immunofluorescence microscopy. *Proc Natl Acad Sci USA* 75:5034, 1978
56. Franke WW, Appelhans B, Schmid F, Freudenstein M, Osborn M, Weber K: Identification and characterization of epithelial cells in mammalian tissues by immunofluorescence microscopy using antibodies to prekeratin. *Differentiation* 15:7, 1979
57. Franke WW, Schmid E, Freudenstein C, Appelhans B, Osborne M, Weber K, Kennan TW: Intermediate-sized filaments of the prekeratin type in myoepithelial cells. *J Cell Biol* 84:633, 1980
58. Franke WW, Schiller DL, Moll R, Winter S, Schmid E, Engelbrecht I, Denk H, Krepler R, Platzer E: Diversity of cytokeratins: Differentiation-specific expression of cytokeratin polypeptides in epithelial cells and tissues. *J Mol Biol* 153:933, 1981
59. Franke WW, Schiller DL, Hatzfeld M, Winter S: Protein complexes of intermediate-sized filaments: Melting of cytokeratin complexes in urea reveals different polypeptide separation characteristics. *Proc Natl Acad Sci USA* 50:7113, 1983
60. Franke WW, Schmid E, Mittnacht S, Grund C, Jorcano JL: Integration of different keratins into the same filament system after microinjection of mRNA for epidermal keratins into kidney epithelial cells. *Cell* 36:813, 1984
61. Friedman L: Congenital cholesteatoma. In: *Pathology of the Ear*, pp 99–103, Blackwell Scientific Publications, Oxford, 1974
62. Fu YS, Perzin K: Non-epithelial tumors of the nasal cavity, paranasal sinuses and nasopharynx: a clinico-pathologic study. VII: Myxoma. *Cancer* 39:195, 1977
63. Fu YS, Perzin K: Non-epithelial tumors of the nasal cavity, paranasal sinuses and nasopharynx: a clinico-pathologic study. VIII: Adipose tissue tumors (lipoma and liposarcoma). *Cancer* 40:1314, 1977
64. Fuchs E, Green H: The expression of keratin genes in epidermis and cultured epidermal cells. *Cell* 15:887, 1978
65. Fuchs E, Green H: Changes in keratin gene expression during terminal differentiation of the keratinocyte. *Cell* 19:1033, 1980
66. Fuchs E, Green H: Regulation of terminal differentiation of cultured human keratinocytes by vitamin A. *Cell* 25:617, 1981
67. Gacek RR: Evaluation and management of primary petrous apex cholesteatoma. *Otolaryngol Head Neck Surg* 88:519, 1980
68. Galankin VN, Livshits GS: Carcinosarcoma of the larynx. *Arch Path Mosk* 38:58, 1976
69. Galle E, Vollmar F, Rüdiger K-D: Beitrag zum Karzinosarkom des Larynx. *HNO* 19:336, 1971
70. Gallivan MVE, Chun B, Rowdwn G, Lack EE: Laryngeal paraganglioma. Case report with ultrastructural analysis and literature review. *Am J surg Path* 3:85, 1979
71. Gannong W: Review of medical physiology. Lange, 1983
72. Garcia-Ibanez E, Garcia-Ibanez JL: Cirugia del conducto auditivo interno. *Acta Otorrhinolaring Esp* 24:324, 1973
73. Garcia-Ibanez E: Communication at the Doctorate Honoris Causa to L Garcia-Ibanez at Ferrara University, Ferrara, Italy, 1980
74. Gauer, Kramer, Jung: Physiologie des Menschen. Band 3, Herz und Kreislauf, Urban & Schwarzenberg, 1972
75. Gauer, Kramer, Jung: Physiologie des Menschen. Band 6, Atmung, Urban & Schwarzenberg, 1975
76. Glassock ME III, Harris PF: Glomus tumors: Diagnosis and treatment. *The Laryngoscope* 84:2006, 1974
77. Glasscock ME III, Jackson CG: Glomus tumors: Diagnosis and surgery. *Rev Laryngol* 100:131, 1979
78. Glenner GG, Grimley PM: Tumors of the extraadrenal paraganglion system (including chemoreceptors), Atlas of Tumor Pathology, second series fasc 9, Washington DC, Armed Forces Inst of Path, 1974
79. Goellner R: Pseudosarcoma of the larynx. *Am J Clin Path* 59:312, 1973
80. Grimelius L: A silver nitrate stain for alpha 2 cells in human pancreatic islet. *Acta Soc Med Upsala* 73:243, 1968
81. Grimley PM, Glenner GG: Histology and ultrastructure of carotid body paragangliomas. Comparison with the normal gland. *Cancer* 20:1473, 1967
82. Guild SR: A hitherto unrecognized structure, the glomus jugularis, in man. *Anat Rec* 79:28, 1941
83. Guild SR: The glomus jugulare, a non-chromaffin paraganglion, in man. *Ann Otol Rhinol Laryng* 62:1045, 1953
84. Haguenauer J-P, Charachon R, Gaillard J, Romanet Ph: Tumeurs glomiques tympano-jugulaires. *Rev Laryng* 100:125, 1979
85. Haid T: Früherkennung des Akustikusneurinoms durch quantitative Neurootologie und radiologische Feindiagnostik. Habilitationsschrift Universität Erlangen-Nürnberg, 1980
86. Hanukoglu I, Fuchs E: The cDNA sequence of a human epidermal keratin: Divergence of sequence but conservation of structure among intermediate filament proteins. *Cell* 31:243, 1982
87. Hanukoglu I, Fuchs E: The cDNA sequence of a type II

cytoskeletal keratin reveals constant and variable structural domains among keratins. *Cell* 33:915, 1983

88. Harnell W: Carotid body tumors, familial and bilateral. *Ann Surg* 171:843, 1970
89. Haubrich J: Carcinomenentstehung an der Oberfläche eines riesenzelligen Tumores des Stimmbandes. *HNO* 14:176, 1960
90. Havens FZ, Parkhill EM: Tumours of the larynx other than squamous cell epithelioma. *Arch ORL Chicago* 34:1113, 1941
91. Heath D, Edwards C, Harris P: Postmortem size and structure of the human carotid body. *Thorax* 25:129, 1970
92. Henschen F: Über Geschwülste der hinteren Schädelgrube, insbesondere des Kleinhirnbrückenwinkels. Fischer, Jena, 1910
93. Henschen E: Zur Histologie und Pathogenese der Kleinhirnbrückenwinkeltumoren. *Arch Psych Nervenkrankheiten* 56:20, 1915
94. Hildmann H: Gutartige Tumoren des Felsenbeines. *Laryng Rhinol Otol* 53:289, 1979
95. Hildmann H, Tiedjen KV: Zur Differentialdiagnose der Glomus-Tumoren. *Laryng Rhinol Otol* 62:502, 1983
96. Himalstein MR, Humphrey TR: Pleomorphic carcinoma of the larynx. *Arch ORL Chicago* 87:389, 1968
97. Hitselberger WE, House WF: Transtemporal bone microsurgical removal of acoustic neuromas. Tumors of the cerebellopontine angle. *Arch Otolaryngol* 80:720, 1964
98. Hitselberger WE, House WF: A combined approach to the cerebellopontine angle. *Arch Otolaryngol* 84:267, 1966
99. Hooper R: Chemodectomata of the glomus laryngicum superior. *Laryngoscope* 82:686, 1972
100. Hornball P, Luggin HM: Carcinosarcomata of the oesophagus. *Ugeskr Laeg* 141:315, 1979
101. House WF, Doyle JB Jr: Early diagnosis and removal of primary cholesteatoma causing pressure to the VIIIth nerve. *Laryngoscope* 72:1053, 1962
102. House HP: An apparent primary cholesteatoma, case report. *Laryngoscope* 63:712, 1953
103. House WF: Monograph: Transtemporal bone micro-surgical removal of acoustic neuromas. *Arch Otolaryngol* 80:597, 1964
104. House WF: Acoustic neuromas, monograph II. *Arch Otolaryngol* 88:644, 1968
105. House JM, Goodman ML, Gacek RR, Green GI: Chemodectomas of the nasopharynx. *Arch Otolaryngol* 96:138, 1972
106. House WF, De la Cruz A, Hitselberger WE: Surgery of the skull base: Transcochlear approach to the petrous apex and clivus. *Otolaryngology, Head Neck Surg* 86:770, 1978
107. Hutton I: Liposarcoma of the thigh. *Proc R Soc Med* 67:655, 1974
108. Invernizzi M: Su di un caso di forma mista di neoplasia laringea. *Min Otol* 9:414, 1959
109. Javit H: Carotid body tumor: Resection or reflection. *Arch Surg* 111:344, 1976
110. Jenkins HA, Fisch U: Glomus tumors of the temporal region. *Arch Otolaryngol* 107:209, 1981
111. Jerger J, Hanford E, Clemis J: The acoustic reflex in eighth nerve disorders. *Arch Otolaryngol* 99:409, 1974
112. Kahler O: Ein Carcino-Sarcom des Recessus Piriformis bei Ekchondrose des Ringknorpels. *Dtsch Med Wschr* 34:614, 1908
113. Kindblon LG, Angervalle L, Jarlstedt J: Liposarcoma of the neck. A clinicopathologic study of 4 cases. *Cancer* 42:774, 1978
114. Kleinsasser O, Glanz H: Sarkomähnliche Gewebsbilder in Larynx-Karzinomen. Pseudokarzinome, Karzinosarkome, Spindelzellenkarzinome, pleomorphe Karzinome. *Z Laryng Rhinol Otol* 57:225, 1978
115. Knowles CHR, Huggil PH: Liposarcoma: with report of a case in a child. *J Path Bact* 68:235, 1954

116. Kohn A: Die Paraganglien. *Arch Mikrosk Anatomie* 62:263, 1903
117. Konaschko PI: Die Arteria auditiva des Menschen und ihre Labyrinthäste. *Z Anat Entwickl-Gesch* 83:241, 1927
118. Kratz RC, Ritterhoff R: Sarcoma of the larynx. *Ann Otol Rhinol Laryng* 70:239, 1961
119. Kubilus J, Baden HP, McGilvray N: Filamentous protein of basal cell epithelioma: Characteristics *in vivo* and *in vitro*. *J Natl Cancer Inst* 65:869, 1980
120. Kupper K, Blessing MH: Carzino-sarkom des Larynxbereiches. *HNO* 22:103, 1974
121. Lack EE: Carotid body hypertrophy in patients with cystic fibrosis and cyanotic congenital heart disease. *Hum Path* 8:39, 1977
122. Lack EE, Cubilla AL, Woodruff JM, Farr HW: Paragangliomas of the head and neck region: a clinical study of 69 patients. *Cancer* 39:397, 1977
123. Lack EE, Cubilla AL, Woodruff JM: Paragangliomas of the head and neck region: A pathologic study of tumors from 71 patients. *Hum Path* 10:191, 1979
124. Lagage R, Jacob S, Seemayer TA: Mixoid liposarcoma: an electronmicroscopic study: Biological and histogenetic considerations. *Virchows Arch (Path Anat)* 384:159, 1979
125. Lane N: Pseudosarcoma (polipoid sarcomalike masses) associated with squamous cell carcinoma of the mouth, fauces and larynx. *Cancer* 10:19, 1957
126. Lang FJ, Krainz W: Carcinosarkom des hypopharynx. *Z Hals Nasen Ohrenh* 5:179, 1923
127. Lang J, Hofmann S, Maier R, Schafhauser O: Über postnatale Wachstumsveränderungen im Bereich der Fossa cranialis posterior. I. Facies posterior partis petrosae (porus et meatus acusticus internus, fossa subarcuata, apertura externa aqueductus vestibuli, apertura externa canaliculi cochlea). *Gogenbaurs morph Jahrb* 127:305, 1981
128. Lang J, Schreiber Th: Über Form und Lage des Foramen jugulare (fossa jugularis), des Canalis caroticus und des Foramen stylomastoideum sowie deren postnatale Lageveränderungen. *HNO* 31:80, 1983
129. Lang J, Hack Ch: Über Lage und Lagevariationen der Kanalsysteme im Os temporale. Teil I. Kanäle der Pars petrosa zwischen Margo superior und Meatus acusticus internus. *HNO* 33:176, 1985
130. Lang J, Hack Ch: Über Lage und Lagevariationen der kanalsysteme im os temporale. Teil II. Kanäle der pars petrosa zwischen meatus acusticus internus und facies inferior partis petrosae. *HNO* 33:279, 1985
131. Lawson W, Zak FG: The glomus bodies (paraganglioma) of the human larynx. *Laryngoscope* 84:98, 1974
132. Lawson W: The neuroendocrine nature of the glomus cell. An experimental ultrastructural and histochemical tissue culture study. Triological Thesis, *Laryngoscope* 90:120, 1980
133. Lawson W: Glomus bodies and tumors. *New York State Journal Medicine*, p 1567, September 1980
134. LeCompte PM: Tumors of the carotid body and related structures (chemoreceptor system). Washington DC, US Armed Forces Inst Path, p 40, 1951
135. Legier JF: Carcinosarcoma of the upper respiratory tract: Report of two cases and review of the literature. *Ann Otol Rhinol Laryng* 71:173, 1962
136. Leopold DA, Gacek RR: Petrous apex tumors. *New York State J Medicine*, pp 1564–1566, September 1980
137. Levit SA, Sheps SG, Espinosa RE, Remine WH, Harrison EG Jr: Catecholamine secreting paraganglioma of glomus jugulare region resembling pheochromocytoma. *New Eng J Med* 281:805, 1969
138. Mafee MF, Valvassori GE, Shugar MA: High resolution and dynamic sequential computed tomography. Use in the evaluation of glomus complex tumors. *Arch Otolaryngol* 109:691, 1983

139. Marchand F: Beiträge zur Kenntnis der normalen und pathologischen Anatomie der Glandula carotica und der Nebennieren: In: *Festschrift R. Virchow.* Internationale Beiträge zur wissenschaftlichen Medizin, Berlin, Hirschwald, 1891

140. McGuirt WF, Stamler F: Pseudosarcoma. *ENT* 55:319, 1976

141. Minckler DS, Meligro CH, Norris HT: Carcinosarcoma of the larynx. Case report with metastases of epidermoid and sarcomatous elements. *Cancer* 26:195, 1970

142. Minnigerode B, Haubrich J: Sarkomaähnliche Srukturmodification eines Kehlkopfkarzinoms als somatisch-stochastischer Strahleneffekt. *Z Laryng Rhinol Otol* 46:695, 1967

143. Miracco C, Santopietro R, Gabrieli C, Gaia F: Liposarcoma mixoide del nasofaringe. *Istocitopatologia* 6:99, 1984

144. Moberg A, Anderson H, Wedemberg E: Disorders of the skull base region. In: *Nobel Symposia,* Almquist, Wiksell 1969

145. Moll R, Franke WW, Schiller DL, Geiger B, Krepler R: The catalogue of human cytokeratin patterns of expression in normal epithelia, tumors and cultured cells. *Cell* 31:11, 1982

146. Moll R, Moll I, Wiest W: Changes in the pattern of cytokeratin polypeptides in epidermis and hair follicles during skin development in human fetuses. *Differentiation* 23:170, 1983

147. Monro RS: The morphology of the branchial glomera and their tumours, with a report of a case of aortico-pulmonary glomus tumor. *Brit J Surg* 38:105, 1950

148. Moore JS: Carcinosarcoma of the vocal cord. *Tex Med* 47:569, 1951

149. Moulonget A, Leroux-Robert J: Epitelioma atipique du larynx a cellules fusiformes. *Ann Otolaryng* 52:1257, 1933

150. Nager GT: Acoustic neuromas. Pathology and differential diagnosis. *Arch Otolaryngol* 89:252, 1969

151. Nelson WG, Battifora H, Santana H, Sun TT: Specific keratins as molecular markers for neoplasms with a stratified epithelial origin. *Cancer Res* 44:1600, 1984

152. New GB: Sarcoma of the larynx. Report of two cases. *Arch ORL* 21:648, 1935

153. Niksic-Ivancic M, Nemanic G, Gjuria B: Lymphknoten im Faszialiskanal als Ursache des Gesichtskrampfes. *Laryngol Rhinol Otol* 59:599, 1980

154. Oldring D, Fisch U: Glomus tumors of the temporal region. *Am J Otolaryngol* 1:7, 1979

155. Olivecrona H: Acoustic tumours. *J Neurol et Psych* 3:141, 1940

156. Olivecrona H: Cholesteatomas of the cerebellopontine angle. *Acta Psychiat et Neurol* 24:639, 1949

157. Paintal AS: Vagal afferent fibers. *Erg Physiol Biol Exp Pharmacol* 52:1969, 1974

158. Panse R: Ein Gliom des Akustikus. *Arch Ohrenh* (*Leipzig*) 61:25, 1904

159. Pearse AG: The cytochemistry and ultrastructure of polypeptide hormone-producing cells of the APUD series and the embryologic, physiologic and pathologic implications of the concept. *J Histochem* 17:303, 1969

160. Pearse AG, Polak JM, Rost RWD, Fontaine J, LeLievre C, LeDouarin N: Demonstration of the neural crest origin of type I (APUD) cells in the avian carotid body, using a cytochemical marker system. *Histochemie* 34:191, 1973

161. Pearse AG: The APUD cell concept and its implications in pathology. In: Sommers SC ed, *Pathology Annual 1974,* New York: Appleton Century Crofts, 1974

162. Pech A, Cannoni M, Pellet W: La voie translabyrinthique. *J Franc Oto-Rhino-Laryng* 30:665, 1981

163. Pfaltz CR: Symptomatology and surgery of the occult petrosal cholesteatoma. *Clin Otolaryngol* 3:508, 1978

164. Phelps PD, Lloyd GAS: Glomus tympanicum tumours: Demonstration by high resolution CT. *Clin Otolaryngol* 8:15, 1983

165. Pietrantoni L: I cosiddetti tumori misti della laringe, della trachea e dei bronchi. *Valsalva* 23:53, 1947

166. Pizzetti F, Leonardelli GB: Sui tumori misti dell' estremo cefalico (con particolare riguardo alle localizzazioni extraparotidee). *Tumori* 36:136, 1950

167. Polli G, Ciabatti PG, Salimbeni C: Su di un caso di paraganglioma branchiomerico non funzionante della laringe. *Riv Ital Otorinolaryngol Audiol Foniatr* 3:123, 1983

168. Portmann M, Cohandon F, Castel JP: A propos de la neurotomie de la 8eme paire cranienne par la fosse temporale. *Ann Chir* 22:1401, 1968

169. Precerutti G, Broich G, Fresa D: L'approccio transcocleare a la fossa cranica media e posteriore. *Il Policlinico sez Chirurgica* 89:687, 1982

170. Precerutti G, Fresa D, Broich G, Brambilla G, Sangiovanni G: L'approccio otoneurochirurgico al neuroma dell' VIII nervo cranico. *Rassegna Clinico Scientifica Lorenzini* 57:3, 1982

171. Randall G, Alonso WA, Ogura JH: Spindle cell carcinoma (pseudosarcoma) of the larynx. *Arch ORL Chicago* 101:63, 1975

172. Rettinger G, Haid T, Wigand ME: Die computertomographische Frühdiagnostik des Akustikusneurinoms durch Luftfüllung des inneren Gehörganges. *HNO* 29:73, 1981

173. Riccardi VM: von Recklinghausen neurofibromatosis. *N Engl J Med* 305:1617, 1981

174. Ricci B: Carcinosarcoma di una corda vocale. *Otolaring Ital* 3:259, 1923

175. Robbins SL, Cotran RS, Kumar V: Pathologic basis of disease. 3rd ed, Philadelphia, Saunders, 1984

176. Rock T, Cabrini G, Rizzi A, Bratena G: Un caso di pseudosarcoma dell' esofago. *Tumori* 61:457, 1975

177. Rolander T, Kim OJ, Shumrick DA: Fibrous xanthoma of the larynx. *Arch Otolaryngol* 96:168, 1972

178. Rosenwasser H: Carotid body tumor of the middle ear and mastoid. *Arch Otolaryngol* 41:64, 1945

179. Rosenwasser H: Glomus jugulare tumors. *Arch Otolaryng* 88:3, 1968

180. Rucco B, Zerneri L: Su di un caso di carcinosarcoma laringeo. Note critiche sugli aspetti sarcomatoidi. *Arch Ital Otol* 76:966, 1965

181. Ruedi L: Cholesteatoma of the attic. *J Laryngol* 72:593, 1958

182. Sandifort: Observationes anatomico-pathologicaes, 1777

183. Saphir O, Vass A: Carcinosarcoma. *Am J Cancer* 33:331, 1938

184. Scalori G: Difficolta' diagnostiche in casi di cancro sottoglottico mascherato da polipi. *Boll Mal Orecchio, Gola, Naso* 73:327, 1955

185. Schadel A, Wadynik A: Einsatz und Problematik der hochauflösenden Computertomographie des Felsenbeines. *HNO* 33:171, 1985

186. Schmidt-Baumler U, Rupp W: Carcinosarcom des Stimmbandes. *Z Laryng Rhinol Otol* 54:772, 1975

187. Schondorf-Seeliger: Maligne Synovialome im Halsbereich. *HNO* 99:101, 1977

188. Schulze W, Kleinsasser O: Intralabyrinthäres und intratympanales Akustikusneurinom. *HNO* 24:16, 1976

189. Shamblin WR, Remine WH, Sheps SG, Harrison EG: Carotid body tumor (chemodectoma). Clinico-pathologic analysis of ninety cases. *Am J Surg* 122:732, 1971

190. Sherwin RP, Strong, MS, Vaughan CW Jr: Polipoid and junctional squamous cell carcinoma of the tongue and larynx with spindle cell carcinoma (pseudosarcoma). *Cancer* 16:51, 1963

191. Shi SR, Bhan AK, Pilch BZ, Chen LB, Goodman ML: Keratin antibody localisation in head and neck tissues and neoplasms. *J Laryng Otol* 98:1241, 1984

192. Siebenmann F: Die Blutgefässe im Labyrinth des menschlichen Ohres. Nach eigenen Untersuchungen an Celloidinkorrosionen und an Schnitten, Wiesbaden, J.F. Bergmann, 1894

193. Smith HJ, Kilman WJ, Corbett DS: Malignant polipoid lesions of the oesophagus. Review and case report. *Rev Interam Radiol* 4:151, 1979
194. Smyth GD: Surgical management of congenital cholesteatoma. *Am J Otol* 3:61, 1981
195. Solcia E, Capella C, Vassallo G: Lead-hematoxylin as a stain for endocrine cells. *Histochemie* 20:116, 1969
196. Spector GJ, Sobol S: Surgery for glomus tumors at the skull base. *Otolaryngol Head Neck Surg* 88:524, 1980
197. Spreter v Kreutenstein H, Harms D: Kurzreferat über Karzinosarkome. *Arch Hals Nasen Ohren Heilkunde* 207:560, 1974
198. Steinert PM, Rice RH, Roop DR, Trus BL, Steven AC: Complete amino acid sequence of a mouse epidermal keratin subunit and implications for the structure of intermediate filaments. *Nature* 302:794, 1983
199. Steinert PM, Parry DAD, Racoosin EL, Idler WW, Steven AC, Trus BL, Roop DR: The complete cDNA and deduced amino acid sequence of a type II mouse epidermal keratin of 60 000 Da: Analysis of sequence differences between Type I and Type II keratins. *Proc Natl Acad Sci USA* 81:5709, 1984
200. Steinert PM, Jones JCR, Goldman RD: Intermediate filaments. *J Cell Biology* 99:22s, 1984
201. Sterker JM, Billet R: Petit tumeurs de l'acoustique. Diagnostics et cure precoce. A propos de 9 cas. *Ann Otolaryngol Chir Cervicofac* 89:323, 1972
202. Sterker JM, Jobert F: Vertiges de meniere traites par neurectomie vestibulaire. Principe, technique, resultats (30 cas). *Rev Neurol* 127:384, 1972b
203. Sterker JM, Jobert F, Pelisse JM: Les vertiges et la neurectomie vestibulaire. *Cah Med* 14:215, 1973
204. Stout AP: Liposarcoma. The malignant tumor of lipoblasts. *Ann Surg* 119:86, 1944
205. Stout AP, Humphreys GH II, Rottenberg LA: A case of carcinosarcoma of the oesophagus. *Am J Roentg* 61:461, 1949
206. Sugarbaker EV, Chretien PB, Jacobs JB: Bilateral familial carotid body tumors: Report of a patient with an occult controlateral tumor and postoperative hypertension. *Ann Surg* 174:242, 1971
207. Sun TT, Green H: Cultured epithelial cells of cornea, conjunctiva and skin: Absence of marked intrinsic divergence of their differentiated states. *Nature* 269:489, 1977
208. Sun TT, Green H: Immunofluorescent staining of keratin fibers in cultured cells. *Cell* 14:469, 1978a
209. Sun TT, Green H: Keratin filaments of cultured human epidermal cells: Formation of intermolecular disulfide bonds during terminal differentiation. *J Biol Chem* 253:2053, 1978b
210. Sun TT, Shih C, Green H: Keratin cytoskeletons in epithelial cells of internal organs. *Proc Natl Acad Sci USA* 76:2813, 1979
211. Sun TT, Eichner R, Nelson W, Tseng SCG, Weiss RA, Jarvinen M, Woodcock-Mitchell J: Keratin classes: Molecular markers for different types of epithelial differentiation. *J Invest Dermatol* 82:109s, 1983
212. Sun TT, Eichner R, Schermer A, Cooper D, Nelson WG, Weiss RA: Classification, expression, and possible mechanisms of evolution of mammalian epithelial keratins: A unifying model. In: *The Cancer Cell*, vol 1, The transformed phenotype, A Levine, W Topp, G Van de Woude and JD Watson (eds), Cold Spring Harbor Lab, NY, 169, 1984
213. Szekely T: Chirurgie der Glomustumoren. *HNO* 32:54, 1984
214. Szimivasan U, Tavalkar GV: True carcinosarcoma of the larynx: a case report. *J Laryngol Otol* 93:1031, 1979
215. Szmurlo: Ein Fall von Coexistenz von Sarkom und Carcinom im Kehlkopf. *Medicyna Warszawa* 29, 1894
216. Taichman LB, Prokop CA: Synthesis of keratin proteins during maturation of cultured human keratinocytes. *J Invest Dermatol* 78:464, 1982
217. Takeda Y, Kaneko R, Suzuki U: Ameloblastic fibrosarcoma in the maxilla, malignant transformation of ameloblastic fibroma. *Virchows Arch (Path Anat)* 404:253, 1984
218. Tange RA, Overtoom TTC, Ludwig JW: A new angiographic technique for asymptomatic hereditary glomus screening. *Arch Otolaryngol* 238:143, 1983
219. Tewfik S: Phonocephalography: A simple, low cost non invasive diagnostic technique. Continued data reporting. *J Laryngol Otol* 97:1133, 1983
220. Traina: Carcinosarcoma del seno mascellare. *Tumori* 1:36, 1924
221. Tseng SCG, Jarvinen M, Nelson WG, Huang HW, Woodcock-Mitchell J, Sun TT: Correlation of specific keratins with different types of epithelial differentiation: Monoclonal antibody studies. *Cell* 30:361, 1982
222. Uhlmann H: Ein echtes Carcinosarcom des Kehlkopfes. *Z Hals Nasen Ohrenh* 1:130, 1922
223. Valdazo A, Schupp C, Houtteville J-P, Rossa Y, Theron J: Le cholesteatome intra-petreux a propos de deux observations. *Rev Otoneuroophthalmol* 52:61, 1980
224. Vassallo G, Capella C, Solcia E: Grimelius silver stain for endocrine cell granules as shown by electron microscopy. *Stain Technol* 46:7, 1971
225. Vetters JM, Toner PG: Chemodectoma of the larynx. *J Path* 68:259, 1970
226. Virchow R: Die krankhaften Geschwülste, Hirschwald Berlin, 1865
227. Weiss RA, Eichner R, Sun TT: Monoclonal antibody analysis of keratin expression in epidermal disease: A 48- and 56-kdalton keraton as molecular markers for hyperproliferative keratinocytes. *J Cell Biol* 98:1397, 1984
228. Wende S, Nakayama N, Schwerdtfeger P: The internal auditory artery (embryology, anatomy, angiography, pathology). *J Neurol* 210:21, 1975
229. White EG: Die Struktur des Glomus caroticum, seine Pathologie und Physiologie und seine Beziehung zum Nervensystem. *Beitr Path Anat* 96:177, 1935
230. Wigand ME, Haid T: Labyrinthäre Durchbrüche des Octavusneurinoms, otochirurgische Aspekte. *Arch Otorhinolaryngol* 213:415, 1976
231. Wigand ME: Der besondere Fall: Isoliertes Neurinom des Labyrinthes. *HNO* 29:140, 1981
232. Wilson H: Carotid body tumors: Familial and bilateral. *Ann Surg* 171:843, 1970
233. Woodcock-Mitchell J, Eichner R, Nelson WG, Sun TT: Immunolocalization of keratin polypeptides in human epidermis using monoclonal antibodies. *J Cell Biol* 95:580, 1982
234. Woods GL, Espinoza CG, Azar HA: Carcinomas with spindle cell (sarcomatoid) component: An immunocytochemical and electron microscopic study. *Lab Invest* 46:91A, 1982
235. Wullstein HL: Pathologie des Mittelohres. Operationen zur Verbesserung des Gehörs, George Thieme Verlag, Stuttgart, 1968
236. Yanagihara N, Matsumoto Y: Cholesteatoma in the petrous apex. *Laryngoscope* 91:272, 1981

SPREADING ON THE COELOMIC (PERITONEAL, PLEURAL AND PERICARDIAL) SURFACE

H.E. KAISER

INTRODUCTION

Carcinomas in general metastasize more frequently via the lymphatic system, sarcomas via the hematogenic system, including many leukemias. The coelom characterizes the animal phyla known as coelomates and is characterized by a body cavity which may be portioned, covered by an endothelial layer. This layer contains a visceral and parietal portion and is according to embryology no true epithelium because it does not derive from ectoderm or entoderm but from mesoderm. These surfaces, covered with a film of fluid, are an ideal place for metastatic seeding. The majority of neoplasms occurring in the coelemic cavities are secondary. The development of neoplasms depends to a great degree on the topography of the host (cf. Chapter 6/Volume I) and this becomes clear if one considers types of tumors in the coelomic cavities. Primary neoplasms of the serosa are characterized by a wide spectrum of growth patterns and biologic aggressiveness. The adenoid tumor is generally benign; the cystic peritoneal mesothelioma shows an intermediate position, exhibits recurrent disease without fatal course whereas the diffuse malignant mesothelioma spreads rapidly (16) and may occur with osseous and cartilaginous differentiation (155).

ORIGIN OF NEOPLASTIC CELLS ENTERING THE COELOMIC CAVITY

Entrance of tumor cells and implantation in serous cavities forming metastases is a frequent event and the major mode of disseminated serosal carcinomatosis. Peritoneal, pleural or pericardial carcinomatosis can easily be traced to direct shedding of mucus and mucus secreting cells from the primary coelomic lesion, from ruptured dermoids or teratomas of the ovaries, or from metastatic lesions. There are also cases with no apparent point of entry as with dispersing from the lymphatics.

Free cells

Often observed are of free tumor cells or fragments in effusions accompanying peritoneal or pleural carcinomatosis. Desquamated mesothelial cells should not be confused with other tumor cells (158). Viable tumor cells can easily be implanted on the serous membranes (66).

Cells emerging from neighboring organs

Primary neoplasms of the coelomic surfaces are rare (cf (143)). Neoplastic cells may emerge as secondary deposits from neighboring organs such as from the lung, the organs of the mediastinum, especially the heart, and from the peritoneum, from the ovaries but also the tubes, uterus and glandular structures of the digestive system, the ureter and the bladder. Direct and metastatic distribution is possible.

Neoplasms from the lymphatic system

The supplying lymph vessels as the tributaries of the bronchomediastinal trunk for pericardium and pleura, and the vessels of such structures as the colic lymph nodes and the mesenteric ones for the peritoneal cavities are the sources of the distribution of malignant cells.

Neoplastic cells from the hematogenic system

Neoplastic cells may escape from the veins of the pericardium and mediastinum and from the veins of the viscera and body wall of the pleural and peritoneal surfaces. Arteries probably play an insignificant role in this regard.

COMPARISON OF PRIMARY AND SECONDARY NEOPLASMS

Pericardium. Primary neoplasms are very rare. Benign neoplasms are fibromatous polyps, lipomas, and also angiomas. In primary malignant neoplasms, sarcomas dominate (round-, spindle-cell sarcomas and angiosarcomas). Mesotheliomas are extremely rare and generally appear in young adults ((140), p. 404). Primary and secondary tumors are recognized site by site (7, p. 650, 30).

Pleura. Primary pleural tumors are rare, but most extend from those of the lung. Nonepithelial tumors of the pleura are the fibromas and lipomas, which are rare. Neurofibromas develop and originate from the sympathicus and the intercostal nerve. The malignant sarcomas are also rare, while fibrosarcomas exhibit a relatively benign progression. Benign epithelial neoplasms also are rare, such as the

K.W. Brunson (ed) Local invasion and spread of cancer.
© 1989, Kluwer Academic Publishers, Dordrecht.

papillomatoses of pleura and peritoneum (154). The malignant epithelial neoplasm is the primary carcinoma of the pleura, generally known as mesothelioma or endothelioma (140, pp. 91–93). Anderson and Scotti (4) list as primary and benign pleural tumors from subpleural tissue the fibromas, lipomas, chondromas, and angiomas (see also 7, pp. 650–52).

Peritoneum. Mesothelioma of the peritoneum is less common than that of the pleura. The localized forms of pleural malignant mesotheliomas are fibrosarcomatous; the diffuse forms are mainly epithelial (93). Fibrous mesothelioma with pleural and peritoneal locations varies due to the ability of mesothelial cells to assume fibroblastic and epithelial-like characteristics ((97); (7), pp. 650–53)(45, 131). Abundant fluid accumulation, possibly containing neoplastic cells, accompanies metastatic tumors, especially ovarian cystadenocarcinomas (4, p. 836).

A native American Pueblo presented with a cluster of malignant mesothelioma (41).

DISTRIBUTION OF PRIMARY AND SECONDARY TUMORS OF SEROSAL SURFACES

There are several pathways of metastases: metastasis from primary tumor by seeding via the lymph and via the blood; and metastasis from the coelomic fluid. Carcinoembryonic antigen is important in the diagnostic distinction between metastatic serosal spread and malignant mesothelioma (47). Intraperitoneal free cancer cells appeared in almost all patients with gastric cancer in whom the area of serosal cancer invasion exceeded 15–20 cm^2; a 5-year survival rate was lower in patients with serosal cancer invasion and free cancer cells than in those without (81).

SPREADING AT PERITONEAL SURFACE

There was an increase in mesothelioma of the peritoneum during the years 1967–82 in England and Wales (53). The number in men increased two-fold compared to that in women, and the geographic pattern coincided with the asbestos-using industry. However, the incidence rate of mesothelioma in British Columbia has increased nearly six times for men for the period 1969 to 1975 but has remained unchanged for women. Nearly all cases could be linked to asbestos (29).

Computed tomographic scans (CT) as well as gallium scans are useful in the evaluation of the extension of abdominal tumors before operation and to follow the progression of the disease after established diagnosis (6, 108).

The role of computed tomography, sonographic and other imaging methods including radiologic examination in the detection of local and distant metastases of patients with newly diagnosed or suspected recurrent gastrointestinal tumors have been evaluated (96, 89, 90).

The patterns of mesotheliomas, particularly of the pleura, have been discussed (54, 159).

Zolenko *et al.* (160) and Zahor *et al.* (156) outlined the history and characteristics of peritoneal mesothelioma and multicystic peritoneal mesothelioma.

Carcinoid neoplasia involving unusual polypoid in-

traperitoneal metastases has been noted (115). Effusions from body cavities can be used for the detection of metastases (106). Irregular or damaged surfaces of ovarian tumors allow more spreading of tumor cells into the peritoneal fluid; the highest amount of spreading occurs in completely malignant tumors, is moderate in semimalignant ones, and lowest in benign tumors (51).

Simple cuboidal epithelium

Positive cytology in the peritoneum is four times as frequent in adenocarcinoma and adenosquamous carcinoma than for squamous carcinoma of the cervix. Peritoneal cytology does not influence prognosis (1). Peritoneal metastases of progressed renal adenocarcinoma may be disclosed by occlusion (15).

Simple columnar epithelium

The overall pattern of spreading of primary adenocarcinomas of the colon exhibits local recurrence, retroperitoneal lymph node metastases, and diffuse peritoneal seeding (135).

Mammary glands

Comparing the metastatic sites of infiltrating duct and infiltrating lobular breast carcinoma showed that peritoneal/retroperitoneal metastases with a characteristic pattern appeared in infiltrating lobular carcinoma (62). Laparoscopy supplemented by biopsy is useful in the diagnosis of disseminated peritoneal tumors (72).

Exocrine portion of pancreas

Adenocarcinoma of the exocrine pancreas showed many cases with peritoneal metastases, but less than the number of hepatic metastases (96).

Pineal gland

Pineal germinoma, a rare tumor in itself, shows in unusual cases metastasis to the peritoneal cavity via the patient's ventriculoperitoneal shunt (38).

Pseudomyxoma peritonei

This lesion is characterized by accumulation of large quantities of epithelial mucus in the peritoneal cavity, resulting from the rupture of benign or malignant cystic neoplasms of the ovary. The definition given by Stedman (129, p. 1161) is somewhat incomplete because a pseudomyxoma peritonei can develop from quite a number of benign or malignant cystic neoplasms if the cysts rupture and expel their mucinous content into the peritoneal cavity. Besides being derived from ovarian neoplasms, pseudomyxoma peritonei results from those of the appendix mucocele or mucogenic carcinoma (100), the bladder and mucinous adenocarcinoma of pancreas and colloid carcinoma of pancreas;

more rarely from colon and stomach, originating from primary mucinous adenocarcinoma (59). The cells were characterized by intracytoplasmic lumina (24). Picard (107) has reviewed the biochemistry of the mucoid substance in pseudomyxoma peritonei. Ultrasound and computed tomography are diagnostic tools for the lesion (49, 61, 69, 70, 73, 94, 142, 153). A pseudomyxoma peritonei, perhaps originating from the appendix, showed a long evolution with distant metastases in the lungs, adrenal glands and lymph nodes. Periodic acid Schiff and Alcian blue were fixed by the mucoid substance; toluidin blue revealed metachromasia; electron microscopy showed nuclear disorganization. The mucoid substance from the pseudomyxoma contained abundant carbohydrates. Pseudomyxoma peritonei is able to produce distant metastasis; EM is important for diagnosis; the mucoid substance is composed of neutral sulfomucins (26). Computed tomography showed peritoneal calcifications after seeding of peritoneal surfaces in a perforated mucinous adenocarcinoma of the appendix (98).

SPREADING AT PLEURAL SURFACE

The pleura may be the source of neoplastic spread from lymphatic or hematogenous metastasis, from effusions, or from direct invasion of neighboring organs; it may itself interact with these structures. A pleural-based mass may lead to rib destruction (21). Rarely, pleural metastases from prostatic carcinoma may appear (128), or from osteosarcoma, as noted by skeletal scintigraphy (122). A similar situation may occur with malignant meningiomas (55). Thoracoscopy is valuable to diagnose solid tumors which extend into the pleural cavity (57) and computer tomography for chest wall tumors (118). Sarcoma of lung and pleura may be diagnosed and treated by pneumonectomy (82), and real-time ultrasonography is applicable to pleural and subpleural lesions (150); see also (50). Asbestos-associated lesions occur worldwide but it would be wrong to overestimate these findings if compared to the frequency of other pleural diseases. Asbestos-associated disease is known from Sri Lanka (138), as well as New South Wales (10) and the industrialized world.

Pseudostratified columnar epithelium

Among thousands of cases of primary bronchogenic carcinoma in the Shanghai Chest Hospital from 1957–1983 were 32 cases with disseminated pleural metastasis and effusion (149). A so-called intravascular bronchioloalveolar tumor of the lung exhibited involvement of the liver, the parietal pleura and the lung (31).

Reticular connective tissue

Chronic lymphatic leukemia may lead to pleural tumor manifestations (121), while a plasmacytoma involving the apical parietal pleura and the adjacent chest wall may be the primary neoplasm in the case of the Pancoast syndrome (25). Transdiaphragmatic extension of invasive thymoma requires estimation of the lesion by computed tomography imaging (119). Chest X-ray and computed tomography of a

patient showed diffuse thickening of both pleurae which was diagnosed as a well-differentiated lymphosarcoma and not a mesothelioma (136).

Fibrous connective tissue

In patients with malignant fibrous pleural tumor, immunofluorescence microscopy showed that the neoplastic cells reacted positively for vimentin and negatively for (cyto)keratin and desmin. Malignant fibrous pleural tumors may not be derived from (cyto)keratin-positive pleural mesothelium but from the submesothelial fibrous tissue. Malignant submesothelial fibrosarcoma would be the proper designation (8). Liposarcomas affect the pleura (147); costal chondrosarcoma can exhibit pleural seeding (105); and in generalized chondromatosis with massive chondroma of the anterior chest wall, the pleura may be invaded (126). Studies with bronchioloalveolar adenomas in mice showed that the highest proportion of lymphocyte-positive tumors occurred on the pleural surface in contact with lymphatics (28).

Mesothelioma ((43, 68, 113) see also Chapter 17/Volume VI).

One cannot assume that all mesotheliomas of pleura. pericardium and peritoneum are caused by asbestos (34). Asbestos is a hazard as known from industrialized countries as the Federal Republic of Germany (146), Italy (14), Denmark (5), Norway (109), Brazil (114); the U.S.A., Great Britain, and others.

Mesothelioma is also an occupational disease of sugar refinery workers (92, 130) and sheet metal workers (161). The relationship between naturally occurring erionite fibers in Central Cappadocia, Turkey and the high incidence of malignant mesothelioma in humans and sheep were investigated. Higher airborne fiber levels in lung tissues were paralleled by an increase of malignancy (9). A combination of historical, gross, light-, electron microscopic and immunocytochemical diagnosis is necessary for a proper evaluation of mesothelioma and topographically related diseases (64). Vimentin does not appear to be a simple discriminatory marker of malignant mesothelioma (75). Benign mesothelioma is known from the pleura (19), as well as the peritoneum (52). Benign appearing mesothelioma cells have been seen in serous effusion (58), and malignant mesothelioma is known from all coelomic cavities, such as pleura and peritoneum (67, 86, 88, 104, 148, 152). There often occur difficulties in the diagnosis of pleural malignant mesothelioma (157) which may be localized to the pleura (76), or combined with follicular thyroid carcinoma (101). Localized pleural mesothelioma may simulate a mediastinal tumor (110); pleural mesothelioma may present a superior vena cava syndrome (111), be complicated by amyloidosis of the internal organs (137); or dysphagia (77) may occur a sarcomatoid pleural mesothelioma (60), may be connected with the syndrome from inappropriate secretion of antidiuretic hormone (123); may cause achalasia of the lower esophageal sphincter (71); may appear in the azygos fissure (13); or may show a connection with the Doege-Potter syndrome (33). Mesothelioma may take a long clinical course (35).

Benign genital mesotheliomas are known to occur particularly in the male genital system in the tail of epididymis (22); the peritoneal tumor may appear as acute appendicitis

(112) or at the greater omentum (44). Mesothelioma is a primary malignant disease requiring for exact diagnosis extensive cytologic evaluation (95), as is the case (light- and electron microscopy) in cystic and papillary tumors of the peritoneum (42).

A malignant mesenchymatous hamartoma (embryonic sarcoma) of the liver led to monomorphic leiomyosarcomatous aspects of the peritoneal metastases and pseudo-tumorous foci abounding in plasmocytes (48). Metastatic spread via the greater omentum may lead to the involvement by secondary tumors of the transverse colon (84). Computed tomography scanning remains a potentially useful adjunct to clinical assessment of patients with intraperitoneal malignancy (46). A combined computed tomography study of the chest, upper abdomen and brain is in most cases a rapid, accurate and practical method for the evaluation of lung cancer (116).

Ovary

Studies of the comparative ultrastructure in the cancer cells of primary large bowel adenocarcinoma and its metastases to the lymph nodes, ovaries and greater omentum indicate a similar cell differentiation in the primary tumor and the metastases (36).

Desmal epithelium

In a patient with a dermoid cyst of the mesentery, computed tomography resulted in visualization of the cystic structure of the tumor (18). A specific protein with an apparent molecular weight of 200 000 and an isoelectric point of 8.7 may be useful as a protein marker between carcinoma and mesothelioma cells in serous effusions (40).

Mesenchyme

Fibrosarcomas of the peritoneum exhibit a highly malignant behavior and a poor prognosis (37, 117).

Reticular connective tissue

Malignant mesenteric tumors include non-Hodgkin's lymphoma, leiomyosarcoma and fibrosarcoma (78). Interferon suppresses the sensitivity of murine lymphomas to natural cell-mediated host resistance (56). Various tumors occurring in the mesentery of the small intestine (39, 103) and the mesentery of the jejunum (32), have been described.

Adipose tissue

An abdominal liposarcoma with peritoneal involvement appeared in a dog (2).

Bone

Pulmonary and mesenteric metastases from telangiectatic osteosarcoma of the proximal fibula occurred in one patient (134).

Smooth musculature

Leiomyomatosis of the peritoneum may be disseminated (132, 139), while leiomyosarcomas of the peritoneum are more common in women than in men (63).

Neurons of the central nervous system

A rare cellular neurinoma of the mesenterium of the small bowel in a patient led to a recurrence along with peritoneal dissemination (102). A multicentric ganglioneuroma with peritoneal involvement was noted in a steer (127).

SPREADING AT PERICARDIAL SURFACE

In children with secondary tumors of the cardiovascular system there were distant metastases in descending frequency: non-Hodgkin's lymphoma, neuroblastoma, soft tissue sarcoma, and bone sarcoma, nephroblastoma and hepatoma involving the myocardium and pericardium (23). Primary neoplasms of the heart are sometimes less frequent than secondary neoplasms. In 12 cardiac sarcomas from 7200 autopsy studies there was one case of pericardial mesothelioma, a tumor with very poor prognosis often followed by cardiac constriction or visceral metastases (27, 83). The analysis of 240 patients with metastases and tumors extending to the heart and pericardium (125) showed the following complex of symptoms accompanying this progression: acute pericarditis (fibrosis, effusional, constrictive); rapid enlargement of the heart shadow, in combination with changes of voltage and ECG complexes, appearance of echo-free spaces; presence of atypical cells in pericardial effusion. The process of tumor extension to the myocardium is characterized by the following findings: progressive refractory cardiac decompensation; steady rhythm disturbances without any dynamic changes; appearance of stenosal murmurs; enlargement and appearance of echo-cardiographic spaces with akinesia and hyperkinesia (see also (120, 145)). Alpha-lactalbumin, an immunohistochemical marker for metastatic carcinomas of the breast, was also found in metastases to the pericardium (87). Cardiac angiosarcomas have a typical location in the right atrium and usually large masses which are rapidly fatal. Kaposi's sarcoma exhibits small cardiac lesions which are asymptomatic, contrary to the symptomatic lesions of the atrial sarcomas, and are restricted to the epicardium or pericardium (74).

NEOPLASTIC EFFUSIONS

These lesions were extensively treated in Chapter 18/Volume VII.

The cytoplasm of the cells from effusions of humans with malignant disease exhibited peculiar ultrastructural features in form of a rod-shaped pentalaminary structure about 25 to 35 nm thick, composed of an outer double membrane, surrounding a central, more dense axis exhibiting transverse striations at about 10 nm intervals (20). Vacuoles of mesothelioma cells and of cells from metastatic carcinomas obtained from pleural fluid showed remarkable differences. The vacuoles were centrally situated, small and of regular size in mesothelioma, but irregular in size, noncentral in location and often positive if treated with mucin stains, in the case of metastatic carcinoma (17). Blind pleural biopsy is a low risk method in differential diagnosis of pleural effusions (11). Pleural fluid carcinoembryonic antigen content is the single most useful measurement for distinction of epithelial malignant tumors from other causes of pleural effusions (65). Solid pleural masses can be more accurately defined by computer tomography (85). Pericardial fluid analysis with cytologic examination is not able to distinguish definitely neoplastic from nonneoplastic disorders in the dog (124). A case of a rare malignant fibrous histiocytoma of the pleura exhibiting malignant effusion with histiocyte-like differentiation of neoplastic cells was reported (150).

SPECIES-SPECIFICITY OF IMPORTANT TUMOR TYPES IN MAN AND ANIMALS

Comparative aspects of neoplasms of the coelomic surfaces in the different animal groups, vertebrates and invertebrates alike, have not been explored. However, a myxosarcoma with peritoneal involvement (91) and a mesothelioma with pleural involvement were seen in cattle (80).

SUMMARY AND CONCLUSIONS

The origin of neoplastic cells found in the coelomic cavity is discussed with a review of primary and secondary neoplasms and their spreading. Although mesothelioma is of great public interest at present, Chapter 16/Volume VI gives an extensive evaluation, especially on the effect of asbestos in the production of this tumor. The topic of neoplastic effusions is treated in Chapter 18/Volume VII. Spontaneous occurrence in animals is rare.

REFERENCES

1. Abu-Ghazaleh S, Johnson W, Cressman WT: The significance of peritoneal cytology in patients with carcinoma of the cervix. *Gynecol Oncol* 17(2):139, 1984
2. Ackerman LJ, Silver JNN: Abdominal liposarcoma in a dog. *Mod Vet Pract* 65(6):470, 1984
3. Amato DA, Borden EC, Shiraki M et al.: Evaluation of bleomycin, chlorozotocin, MGBG, and bruceantin in patients with advanced soft tissue sàrcoma, bone sarcoma, or mesothelioma. *Invest New Drugs* 3(4):397, 1985
4. Anderson WAD, Scotti TM: Synopsis of Pathology (9th edition). St. Louis, MO: CV Mosby, 1976
5. Andersson M, Olsen JH: Malignant mesotheliomas in Denmark 1943–1980. Cancer statistics 9. *Ugeskr Laeger* 146(14):1085, 1984
6. Armas RR, Goldsmith S: Gallium scanning in peritoneal mesothelioma. *AJR* 144(3):563, 1985
7. Ashley DJB: Evans' Histological Appearance of Tumours (3rd edition). Edinburgh–London–New York: Churchill Livingstone, 1978
8. Bader H, Altmannsberger M, Osborn M: Typing of intermediate filaments in malignant fibrous pleural tumors. *J Cancer Res Clin Oncol* 107(1):42, 1984
9. Baris I, Simonaio L, Artvini M: Epidemiological and environmental evidence of the health effects of exposure to erionite fibres: a four-year study in the Cappadocian region of Turkey. *Int J Cancer* 39(1):10, 1987
10. Barnes R: Compensable asbestos-related disease in New South Wales. *Med J Aust* 2(5):221, 1983
11. Barthel E, Krecklow B: Results of combined blind pleural biopsy and cytology in the differential diagnosis of pleural effusions. *Z Erkr Atmungsorgane* 163(1):61, 1984
12. Beneke R: *Dtsch Arch klin Med* 64:237, 1899
13. Bhatt RC, Flanagan PM, Walls IP: Mesothelioma in the azygos fissure. *Br J Radiol* 57(676):336, 1984
14. Biava PM, Fiorito A, Canciani L, Bovenzi M: Epidemiology of pleural mesothelioma in the Province of Trieste: the role of occupational exposure to asbestos. *Med Lav* 74(4):260, 1983
15. Billebaud T, Foulques H, Alexandre JH: Late ileal and peritoneal metastases of renal adenocarcinoma disclosed by occlusion. *Presse Med* 13(40):2457, 1984
16. Bolen JW: Tumors of serosal tissue origin. *Clin Lab Med* 7(1):31, 1987
17. Boon ME, Veldhuizen RW, Ruinaard C et al.: Qualitative distinctive differences between the vacuoles of mesothelioma cells and of cells from metastatic carcinoma exfoliated in pleural fluid. *Acta Cytol (Baltimore)* 28(4):443, 1984
18. Buonanno G, Gonnella F, Pettinato G, Castaldo C: Autoimmune hemolytic anemia and dermoid cyst of the mesentery. A case report. *Cancer* 54(11):2533, 1984
19. Burrig KF, Kastendieck H, Husselmann H: Localized fibrous pleural tumor (benign mesothelioma). Clinico-pathological study of 24 cases for classification, morphogenesis and prognosis. *Pathologe* 4(3):120, 1983
20. Cappelli-Gotzos B, Gotzos V, Conti G: Peculiar ultrastructural features in the cytoplasm of cells from human effusions associated with malignant disease. *Ultrastruct Pathol* 5(2–3):243, 1983
21. Catz EG, Chaudhary BA, Speir WA: Pleural-based mass with rib destruction. *Chest* 85(3):409, 1984
22. Chahla Y: Benign genital mesothelioma. Two case reports. *Eur Urol* 11(4):285, 1985
23. Chan HS, Sonley MJ, Moes CA et al.: Primary and secondary tumors of childhood involving the heart, pericardium, and great vessels. A report of 75 cases and review of the literature. *Cancer* 56(4):825, 1985
24. Chejfec G, Rieker WJ, Jablokow VR, Gould VE: Pseudomyxoma peritonei associated with colloid carcinoma of the pancreas. *Gastroenterology* 90(1):202, 1986
25. Chen KT, Padmanabhan A: Pancoast syndrome caused by extramedullary plasmacytoma. *J Surg Oncol* 24(2):117, 1984
26. Chevillotte G, Choux R, Spik et al.: Pseudomyxoma peritonei: a case with multiple metastases. Ultrastructural study and chemical analysis of the mucoic substance. *Gastroenterol Clin Biol* 7(5):445, 1983
27. Chomette G, Auriol M, Cabrol C, Tranbaloc P: Primary malignant tumors of the heart. Anatomo-clinical study of 12 cases. *Ann Med Interne (Paris)* 36(4):301, 1985
28. Choudhury C, Kauffman SL, Seravalli E et al.: Lymphocytic infiltration of bronchioloalveolar adenomas in mice. *Cancer Lett* 20(3):299, 1983
29. Churg A: Malignant mesothelioma in British Columbia in 1982. *Cancer* 55(3):672, 1985
30. Churg J, Rasen SH, Moolten S: Histological characteristics of mesothelioma associated with asbestos. *Ann NY Acad Sci* 132:614, 1965
31. Corrin B, Harrison WJ, Wright DH: The so-called intravascular bronchioloalveolar tumour of lung (low grade sclerosing angiosarcoma): presentation with extrapulmonary deposits. *Diagn Histopathol* 6(3–4):229, 1983

32. Daniel, S, Lazarevic B, Attia A: Lymphangioma of the mesentery of the jejunum: report of a case and a brief review of the literature. *Am J Gastroenterol* 78(11):726, 1983

33. Dao MT, Jehan A, Borel B et al.: Doege-Potter syndrome. Apropos of a case of hypoglycemic pleural mesothelioma. *LARC Med* 4(2):85, 1984

34. Davies D: Are all mesotheliomas due to asbestos? *Br Med J (Clin Res)* 289(3):1164, 1984

35. de Juan Barquin A, de Juan Martin M: Peritoneal mesothelioma with a long clinical course. *Rev Clin Esp* 170(1–2):79, 1983

36. Delektorskaia VV, Perevoshchikov AG: Electron microscopic study of cellular differentiation in metastases of cancer of the large intestine in man. *Arkh Patol* 46(3):38, 1984

37. Delpero JR, Lieutaud R, Dominguez C et al.: Primary pedunculated fibrosarcoma of the peritoneum: a case report. *J Surg Oncol* 25(3):178, 1984

38. Devkota J, Brooks BS, el Gammal T: Ventriculoperitoneal shunt metastasis of a pineal germinoma. *Comput Radiol* 8(3):141, 1984

39. Dmytriv LI, Vavrik ZhM, Koshik TF: Large cavernous lymphangioma of the small intestine mesentery. *Klin Khir* (5):38, 1983

40. Donna A, Betta PG, Marchesini A: Isolation and characterization of a possible new protein marker for differential diagnosis between metastatic carcinoma and mesothelioma cells in serous effusions: preliminary findings. *Cancer Detect Prev* 8(1–2):255, 1985

41. Driscoll RJ, Mulligan WJ, Schultz D, Candelaria A: Malignant mesothelioma. A cluster in a native American Pueblo. *N Eng J Med* 318(22):1437–8, 1988

42. Dumke K, Schnoy N, Specht G, Buse H: Comparative light and electron microscopic studies of cystic and papillary tumors of the peritoneum. *Virchows Arch (A)* 399(1):25, 1983

43. Dunnill MS: Pleural mesothelioma (editorial). *Eur J Respir Dis* 65(3):159, 1984

44. Egorov VP: Cystic mesothelioma of the greater omentum. *Khirurgiia (Mosk)* (9):118, 1983

45. Ehrenhaft JL, Serisenig DM, Lawrence MS: Mesothelioma of the pleura. *J Thor Cardiovasc Surg* 40:393, 1960

46. Epstein RJ, Oliver B, Macintosh PK, Levi JA: Computed tomography of intraperitoneal malignancy. *Aust NZ J Med* 14(1):13, 1984

47. Faravelli B, D'Amore E, Nosenzo M et al.: Carcinoembryonic antigen in pleural effusions. Diagnostic value in malignant mesothelioma. *Cancer* 53(5):1194, 1984

48. Fievez M, Jacques P, Guiot F, Golaire MC: Malignant mesenchymatous hamartoma of the liver in adults. Apropos of a case. *Sem Hop Paris* 59(21):1625, 1983

49. Foster DR: Ultrasound findings in pseudomyxoma peritonei. *Australas Radiol* 29(1):39, 1985

50. Friedman PJ, Feigin DS, Liston SE et al.: Sensitivity of chest radiography, computed tomography, and gallium scanning to metastasis of lung carcinoma. *Cancer* 54(7):1300, 1984

51. Fujimaru J, Sato S: A cytological study of peritoneal fluid obtained in gynecological laparotomies – with special reference to the diagnosis of ovarian malignancy. *Nippon Sank Fujinka Gakkai Zasshi* 36(6):917, 1984

52. Galil-Ogly GA, Ivanov ED, Bershchanskaia AM: Benign cystic mesothelioma of the peritoneum. *Arkh Patol* 47(12):68, 1985

53. Gardner MJ, Jones RD, Pippard EC et al.: Mesothelioma of the peritoneum during 1967–82 in England and Wales. *Br J Cancer* 51(1):121, 1985

54. Giampalmo A, Buffa D, Quaglia AC et al.: Proposed outline of the most likely pathogenetic patterns in mesotheliomas, especially of the pleura. *Pathologia* 76(1044):437, 1984

55. Granata F, Bracale C, Longhi P et al.: Malignant meningiomas. Anatomo-clinical considerations of 2 cases. *Riv Neurobiol* 29(4):566, 1983

56. Greenberg AH, Miller V, Jablonski T, Pohajdak B: Suppression of NK-mediated natural resistance by interferon treatment of murine lymphomas. *J Immunol* 132(4):2129, 1984

57. Guerin JC, Biron E, Kalb JC: Value of thoracoscopy in the diagnosis of solid tumors extending into the pleural cavity. *Poumon Coeur* 39(1):37, 1983

58. Guffanti MC, Faleri ML: Benign-appearing mesothelioma cells in a serous effusion. *Acta Cytol (Baltimore)* 29(1):90, 1985

59. Gustafson KD, Karnaze GC, Hattery RR et al.: Pseudomyxoma peritonei associated with mucinous adenocarcinoma of the pancreas: CT findings and CT-guided biopsy. *J Comput Assist Tomogr* 8(2):335, 1984

60. Hammar SP, Bolen JW: Sarcomatoid pleural mesothelioma. *Ultrastruct Pathol* 9(3–4):337, 1985

61. Hann L, Love S, Goldberg RP: Pseudomyxoma peritonei: preoperative diagnosis by ultrasound and computed tomography. A case report. *Cancer* 52(4):642, 1983

62. Harris M, Howell A, Chrissohou M et al.: A comparison of the metastatic pattern of infiltrating lobular carcinoma and infiltrating duct carcinoma of the breast. *Br J Cancer* 50(1):23, 1984

63. Hashimoto H, Tsuneyoshi M, Enjoji M: Malignant smooth muscle tumors of the retroperitoneum and mesentery: a clinicopathologic analysis of 44 cases. *J Surg Oncol* 28(3):177, 1985

64. Herrera GA, Alexander CB, Jones JM: Ultrastructural characterization of pulmonary neoplasms. II. The role of electron microscopy in characterization of uncommon epithelial pulmonary neoplasms, metastatic neoplasms to and from lung, and other tumors, including mesenchymal neoplasms. *Surv Synth Pathol Res* 4(2):163, 1985

65. Hesdorffer C, Derman DP, Bezwoda WR: The value of pleural fluid carcinoembryonic antigen estimation in the diagnosis of malignant tumours of the pleural cavity. *S Afr Med J* 66(2):54, 1984

66. Hickling RA: Vital staining of malignant cells in peritoneal effusion. *J Path Bact* 34:789, 1931

67. Higami T, Tsubota N, Nishiyama N et al.: A case of malignant localized pleural mesothelioma. *Kyobu Geka* 37(10):814, 1984

68. Hillerdal G: Malignant mesothelioma 1982: review of 4710 published cases. *Br J Dis Chest* 77(4):321, 1983

69. Hopper KD: Ultrasonic findings in pseudomyxoma peritonei. *South Med J* 76(8):1051, 1983

70. Horgan JG, Chow PP, Richter JD et al.: CT and sonography in the recognition of mucocele of the appendix. *AJR* 143(5):959, 1984

71. Hostein J, Gignoux C, Roget et al.: Achalasia of the lower esophageal sphincter caused by pleural mesothelioma. *Gastroenterol Clin Biol* 8(11):880, 1984

72. Ishida H, Dohzono T, Furukawa Y et al.: Laparoscopy and biopsy in the diagnosis of malignant intra-abdominal tumors. *Endoscopy* 16(4):140, 1984

73. Itoh H, Seki T, Hagiri M et al.: Computed tomography and ultrasonic diagnosis of pseudomyxoma peritonei: report of a case. *Rinsho Hoshasen* 29(8):921, 1984

74. Janigan DT, Husain A, Robinson NA: Cardiac angiosarcomas. A review and a case report. *Cancer* 57(4):852, 1986

75. Jasani B, Edwards RE, Thomas ND, Gibbs AR: The use of vimentin antibodies in the diagnosis of malignant mesothelioma. *Virchows Arch (A)* 406(4):441, 1985

76. Jin CN: Localized mesothelioma of the pleura. *Chung Hua Chung Liu Tsa Chih* 5(1):66, 1983

77. Johnson CE, Wardman AG, McMahon MJ, Cooke NJ: Dysphagia complicating malignant mesothelioma. *Thorax* 38(8):635, 1983

78. Kida H, Kunii Y, Kajima T et al.: Four cases of malignant mesenteric tumor. *Gan No Rinsho* 30(1):86, 1984

79. Kimura N, Namiki J, Wada J, Sasano N: Peritoneal implantation of endodermal sinus tumor of the pineal region via a ventriculoperitoneal shunt. Cytodiagnosis with immunocytochemical demonstration of alpha-fetoprotein. *Acta Cytol* 28(2):143, 1984

80. Klopfer U, Brenner G, Nobel TA et al.: Mesothelioma in cattle – a rare or an unidentified tumor? *Zentralbl Veterinarmed (B)* 30(10):785, 1983

81. Koga S, Kaibara N, Iitsuka Y et al.: Prognostic significance of intraperitoneal free cancer cells in gastric cancer patients. *J Cancer Res Clin Oncol* 108(2):236, 1984

82. Kolarov I, Balevski M, Petrov D, Ianakiev D: Diagnosis and treatment of sarcoma of the lungs and pleura. *Khirurgiia (Sofiia)* 38(3):13, 1985

83. Kononenko LG, Goncharova LS, Stepanenko AA: Pericardial mesothelioma. *Sov Med* (9):117, 1985

84. Krestin GP, Beyer D, Lorenz R: Secondary involvement of the transverse colon by tumors of the pelvis: spread of malignancies along the greater omentum. *Gastrointest Radiol* 10(3):283, 1985

85. Kurtz B, Schmitt WG: Ultrasonic diagnosis of pleural shadows compared to computer tomography. *ROFO* 138(5):577, 1983

86. Leblanc P, Desmeules M: Malignant pleural mesothelioma: clinical aspects and results of treatment. *Union Med Can* 113(11):968, 1984

87. Lee AK, DeLellis RA, Rosen PP et al.: Alpha-lactalbumin as an immunohistochemical marker for metastatic breast carcinoma. *Am J Surg Pathol* 8(2):93, 1984

88. Liu GG: Report of 30 cases of pleural mesothelioma. 6(2):89, 1983

89. Lorenz R, Beyer D: Ultrasonography of peritoneal tumors and carcinomatosis (Meeting abstract) 5th Congr Europ Fed of Soc for Ultrasound in Medicine and Biology, Strasbourg, France, p. 12, 1984

90. Lorenz R, Beyer D, Friedman G, Hensen L: Sonographic diagnosis of peritoneal carcinosis. *Rofo* 140(2):168–72, 1984

91. Loupal G, Baumgartner W: Myxosarcoma in a heifer. *Tierärztl Prax* 12(2):173, 1984

92. Malker HR, Malker BK, Blot WJ: Mesothelioma among sugar refinery workers. *Lancet* 2(8354):858, 1983

93. Martini N, McCormack PM, Bains MS et al.: Pleural mesothelioma. *Thorac surg* 43(1):113, 1987

94. Masaryk TJ, Chilcote WA: CT of pseudomyxoma peritonei: case report. *Comput Radiol* 8(1):43, 1984

95. Matzel W: Biochemical and cytological features of diffuse mesotheliomas of the pleura. *Arch Geschwulstforsch* 55(4):259, 1985

96. Mauro MA, Vincent LM, Mandell VS et al.: Gas within pelvic pseudotumors: CT demonstration. *J Comput Assist Tomogr* 8(3):473, 1984

97. Maximow AA: Über das Mesothel (Deckzellen der serosen Haute) und die Zellen der serosen Exsudate. Untersuchungen an entzundetem Gewebe und an Gewebskulturen. *Archiv exp Zellforsch* 4:1, 1927

98. Miller DL, Udelsman R, Sugerbaker PH: Calcification of pseudomyxoma peritonei following intraperitoneal chemotherapy: CT demonstration. *J Comput Assist Tomogr* 9(6):1123, 1985

99. Moreaux J, Catala M, Marzano L: Results of the surgical treatment of pancreatic cancer. Study of a series of 96 surgically treated patients. *Gastroenterol Clin Biol* 8(1):11, 1984

100. Muller G, Dirschmid K, Breitfellner G, Zimmermann G: Clinical aspects of pseudomyxoma peritonei. *Chirurg* 55(1):32, 1984

101. Nakano T, Maebo A, Moriwaki Y et al.: A case report of diffuse malignant pleural mesothelioma combined with follicular thyroid carcinoma, and a biochemical study on its glycosaminoglycans. *Nippon Kyobu Shikkan Gakkai Zasshi* 21(11):1117, 1983

102. Okhovskaia IG, Sokolova IN, Patiutko IuI: Neurinoma with peritoneal dissemination. *Arkh Patol* 47(9):82, 1985

103. Orzechowski H, Wodarczyk K: Liposarcoma of the small-intestinal mesentery as a cause of acute peritonitis. *Wiad Lek* 37(5):385, 1984

104. Pandolfo I, Scribano E, Gaeta M et al.: A rare cause of air bronchogram: malignant pleural mesothelioma. Apropos of a case. *Ann Radiol (Paris)* 28(1):73, 1985

105. Pandolfo I, Gaeta M, Blandino A et al.: Costal chondrosarcoma with pleural seeding: CT findings. *J Comput Assist Tomogr* 9(2):408, 1985

106. Pfitzer P et al.: Nachweis von Metastasen in Ergüssen der Körperhöhlen. *Pathologe* 5:252, 1984

107. Picard J, Paul A: Biochemistry of the mucoid substance in pseudomyxoma peritonei. *Gastroenterol Clin Biol* 7(5):441, 1983

108. Picus D, Glaser HS, Levitt RG et al.: Computed tomography of abdominal carcinoid tumors. *AJR* 143(3):581, 1984

109. Pillgram-Larsen J, Urdal L, Birkeland S, Smith-Meyer R: Pleural mesothelioma in Oslo. *Tidsskr Nor Laegeforen* 104(19–21):1306, 1984

110. Przystasz T, Badowski A, Dumanski Z: A case of localized pleural mesothelioma simulating mediastinal tumor. *Pneumonol Pol* 52(8):393, 1984

111. Ragalie GF, Varkey B, Choi H: Malignant pleural mesothelioma presenting as superior vena cava syndrome. *Can Med Assoc J* 128(6):689, 740, 1983

112. Ramaswamy G, Shah UB, Tohertkoff V: Diffuse malignant peritoneal mesothelioma presenting as acute appendicitis. *NY State J Med* 84(3 Pt 1):125, 1984

113. Raptopoulos V: Peritoneal mesothelioma. *CRC Crit Rev Diagn Imaging* 24(4):293, 1985

114. Riani Costa JL, Ferreira YM Jr, Mendes R: Asbestos and disease: introduction to the problem in Brazil. *AMB* 29(1–3):18, 1983

115. Robb JA, Kuster GG, Bordin GM et al.: Polypoid peritoneal metastases from carcinoid neoplasms. *Human Pathol* 15(10):1002, 1984

116. Rossi A, Ferrozzi F, Ferrozzi G et al.: CT in the evaluation of the extension of bronchogenic carcinoma. *Acta Biomed Ateneo Parmense* 56(4–5):213, 1985

117. Roth A: Recurrent mesenchymoma of the peritoneum with hepatic metastasis in an 8-year-old child. *Arch Anat Cytol Pathol* 32(3):170, 1984

118. Rotte KH, Kriedemann E: The value of computer tomography in the diagnosis of chest wall tumors. *Arch Geschwulstforsch* 53(5):441, 1983

119. Scatarige JC, Fishman EK, Zerhouni EA, Siegelman SS: Transdiaphragmatic extension of invasive thymoma. *AJR* 144(1):31, 1985

120. Schoen FJ, Berger BM, Guerina NG: Cardiac effects of noncardiac neoplasms. *Cardiol Clin* 2(4):657, 1984

121. Seibold H, Mohr W, Schongen AP, Sigel H: Pleural tumor manifestations in chronic lymphatic leukemia. *MMW* 125(24):523, 1983

122. Shore RM, Frye TR, Weis LD, Mulne AF: Pleural metastasis with osteosarcoma. Dramatic presentation on skeletal scintigraphy. *Clin Nucl Med* 9(11):622, 1984

123. Siafakas NM, Tsirogiannis K, Filaditaki B et al.: Pleural mesothelioma and the syndrome of inappropriate secretion of antidiuretic hormone. *Thorax* 39(11):872, 1984

124. Sisson D, Thomas WP, Ruehi, WW, Zinki JG: Diagnostic value of pericardial fluid analysis in the dog. *J Am Vet Med Assoc* 184(1):51–5, 1984.

125. Skhvatsabaja LV: Secondary malignant lesions of the heart and pericardium in neoplastic disease. *Oncology* 43(2):103, 1986

126. Skobkarev IuD, Rabinovich SM, Polushkina EE: Case of generalized chondromatosis with massive chondroma of the

anterior chest wall invading the pleural cavity. *Grudn Khir* (3):80, 1984

127. Sokale EO, Ladds PW: Multicentric ganglioneuroma in a steer. *Vet Pathol* 20(6):767, 1983

128. Spreen KA, Edell SL: Pleural metastases secondary to prostatic carcinoma: an unusual presentation. *Del Med J* 56(7):417, 1984

129. Stedman's Medical Dictionary (24th edition): Baltimore–London: Williams & Wilkins, 1982

130. Steineck G, Carstensen J, Wiklund K, Eklund G: Mesothelioma among sugar refinery workers. *Lancet* 2(8365–66):1503, 1983

131. Stout AP, Himadi GM: Solitary (localized) mesothelioma of the pleura. *Ann of Surg* 133:50, 1951

132. Tabbara WS, Abboud J, Abul Hosn A: Disseminated peritoneal leiomyomatosis. Apropos of 2 new cases. *Arch Anat Cytol Pathol* 33(3):140, 1985

133. Takahashi Y, Mai M, Ogino T et al.: The metastatic patterns of gastric cancer from its histopathological characteristics in the primary lesion – particularly in relation to peritoneal dissemination and liver metastases. *Gan No Rinsho* 31(14):1792, 1985

134. Takaue Y, Slopis JM, Anzai T et al.: Successful treatment of pulmonary and abdominal metastatic osteosarcoma. *Med Pediatr Oncol* 13(3):126, 1985

135. Tong D, Russell AH, Dawson LE, Wisbeck W: Second laparotomy for proximal colon cancer. Sites of recurrence and implications for adjuvant therapy. *Am J Surg* 145(3):382, 1983

136. Tsujimura T, Kobayashi Y, Yoshioka H: Malignant thymoma with diffuse extensive growth on the pleura. *Gan No Rinsho* 29(5):443, 1983

137. Tyrkasova VM, Gubenko TV, Podlubnaia LS, Bolgarina AI: Case of pleural mesothelioma complicated by amyloidosis of the internal organs. *Klin Med (Mosk)* 62(10):126, 1984

138. Uragoda CG, Sheriffdeen AH, Amerasinghe A: A case of asbestos associated disease in Sri Lanka. *Ceylon Med J* 28(4):247, 1983

139. Valente PT: Leiomyomatosis peritonealis disseminata. A report of two cases and review of the literature. *Arch Pathol Lab Med* 108(8):669, 1984

140. von Albertini A: Histologische Geschwulstdiagnostik. Stuttgart: George Thieme Verlag (2nd edition), 1974

141. Wackym PA, Gray GF Jr: Tumors of the appendix: I. Neoplastic and nonneoplastic mucoceles. *South Med J* 77(3):283, 1984

142. Weigert F, Lindner P, Rohde U: Computed tomography and magnetic resonance of pseudomyxoma peritonei. *J Comput Assist Tomogr* 9(6):1120, 1985

143. Willis RA: Pathology of Tumours (3rd edition), p. 185. London: Butterworth, 1962

144. Willis RA: The Spreading of Tumours in the Human Body (3rd edition). London: Butterworth, 1973

145. Wishnitzer R, Eliraz A, Mashiah A, Shani A: Cardiac tamponade as a presentation of metastatic extracardiac malignancy. *Harefuah* 108(7):342, 1985

146. Woitowitz HJ, Lange HJ, Beierl L et al.: Mortality rates in the Federal Republic of Germany following previous occupational exposure to asbestos dust. *Int Arch Occup Environ Health* 57(3):161–71

147. Wouters EF, Greve LH, Visser R, Swaen GJ: Liposarcoma of the pleura. *Neth J Surg* 35(5):192, 1983

148. Wouters EF, Havenith MG, Vermeulen A, Greve LH: Malignant mesothelioma presenting in the pleura and peritoneum. *Neth J Med* 27(6):213, 1984

149. Wu SF, Huang OL, WU HS et al.: Critical evaluation of results of extension of indication for surgery for primary bronchogenic carcinoma. *Semin Surg Oncol* 1(1):23, 1985

150. Yang HY, Weaver LL, Foti PR: Primary malignant fibrous histiocytoma of the pleura. A case report. *Acta Cytol (Baltimore)*. 27(6):683, 1983

151. Yang PC, Sheu JC, Luh KT et al.: Clinical application of real-time ultrasonography in pleural and subpleural lesions. *Taiwan I Hsueh Hui Tsa Chih* 83(7):646, 1984

152. Yano T, Ichikawa Y, Tanaka F et al.: A case of bilateral diffuse malignant pleural mesothelioma with patchy and reticular shadows on the chest X-ray film. *Nippon Kyobu Shikkan Gakkai Zasshi* 22(8):690, 1984

153. Yeh HC, Shafir MK, Slater G et al.: Ultrasonography and computed tomography in pseudomyxoma peritonei. *Radiology* 153(2):507, 1984

154. Yoshida T: Gleichzeitige Papillomatose der Pleura und des Peritoneums, zugleich ein Beitrag zur Frage des primären Carcinomas der serösen Häute. *Virchows Arch* 299:363, 1937

155. Yousem SA, Hochholzer L: Malignant mesothelioma with osseous and cartilaginous differentiation. *Arch Pathol Lab Med* 111(1):62, 1987

156. Zahor Z, Povyril C, Smat V et al.: Multicystic peritoneal mesothelioma. *Cas Leki Ceski* 123(38–39):1205, 1984

157. Zakharychev VD: Difficulties and errors in the diagnosis of malignant pleural mesothelioma. *Sov Med* (12):91, 1985

158. Zemansky AP Jr: Examination of fluids for tumor cells; analysis of 113 cases checked against subsequent examination of tissue. *Am J Med Sci* 175:489, 1928

159. Zerbino DD, Dmitruk JM: Etiology, pathogenesis and clinico-morphological characteristics of mesotheliomas: a review of the literature. *Vrach Delo* (10):4, 1984

160. Zolenko D, Lamy V, Geets L, Meisse R: Peritoneal mesothelioma, natural history. *Acta Gastroenterol (Belg)* 47(4):360, 1984

161. Zoloth S, Michaels D: Asbestos disease in sheet metal workers: the results of a proportional mortality analysis. *Am J Ind Med* 794):315, 1985

4

SPREADING BY IMPLANTATION ON EPITHELIAL SURFACES AND IATROGENIC SPREADING BY IMPLANTATION*

H.E. KAISER

Neoplastic fragments, due to the low adhesion of neoplastic cells and easier detachment of such cells, have been transmitted to various epithelial surfaces as implantation metastases. These cells experience fewer rejections than cells from foreign donors. The metastatic principle is the same as in the other types of metastasis, although the occurrence of this type of metastasis is rare and can even be considered as among artificial types of metastasis. Therapeutically, the principle applies in tissue grafting and organ transplantation, described in Chapter 16/Volume VI. Involuntary seeding, implantation or transplantation of tumor cells is known, it will be described within the framework of this chapter as iatrogenic tumor cell implantation or transplantation. This term, implantation, is used to distinguish the processes involved from therapeutic grafting and transplantation. Implantation metastasis may represent the peak of metastatic inefficiency. It is obvious that the tumor/host interaction plays an important indirect role by such occurrences of penetration of tissue spaces, circulatory, and lymphatic systems (see (10)). The especially significant phase of these processes of implantation metasasis are the initial stages. Irritation of the normal soil epithelium by rubbing of neoplastic tissues upon an originally healthy, but more tender surface, with resultant problems of wound processes, may appear in such cases as implantation metastasis from a cancer of the scrotum to the skin of the thigh (9); or a carcinoma of a female breast, which rubs against the skin of the thoracic wall. A well-differentiated, endometrial adenocarcinoma was observed in an abdominal wound, but was confined to a polyp (3).

Some characteristic of epithelial surfaces which may play a role in the process of such implantation metastases are summarized in Table 1.

Some of the facts, as set forth in Table 1, support the conclusion that implantation metastasis in many cases should be considered as improbable. "The presence of rich bacterial flora on skin and on alimentary and respiratory mucous membranes, the presence of digestive enzymes and mucus in the alimentary tract and of mucus in the respiratory tract, the certainly enfeebled vitality of fragments of tumor detached from ulcerating growth, and the absence of breaches in healthy epithelial surfaces; all these considerations should give pause to a too facile assumption of implantation metastasis" (55).** As described in other chapters of Volume VIII, it is well-recognized that metastasizing cells are equipped with enzymes to penetrate the unbroken epithelium. "The intrinsic improbability of obtaining successful tissue grafts on intact surfaces bathed by fluids rich in digestive enzymes, mucus and bacteria justifies great stringency in passing judgment on alleged cases of tumor implantation within the alimentary tract" (55).

"Because the respiratory tract contains no digestive enzymes and fewer bacteria than the alimentary tract, the occurrence of implantation metastasis is intrinsically more probable in the bronchi and the lungs than in the stomach and the intestines. Nevertheless, decidedly unfavourable to tumor grafting in this situation must be the mucoid character of bronchial secretion, the presence of an appreciable bacterial flora, and the mechanical hindrances to the effective lodgment of foreign particles afforded by the respiratory movements and the ciliary activity of the respiratory epithelium. It is, then, not surprising to find that most of the alleged instances of implantation metastasis by way of the air passages are caused by other explanations" (55).

"... since the cavities of the healthy uterus and tubes are bacteria-free, and since they contain no lytic secretions and but little mucus, tumor implantation in the tubal mucosa or the endometrium must be regarded as probable. In the vagina or vulva, on the contrary, the conditions must be highly unfavorable to successful implantation. It is important to recognize that in this territory local metastasis via lymphatic and venous channels is a frequent event, and that many instances of implantation may equally well be attributed to spread by these familiar routes" (55).

Willis stated that he believed, from the study of recorded cases, that genuine implant metastases from ovarian and tubal tumors probably do occur in the endometrium.

Autopsies of 532 cases of ovarian malignancies showed a very frequent dissemination of the tumors into the parietal and visceral peritoneum (93.9%), greater omentum (73.6%), lymph nodes (82.2%), pleura (31.5%), and liver (25.4%). Implantation was the most common mode of spread; it enjoyed highest clinical significance, due to rapid growth and determination of the clinical course. By way of contrast, lymphogenous and hematogenous metastases were of lesser importance because they developed much more slowly (51).

"In health the urinary passages are sterile and almost devoid of mucus, conditions which are favorable to successful tissue grafting. The chemical and osmotic properties of urine cannot be regarded as disadvantageous to detached fragments of urinary epithelial growths, for urine is the

---

*Implantation metastasis, inoculation metastasis, contact cancer.
**Historic references cited after Willis (55).

K.W. Brunson (ed) Local invasion and spread of cancer.
© 1989, Kluwer Academic Publishers, Dordrecht.

Table 1. Observed regions where implantation metastasis occurs.*

Neoplasm	Tumor in primary location	Tumor in secondary location
Skin cancer	one skin region	opposite skin region
Carcinoma of eyelid	eyelid	conjunctiva of eye-bulb
Carcinoma of lip	one lip	other lip
Carcinoma of tongue	tongue	cheek
Carcinoma of vocal cord	one vocal cord	opposite vocal cord
Carcinoma of upper respiratory tract	upper respiratory passages	lung
Carcinoma of lung	one lung	opposite lung
Carcinoma of alimentary tract	one segment of alimentary tract	another segment of alimentary tract
Carcinoma of gallbladder	gallbladder	intestines
Ovarian carcinoma	from ovary via tube	uterus
Carcinoma of renal pelvis	renal pelvis	bladder
Carcinoma of ureter	ureter	bladder
Carcinoma of uterine corpus	Fallopian tube, ovary, peritoneum	generally ovary, less often uterus
Carcinoma of cervix	cervix	vagina
Carcinoma of vagina	vaginal wall	opposing wall
Carcinoma of vulva	one side of vulva	opposite side

*Implantation metastases occur frequently at the same level from right to left, or left to right on the one hand or from anterior to posterior, or posterior to anterior on the other. A second trend of implantation metastases is the occurrence in caudal direction.

normal habitat of these growths and of the epithelium from which they derived. There are then no prima faciae objections to the possibility of metastasis by implantation in the urinary tract" (55) (see Table 2). These summaries of the organ receptivity lead to the possible determination of the degree of frequency.

Blood derived from major head and neck resections exhibited, in one of six such preparations, the presence of viable, colony-forming tumor cells. It was demonstrated that blood bathing the raw, open surgical field contains tumor cells capable of initiating new neoplastic growth (2).

Immunosuppressive conditions may further implantation metastasis, especially to membranes of the serous lining, as in the large body cavities.

Kaposi's sarcoma was previously described in elderly Caucasian men of Mediterranean or Ashkenazic, Jewish origin, and also in young Central African males. The disease also occurs following renal transplantations or immunosuppressed on an iatrogenic basis. Kaposi's sarcoma has been observed as spontaneously regressing in transplant patients in whom immunosuppressive therapy was discontinued. A close relationship has been noted between cellular immunity, infection with cytomegalovirus, and Kaposi's sarcoma in combination with AIDS (20). Involuntary implantation of tumor seeds by organ transplantation can be viewed as a facet of iatrogenic implantation, comparable to tumor cell transfer by operation. Surgeons should therefore continue to employ en bloc resection of tumors, as well as other methods, to minimize iatrogenic dissemination (18, 46).

Table 2. Receptivity degrees to implantation metastasis.

Organ system	Organ(s)	Degrees
Urinary tract	Kidney, renal pelvis, ureter bladder	I
Female genital tract	Tubes, uterus	II
	Vagina, vulva	VI
Respiratory tract	Trachea, bronchi	III
Skin	–	IV
Alimentary tract	–	V

As a result of treatment of renal tumors by combined therapy, chronic inflammation, ulceration and formation of fistulae may be promoted, as may occur similarly in other tumors following implantation of neoplastic cells (50). If these cases are considered iatrogenic implantation or iatrogenic transplantation is a matter of selection, so it is done by chance, and unintentionally I prefer the first assumption. Bladder carcinoma arising from regenerated urothelium over lyophilized dura patch indicates that implantation of tumor cells occurs during the recurrence of superficial bladder cancer (45). Tuchmann and co-workers in 1986 (49) studied the effect of the use of the scalpel and CO_2 laser in animal experiments investigating tumor inoculation with the C57B1/6 mouse and Lewis lung carcinoma. The laser-operated animals showed a significantly longer survival and the interval without recurrence was longer for all tumor sizes when the laser was used (p less than 0.005).

The laser produced a high rate of cell destruction and seems to have some importance in those cases where the tumor is excised with a narrow margin. The progression of tumors in experimental animals is enhanced by injecting tumor cells together with fibroblasts (36). Inoculation metastasis must be carefully distinguished from multiple primary neoplasms or hematogenous lymphatic or contiguous metastases. Metachronous occurrence, as in the skin and mucous membranes is an especially important consideration. The distribution of multifocal neoplasms is mostly associated with a location which can be considered scattered, whereas inoculation metastases occur one-sided, and often caudally from the seeding growth.

SUMMARY AND CONCLUSION

Implantation metastasis, as reported in earlier decades of this and of the 19th century, exhibited a more limited occurrence. At the present time, immunosuppression, as a modality of treatment, may exhibit a higher degree of frequency in implantation metastasis and may lend a greater importance

Table 3. Conditions of epithelial surfaces, important (positive or negative) for inoculation metastasis.

Organ group or system	Organ	Positive aspects for inoculation	Negative aspects for inoculation metastasis	Degree	Comments
	Skin	Readily accessible	Rich bacterial flora, absence of breaches if surface is healthy	IV	Enfeebled vitality of tumor fragments
Alimentary tract	–	Extended epithelial surface	Rich bacterial flora, digestive enzymes and mucus, absence of breaches in healthy surface	V	Occasional diagnosis during autopsy, difficult to demonstrate
Respiratory tract	–	Fewer bacteria than	Rich bacterial flora, mucus, absence of breaches in healthy surface, movement of cilia	III	Movement of cilia renders implantation metastasis highly unlikely
Female genital tract	Tubes	Bacteria-free, no lytic reactions, little mucus	Mucus movement	II	
	Uterus	–		II	
	Vagina	Contacts with walls	Acidic environment,	IV	
	Vulva	Contacts with surfaces	Rich microbial flora	VI	
Urinary tract		Sterile environment devoid of mucus; implanting cells remain in customary environment		I	

Table 4. Selected cases of implantation metastasis, 1869–1958.

Structure of implantation	Tumor as source of implantation	Comments	References
Skin of thigh	Carcinoma of scrotum	Contact	(9)
Left thigh	Carcinoma of right thigh	Contact	(54)
Nose	Cancer of lower lip	Rubbing with hand	(5)
Bulb conjunctiva	Squamous carcinoma of eyelid	Contact	(14)
Mucosa of cheek	Carcinoma of tongue	Contact	(7)
Conjunctiva	Squamous cell cancer of hand	Rubbing	(26)
Trachea	Esophageal cancer	Inhalation	(31)
Lung	Carcinoma of tongue	Inhalation	(19)
Bronchi	Adamantinoma of maxilla	Inhalation	(52)
Bronchi	Laryngeal carcinoma	Inhalation	(56)
Lung	Basal cell carcinoma of face and mouth	Aspiration	(37)
Tube	Gastric carcinoma		(27)
Tube	Uterine cancer	Retrograde passage	(29, 33, 40–42, 53)
Vulva	Carcinoma of cervix uteri	Contact w/cancer of prolapsed uterus	(1)
Vulva	Carcinoma of vulva	Contact cancer	(39)
Ureter	Carcinoma of renal parenchyma		(30)

to this problem. This historic change may be ascribable to the higher survival rate of cancer patients as a result of therapy.

REFERENCES

1. Andrews HR: Carcinoma of the cervix of a prolapsed uterus in a patient aged 86, with a contact-carcinoma on one of the labia, vaginal hysterectomy. *Proc Roy Soc Med (Lond)* 3(6) Obstet Sect 161, 1910

2. Atiyah RA, Krespi YP, Hidvegi D et al.: The mechanical spread of viable tumor during surgery. *Otolaryngol Head Neck Surg* 94(3):278, 1986
3. Barter JF, Hatch KD, Orr JW Jr et al.: Isolated abdominal wound recurrence of an endometrial adenocarcinoma confined to a polyp. *Gynecol Oncol* 25(3):371, 1986
4. Brausi M, Latini A, Palladini PD: Local seeding of anaplastic carcinoma of prostate after needle biopsy. *Urology* 27(1):63, 1986
5. Butlin HT: Address in surgery on the contagion of cancer in human beings: autoinoculation. *Brit Med J* 2:255, 1907
6. Campins M, Madrenas J, Biosca M et al.: Extra-uterine mul-

lerian carcinosarcoma. *Acta Obstet Gynecol Scand* 65(7):811, 1986

7. Caan A: Beitrag zur Frage der Abklatschcarcinome. *Beitr Klin Chir* 68:717, 1910
8. Carr RJ, Gilbert PM: Tumour implantation to a temporalis muscle flap donor site. *Br J Oral Maxillofac Surg* 24(2):102, 1986
9. Cookson HA, Pullar TH: Contact spread of epithelioma from scrotum to thigh. *Lancet* 2:1273, 1932
10. Crissman JD: Tumor-host interactions as prognostic factors in the histologic assessment of carcinomas. *Pathol Annu* 21 Pt 1:29, 1986
11. Cutherell L, Wanebo HJ, Tegtmeyer CJ: Catheter tract seeding after percutaneous biliary drainage for pancreatic cancer. *Cancer* 57(10):2057, 1986
12. Emmerova M, Malkusova I, Barcal R: Implantation of skin metastases due to pericardial puncture. *Vnitr Lek* 32(3):286, 1986
13. Emtage JB, Perez-Marrero R: Extension of carcinoma of prostate along perineal needle biopsy tract. *Urology* 27(6):548, 1986
14. Eymann L: Kontaktkarzinom der Conjunctiva palpebrae und der Kornea. *Klin Mbl Augenheilk* 55:339, 1915
15. Fermor B, Umpleby HC, Lever JV et al.: Proliferative and metastatic potential of exfoliated colorectal cancer cells. *JNCI* 76(2):347, 1986
16. Freeman CR, Shustik C, Brisson ML et al.: Primary malignant lymphoma of the central nervous system. *Cancer* 58(5):1106, 1986
17. Fröhlich E, Frühmorgen P, Seeliger H: Cutaneous implantation metastasis after fine needle puncture of a pancreatic cancer (published erratum appears in *Ultraschall Med 1986* 7(6):309). *Ultraschall Med* 7(3):141, 1986
18. Georgi A: Diagnosis problems in metastasis – a round table. In: Metastasen Huebner (ed.). Stuttgart: Gustav Fischer Verlag, pp. 164–85, 1983
19. Godlee RJ: *Trans Path Soc Lond* 25:18, 1874
20. Groopman J, Mitsuyasu R: Kaposi's sarcoma and AIDS (meeting abstract). *J Cell Biochem* (Supple 8A):9, 1984
21. Habscheid W, Kirchner T: Skin metastases following ultrasound-guided fine-needle puncture of pancreatic cancer (letter). *Dtsch Med Wochenschr* 112(7):283, 1987
22. Haddad FS, Haddad L, Griffin EE 2d et al.: Doubling time and annual doubling rate of human prostatic cancer. *Urology* 29(1):35, 1987
23. Hsui JG, Given FT Jr, Kemp GM: Tumor implantation after diagnostic laparoscopic biopsy of serous ovarian tumors of low malignant potential. *Obstet Gynecol* 68(3 Suppl):905, 1986
24. Irwin BC, Hendrickse WA, Pincott JR et al.: Juvenile laryngeal papillomatosis. *J Laryngol Otol* 100(4):435, 1986
25. Kalifat R, Baup H, Freitag S et al.: Gliomas of the uterus. Apropos of 3 cases and review of the literature. *J Gynecol Obstet Biol Reprod* (Paris) 15(5):627, 1986
26. Kaufmann C: Ueber Multiplizitaet des primaeren Carcinomas. *Virchows Arch* 75:317, 1879
27. Kaufmann C: Pathology (translation by Reimann SP of the Lehrbuch der Pathologischen Anatomie). Philadelphia: Saunders, 1929
28. Kiser GC, Totonchy M, Barry JM: Needle tract seeding after percutaneous renal adenocarcinoma aspiration. *J Urol* 136(6):1292, 1986
29. Kundrat R: Zwei Faelle von primaeren Tubencarcinomen: Untersuchung ueber Metastasen in den Tuben bei Carcinomen des Collum und des Corpus uteri. *Arch Gnäk* 80:384, 1906
30. Macalpine JB: Implantation of secondaries from renal carcinoma (hypernephroma) within ureteric lumen. *Br J Surg* 36:164, 1948
31. Moxon W: *Trans path Soc Lond* 20:28, 1869
32. Muller NL, Bergin CJ, Miller RR et al.: Seeding of malignant cells into the needle track after lung and pleural biopsy. *J Can Assoc Radio* 37(3):192, 1986
33. Offutt SR: Relationship of carcinoma of body of uterus and of ovaries. *Surg Gynec Obstet* 54:490, 1932
34. Olsen KD: The parotid lump – don't biopsy it! An approach to avoiding misadventure. *Postgrad Med* 81(4):225, 232, 1987
35. Oni OO: Mechanisms of cancer metastasis to bone (letter). *J Bone Joint Surg* (Am) 69(2):309, 1987
36. Picard O, Rolland Y, Poupon MF: Fibroblast-dependent tumorigenicity of cells in nude mice: implication for implantation of metastases. *Cancer Res* 46(7):3290, 1986
37. Pickren JW, Katz AD: Aspiration metastases from basal cell carcinoma. *Cancer* 11:783, 1958
38. Rashleigh-Belcher HJ, Russell RC: Cutaneous seeding of pancreatic carcinoma by fine-needle aspiration biopsy. *Br J Radiol* 59(698):182, 1986
39. Rentschler CB: Primary epithelioma of vulva; analysis of 71 cases. *Ann Surg* 89:709, 1929
40. Sampson JA: Benign and malignant endometrial implants in peritoneal cavity, and their relation to certain ovarian tumors. *Surg Gynec Obstet* 38:287, 1924
41. Sampson JA: Carcinoma of the tubes and ovaries secondary to carcinoma of the body of the uterus. *Am J Path* 14:385, 1934
42. Sampson JA: Implantation carcinoma of the tubal mucosa secondary to carcinoma of the ovary. *Am J Path* 14:385, 1938
43. Samsonov VA: Metastases of kidney cancer (based on autopsy data). *Vopr Onkol* 32(2):78, 1986
44. Sarabia M, Millan JM, Escudero L et al.: Intracranial seeding from an intramedullary malignant astrocytoma. *Surg Neurol* 26(6):573, 1986
45. Selli C, Carcangiu ML, Carini M: Bladder carcinoma arising from regenerated urothelium over lyophilized dura patch. *Urology* 27(1):53, 1986
46. Sugarbaker EV, Ketcham AS: Mechanisms and prevention of cancer dissemination: an overview. *Semin Oncol* 4(1):19, 1977
47. Suzuki K, Kimula Y, Ogata T et al.: Bronchial carcinoid with multiple aerogenous implanted foci. *J Surg Oncol* 34(3):211, 1987
48. Tersigni R, Rossi P, Bochiochio O et al.: Tumor extension along percutaneous transhepatic biliary drainage tract. *Eur J Radiol* 6(4):280, 1986
49. Tuchmann A, Fischer PL, Bauer P et al.: Scalpel and CO_2 laser in the animal experiment. A comparative study of inoculation tumors of the mouse. *Langenbecks Arch Chir* 368(2):125, 1986
50. Vieweg G, Fröhlich D: Contribution on diagnosis and therapy of iatrogenic complications after combined therapy of malignant renal tumors. *Z Arztl Fortbild* (Jena) 75(22):1045, 1981
51. Vinokurov VL, Irzhanov SI, Zeldovich DR et al.: Patterns in the metastasis of malignant ovarian tumors based on autopsy data. *Vopr Onkol* 31(12):62, 1985
52. Vorzimer J, Perla D: An instance of adamantinoma of the jaw with metastases in the right lung. *Am J Path* 8:445, 1932
53. Werner P: Ueber gleichzeitiges Vorkommen von Carcinomen im Uterus und in den Adnexen. *Arch Gynaek* 101:725, 1913
54. Williams A: Inoculability of cancer. *Br Med J* 2:1369, 1987
55. Willis RA: The Spread of Tumours in the Human Body. 3rd edition. London: Butterworth, 1973
56. Zalka von E: Ueber Aspirations-(Implantations-) Metastasen in den Bronchien und der Lunge im Falle von Kehlkopfkrebs. *Arch Ohr usw Heilk* 138:164 1934 (abstract *Am J Cancer* 1935, 24:182)

PROGRESSION OF EMBRYONAL AND MIXED NEOPLASMS

H.E. KAISER

INTRODUCTION

Embryonal and mixed neoplasms are a heterogeneous group that in certain aspects possess a common background. The body of the eumetazoan animals, from platyhelminths to chordates, including the vertebrates, has three germ layers. Only two germ layers are present in coelenterates and cteno-phorans. In general, cancers develop from ectoderm and entoderm. One exception, the epithelial covering (endo-thelium) of the inside of the blood vessels, is derived from the mesoderm. Embryonal tissues differentation shows vari-able aspects in animals and plants. In animals, the adult cells of the tissues are no longer totipotent; they are only able to dedifferentiate. In contrast, the cells in plants, especially vascular plants, can undergo embryonalization and are able to become totipotent, and such a cell is capable of giving rise to a total new plant. These are the reasons why embryonal and mixed tumors of the same value do not occur in plants as in animals. Additional factors are the lack of floating cells in body fluids and the firm cell walls of the plants.

Neoplasms are able to develop in each phase of an eumetazoan organism (47, pp. 243–66). Embryonal neoplasms are those tumors which develop from the primor-dium of one or more organs during the embryonal develop-ment of an organism or from embryonal cell residues, name-ly, the dictyoma, embryonal carcinoma, hepatoblastoma, medulloblastoma, nephroblastoma, neuroblastoma, pulmo-blastoma, retinoblastoma, botryoid rhabdomyosarcoma, and testicular adenocarcinoma of infants, which seem to be related to the parental tissues.

Mixed neoplasms are those which are composed of two or more tissues as descendants of two or more germ layers. Mixed epithelial tumors occur in the bladder, the bronchus, the epididymis, the larynx, the salivary glands, the skin, the thyroid gland, and the trachea. Mixed connective tissue tumors are also known. Teratomas are mixed tumors which are composed of unrelated morphologic structures in one area deriving from a mixture of germ layers, mainly the ovary, the testis, and the pineal gland.

A collision tumor is one composed of two tissues (squa-mous cell and columnar epithelium) which began to grow as separate units and intermingled during progression; representatives of this type are the adenosquamous carcino-mas. The embryonal tumors, mixed tumors and teratomas have one characteristic which is more or less pronounced in the different groups: these neoplasms not only appear in early developmental stages or from remaining embryonic rests but they all show a more or less pronounced mixture of tissues ranging from an ability for differentiation only to combination of tissues from all three germ layers, as occurs in typical teratomas.

EMBRYONAL TUMORS*

Review of embryonal tumors: selected aspects

Nephroblastoma (syn. Wilms' tumor of kidney, adenosarcoma, embryonal nephroma, "mixed" tumor of kidney)

Approximately 20% of all childhood tumors are nephro-blastomas, and most develop in children up to one year of age. The peak occurs by age three; 1% of deaths in children from birth to 14 years are due to this tumor; boys are more susceptible than girls. During development a nephroblas-toma arises as solitary growth in the tissues of the kidney; rapid growth is characteristic. Nephroblastoma is highly malignant but also radiosensitive. Due to the second fact, nephroblastoma is "curable" through surgery and radiation (4, pp. 808–9).

Primary tumors and metastases of nephroblastoma have stemlines in the diploid and low aneuploid (hyperdiploid) range of blastema as detected by cytometric DNA-ploidy determinations. The blastema seems to be the most likely component of metastasis in contrast to epithelial and stro-mal elements which are rarely if at all represented in metas-tasis. Blastema exhibits high sensitivity to therapy and plays a central role in prognosis (114).

Koriakina (55) reported recently on cytologic characteris-tics of nephroblastoma. Rhabdoid tumor of kidney is able to simulate other renal neoplasms in children but exhibits a characteristic clinical course with a high frequency of in-tracranial neoplasms (77). Intermediate filament proteins can be used to study the heterogeneic characters of tumors (91), and molecular aspects of cytogenetic abnormalities in cancer cells are important for an understanding of oncogene activation in man (11). Computed tomography is useful for evaluation of renal masses and staging of malignant tumors of the kidney (62; see also 51). Antibodies to desmoplakins are of value in tumor cell typing and diagnosis of nephro-blastoma (21). Ultrasound is the method for the diagnosis of Wilms' tumor in most patients (20). Many patients with nephroblastoma showed congenital abnormalities and some

---

The arrangement of the tumors follows the sequence of tissues ((47), p. 653).

K.W. Brunson (ed) Local invasion and spread of cancer.

had more than one abnormality; 70% survived more than 5 years (83).

Cultured cells of bilateral nephroblastoma in a child exhibited cytogenetically a new translocation not reported previously: 46,XY,t(3;17) (104). It is assumed that Wilms' tumor is preceded by two mutations at both alleles of a critical gene located within p13 band of chromosome 11. A new mapping of chromosome 11p confirmed these results (90). Studies by Michalopoulos *et al.* (76) showed the deletion of the affected chromosome in an aniridia-Wilms' tumor association includes band 11p13, but does not extend to calcitonin or other genes thought to be located in the distal half of chromosome 11p. However, a child with nephroblastoma not associated with aniridia had several chromosome abnormalities including a t(2;7)(q33;p22) in 6% of the lymphocytes (93).

Embryonic tumors of liver (syn. embryonal mixed tumor of liver, embryonic hepatoma, hepatoblastoma)
These tumors, a heterogeneous group, are characterized by embryonic cells. Differentiated and undifferentiated epithelial and mesenchymal cells occur side by side. The tumors are rare (see Chapter 7/Volume VII), and are most common in infants and children but have also been observed in adults (4, pp. 592–3). In the adult, hepatoblastoma is one of the least common liver tumors (49).

The appearance of other tissues such as bone or osteoid in hepatoblastoma is well known; even teratoid features may occur (66). Fetal hepatoblastoma may metastasize to the placenta (94) or the liver. Another hepatoblastoma appeared together with Aicardi syndrome with severe brain malformation in an infant (110). One case of hepatoblastoma exhibited a sarcoid reaction, but no strong correlation between histological pattern and prognosis was established (99).

Chemically transformed cells of cultured rat liver produced various clonal subpopulations with remarkable variability and a high embryonal potential (112). Hepatoblastoma occurs spontaneously and experimentally induced in mice.
Pulmoblastoma: This embryonic tumor of the lung occurred in a child (65).

Embryonal carcinoma (syn. embryoma, teratocarcinoma, trophocarcinoma)
Mainly epithelial in character, they also contain teratomatous elements; 20% of germinal tumors are composed of this highly malignant tumor. The parenchyma consists of broad epithelial sheaths or syncytial masses and a connective tissue stroma (4, pp. 765–6).

Tumor patterns reflecting the stages of differentiation can be placed in chronological order with respect to embryogenesis (45). One from 4 human embryonal carcinoma cell lines differed from the others due to its rapid growth, high tumorigenic potential, formation of solid cell aggregates, and less differentiated solid histologic pattern. This indicates that there are different cell lines of human embryonal carcinoma (102). There was a heterogeneity among stem cells derived from a single human teratocarcinoma (3). The presence of a 54 K keratin polypeptide distinguished the benign and malignant trophoblastic cells from human embryonal carcinoma cells and a yolk sac carcinoma cell line

(17). Some cells of embryonal carcinoma were unaffected by lengthy exposures of retinoic acid whereas the growth of their progeny was inhibited. Embryonal carcinoma cells may become epigenetically refractory to retinoic acid (103). Tumor tissue can be localized by carcino-embryonic antigen and pregnancy-specific beta-1-glycoprotein using specific antibodies, radiolabeled or conjugated to antineoplastic drugs (46). Embryonal proliferation may be controlled by interaction between primitive ectoderm cells and their differentiated derivatives, mediated by specific soluble growth factors (40). The isolation of clonal embryonal carcinoma cell derivatives which are stable, heritable differentiation variants provides resources for somatic-cell genetic analysis of stem-cell pluripotency (28). Mice which have been immunized against H-2 class I antigens on transfected L cells reject transplanted embryonal carcinoma cells (81). Wobus *et al.* (116) characterized the pluripotent mouse teratocarcinoma cell line TCE.

Embryonal carcinoma of the salivary glands is rare in children and adolescents (101), while in adults such tumors originate in the kidney, bladder, prostate, and testis (41). A metastatic embryonal carcinoma of the testis regressed spontaneously with a 22-year follow-up (43).

Testicular adenocarcinoma of infancy (syn. orchioblastoma, endodermal sinus tumor, yolk-sac tumor, infantile embryonal carcinoma)
This tumor is the most common one of infancy, appears before 3 years of age, and is often curable by orchiectomy. It is composed of differentiated and undifferentiated epithelial elements (4, p. 770). The peritoneum, diaphragm and pleura can be involved by this type of tumor (95).

Embryonic (botryoid) rhabdomyosarcoma
These neoplasms originate in close relationship to the mucosa of a hollow organ of the body cavity and develop into large grape-like masses and grow into large oedomatous masses. In children up to 5 years old, vagina, urethra, bladder in the female and vesicourethral region and prostate and bladder in the male infant, are typical locations. In children up to 10 years, embryonic rhabdomyosarcomas have been seen in the orbit, head and neck, ear, nasopharynx, common bile duct, retroperitoneum extremities, and even in the mitral valve (35). The tumors are composed of a mesenchymal blastoma; differentiation varies (Ashley, 1978, p. 47). One child exhibited embryonal botryoid rhabdomyosarcoma of the mitral valve (35).

Another child with Dandy-Walker syndrome had the rare combination of bilateral cystic nephroblastomas and botryoid sarcoma (50).

Dictyoma (syn. medulloepithelioma)
This rare neoplasm of the ciliary body is related to retinoblastoma in that it shares an origin from embryonic retinal elements. The lesion is solitary and unilateral, usually arising in children from 1 to 8 years of age. The epithelium is single or multilayered, the stroma scanty or missing. Andersen (2) regarded the slow-growing tumor as a hamartoma. One ditokyma exhibited glial differentiation (48), and a retinal dictyoma metastasized to the submandibular lymph nodes (31).

Medulloepithelioma,   desmoplastic   infantile   ganglioglioma, pineoblastoma and medulloblastoma are multipotential tumors in regard to differentiation. Aberrant developmental regulatory mechanisms may be involved in the behavior of these tumors (113).

Retinoblastoma (syn. neuroblastoma retinae; glioma retinae, neuroepithelima of the retinae; ependymoma retinae) (36, 69, 97).

This embryonic neoplasm occurs from 1 to 10,000 births to 1 in 34,000 births. The neoplasm is generally recognized directly after birth or in the first two years but may occur later in life. The neoplasm is densely cellular and the supporting tissue consists of delicate, richly vascular stroma. The retinoblastoma gene seems to be located on chromosome 15, according to chromosome studies (see Chapter 14/ Volume III; 4, p. 462). Survivors of retinoblastoma have a tendency to develop other neoplasms (84).

Oncogenes in retinoblastoma and neuroblastoma were compared (62). Retinoblastoma belong to the somatostatin-producing tumors (8). Neoplasms in the perinatal period are remarkably different from those in older children and adolescents, both by biological behavior and response to therapy (44). Cytogenetic analysis of 27 retinoblastomas showed gross aneuploidy of chromosome arms 6p and 1q as very common, whereas chromosome 13 was rarely missing. Nonrandom translocations at three break points occurred as follows: 14q32, 17p12, and 10q25; 14q32 is not the same sequence used in certain Burkitt's lymphomas. One line had double minute chromosomes. The common patterns indicate an early advantage to malignant cells rather than induced malignant transformation (63, 105, 106). The chromosomal region 13q14 with the Rb susceptibility gene represents one of a class of recessive human cancer genes that can be contrasted to known oncogenes functioning following amplification, aberrant insertion, or base substitutions at key sites within their gene. Loss of function of both Rb alleles seems to characterize the mechanism by which the Rb gene produces tumors, which may also include the second primary malignancies seen with high frequency in patients with the hereditary form of retinoblastoma (7). Retinoblastoma is known in hereditary, non-hereditary and chromosomal deletion forms. It is a frequent experience that children who were treated earlier for retinoblastoma develop secondary bone sarcomas (99).

Inactivation of the retinoblastoma susceptibility gene has been implicated in the genesis of retinoblastoma, certain breast cancers, small cell lung cancer and carcinoid of the lung. Growth inhibition may be as important in development of malignancies as growth stimulation. This effect of inhibition may be an initiating stage of carcinogenesis. Survivors of retinoblastomas tend to develop sarcomas such as osteosarcomas and their mothers have a higher risk of developing breast cancer (37, 60, 71).

The first reported primary malignant rhabdoid tumor of the CNS (subarachnoid space and cerebellum) was composed of highly cellular monomorphic polygonal cells with roughly ovoid vesicular nuclei and conspicuous nucleoli. This aggressive type of tumor occurs most frequently in association with neoplasms of the kidney, the liver and other sites (9).

Neuroblastoma (syn. sympathicoblastoma)

This tumor occurs in the fetus, the newborn and infants a few weeks old (4, pp. 312–17). Therefore it can be seen as an embryonic neoplasm. Neuroblastoma may major to gangliomyoma. Regression appears with a certain frequency; the age ranges from the fetus to 10 years and the peak occurs in the first two years of life. Most of the tumors originate in the abdomen, mainly the adrenal glands and related sympathetic ganglia in the lumbar region, pelvis, posterior mediastinum, and sometimes in the cervical sympathetic chain. In the CNS, olfactory neuroblastoma is more or less an exception. Tumors originating from the adrenals are more malignant than the nonadrenal counterparts.

MR imaging seems to be a reliable technique for diagnosis, staging, and follow-up of children with neuroblastoma (23). The most useful technique for staging of neuroblastoma is scintigraphy with II31-meta-iodobenzyl-guanidine (MLBG) (29); the compound is also effectively used for treatment (42).

Chromosomal translocation t(2;?)(p24;?) may be related to the activation and following amplification of the N-*myc* oncogene (16). More aggressive treatment of these neoplasms may lead to secondary tumors in the future (100). Chemotherapy including high-dose melphalan is promising when used as consolidation therapy in patients who have already attained complete remission with conventional therapies (39).

Medulloblastoma

This neoplasm variably occurs in the cerebellum in infants to children over 15 years (median peak 5 to 9 years) with a second small peak at 20 to 25 years (4, pp. 457–60). In the older patients, the tumor occurs more laterally. Medulloblastoma of children comprises approximately 28% of all intracranial neoplasms of the first decade of life and there is a preponderance in boys. Neoplasms in the young are more aggressive than those in the adults. Serial analysis of specific biochemical markers (CSF polyamines) in cases of medulloblastoma may be possible (58).

Mixed differentiation of neoplasms has important clinical implications (74). Cerebellar medulloblastomas seen at one hospital exhibited a seasonal peak between September and December (67). Immunocytochemical techniques can only supplement but not replace classical histopathologic evaluation. The desmoplastic variety of medulloblastomas shows frequent glioneuronal differentiation (12). Cerebral tumors consisted of larger or smaller amounts of primitive embryonal cells. The tumors showed certain similarities to posterior fossa medulloblastomas but also important differences in histology, immunohistology, natural history and response to treatment. The proper term for these tumors is "primitive neuroectodermal tumor". An indirect immunoperoxidase method using an antibody to aldolase C for the localization of aldolase C isozyme showed no positive staining in medulloblastomas (56). The majority of malignant cells in primitive childhood brain tumors lacked any intermediate filament protein reactivity (111). Medulloblastomas are generally negative for vimentin and glial fibrillary acidic protein (34, 117), but some cases showed positive immunostaining for glial fibrillary acidic protein. Glial fibrillary acidic protein is specific for astrocytes, which suggests astrocytic differentiation in the tumor cells of medulloblastomas (57).

A boy with medulloblastoma and grade IV spinal cord involvement survived almost 3 years after the spinal cord metastases (107).

The 2A6 and 81C6 monoclonal antibodies can be used for

investigations of the extracellular matrix of malignant neuroepithelial neoplasms (73). The levels of L-ornithine decarboxylase are a more reliable indication of the grade of malignancy in medulloblastoma than the levels of S-adenosyl-L-omethionine decarboxylase (96).

MIXED NEOPLASMS

Mixed neoplasms of skin (4, pp. 353–54): Various cases of cutaneous malignant mixed tumors have been described (13, 38). One of the rarest types of sweat gland origin is the so-called malignant chondroid syringoma or malignant mixed tumor of the skin (87, 92).

A number of tumors deriving from sweat glands resemble the mixed tumors of salivary glands. The lesions are mostly located on the face and head of persons older than 35 years. More infrequently they are found on the trunk and extremities and also at palmar and plantar surfaces. Growth is slow and malignant conversion rare. The mixed elements of the tumor consist of epithelial structures and parts of cartilage, chondroid and mixoid tissue. Gallager *et al.* (32) described a tumor (perhaps a mucoepidermoid carcinoma) of the foot composed of squamous and mucine-containing signet-like cells. Metastases had spread to the heart, liver, kidney, spleen, adrenals, pancreas, skin, regional and distant lymph nodes. Mixed tumors of the lacrimal gland have been described (10, 86).

Mixed tumors of the salivary glands (syn. composite tumors; polymorphic adenomas; adenomes metaplastiques polymorphes; enclavomas)
The majority of salivary gland neoplasms are mixed tumors and comprise approximately 28% of all salivary gland neoplasms. The size may span from a few millimeters to many centimeters in diameter. The tumors are composed of epithelial and myoepithelial tissues. These are monomorphic adenomas, basal cell adenoma, oxophylic adenoma (syn. oncocytoma), adenolymphoma (syn. papillary cystadenoma lymphomatosus; oncocytoma; Warthin's tumor; branchioma; orbital inclusion cyst; branchiogenic adenoma) acinic or acinous-cell carcinoma, adenocystic carcinoma (syn. cylindroma), mucoepidermoid tumors, epidermoid carcinoma, salivary-duct carcinoma, anaplastic small cell tumor of salivary glands, benign lympho-epithelial lesion.

"Mixed Tumors" of the thyroid gland as reported by Willis (115) are extremely rare and composed of hyperplastic or neoplastic thyroid parenchyma with neoplastic mesenchymal components which are generally osteosarcomatous or chondrosarcomatous (4, p. 266). Mixed tumors of the trachea are very rare (4, p. 632), as well as mixed cardiac tumors (5).

Mixed tumors of the mediastinum involving a primary embryonal carcinoma and carcinoma and choriocarcinoma of the mediastinum have been noted (54). The "chondroma" or chondromatous hamartoma (syn. chondro-adenoma) was considered in 1962 by Willis as a mixed neoplasm of the bronchial wall whereas other experts see it as a hamartoma (4, p. 648).

A primary malignant mixed mesodermal tumor of the gallbladder with osteosarcomatous regions in this organ was described (1). Mixed mesodermal tumors of the urinary bladder with malignant epithelial and mesenchymal elements were noted (6) while another case showed undifferentiated mesenchymal cells and those with chondroblastic differentiation (25).

A mixed tumor of the Fallopian tube resembling an adenoacanthocarcinosarcoma contained atypical cartilage (26).

Mixed tumors in the bladder occur as combinations of transitional cell carcinoma and adenocarcinoma or transitional cell carcinoma and squamous cell carcinoma or all three types together (82).

A benign mixed tumor of the vagina was described by Chen (15) and two mixed tumors of the vulva of the salivary gland type seem to have developed from Bartholin's gland. In one of the benign tumors a carcinoma arose (85). Mixed tumors of the epididymis are the rarest lesions in this organ (4, p. 779).

Benign and malignant mixed tumors of connective tissue occur. To the first group belong the benign mesenchymoma and the benign mixed mesodermal tumors of the uterus; to the second group, the malignant mesenchymoma and the malignant mixed mesodermal tumors of the uterus.

Carcinosarcomas (syn. collision tumors)
These rare neoplasms are composed of a mixture of epithelial and mesenchymal elements; both components are malignant. These tumors occur most often in the bladder and the breast but have also been found in the uterus, stomach, larynx, lung, and gallbladder. The carcinosarcomas can be divided according to Meyer (75) into collision tumors (invading each other if growing in the same region), combination tumors (arising from multipotent cells) and composition tumors (arising in the same tissue). Of diagnostic importance is the appearance of both tissue types in the metastases (4, p. 154).

Uterine mesodermal mixed neoplasms (4, p. 719)
Carcinosarcoma of the Fallopian tube is a rare neoplasm (88).

In endometrial carcinosarcomas, the most frequent metastatic site was the lung (72, 89).

A carcinosarcoma of the esophagus was reported by Ganul *et al.* (33).

Stomach (4, p. 562): Carcinosarcoma of the stomach is exceedingly rare (19).

Gallbladder: Only two cases have been reported (68). The tumor is highly anaplastic and rapidly fatal.

Larynx (4, p. 627): The carcinosarcoma of the larynx is difficult to diagnose because also other malignancies of the larynx exhibit stromal overgrowth. One case showed the mixture of epithelial and mesenchymal tissues in the primary as well as in the metastatic lesions of the tumor (80).

Lung (4, p. 650): Carcinosarcomas of the lung are occasionally seen and Ashley gives some reference citations on such cases. They were divided into an endobronchial type with squamous carcinomatous component in most cases and a peripheral type in which it is glandular in 50% of cases (18).

Bladder (4, p. 838): In the bladder, carcinosarcomas generally exhibit as the carcinomatous component transitional cell epithelium whereas the mesenchymal part may be composed of undifferentiated, myosarcomatous, cross-striated muscular cartilage or bony elements.

Breast (4, p. 381): Carcinosarcomas of the breast are rare and when they spread they mimick the tissue mixture of the primary neoplasm in certain cases. Metastasis occurs to the regional lymph nodes. The epithelial elements exhibit only rarely keratinization. Fibroblastic cartilaginous and bony elements may appear.

Walker carcinosarcoma of the rat is an important experimental model widely used in cancer research. The cellular proliferation of carcinosarcoma and metastases showed that the cell cycle of metastases is shorter and the labeling index is higher than in primary tumors (52).

TERATOMAS (4, pp. 843–57)

Teratomas contain tissue components in an arrangement that does not exist normally. The tissue types present in teratoma vary and malignant spreading may involve all parts of the structure or may differ. Metastatic spreading has been treated in Chapter 22/Volume VIII; therefore, in this chapter only a few comments on the most recent literature are given (4, pp. 845–55).

Teratomas are important gonadal neoplasms but also occur in extragonadal sites such as the mediastinum, parapineal and sacrococcygeal areas and retroperitoneum. In the testis, they compose 90% of all tumors of the testicle and 99% of them are malignant. In the ovary, they compose around 20% and 90% of them are mature cystic teratomas and benign. Malignant testicular teratomas are ten times more common than ovarian and 20 times more common than their extragonadal counterparts. The malignant teratomas are mainly found in children and young adults. Germ cell tumors of the testis occur frequently in western and northern Europe in contrast to southern and eastern Europe. They are rare in Africa and in this country are uncommon in blacks when compared to whites. Ovarian or extragonadal germ cell tumors do not exhibit these significant differences (109). It is assumed that differentiation of the carcinomatous stem cells produces forms which are transitional between seminomatous and non-seminomatous tumor types (53). Computed tomography enables diagnosis and staging of teratomatous lesions of the mediastinum (84). (See also Takakura, (108) for intracranial germ cell tumors; Marsh (70) for shunting and irradiation of tumors of the pineal; Cavanagh (14) for teratomas of the ovary; and Morley (79) for cellular iron uptake.

The presence of true desmosomes together with scanty vimentin filaments in most tumor cells makes seminomas different from most other germ cell and nongerm cell tumors. Seminal cells can be heterogenous in their cytoskeletal complement and may include cells with cytokeratin expression, which indicates a multipotential character of the initially transformed cell(s) (22). Syncytiotrophoblastic cells in testicular tumors are signs of a worse prognosis than otherwise indicated (24).

SUMMARY AND CONCLUSIONS

The three groups of embryonal tumors, mixed tumors and teratomas have one common characteristic. These neo-plasms not only appear often in early developmental stages or from remaining embryonic nests, but they all show a more or less pronounced mixture of tissues which range from a variability in differentiation only, to a combination of components from all three germ layers as is the case in typical teratomas. If embryonic, they are able to develop from their stem cells into various differentiations.

REFERENCES

1. Aldovini D, Piscioli F, Togni R: Primary malignant mixed mesodermal tumor of the gallbladder. Report of a case and critical review of diagnostic criteria. *Virchows Arch (Pathol Anat)* 396(2):225, 1982
2. Andersen SR: Medullo-epitheliomas, diktyoma and malignant epithelioma of the ciliary body. *Acta Ophthalmologica (Copenhagen)* 26:313, 1948
3. Andrews, PW, Damjanov I, Simon D, Dignazio M: A pluripotent human stem-cell clone isolated from the TERA-2 teratocarcinoma line lacks antigens SSEA-3 and SSEA-4 *in vitro*, but expresses these antigens when grown as a xenograft tumor. *Differentiation* 29(2):127, 1985
4. Ashley DJB: Evans' Histological Appearances of Tumours. (3rd edition) vols. I and II. Edinburgh–London–New York: Churchill Livingstone, 1978
5. Astafev VI, Zheltovskii IuV, Kanonenko VN et al.: Case of a mixed cardiac tumor. *Grudn Khir* (2):81, 1981
6. Babaian RJ, Johnson DE, Manning J, Ayala A et al.: Mixed mesodermal tumors of urinary bladder: prognosis and management. *Urology* 15(3):261, 1980
7. Benedict WF: Retinoblastoma gene: a human cancer recessive (regulatory?) susceptibility gene. *Carcinog Compr Surv* 10:403, 1985
8. Berelowitz M: Somatostatin-producing tumors. *Adv Exp Med Biol* 188:475, 1985
9. Biggs PJ, Garen PD, Powers JM et al.: Malignant rhabdoid tumor of the central nervous system. *Hum Pathol* 18(4):332, 1987
10. Bourgeois H, Maille M, Maurin F, Jacob H: A case of mixed tumor of the lacrimal gland: histologic and prognostic discussion. *Bull Soc Ophtalmol Fr* 82(3):313, 1982
11. Brodeur GM: Molecular correlates of cytogenetic abnormalities in human cancer cells: implications for oncogene activation. *Prog Hematol* 14:229, 1985
12. Budka H: Pathology of midline brain tumors. Immunocytochemical tumor markers and classificatory aspects. *Acta Neurochir (Suppl) (Wien)* 35:23, 1985
13. Carapeta FJ, Martin J, Grasa MP et al.: Mixed tumor of the skin. Apropos of 5 cases. *Actes Dermosilifiliogr* 72(11–12):571, 1981
14. Cavanagh D, Marsden DE, Ruffolo EH: Primary nonepithelial cancers of the ovary. *Obstet Gynecol Annu* 14:344, 1985
15. Chen KT: Benign mixed tumor of the vagina. *Obstet Gynecol* 57(6 Suppl): 895, 1981
16. Christiansen H, Franke F, Bertram CR et al.: Evolution of tumor cytogenetic aberrations and N-*myc* oncogene amplification in a case of disseminated neuroblastoma. 26(2):235, 1987
17. Clark RK, Damjanov I: Intermediate filaments of human trophoblast and choriocarcinoma cell lines. *Virchows Arch (A)* 407(2):203, 1985
18. Cohen-Salmon D, Michel RP, Wang NS et al.: Pulmonary carcinosarcoma and carcinoma: report of a case studied by electron microscopy, with critical review of the literature. *Ann Pathol* 5(2):115, 1985
19. Dawson EK: (cited after Ashley), 1965
20. De Campo JF: Ultrasound of Wilms' tumor. *Pediatr Radiol* 1691):21, 1986

21. Denk H, Weybora W, Ratschek M, Schar R et al.: Distribution of vimentin, cytokeratins, and desmosomal-plaque proteins in human nephroblastoma as revealed by specific antibodies: coexistence of cell groups of different degrees of epithelial differentiation. *Differentiation* 29(1):85, 1985
22. Denk H, Moll R, Weybora W et al.: Intermediate filaments and desmosomal plaque proteins in testicular seminomas and non-seminomatous germ cell tumours as revealed by immunohistochemistry. *Virchows Arch (A)* 410(4):295, 1987
23. Dietrich RB, Kangarioo H, Lenarsky C, Feig SA: Neuroblastoma: the role of MR imaging. *AJR* 148(5):937, 1987
24. Dressler K, Lauke H, Holstein AF: Morphology of syncytiotrophoblast cells in testicular tumors. *Urologe (A)* 26(1):38, 1987
25. Duong HD, Jackson AG, Kovi J et al.: Mixed mesodermal tumor of urinary bladder: a light and electron microsomic study. *Urology* 17(4):377, 1981
26. Egorov VP: Heterotopic mesodermal tumor of the Fallopian tube. *Arkh Patol* 44(2):54, 1982
27. Elbers JR, Wagenaar SS: Malignant mixed mesodermal tumor of the ovary. *Eur J Obstet Gynaecol Reprod Biol* 10(1):47, 1980
28. Felix JS: Derivation of a nondifferentiating clone from multipotential PSA1 embryonal carcinoma cells. *Differentiation* 29(3):254, 1985
29. Ferris J, Caballero O, Verdeguer A et al.: 131I-MIBG-metaiodobencylguanidine (131I-MIBG) in the study of neuroblastoma. *An Esp Pediatr* 26(3):164, 1987
30. Gaffney CC, Sloane JP, Bradley NJ et al.: Primitive neuroectodermal tumours of the cerebrum. Pathology and treatment. *J Neurooncol* 3(1):23, 1985
31. Galimova RZ, Ozhanavbaeva PN: Retinal diktyoma with metastasis to the submandibular lymph nodes. *Vestn Oftalmol* 101(4):72, 1985
32. Gallager HS, Miller GV, Grampa G: Primary mucoepidermoid carcinoma of the skin. Report of a case. *Cancer* 12:286, 1959
33. Ganul VL, Okulov LV, Kirkilevskii SI et al.: Carcinosarcoma and pseudosarcoma of the esophagus. *Klin Khir* (10):60, 1985
34. Gottschalk J, Martin H, Kretschmer B et al.: Significance of immunohistochemistry in neuro-oncology. I. Demonstration of glial fibrillary acid protein (GFAP) in extracranial metastases from primary brain tumors. *Zentralbl Allg Pathol* 130(5):391, 1985
35. Hajar R, Roberts WC, Folger GM Jr: Embryonal botryoid rhabdomyosarcoma of the mitral valve. *Am J Cardiol* 57(4):376, 1986
36. Hamerski W: Tumors of the retina. *Pieleg Polozna* (9):2–3, 19, 1985
37. Harbour JW, Shinn-Liang L, Whang-Peng J et al.: Abnormalities in structure and expression of the human retinoblastoma gene in SCLC. *Science* 241:353, 1988
38. Harrist TJ, Aretz TH, Mihm MC Jr et al.: Cutaneous malignant mixed tumor. *Arch Dermatol* 117(11):719, 1981
39. Hartmann O, Kalifa C, Benhamou E, Patte C et al.: Treatment of advanced neuroblastoma with high-dose melphalan and autologous bone marrow transplantation. *Cancer Chemother Pharmacol* 16(2):165, 1986
40. Heath JK, Rees AR: Growth factors in mammalian embryogenesis. *Ciba Round Syng* 116:3, 1985
41. Hecht F: Embryonal origin of adult tumors: carcinomas of kidney, bladder, prostate, and testicle (editorial). *Cancer Genet Cytogenet* 24(1):189, 1987
42. Hoefnagel CA, Voute PA, de Kraker J et al.: Radionuclide diagnosis and therapy of neural crest tumors using iodine-131 metaiodobenzylguanidine. *J Nucl Med* 28(3):306, 19087
43. Husseini S, Krauss DJ, Rullis I: Spontaneous regression of metastatic embryonal testicular carcinoma: 22-year follow-up. *J Urol* 136(1):119, 1985
44. Isaacs H Jr: Perinatal (congenital and neonatal) neoplasms: a report of 110 cases. *Pediatr Pathol* 3(2–4):165, 1985
45. Jacobsen GK: Histogenetic considerations concerning germ cell tumours. Morphological and immunohistochemical comparative investigation of the human embryo and testicular germ cell tumours. *Virchows Arch (A)* 408(5):509, 1986
46. Jacobsen GK, Olsen J: Residual retroperitoneal tumour tissue in patients treated for metastatic non-seminomatous testicular germ cell tumours: an immunohistochemical investigation. *Tumour Biol* 6(1):25, 1985
47. Kaiser HE (ed): Neoplasms – Comparative Pathology of Growth in Animals, Plants, and Man. Baltimore: Williams & Wilkins. 1981
48. Kasantikul V: Vatanatumrak B: Rutnin U: Medulloepithelioma (diktyoma) with glial differentiation. *J Med Assoc Thai* 67(10):580, 1984
49. Kawarada Y, Uehara S, Noda M, Yatani R et al.: Non-hepatocytic malignant mixed tumor primary in the liver. Report of two cases. *Cancer* 55(8):1790, 1985
50. Kinoshita T, Nakamura Y, Kinoshita M et al.: Bilateral cystic nephroblastomas and botryoid sarcoma in a child with Dandy-Walker syndrome. *Arch Pathol Lab Med* 110(2):150, 1986
51. Kirks DR, Rosenberg ER, Johnson DG, King LR: Integrated imaging of neonatal renal masses. *Pediatr Radiol* 15(3):147, 1985
52. Kiseleva EG: Cellular proliferation kinetics of Walker carcinosarcoma, Zajdela's ascitic hepatoma and their metastases to the lymph nodes. *Eksp Onkol* 7(5):42, 1985
53. Kiss F, Juhasz J: Testicular germ cell tumours. Current problems of histogenesis and classification. *Int Urol Nephrol* 17(1):85, 1985
54. Knapp RH, Fritz SR, Reiman HM: Primary embryonal carcinoma and choriocarcinoma of the mediastinum. A case report. *Arch Pathol Lab Med* 106(10):507, 1982
55. Koriakina RF: Cytologic characteristics of nephroblastoma. *Lab Delo* (2):81, 1985
56. Kumanishi T, Watabe K, Washiyama K: An immunohistochemical study of aldolase C in normal and neoplastic nervous tissues. *Acta Neuropathol (Berl)* 67(3–4):309, 1985
57. Kumanishi T, Washiyama K, Watabe K, Sekiguchi K: Glial fibrillary acidic protein in medulloblastomas. *Acta Neuropathol (Berl)* 67(1–2):1, 1985
58. Kun LE, D'Souza B, Tefft M: The value of surveillance testing in childhood brain tumors. *Cancer* 56(7 Suppl):1818, 1985
59. Lapis P, Kopper L, Bodrogi I et al.: Characteristics and chemotherapeutic sensitivity of a human testicular cancer grown in artificially immunosuppressed mice. *Oncology* 42(2):112, 1985
60. Lee EY-HP, To H, Shew J-Y et al.: Inactivation of the retinoblastoma susceptibility gene in human breast cancers. *Science* 241:218, 1988
61. Lee WH, Murphee AL, Benedict WF: Comparison studies of oncogenes in retinoblastoma and neuroblastoma. *Prog Clin Biol Res* 175:131, 1985
62. Levine E: Computed tomography of renal masses. *CRC Crit Rev Diagn Imaging* 24(2):91, 1985
63. Lund OE, Murken JD: The 13q14 delation syndrome. *Fortschr Ophthalmol* 82(4):385, 1985
64. Mackillop WJ, Blundell J, Steele P: Short-term culture of pediatric brain tumors. *Childs Nerv Syst* 1(3):163, 1985
65. Mahnke PF, Weidenbach H: Morphology, histogenesis and dignity of pulmoblastoma with special regard to the pulmoblastoma in childhood. *Zentralbl Allg Pathol* 124(6):540, 1980
66. Manivel C, Wick MR, Abenoza P et al.: Teratoid hepatoblastoma. The nosologic dilemma of solid embryonic neoplasms of childhood. *Cancer* 57(11):2168, 1986

67. Manshande JP, Van Tornout J, Coppens M et al.: Seasonal variation in incidence of cerebellar medulloblastoma. *Brain Dev* 7(5):525, 1985

68. Mansori KS, Cho SY: Malignant mixed tumor of the gallbladder. *Am J Clin Pathol* 73(5):709, 1980

69. Marco M, Chaques V, Serra I: Retinoblastoma: clinical and therapeutic study. *Bull Mem Soc Fr Ophtalmol* 96:410, 1985

70. Marsh WR, Laws ER Jr: Shunting and irradiation of pineal tumors. *Clin Neurosurg* 32:384, 1985

71. Marx JL: Eye cancer gene linked to new malignancies. *Science* 241:293, 1988

72. Mastilovic M, Draca P, Budakov P et al.: Primary multiple synchronous homologous malignant tumors of the endometrium. *Med Pregl* 38(3–4):157, 1985

73. McComb RD, Bigner DD: Immunolocalization of monoclonal antibody-defined extracellular matrix antigens in human brain tumors. *J Neurooncol* 3(2):181, 1985

74. Mendelsohn G, Maksem JA: Divergent differentiation in neoplasms. Pathologic, biologic, and clinical considerations. *Pathol Annu* 21 Pt 1:91, 1986

75. Meyer R: Beitrag zur Verständigung über die Namensgebung in der Geschwulstlehre. *Zentralbl. Allg Pathologie* 30:291, 1920

76. Michalopoulos EE, Bevilacqua PJ, Stokoe N et al.: Molecular analysis of gene deletion in aniridia–Wilms' tumor association. *Hum Genet* 70(2):157, 1985

77. Montgomery P, Kuhn JP, Berger PE: Rhabdoid tumor of the kidney: a case report. *Urol Radiol* 7(1):42, 1985

78. Moore AV, Silverman PM, Putnam CE: Current concepts in computerized tomography of the mediastinum. *CRC Crit Rev Diagn Imaging* 24(1):1, 1985

79. Morley CG, Bezkorovainy A: Cellular iron uptake from transferrin: is endocytosis the only mechanism? *Int J Biochem* 17(5):553, 1985

80. Minckler DS, Meligro CH, Norris HT: Carcinosarcoma of the larynx. Case report with metastases of epidermoid and sarcomatous elements. *Cancer* 26:195, 1970

81. Moser AR, Johnson LL, Dove WF: Mice coisogenically immunized against H-2 class I antigens on transfected L cells reject transplanted embryonal carcinoma cells. *Immunogenetics* 22(6):533, 1985

82. Mostofi FK, Thompson RV, Dean AL: Mucous adenocarcinoma of the urinary bladder. *Cancer* 8:741, 1955

83. Nakissa N, Constine LS, Rubin P, Strohl R: Birth defects in three common pediatric malignancies: Wilms' tumor, neuroblastoma and Ewing's sarcoma. *Oncology* 42(6):358, 1985

84. Ngo RS, Ronan SG, Manaligod JR: Cutaneous malignant melanoma and bilateral retinoblastomas: a case report and review of the literature. *Pediatr Pathol* 6(2–3):227, 1986

85. Ordonez NG, Manning JT, Luna MA: Mixed tumor of the vulva: a report of two cases probably arising in Bartholin's gland. *Cancer* 48(1):181, 1981

86. Ossoff RH, Jones JA, Bytell DE: Recurrent benign mixed tumor of lacrimal gland: report of a case with intracranial extension. *Otolaryngol Head Neck Surg* 89(4):599, 1981

87. Potter GK, Baldinger HG, Boxer MC: Chondroid syringoma in a toe. *Cutis* 30(3):339, 1982

88. Punnonen R, Lauslahti K, Pystynen P: Primary malignancies of the Fallopian tube. *Ann Chir Gynaecol* (Suppl) 197:15, 1985a

89. Punnonen R, Lauslahti K, Pystynen P, Kauppila O: Uterine sarcomas. *Ann Chir Gynaecol* (Suppl) 197:11, 1985b

90. Raizis AM, Becroft DM, Shaw RL, Reeve AE: A mitotic recombination in Wilms' tumor occurs between the parathyroid hormone locus and 11p13. *Hum Genet* 70(4):344, 1985

91. Ramaekers FC, Moesker O, Huysmans A, Schaart G et al.: Intermediate filament proteins in the study of tumor heterogeneity: an in-depth study of tumors of the urinary and respiratory tracts. *Ann NY Acad Sci* 455:614, 1985

92. Redono C, Rocamora A, Villoria F, Garcia M: Malignant mixed tumor of the skin: malignant chondroid syringoma. *Cancer* 49(8):1690, 1982

93. Rivera H, Ruiz C, Garcia-Cruz D et al.: Constitional mosaic t (2;7)(q33;q22) and other rearrangements in a girl with Wilms' tumor. *Ann Genet (Paris)* 28(1):52, 1985

94. Robinson HB Jr, Bolande RP: Case 3. Fetal hepatoblastoma with placental metastases. *Pediatr Pathol* 4(1–2):163, 1985

95. Sarria JA, Spitale L: Endothermal sinus tumor. *Eur J Gynaecol Oncol* 7(1):36, 1986

96. Scalabrino G, Ferioli ME: Degree of enhancement of polyamine biosynthetic decarboxylase activities in human tumors: a useful new index of degree of malignancy. *Cancer Detect Prev* 8(1–2):11, 1985

97. Scheithauer BW: Neuropathology of pineal region tumors. *Clin Neurosurg* 32:351, 1985

98. Schlienger P, Calle R, Haye C, Vilcoq JR: Bone sarcoma and malignant tumors of the retina. *Bull Cancer* (Paris) 72(1):16, 1985

99. Schmidt D, Harms D, Lang W: Primary malignant hepatic tumours in childhood. *Virchows Arch (A)* 407(4):387, 1985

100. Schneider K, Dickerhoff R, Bertele RM: Malignant gastric sarcoma – diagnosis by ultrasound and endoscopy. *Pediatr Radiol* 16(1):69, 1986

101. Seifert G, Okabe H, Casellitz J: Epithelial salivary gland tumors in children and adolescents. *ORL J Otorhinolaryngol Relat Spec* 48(3):137, 1986

102. Sekiya S, Kawata M, Iwasawa H et al.: Characterization of human embryonal carcinoma cell lines derived from testicular germ-cell tumors. *Differentiation* 29(3):259, 1985

103. Sherman MI, Gubler ML, Barkai U et al.: Role of retinoids in differentiation and growth of embryonal carcinoma cells. *Ciba Found Symp* 113:42, 1985

104. Soulie J, Rousseau-Merck MF, Mouly H et al.: Bilateral nephroblastoma associated with a 3;17 translocation. *Cytogenet Cell Genet* 39(1):64, 1985

105. Sparkes RS: The genetics of retinoblastoma. *Biochim Biophys Acta* 780(2):95, 1985

106. Squire J, Gallie BL, Phillips RA: A detailed analysis of chromosomal changes in heritable and non-heritable retinoblastoma. *Hum Genet* 70(4):291, 1985

107. Stevering CJ, Gabreels FJ, Lippens RJ et al.: Treatment of leptomeningeal dissemination of medulloblastoma. Report of a case with a long-term survival. *Clin Neurol Neurosurg* 87(4):291, 1985

108. Takakura K: Intracranial germ cell tumors. *Clin Neurosurg* 32:429, 1985

109. Talerman A: Germ cell tumours. *Ann Pathol* 5(3):145, 1985

110. Tanaka T, Takakura H, Takashima S, Kodama T et al.: A rare case of Aicardi syndrome with severe brain malformation and hepatoblastoma. *Brain Dev* 7(5):507, 1985

111. Tremblay GF, Lee VM, Trojanowski JQ: Expression of vimentin, glial filament, and neurofilament proteins in primitive childhood brain tumors. A comparative immunoblot and immunoperoxidase study. *Acta Neuropathol (Berl)* 68(3):239, 1985

112. Tsao MS, Grisham JW: Hepatocarcinomas, cholangiocarcinomas, and hepatoblastomas produced by chemically transformed cultured rat liver epithelial cells. A light- and electron-microscopic analysis. *Am J Pathol* 127(1):160, 1987

113. Vandenberg SR, Herman MM, Rubinstein LJ: Embryonal central neuroepithelial tumors: current concepts and future challenges. *Cancer Metastasis Rev* 5(4):343, 1987

114. van Leeuwen EH, Postma A, Oosterhuis JW et al.: An analysis of histology and DNA-ploidy in primary Wilms' tumors and their metastases and a study of the morphological effects of therapy. *Virchows Arch (A)* 410(6):487, 1987

115. Willis RA: Pathology of tumours, 3rd ed., pp. 613, 616. London: Butterworth, 1973

116. Wobus AM, Holzhausen H, Bloch C et al.: Establishment and characterization of the pluripotent mouse teratocarcinoma cell line TCE. *Biomed Biochim Acta* 44(11–12):1609, 1985

117. Yung WK, Luna M, Borit A: Vimentin and glial fibrillary acidic protein in human brain tumors. *J Neurooncol* 3(1):35, 1985

MULTICENTRIC PARAGANGLIOMAS AND ASSOCIATED NEUROENDOCRINE TUMORS

PHILIP M. GRIMLEY*

INTRODUCTION

The paraganglia comprise the adrenal medullae and a system of dispersed cell groups which are embryologically co-derived from the neural crest. Extra-adrenal paraganglia are located throughout the distribution of the visceral autonomic nervous system and are allied closely with sympathochromaffin ganglia (37, 71, 105). In essence, they represent a functional extension of the autonomic nervous system into the retroperitoneum and the linings or coats of the thoracic, abdominal and genitourinary viscera.

Paraganglia are richly innervated by autonomic nerve fibers. The parenchymal chief cells synthesize catecholamines from tyrosine (see 26) are supported by sustentacular elements analogous to peripheral nerve Schwann cells (79, 105). Cells of the sustentacular network express S-100 protein and can be highlighted immunocytochemically (76, 123). In extra-adrenal paraganglia, the sustentacular cells delineate a characteristic cell nest or "Zellballen" pattern of the chief cells which can be observed both in normal and neoplastic tissues (33, 71, 157).

Neuroendocrine phenotype

Biologically, the paraganglia constitute one of the major functional subsets amongst the multiple groups of topographically dispersed neuroendocrine cells. The operational definition of a "neuroendocrine" phenotype is based upon a conjunction of cytoarchitectural, biosynthetic and cytofunctional criteria (76, 77). These include polyprotein gene expression with an overlapping biosynthetic profile (47, 52, 158, 205), product storage in argyrophilic, dense-core secretory granules (13, 143); physiologic activity in monoamine precursor uptake and decarboxylation (144), and functional capacities to amplify or generate neural signals either by means of humoral stimulation (26, 145) or by biochemical transduction of microenvironmental perturbations (198).

The oligopeptide or monoamine molecules secreted by paraganglion and other neuroendocrine cells can effect a multiplicity of bioregulatory actions. These actions can be systemic (endocrine function), local on adjacent neuroendocrine cells (paracrine function), or self-regulatory (autocrine

function). Such physiologic variation amongst neuroendocrine cell groups provides a sophisticated, multilevel feedback mechanism for modulating microcirculatory dynamics and hormonal responses in target organs (52, 151, 176). For example, paracrine oligopeptide secretions of some neuroendocrine cells regulate local biosynthetic activity in the gastrointestinal tract (115); while paracrine or autocrine interactions of monoamines are thought to underlie the mechanism of chemoreception in certain extra-adrenal paraganglia (108). A role of neuroendocrine cells in function of the immune system has recently been suggested (5).

Biosynthetic profile

The biosynthetic products of paraganglia (Table 1) resemble other neuroendocrine cells. They include biologically active monoamines and regulatory oligopeptides as well as a host of common enzymes, structural proteins such as neurofila-

Table 1. Biosynthetic products of paraganglion neuroendocrine cells.

Monoamines
  Dopamine[a]
  Norepinephrine[a]
  Epinephrine[a]
  Serotonin

Oligopeptides[b]
  Adrenocorticotropin (ACTH)
  Opioid peptides (enkephalins)
  Calcitonin
  Somatostatin
  Vasoactive intestinal peptide (VIP)

Enzymes
  Neuron specific enolase (NSE)[b]
  Tyrosine hydroxylase
  DOPA decarboxylase
  Dopamine beta hydroxylase
  Phenylethanolamine N-methyltransferase

Structural proteins
  Cytochrome B(561)
  Chromogranins A and B[b]
  Intermediate filaments[b]
  Neurofilaments[b]

[a] Secretory products
[b] Immunoreactive substances

---

* The opinions or assertions expressed herein are private views of the author and should not be construed as official or as necessarily reflecting views of the Department of Defense or of the Uniformed Services University.

K.W. Brunson (ed) Local invasion and spread of cancer.
© 1989, Kluwer Academic Publishers, Dordrecht.

ments (192) or intermediate filaments (172) and surface membrane antigens (see 6, 26, 74, 76). Cytosecretory products may be stored and later released. Many of the biosynthetic products now can be specifically identified in tissue sections with monoclonal antibodies (e.g. 76, 87, 124, 163, 172, 192, 197). Very recently it has become feasible to identify peptide messenger RNAs of neuroendocrine cells *in situ*, by using labelled nucleic acid probes (205).

All neuroendocrine cells contain high levels of an enolase enzyme which is characteristic of neural tissues (170). Enolase isoenzymes are products of three independent gene loci: alpha, beta and gamma. The gamma gene is expressed at highest levels in brain neurons and peripheral neuroendocrine cells (125). It is often designated "neuron specific" and can be detected immunocytochemically within the cytoplasmic compartment using monoclonal antibodies (125, 188).

Secretory granules

The biosynthetic products of paraganglia are stored within relatively homogeneous cytoplasmic granules of a size range near the limits of conventional light microscopic resolution (0.5–2 μM). These granules are highlighted by nonspecific chromaffin, argyrophil or argentaffin reactions (32, 37, 175). Ultrastructurally, the granules are membrane-delimited and their cores are usually electron-dense in osmicated tissues (79, 143). This is probably due to the internal concentration of monoamines and associated nucleotides in addition to enkephalins (120) and other oligopeptides. The matrix contains a large proportion of acid soluble proteins categorized as *chromogranins* (138). These can be identified immunocytochemically in normal or neoplastic neuroendocrine cells with specific polyclonal or monoclonal antibodies (13, 100, 138, 203).

Specialization of paraganglia

Biochemical studies, including peptide analyses and molecular genetic studies indicate that intracellular control of polyprotein gene expression in neuroendocrine cells can be exerted at several levels: transcription, post-transcription, translation or post-translation (52). As defined above, all of the neuroendocrine cells are endowed with the potential to synthesize or store a remarkably broad spectrum of biosynthetic products, some of which resemble neurotransmitter substances of the central nervous system (48, 77, 151, 159, 176, 189, 205).

Paraganglion cells are recognized as an ontogenetically discrete subset of neuroendocrine cells which differentiate from the neural crest (76). Neuritic processes are reminiscent of this origin (79, 191). A consistent range of biosynthetic expression and functional activity is characteristic: the parenchymal cells produce, store or secrete catecholamines (37, 71). This is associated with the presence of catechol-amine-related hydroxylase and decarboxylase biosynthetic enzymes (6, 26). Typically, the storage granules contain abundant opiate peptides (44, 100, 120, 124).

A particular physiologic response of paraganglion parenchymal cells is their exquisite sensitivity to local hypoxia and consequent rapid release of catecholamines when blood flow or oxygen tension is reduced (26). Two major groups of

paraganglia which have been accessible to direct experimental investigations (intra-adrenal and extra-adrenal paraganglia) exhibit further subspecialization: (1) The intra-adrenal paraganglia (adrenal medullae) respond to efferent autonomic stimuli by liberating increased quantities of catecholamines into the venous circulation. In this respect, these parenchymal cells resemble sympathetic neurons and contribute to the mobilization of cardiac, hepatic, and other systemic organ responses to somatic injury or stress. Indeed, the adrenal medullae are viewed as an integral functional element of the sympathetic nervous system (26). (2) The intercarotid and aorticopulmonary paraganglia exemplify extra-adrenal paraganglia which transduce chemical changes in the partial pressure of arterial oxygen, carbon dioxide, or pH into afferent nervous signals which stimulate ventilation. The exact mechanisms of such chemosensory transduction remain controversial, but probably involve complementary activities of one or more catecholamines in feedback loops which modulate both internal capillary blood flow and thresholds for afferent neural stimulation (108, 198).

Functions of other extra-adrenal paraganglia presumably imitate those of the intercarotid bodies or of the adrenal medullae and peripheral sympathetic neurons, but have not been directly probed. Curiously, many extra-adrenal paraganglia are more conspicuous during fetal life or infancy than in the normal adult (37, 105).

TOPOGRAPHY AND HISTOGENESIS OF NEUROENDOCRINE CELL SUBSETS

Paraganglia and other major subsets of the neuroendocrine cells are distinguished empirically, based upon both topography and histogenesis (see 76).

Paraganglion cells. The paraganglion cells occur as macroscopically cohesive units in the adrenal medullae and in

Table 2. Major families of extra-adrenal paraganglia and related paragangliomas.

Family	Sites of paragangliomas
Branchiomeric	Jugulotympanic (middle ear)
	Inter-carotid (carotid bodies)
	Intrathyroid
	Laryngeal
	Aortico-pulmonary (superior mediastinum)
	Coronary-interatrial (heart base)
Intravagal	Ganglion nodosom
	nasopharynx
	angle of mandible
	Inferior vagus nerve distribution
Aortico-Sympathetic	Paravertebral
	intrathoracic
	retroperitoneal
	Organ of Zuckerkandl
Visceral-Autonomic	Gastroduodenal region
	Porta hepatis
	Genital tract
	Urinary bladder
	Cauda equina

some major extra-adrenal locations (37). During embryonic development the ancestral stem cells of paraganglia migrate from the ventral neural crest (104, 118, 166). Topographically, they remain associated principally with cervical and mediastinal tissues of ontogenetic gill arch derivation with the paravertebral sympathochromaffin ganglia, or with peripheral elements of the ortho and parasympathetic nervous systems located in the viscera or cerebrospinal axis (71, 122). Anatomically constant groups of extra-adrenal paraganglia thus can be grouped into several broad "families" (Table 2): branchiomeric; intravagal, aortico-sympathetic, and visceral autonomic (see 71, 105).

Specialized functional features of paraganglion cells were discussed above.

Thyroid gland C-cells. C-cells, characterized by production of calcitonin, are found within the follicles of the thyroid gland. Embryogenetic studies indicate an origin of C-cells from the neuroectoderm or neural crest (see 4, 146), but some developmental and oncological observations have raised the possibility of an endodermal or a combined endodermal and neural crest origin (58, 101).

Bronchopulmonary neuroendocrine cells. Neuroendocrine cells are widely distributed within the bronchopulmonary system, both singly and as tight clusters which have been referred to as "neuroepithelial bodies" (181, 186). They appear during first trimester differentiation of the fetal lung (182). Origins of pulmonary neuroendocrine cell groups both from neuroectoderm and gut-endoderm have been suggested by immunohistochemical studies as well as patterns of neoplasia (21, 73, 127).

Gastrointestinal and pancreatic neuroendocrine cells. These cells localize within the mucosa of the stomach or the intestine. In the pancreas, they form both the classical islets and extra-insular collections of hormonally active cells. Subtle differences in the spectrum of regulatory peptide biosynthesis may be related to specific anatomic distribution within the gastrointestinal tract (21, 42). Neuroendocrine cells appear during early differentiation of the gastroenteric pancreatic axis both in normal embryos (4, 173) and in teratomas (21). Other pathobiologic evidence also supports an origin from pluripotential foregut precursors (38, 42).

Genitourinary tract neuroendocrine cells. Some groups of neuroendocrine cells which are associated with intramural neural plexi in the bladder or vagina probably represent visceral-autonomic paraganglia. Plausibly, these have been related to the sacral-parasympathetic limb of the autonomic nervous system (71).

Argyrophilic cells which are immunoreactive for serotonin, somatostatin and nonspecific enolase have been demonstrated in the prostatic urethra, prostatic ductules and prostate acini (51). These are possibly of endodermal (perhaps hindgut) origin (50).

Neuroendocrine cells are found in the normal female genital tract and some ovarian neoplasms (171). Pathways of normal development indicate that some of the latter could arise from coelomic epithelium (171). Intrauterine paragangliomas very rarely have been reported (208).

TOPOGRAPHY OF PARAGANGLIOMAS

Anatomic distribution

Solitary or multicentric paragangliomas may arise in relationship to any of the topographic families of paraganglia listed under Table 2. Overall, approximately 90% of paragangliomas arise within the adrenal gland, and are alternatively classified as "pheochromocytomas" in this location (141).

Extra-adrenal paragangliomas are most common in jugulotympanic, intercarotid, superior mediastinal and retroperitoneal paravertebral sites. The majority arise in the head and neck (14, 71, 110), where they are allied to anatomic structures of branchial arch ontogeny (branchiometric paraganglia) or are associated with the vagus nerve. Within the branchiomeric family, intercarotid and jugulotympanic paragangliomas are most common, laryngeal paragangliomas are relatively uncommon and intrathyroid paragangliomas are rare (25, 65, 71, 110).

Vagal paraganglioma may arise at the level of the ganglion nodosum or in more inferior portions of the vagus nerve. They typically present in the angle of the mandible or near the fossa of Rosenmuller in the posterior pharynx (33, 93, 102, 149, 185).

In the thorax, paragangliomas represented 4% of cases in a large series of neural tumors (154). Lack *et al.* (113) reviewed 36 cases of intrathoracic paragangliomas. Mediastinal supra-aortic, aorticopulmonary or coronary-interatrial paragangliomas may impinge upon the atrial walls or upon the base of the heart and the great vessels. Posterior mediastinal tumors may arise from the paravertebral sympathetic trunk (64, 100, 140).

Paragangliomas are probably more common in the retroperitoneum than in the mediastinum (71, 111, 131). They occur less commonly in visceral locations supplied by orthosympathetic or craniosacral parasympathetic elements: the orbit (187), duodenum (148), hepatic ducts (133), bladder wall (117), genitourinary tract, or cauda equina (121). Urinary bladder and cauda equina tumors are probably the most frequent of the latter group. The urinary bladder paragangliomas are often functional and resemble adrenal medullary pheochromocytomas both histologically and cytochemically: there is often a positive tissue chromaffin reaction (1).

Bronchopulmonary neuroendocrine cell neoplasms usually present as carcinoid tumors or small cell anaplastic ("oat cell") tumors (73). True intrapulmonary paragangliomas are extremely rare (31). Multicentric "minute paragangliomas", which are incidental autopsy or surgical findings, lack clinical significance (96) and actually may be of pleural origin (36).

Multicentric presentation

In up to 10% of cases, paragangliomas are bilateral, ipsilateral or multicentric (149, 152, 200). Intra-adrenal paraganglioma is more frequently bilateral in familial than in sporadic cases; (199) and the same is probably true for extra-adrenal paragangliomas (see below).

The finding of a paraganglioma in any one anatomic site always signals the possibility of other paragangliomas: multiple paragangliomas may arise synchronously or metachronously with intervals of many years (103). Presymptomatic recognition of multiple tumors permits prompt excision and can avert the problem of local infiltration.

Multicentric paragangliomas typically involve the adrenal glands or the intercarotid paraganglia and one or more extra-adrenal sites (77). Intercarotid paragangliomas were bilateral in up to 5% of cases analyzed retrospectively (56); however, the true incidence of multicentricity probably would be higher in prospective studies with complete reporting of metachronous cases (see 97, 147, 155, 204). Multiple ipsilateral head and neck paragangliomas (102, 137) and combinations of thoracic and abdominal extra-adrenal paragangliomas have been reported (19, 64, 92, 113, 183). Multicentric paragangliomas often involve the remnant organ of Zuckerkandl (18, 39, 70, 131). The occurrence of disseminated extra-adrenal paragangliomatosis has been well documented in several cases (103), and can be associated with Carney's triad of gastric leiomyosarcoma and pulmonary chondroma (27). Extra-adrenal and adrenal paragangliomas concur in sporadic cases (164). They also have been associated in developmental dysplasias involving the central nervous system (92, 124, 209).

FAMILIAL PARAGANGLIOMAS

Families with a high frequency of single or multiple paragangliomas have been reported (81, 102, 142, 152, 193, 204, 209). There is an increased incidence of bilateral intercarotid paragangliomas in these cases (71, 147, 204, 206). In one series of extra-adrenal paragangliomas, Parry *et al.* (142) obtained evidence for an autosomal dominant mode of inheritance in up to 7% of cases. As discussed above, the overall incidence of familial paragangliomas is probably higher, since many small tumors are never detected by conventional examinations (97) and metachronous tumors may not be correlated in horizontal studies.

A female sex predominance has been noted in some series of extra-adrenal paragangliomas (71, 109, 139, 142, 162), but this is not consistent and sex-related differences in genetic penetrance of the susceptibility to paraganglioma development have been postulated (193). Familial intercarotid paragangliomas tend to arise at an earlier age than sporadic tumors (142).

CLINICAL MANIFESTATIONS OF PARAGANGLIOMAS

Functional paragangliomas

Paragangliomas may be detected relatively early if signs related to excess catecholamine secretion can be promptly recognized. Collectively, those paragangliomas which reveal themselves clinically by the production of excess catecholamines have been estimated to be prevalent in 0.04–0.2% of the United States population for a current total of approximately 40,000 cases (66). The adrenal medullae are the major sites of functionally active neoplasms in the paraganglion system: intra-adrenal paragangliomas (pheochromocytomas), account for at least 90% of all catecholamine secreting neoplasms. Functional tumors of the extra-adrenal paraganglia account for the remainder. These typically arise in association with aorticosympathetic paraganglia of the thorax (up to 48% of intrathoracic cases) (91, 113) or of the abdominal retroperitoneum (up to 25% of retroperitoneal cases) (70, 111, 136). Intercarotid, jugulotympanic or intravagal paragangliomas infrequently produce symptoms or signs related to excess catecholamine production (40, 71, 119, 131, 149, 185).

Symptoms of labile hypertension or laboratory findings related to excessive catecholamine production are the most common presenting evidence of functional paragangliomas. In 99% of cases the manifestations include at least one symptom in the triad of excessive diaphoresis, headache and palpitation or tachycardia (22). The paroxysmal effects of excess catecholamine production on the cardiovascular system remain life-threatening until functional tumors are excised. Intraoperative or postoperative hypotension are serious risks for which the surgeon and anesthesiologist always must be prepared even when there are no overt functional signs or symptoms.

Other functional manifestations of paragangliomas may rarely be related to abnormal secretion of neuroendocrine peptides. Reports include abnormal serum levels of biologically active calcitonin (202); ACTH (7, 80), vasoactive intestinal peptide and somatostatin (163) and possibly serotonin (57). Immunoreactive oligopeptides such as calcitonin (87) somatostatin (161) or VIP may be detected in paraganglion tumor cells (191) without evidence of serum elevations or clinical activity.

Laboratory tests

In the appropriate clinical settings, biochemical tests of serum or urine can be extremely valuable adjuncts for the diagnosis of paragangliomas (129). Laboratory tests are not advocated as general screening tools; even with maximal levels of sensitivity and specificity the predictive value remains less than 2% due to an extremely low prevalence of neuroendocrine cell tumors in the average population.

The predictive value of serum or urine biochemical tests is significantly enhanced in family groups and other populations known to be at medically high risk for paragangliomas or other neuroendocrine lesions (e.g. 62, 85, 139). Thus, recognition of genetic or developmental factors predisposing to the pathogenesis of paragangliomas or other neuroendocrine cell tumors deserves primary emphasis (77). Presymptomatic biochemical screening or provocative testing of subjects at suspected risk should be considered only in the appropriate family settings (23, 126).

When symptoms or signs raise the suspicion of a functional paraganglioma, follow-up laboratory testing is clearly indicated. At the minimum, biochemical screening should include a battery of 24 hour urine biochemistries: metanephrines, vanillylmandelic acid (sequential degradation products of norepinephrine or epinephrine) and free catecholamines. Results of these determinations may vary due to differences in tumor cell levels of catechol-O-methyl transferase and monoamine oxidase which are involved in the sequential catabolic steps, so that reliance on a single test is not advisable (129).

Epinephrine may be the predominant catecholamine in pheochromocytoma or paragangliomas of the abdominal retroperitoneum. Paragangliomas of other extra-adrenal sites usually secrete an excess of norepinephrine. Plasma catecholamines measured in fasting patients can be the most sensitive and specific test for excess catecholamine production; and pretreatment with clonidine to suppress physiologic catecholamine elevation in apprehensive or stressed patients increases the specificity (22). In patients with pheochromocytomas related to multiple endocrine neoplasia, an increase in the fraction of epinephrine may be an early sign of adrenal medullary hyperplasia (63, 85).

Nonfunctional paragangliomas

Paragangliomas in confined locations, such as within the middle ear, paranasal sinuses, inferior vagal nerve, or paravertebral sulcus may produce neurologic signs or symptoms relatively early. Unfortunately, many extra-adrenal paragangliomas are physiologically silent during early stages of hyperplasia and neoplastic growth. They eventually come to clinical attention for a variety of reasons: (a) palpation of a mass in the head and neck region (intercarotid or intravagal paragangliomas), (b) pulsation of a mass, (c) otorhinologic symptoms or signs (jugulotympanic or intravagal paragangliomas), (d) dysphonia, dysphagia (intravagal or aortico-sympathetic paragangliomas) or superior vena caval syndrome (aorticopulmonary paragangliomas), (e) incidental radiographic finding of an intrathoracic, or retroperitoneal mass, (f) signs of local expansion or infiltration of a mass, including neural or vascular infiltration or compression with neuritis, pain or hemorrhage. Thus, the importance of simple physical findings including cranial nerve palsies, auditory deficits, nasal blockage, or difficulty in deglutition should not be neglected in the detection of head and neck paragangliomas.

Radiography

Diagnostic radiography is a major tool in confirming the diagnosis of catecholamine secreting neoplasms and fixing their locations. Ultrasound examination of the cervical region (72) combined with chest films and computed axial tomography of the thorax and abdomen can provide a thorough screen for multicentric paragangliomas. High resolution abdominal CT scan can even resolve early increases in size of the adrenal medullae (153, 163). The medullary tissue is normally concentrated in the head and body of the gland, so that expansion of the tail can be an early sign of hyperplasia/neoplasia (23). Multiple chest films are essential when extra-adrenal paraganglioma of the heart base or posterior mediastinum is suspected (154).

Paragangliomas typically are highly vascularized and therefore particularly well visualized after injection of radiocontrast material (97, 149). Radionuclide scintigraphy is a valuable adjunct for screening, diagnosis or staging of paragangliomas (e.g. 153, 160, 174, 196).

TISSUE DIAGNOSIS

Histopathologic diagnosis of paragangliomas usually is not difficult. Intra-adrenal tumors and some extra-adrenal paragangliomas are typified by highly vascularized sheets of syncytial lightly eosinophilic cells with abundant, finely granular cytoplasm. Nuclei are generally round and regular with some scattered hyperchromatic or polyploid giant forms. Extra-adrenal paragangliomas typically retain a tendency to grow in compartmentalized cell clusters referred to as "Zellballen" (78). Mixed syncytial and Zellballen patterns occur in both the adrenal gland and extra-adrenal locations (77). Admixture of gangliocytic or neuroblastic cells is sometimes noted in paragangliomas especially in the duodenum (148) or retroperitoneum. This may reflect multidirectional differentiation (see 45, 165).

Differentiation of extra-adrenal paraganglioma from hemangiopericytoma, clear cell renal carcinoma or epithelioid meningioma of the spinal roots sometimes poses a diagnostic challenge. In the mediastinum paraganglioma can be particularly difficult to distinguish from carcinoid or small cell anaplastic tumors (77), and the pattern of well defined cell nests may be lost when there is extensive infiltration of adipose tissue. The pattern of growth of intravagal paragangliomas is often distorted by nerve sheath compression and fibrous reaction (71).

Silver stains for cytoplasmic granules (argyrophil reaction, see 175), electron microscopy (e.g. 13, 143) and specific immunocytochemical techniques for detection of biosynthetic products (see above) verify the tissue diagnosis. Biois. Biochemical analysis of tissue samples (e.g. 40) or catecholamine-induced fluorescence of touch preparations (see 41, 42) are useful methods for assessing catecholamine content, but not routinely available.

Fine needle aspiration biopsy of superficial extra-adrenal paraganglioma has been successful in some cases (16, 55). More frequent employment of this technique should be encouraged and it could be effectively utilized even for deep lesions if combined with fluorography or computerized tomographic guidance. A panel of currently available immunocytochemical reagents can serve to verify cytodiagnostic accuracy. Moreover, rapid detection of neuroendocrine cells may soon become practicable using nucleic acid probes (205).

PARAGANGLIOMAS AND MULTISYSTEM TUMORS

Unicentric or multicentric paragangliomas may be associated with tumors of other organ systems in recurrent familial or sporadic patterns. Such multisystem neoplasms typically include other tumors of neuroendocrine phenotype, classical endocrine tumors of the pituitary, thyroid or parathyroid glands, or tumors arising in the peripheral or central nervous systems (77). Some repetitive associations of paragangliomas with connective tissue tumors or hamartomas have also been noted (27).

Major familial patterns of multisystem and multicentric neuroendocrine neoplasms are well recognized and there are stable familial variations in the patterns of tumor expression (12, 183). Repetitive association of paragangliomas with tumors of endocrine glands has been particularly well documented in families with syndromes of multiple endocrine neoplasia (MEN) (47).

MEN Type I

This type of multiple endocrine neoplasia is inherited as an autosomal dominant with penetrance of up to 80%. The multisystem proliferative lesions or neoplasms typically involve the parathyroid glands, anterior hypophysis, and/or pancreatic islets. Proliferative lesions of thyroid gland follicles can also occur. The parathyroids are most commonly involved and nodular parathyroid hyperplasia may be the common underlying abnormality in all families (194) Paragangliomas are rare (27).

MEN Type IIA(II)

This entity is characterized by parathyroid tumors, medullary carcinoma of the thyroid gland C-cells and intra-adrenal paragangliomas. The association of thyroid medullary carcinoma and intra-adrenal paragangliomas is particularly striking (168, 183). Intra-adrenal paraganglioma (pheochromocytoma) is bilateral in 70% of cases of MEN type IIA, and often is preceded by nodular hyperplasia of the adrenal medullae (199). Retroperitoneal or intercarotid paragangliomas can occur (183).

Inheritance is governed by an autosomal dominant trait with high penetrance and variable expression (12, 183). Hyperparathyroidism occurs in a high proportion of patients and is related to diffuse or nodular hyperplasia of the parathyroid glands (194); serum calcium and parathormone elevations often precede evidence of the thyroid disease.

MEN Type IIB(III)

Clinically and pathologically this syndrome closely parallels MEN Type IIA; however, the genetic trait is separate. A major distinction of MEN type IIB is the development of multiple mucosal neuromas or intestinal ganglioneuromatosis and dysfunctional obstipation (49, 168). Indeed, the clinical and radiological presentation may resemble Hirschsprung's disease. Histologically there is a massive dysplasia of the myenteric plexus rather than aganglionosis. Elevated nerve growth stimulating activity may occur (49). Some patients exhibit musculoskeletal abnormalities and a Marfanoid habitus (28).

This multiple endocrine neoplasia entity is characterized by parathyroid tumors, medullary carcinoma of the thyroid gland C-cells and intra-adrenal paragangliomas. The association of thyroid medullary carcinoma and intra-adrenal paragangliomas is particularly striking (168, 183). Intra-adrenal paraganglioma (pheochromocytoma) is bilateral in 70% of cases of MEN type IIA, and often is preceded by nodular hyperplasia of the adrenal medullae (199).

Mixed MEN syndromes

Mixed syndromes in which well recognized elements of the

defined MEN entities are recombined have been recognized by a number of clinicians (see 77). In a Mexican family, extra-adrenal paragangliomas were associated with multiple endocrine gland neoplasias (114). Paragangliomas also have been reported in association with pituitary adenomas (17), and some of these patients manifest parathyroid disease with hypercalcemia (3).

Kindreds with adrenal medullary paragangliomas and pancreatic islet cell tumors have been followed by several groups and genetic studies have demonstrated a probable autosomal dominant mode of inheritance (29, 95, 135). Associations of intra-adrenal paragangliomas with carcinoid tumors of the gastrointestinal tract are rare, but theoretically noteworthy with respect to postulating common pathogenetic factors in neuroendocrine neoplasms (see (75, 86, 134)). Duodenal carcinoids have been associated both with neurofibromatosis and adrenal medullary paragangliomas (75). In the latter cases, the carcinoid tumors were composed predominantly of cells synthesizing somatostatin (43, 75).

Paragangliomas and "neurocristopathies"

Multisystem associations of neoplasms which evidently originate in neuroendocrine cells of differing histogenesis and embryonic lineages pose important questions regarding possible linkages in development or function. Bolande (20) coined the term *neurocristopathies* to denote complexes of concerted dysplasias or neoplasms arising in multiple tissues and organs derived from neural crest stem cells. Paragangliomas have been associated with several constellations of developmental dysplasias involving more than one neural crest element, including von Recklinghausen's syndrome (10, 92, 104, 124, 167, 209) and the Von Hippel–Lindau syndrome (92, 95, 183, 209).

Screening for multisystem tumors

In families with recognized MEN, annual laboratory screening of kindred has included serum calcium measurements and radioimmunoassay for parathyroid hormone to detect early parathyroid lesions and radioimmunoassay for gastrin to detect early islet cell hyperactivity at all ages between 10 and 65 (23, 126). Serum levels of pancreatic polypeptide also can be useful (62, 139). Elevation of serum prolactin or other pituitary gland hormones may reveal early proliferative lesions or adenomas of the anterior hypophysis (139). Monitoring for increase of the urinary sepinephrine fraction may be useful in early detection of adrenal medullary paraganglioma (63, 85). Paroxysms associated with intra-adrenal paragangliomas can be fatal (183) so that lifetime surveillance for adrenal medullary hyperplasia or neoplasia is considered essential (23, 126).

Genetic mapping, based upon recognition of familial patterns of DNA polymorphism associated with tumor predilection will probably be developed in the near future. This technique has been pioneered in families with Huntingdon's chorea (82).

PROGRESSIVE GROWTH OF PARAGANGLIOMAS

Growth of paragangliomas is typically indolent with a natural evolution over many years. The majority of paragangliomas are neither histologically nor cytologically malignant. Their predilection for local invasion, distant metastasis or systemic hormone activity cannot be predicted solely upon morphologic grounds, although necrosis, invasion and frequent mitoses are more often associated with malignancy.

Pre-neoplastic lesions

Intra-adrenal paragangliomas of either the sporadic or familial types may be preceded by nodular hyperplasia (48, 131). In familial cases, this may be accompanied by a shift in the fraction of epinephrine to norepinephrine production (63, 85). Epinephrine biosynthesis depends upon the enzyme phenylethanolamine-N-methyl transferase and reflects a higher level of differentiation (129). Hyperplasia of extra-adrenal paraganglia primarily involves supportive neural elements (60, 99) and does not appear to be directly related to subsequent autonomous growth of the parenchymal cells (157).

Silent growth and local infiltration

In a series of 107 intra-adrenal paragangliomas, Melicow (131) found that 17 were clinically silent and detected incidentally during laporotomy or autopsy.

Local infiltration of extra-adrenal paragangliomas can be insidious and very dangerous, especially if major vessels, base of the skull, the heart base or atrial walls (100) are involved. Jugulotympanic paragangliomas can infiltrate the temporal bone (179) and recurrence rates are particularly high (110). An analogy can be drawn to basal cell carcinoma, where the lesion does not usually metastasize systemically, but initial wide excision is imperative to avoid disastrous local complications. Local infiltration can be restrained by irradiation (68, 93, 149, 178). This is probably due to induction of fibrosis rather than specific cytotoxicity (178).

Extra-adrenal paragangliomas of the thorax and retroperitoneum often achieve a relatively large mass before they are detected and thus carry a proportionately greater risk of invasion and metastasis. Asymptomatic extra-adrenal paragangliomas are an especially ominous problem in the heart base and the retroperitoneum where local extension and vascular invasion may defy surgical excision (64, 100, 111).

Systemic metastasis

The metastatic potential of paragangliomas is less than 10% overall, but up to 30% of cases with lymph node metastasis have been reported in some series (68, 111). In a given case metastatic potential generally cannot be gauged on the basis of cytologic criteria. Most tumors, including those which metastasize fail to exhibit dramatic cytologic atypia. On the other hand, cases in which sections display necrosis of cell nests, vascular invasion and numerous mitoses or enlarged atypical nuclei are statistically more likely to metastasize. The incidence of systemic malignancy is evidently highest in intravagal paragangliomas which tend to recur (102, 110, 149) and in mediastinal or retroperitoneal paragangliomas (111, 141), with relatively large mass at the time of detection. Massive intercarotid paragangliomas also appear to metastastize more frequently (68).

Metastasis to regional lymph nodes is not consistently followed by systemic dissemination. Systemic metastases can involve the lungs, liver or bones of the skull, vertebrae or pelvis (84, 130). Immediate extirpation of metastatic nodules is optimal, since recurrence may be very slow and some patients are essentially cured (177). Thus far, systemic chemotherapy has not proven successful (177). Clinically, it can be crucial to distinguish multiple synchronous or metachronous paragangliomas from true metastases. The importance of early detection and complete surgical extirpation of lesions cannot be overemphasized.

PATHOGENESIS OF PARAGANGLIOMAS AND MULTICENTRIC-MULTISYSTEM NEUROENDOCRINE TUMORS

Paragangliomas occur both sporadically and in familial patterns. Both environmental and genetic factors have been implicated in their pathogenesis. Somatic defects or carcinogenic events manifesting at common stages in the development or maturation of neuroendocrine cells could explain the relatively high frequency of multicentric paragangliomas as well as their multisystem tumor associations.

Environmental factors

A role of chronic hypoxemia leading to compensatory hyperplasia of chemosensitive paraganglia (inter-carotid bodies) and subsequent development of paraganglioma has been suggested clinically both by human (see (112)) and veterinary studies (88). The chronic hypoxemia may be produced by high altitude (8, 9, 54, 68, 162), chronic pulmonary disease (53, 109) including cystic fibrosis (112), or congenital cyanotic heart disease (18, 112). Cyanotic cardiac malformations have been associated with pheochromocytomas (61) and retroperitoneal paragangliomas (18).

Cytogenetic alterations

Recent cytogenetic studies indicate significant chromosomal instability in members of families with multiple endocrine neoplasia syndromes (83, 94, 184). Consistent minor deletions in the short arm of chromosome 20 were reported in patients with MEN type II (11). As in neural tumors (201) it is conceivable that chromosomal translocations lead to activation of oncogenes. Location on chromosome 20 of the *c-src* proto-oncogene which encodes for tyrosine kinase is of particular interest (11). In an experimental system, *v-src* expression appeared to have an inductive effect on rat chromaffin cell differentiation (2).

Experimental hypotheses

The central significance of a neuroendocrine phenotype in relationship to oncogenesis and the syndromes of multiple neuroendocrine neoplasia could be explained by a number of mechanisms (76). For example, some common aberration in functional differentiation or maturational "switching" with perturbation in the regulation of oncogenes. Studies in which foreign DNA were introduced into the genome of mice show that reproducible patterns of multiple tumor development can be manipulated by minor changes in construction of a single gene (132). In children with a congenital syndrome, it has been shown that three embryonal tumors may have a common pathogenesis related to pleiotropic expression of a recessive mutant allele, which is "unmasked" by a somatic chromosomal alteration at defined times specific to the development of diverse tissues (107).

Several investigators have proposed two-step mutational models in the pathogenesis of multicentric neuroendocrine neoplasms (15, 90, 106). This may be related to the many observations of hyperplastic or proliferative lesions preceding neuroendocrine cell neoplasia in man (30, 46, 131, 206) and in experimental animals (48, 101). In familial medullary carcinoma, Baylin *et al.* (15) found that individual tumor nodules were monoclonal with respect to glucose-6-phosphate dehydrogenase isoenzymes, suggesting that they arose as a final monoclonal mutation from hyperplastic and polyclonal C-cells. Hereditary neurofibromas appear to have a similar multicellular origin (59).

Ontogenetic basis for multicentricity and multisystemic associations of paragangliomas

Involvement of histogenetically diverse neuroendocrine elements in neoplastic processes, and indeed the common phenotype of neuroendocrine cells in multiple locations, might be explained by ontogenetic transpositions of contiguous chromosomal elements (see (35, 69)) leading to evolution of common control mechanisms for regulation of gene expression.

Tissues derived from the neural crest have exercised a crucial role in the evolution of vertebrates (67). Phylogenetic specialization of neural crest derivatives resulted in the development not only of neurosensory and motor structures, but also of essential craniopharyngeal modifications dependent upon the expression of mesodermal functions. Ontogenetically, pluripotential stem cells which form the neural crest in avians or mammals segregate early into dorsally migrating melanoblasts and ventrally migrating gangliosympathetic neuroblasts. Both elements then undergo a complex anatomic diaspora which has been demonstrated by means of somatic hybridization (e.g. 98) or neural crest ablation experiments (118, 150). In the case of gangliosympathicoblasts this migration is accompanied by a remarkable plasticity in phenotypic maturation as well as a divergence in the predominant patterns of neurosecretory hormone biosynthesis.

The ventrally migrating stem cells differentiate into at least four distinct tissue components: (1) the vascular mesenchyme involved in specialization of the gill arches and associated branchiomeric derivatives, (2) the dorsal root sensory ganglia, (3) the autonomic ganglia and codispersed paraganglion cells which have become specialized for different levels of sensory, effector or regulatory functions, and (4) the associated neurosupportive elements including peripheral nerve Schwann cells, ganglionic satellite cells and paraganglion sustentacular cells. Many paraganglia are relatively more conspicuous and perhaps most fully developed during fetal life (105), and evidently diminish in functional relevance after birth. It appears likely that some neoplasms arise in loci of regressed paraganglia such as the retroperitoneal organs of Zuckerkandl. Indeed, this probably accounts for the wider topographic distribution of extra-adrenal paragangliomas than might be anticipated from the obvious gross locations of paraganglia in normal adults (71).

The origin of neural crest from neuroectoderm at the earliest stages of embryonic differentiation and a close association with epidermal placodes provides a spatial and temporal scenario for carcinogenic events to impact a number of developmentally interrelated but histogenetically distinct cells or tissues. Coincident developmental or maturational events would best account for the associations of neuroendocrine cell neoplasms in tissues of neural crest ancestry with neuroblastoma, neurofibromatosis, ganglioneuromatosis, cerebellar or retinal hemangiomas and mucosal neuromas (10, 75, 92, 95, 104, 164, 168, 183).

ANIMAL MODELS OF PARAGANGLIOMA AND RELATED TUMORS

Canines

Brachycephalic breeds of male dogs are particularly susceptible to development of intercarotid or paraaortic paragangliomas (88, 89, 156). This may be related to chronic respiratory disease (88).

Bovines

Adrenal medullary paragangliomas and neoplasms of thyroid gland C-cells have been noted in bulls (207) and may be hereditary in certain bovine breeds (180). Enlargement of the carotid bodies and an increased frequency of paragangliomas occurred in bulls dwelling at very high altitudes in the Andes (8).

Rodents and guinea pigs

Spontaneous neuroendocrine tumors arise in ageing rats (24). Van Zwieten *et al.* (195) described aorticopulmonary paragangliomas in ageing rats of several strains. In rats of the Long-Evans strain, spontaneous C-cell proliferative lesions occur in the thyroid gland and are frequently accompanied by diffuse and nodular hyperplasias of the adrenal medulla, by anterior pituitary proliferative lesions and by parathyroid hyperplasia (190). Hyperplasias or neoplasias were more frequent in females of the WAG/Rij strain and more frequent in males of the BN/Bi strain or of the (WAG × BN) F1 hybrid (116). Edwards *et al.* (54) reported hyperplasia of the carotid body in guinea pigs at high altitudes.

Fish

The existence of multiple neural crest tumors in the bicolor damselfish is of related interest to other animal models, although paragangliomas were not specifically identified (169).

REFERENCES

1. Albores-Saavedra J, Maldonado ME, Ibarra J, Rodriguez HA: Pheochromocytoma of the urinary bladder. *Cancer* 23:1110, 1969
2. Alema S, Casalbore P, Agostini E, Tato F: Differentiation of PC12 phaeochromocytoma cells induced by v-*src* oncogene. *Nature* 316:557, 1985
3. Anderson RJ, Lufkin EG, Sigenore GW, Carney JA, Sheps SG, Silliman YE: Acromegaly and pituitary adenoma with pheochromocytoma: A variant of multiple endocrine neoplasia. *Clin Endocrin* 14:605, 1981
4. Andrew A: APUD cells, apudomas and the neural crest. *S Afr Med J* 50:890, 1976
5. Angeletti RH, Hickey WF: A neuroendocrine marker in tissues of the immune system. *Science* 230:89, 1986
6. Angeletti RH, Nolan JA, Zaremba S: Catecholamine storage vesicles: topography and function. *Trends Biochem Sci* 10:240, 1985
7. Apple D, Kreines K: Cushing's syndrome due to ectopic ACTH production by a nasal paraganglioma. *Amer J Med Sci* 283:32, 1982
8. Arias-Stella J, Bustos F: Chronic hypoxia and chemodectomas in bovines at high altitudes. *Arch Path Lab Med* 100:636, 1976
9. Arias-Stella J, Valcarcel J: Chief cell hyperplasia in the human carotid body at high altitudes. Physiology and pathologic significance. *Hum Pathol* 7:361, 1976
10. Avsare SS, Prabhu SR, Vengsarkar US, Manghani DK, Dastur DK: Von Recklinghausen's disease with a malignant meningeal, cerebral and optic nerve tumour and bilateral vagal schwannomas. *J Neurological Sciences* 54:427, 1982
11. Babu VR, Van Dyke DL, Jackson CE: Chromosome 20 deletion in human multiple endocrine neoplasia types 2A and 2B: A double-blind study. *Proc Natl Acad Sci USA* 81:2525, 1984
12. Ballard HS, Frame B, Hartsock RJ: Familial multiple endocrine adenoma-peptic ulcer complex. *Medicine* 43:481, 1964
13. Balsera E, Lloyd RV, Livingston SK, Lavallee M, Azar HA: Immunohistochemistry and electron microscopy of neuroendocrine neoplasms. *Lab Invest* 54:4A, 1986
14. Batsakis JD: Paragangliomas of the head and neck. In: *Tumors of the head and neck*, edited by Batsakis JD, Baltimore: Williams & Wilkins, 369, 1980
15. Baylin SB, Hsu SH, Gann D, Smallridge R, Wells S: Inherited medullary thyroid carcinoma: A final monoclonal mutation in one of multiple clones of susceptible cells. *Science* 199:429, 1978
16. Berg B, Biorklund A, Grimelius L, Ingemansson S, Larsson L-I, Stenram U, Akerman M: New pattern of multiple endocrine adenomatosis. Chemodectoma, bronchial carcinoid, GH-producing pituitary adenoma and hyperplasia of the parathyroid glands, and antral and duodenal gastrin cells. *Acta Med Scand* 200:321, 1976
17. Blumenkopf B, Boekelheide K: Neck paraganglioma with a pituitary adenoma. Case report. *J Neurosurg* 57(3):426, 1982
18. Bockelman HW, Arya S, Gilbert EF: Cyanotic congenital heart disease with malignant paraganglioma. *Cancer* 50:2513, 1982
19. Bogdasarian RS, Lotz PR: Multiple simultaneous paragangliomas of the head and neck in association with multiple retroperitoneal pheochromocytomas. *Otolaryngol Head Neck Surg* 87(5):648, 1979
20. Bolande RP: The neurocristopathies: A unifying concept of disease arising in neural crest maldevelopment. *Hum. Biol* 5:409, 1974
21. Bosman FT, Louwerens J-WK: APUD cells in teratomas. *Am J Pathol* 104:174, 1981
22. Bravo EL, Gifford RW Jr: Pheochromocytoma: Diagnosis, localization and management. *New Engl J Med* 1298, 1984
23. Brennan MF: Cancer of the endocrine system. In: *Cancer: Principles and Practice of Oncology*, 2nd Edn, edited by Vincent T DeVita Jr, Samuel Hellman, and Steven A Rosenberg, Lippincott, Philadelphia, 1985
24. Burek JD: Pathology of aging rats. CRC Press, West Palm Beach, Florida, 29, 1978
25. Buss DH, Marshall RB, Baird FG, Myers RT: Paraganglioma of the thyroid gland. *Am J Surg Pathol* 4:589, 1980
26. Carmichael S, Winkler H: The adrenal chromaffin cell. *Scientific American* 253(2):40, 1985
27. Carney JA: The triad of gastric epithelioid leiomyosarcoma, pulmonary chondroma, and functioning extra-adrenal paraganglioma: A five-year review. *Medicine* 62:159, 1983
28. Carney JA, Bianco AJ Jr, Sizemore GW, Hayles AB: Multiple endocrine neoplasia with skeletal manifestations. *J Bone Joint Surg* 63:405, 1981
29. Carney JA, Go VL, Gordon H, Northcutt RC, Pearse AGE, Sheps SG: Familial pheochromocytoma and islet cell tumor of the pancreas. *Am J Med* 68:515, 1980
30. Carney JA, Sizemore GW, Sheps SG: Adrenal medullary disease in multiple endocrine neoplasia, type 2. Pheochromocytoma and its precursors. *Amer J Clin Path* 66:279, 1976
31. Carter D, Eggleston JC: Tumors of the lower respiratory tract, fascicle 17, Atlas of Tumor Pathology (2nd Series), Armed Forces Institute of Pathology, Washington, DC, 1979
32. Chambers RC, Bowling MC, Grimley PM: Glutaraldehyde fixation in routine histopathology. *Arch Path* 85:18, 1968
33. Chaudhry AP, Haar JG, Koul A, Nickerson PA: A nonfunctioning paraganglioma of vagus nerve. *Cancer* 43:1689, 1979
34. Cheville NF: Ultrastructure of canine carotid body and aortic body tumors. Comparison with tissues of thyroid and parathyroid origin. *Vet Path* 9, 166, 1972
35. Cohen SN, Shapiro JA: Transposable genetic elements. *Scientific American* 242(2):40, 1980
36. Costero I, Barroso-Moguel R, Martinez-Palomo A: Pleural origin of some of the supposed chemodectoid structures of the lung. *Beitr Pathol* 146:351, 1972
37. Coupland RE: The Natural History of the Chromaffin Cell. London, Longmans, p. 1, 1965
38. Cox WF, Pierce GB: The endodermal origin of the endocrine cells of an adenocarcinoma of the rat. *Cancer* 50:1530, 1982
39. Cragg RW: Concurrent tumors of the left carotid body and both Zuckerkandl bodies. *Arch Pathol* 18:635, 1934
40. Crowell WT, Grizzle WE, Siegel AL: Functional carotid paragangliomas: Biochemical, ultrastructural and histochemical correlation with clinical symptoms. *Arch Pathol Lab Med* 106:599, 1982
41. Dalal BI, Slinger RP: Formalin-induced fluorescence in melanomas and other lesions. *Arch Pathol Lab Med* 109:551, 1985
42. Dayal Y: Endocrine cells of the gut and their neoplasms, pp. 267–302. In: *Pathology of the Colon, Small Intestine and Anus.* Norris HT (Ed) New York: Churchill Livingstone, 1983
43. Dayal Y, Tallberg K, DeLellis RA, Wolfe HJ: Duodenal carcinoids in patients with and without neurofibromatosis. A comparative study. *Lab Invest* 52:18A, 1985
44. DeLellis RA, Tischler AS, Lee AK, Blount M, Wolfe HJ: Leu-enkephalin-like immunoreactivity in proliferative

lesions of the human adrenal medulla and extra-adrenal paraganglia. *Am J Surg Path* 7:29, 1983

45. DeLellis RA, Tischler AS, Wolfe HJ: Multidirectional differentiation in neuroendocrine neoplasms. *J Histochem Cytochem* 32:399, 1984

46. DeLellis RA, Wolfe HJ, Gagel RF, Friedman ZT, Miller HH, Gang DL, Reichlin S: Adrenal medullary hyperplasia: A morphometric analysis in patients with familial medullary thyroid carcinoma. *Am J Pathol* 83;177, 1976

47. DeLellis RA, Wolfe HJ: The polypeptide hormone-producing neuroendocrine cells and their tumors. *Meth Achiev Exp Pathol* 10:190, 1981

48. DeLellis RA, Dayal Y, Tischler AS, Lee AK, Wolfe HJ: Multiple endocrine neoplasia (MEN) syndromes: Cellular origins and interrelationships. *Int Rev Exp Pathol* 28:163, 1986

49. DeSchryver-Kecskemeti K, Clouse RE, Goldstein MN, Gersell D, O'Neal L: Intestinal ganglioneuromatosis. A manifestation of overproduction of nerve growth factor. *N Engl J Med* 308:635, 1983

50. Di Sant'Agnese PA, de Mesy Jensen KL: Somatostatin and/or somatostatinlike immunoreactive endocrine-paracrine cells in the human prostate gland. *Arch Pathol Lab Med* 108:693, 1984

51. Di Sant'Agnese PA, deMesy Jensen KL, Churukian CJ, Agarwal MM: Human prostatic endocrine-paracrine (APUD) cells. *Arch Pathol Lab Med* 109:607, 1985

52. Douglass J, Civelli O, Herbert E: Polyprotein gene expression: Generation of diversity of neuroendocrine peptides. *Ann Rev Biochem* 53:665, 1984

53. Edwards C, Heath D, Harris P: The carotid body in emphysema and left ventricular hypertrophy. *J Pathol* 104:1, 1971

54. Edwards C, Heath D, Harris P: Ultrastructure of the carotid body in high-altitude guinea-pigs. *J Pathol* 107:313, 1972

55. Engzell U, Franzen S, Zajicek J: Aspiration biopsy of tumors of the neck. II. Cytologic findings in 13 cases of carotid body tumor. *Acta Cytologica* 15:25, 1971

56. Farr HW: Carotid body tumors: A 40-year study. *CA-A Cancer Journal for Clinicians* 30:260, 1980

57. Farrior III JB, Hyams VJ, Benke RH, Farrior JB: Carcinoid apudoma arising in a glomus jugulare tumor: Review of endocrine activity in glomus jugulare tumors. *Laryngoscope* 90:110, 1980

58. Fernandes BJ, Bedard YC, Rosen I: Mucus-producing medullary cell carcinoma of the thyroid gland. *J Clin Pathol* 78:536, 1982

59. Fialkow PJ, Sagebiel RW, Gartler SM, Rimoin DL: Multiple cell origin of hereditary neurofibromas. *New Engl J Med* 284:298, 1971

60. Fitch R, Smith P, Heath D: Nerve axons in carotid body hyperplasia. *Arch Pathol Lab Med* 109:234, 1985

61. Folger GM Jr, Roberts WC, Mehrizi A, Shah KD, Glandy DL, Carpenter CCJ, Esterly JR: Cyanotic malformations of the heart with pheochromocytoma. A report of five cases. *Circulation* 29:750, 1964

62. Friesen SR, Tomita T, Kimmel JR: Pancreatic polypeptide update: Its roles in detection of the trait for multiple endocrine adenopathy syndrome, type I and pancreatic polypeptide-secreting tumors. *Surgery* 94:1028, 1983

63. Gagel RF, Melvin KEW, Tashjian AH Jr, Miller HH, Feldman ZT, Wolfe HJ, DeLellis RA, Cervi-Skinner S, Reichlin S: Natural history of the familial medullary carcinoma-pheochromocytoma syndrome and the identification of preneoplastic stages by screening studies: A five-year report. *Trans Assoc Am Phys* 88:177, 1975

64. Gallivan MVE, Chun B, Rowden G, Lack EE: Intrathoracic paravertebral malignant paraganglioma. *Arch Pathol Lab Med* 104:46, 1980

65. Gallivan MVE, Chun B, Rowden G, Lack EE: Laryngeal paraganglioma. Case report with ultrastructural analysis and literature review. *Am J Surg Path* 3:85, 1979

66. Gambino R: Laboratory diagnosis of pheochromocytoma. *Lab Report for Physicians* 4:75, 1982

67. Gans C, Northcutt RG: Neural crest and the origin of vertebrates: A new head. *Science* 220:268, 1983

68. Gaylis H, Mieny CJ: The incidence of malignancy in carotid body tumors. *Br J Surg* 64:885, 1977

69. Gilbert W: Genes-in-pieces revisited. *Science* 228:823, 1985

70. Glenn F, Gray GF: Functional tumors of the organ of Zuckerkandl. *Ann Surg* 183:578, 1976

71. Glenner GG, Grimley PM: Tumors of the extra-adrenal paraganglion system (including chemoreceptors), Fascicle 9, Atlas of Tumor Pathology (2nd series), Armed Forces Institute of Pathology, Washington, DC, 1974

72. Gooding GAW: Gray-scale ultrasound detection of carotid body tumors: report of two cases. *Radiology* 132:409, 1979

73. Gould VE, Linnoila RI, Memoli VA, Warren WH: Biology of Disease. Neuroendocrine components of the bronchopulmonary tract: hyperplasias, dysplasias, and neoplasms. *Lab Invest* 5:519, 1983

74. Gould VE, Wiedenmann R, Schwechheimer K, Dockhorn-Dworniczak B, Radosevich JA, Moll R, Franke WW: Synaptophysin expression in neuroendocrine neoplasms as determined by immunocytochemistry. *Am J Pathol* 126:243, 1987

75. Griffiths DFR, Williams GT, Williams ED: Multiple endocrine neoplasia associated with von Recklinghausen's disease. *Brit Med J* 287:1341, 1983

76. Grimley PM, Albores-Saavedra J: Neoplasms with neuroendocrine differentiation: Implications of molecular pathology. *J Exp Pathol* 3:155–176, 1987

77. Grimley PM, DeLellis RA: Multisystem neuroendocrine neoplasms. In: *Pathology of Incipient Neoplasia* (Albores-Saavedra J, Henson D, editors) pp. 25–454, Philadelphia, W.B. Saunders, 1986

78. Grimley PM, Glenner GG: Histology and ultrastructure of carotid body paragangliomas: Comparison with the normal gland. *Cancer* 20:1473, 1967

79. Grimley PM, Glenner GG: Ultrastructure of the human carotid body. A perspective on the mode of chemoreception. *Circulation* 37:648, 1968

80. Grizzle WE, Tolbert L, Pittman CS, Siegel AL, Aldrete JS: Corticotropin production by tumors of the autonomic nervous system. *Arch Pathol Lab Med* 108:545, 1983

81. Gruffman G, Gillman MW, Pasternak LR et al: Familial carotid body tumor; case report and epidemiologic review. *Cancer* 46:2116, 1980

82. Gusella JF, Wexler NS, Conneally PM, Naylor SL, Anderson MA, Tanzi RE, Watkins PC, Ottina K, Wallace MR, Sakaguchi AY, Young AB, Shoulson AB, Bonilla E, Martin JB: A polymorphic DNA marker genetically linked to Huntington's disease. *Nature* 306:234, 1983

83. Gustavson K-H, Jansson R, Oberg K: Chromosomal breakage in multiple endocrine adenomatosis (types I and II). *Clin Genetics* 23:143, 1983

84. Gustilo RB, Lober PH, Salovich EL: Chemodectoma (carotid-body tumor) metastasizing to bone: Case report. *J Bone Joint Surg (Am)* 47:155, 1965

85. Hamilton BR, Landsberg L, Levine RJ: Measurement of urinary epinephrine in screening for pheochromocytoma in multiple endocrine neoplasia type II. *Amer J Med* 65:1027, 1978

86. Hansen OP, Hansen M, Hansen HH, Rose B: Multiple endocrine adenomatosis of mixed type. *Acta Med Scand* 200:327, 1976

87. Hassoun J, Monges G, Giraud P, Henry JF, Charpin C, Payan H, Toga M: Immunohistochemical study of pheochromocytomas. An investigation of methionine-enkephalin, va-

soactive intestinal peptide, somatostatin, corticotropin, -endorphin, and calcitonin in 16 tumors. *Am J Pathol* 114:56, 1984

88. Hayes HM Jr: An hypothesis for the aetiology of canine chemoreceptor system neoplasms, based upon an epidemiologic study of 73 cases among hospital patients. *J Small Anim Pract* 16:337, 1975

89. Hayes HM, Fraumeni JF: Chemodectomas in dogs: Epidemiologic comparisons with man. *J Natl Cancer Inst* 52:1455, 1974

90. Hermann J: Delayed mutation model: Carotid body tumors and retinoblastoma. Genetics of human cancer. Mulvihill JJ, Miller RW (Eds), Raven Press, New York, 417–437, 1977

91. Hodgkinson DJ, Telander RL, Shepps SG, Gilchrist GS, Crowe JK: Extra-adrenal intrathoracic functioning paraganglioma (pheochromocytoma) in childhood. *Mayo Clin Proc* 55:271, 1980

92. Hoffman RW, Gardner DW, Mitchell FL: Intrathoracic and multiple abdominal pheochromocytomas in Von Hippel-Lindau disease. *Arch Intern Med* 142:1962–1965, 1982

93. House JM, Goodman ML, Gacek RR, Green GL: Chemodectomas of the nasopharynx. *Arch Otolaryng* 96:38, 1972

94. Hsu TC, Pathak S, Samann N, Hickey RC: Chromosome instability in patients with medullary carcinoma of the thyroid. *J Amer Med Assoc* 246:2046, 1981

95. Hull MT, Roth LM, Glover JL, Walker PD: Metastatic carotid body paraganglioma in Von Hippel-Lindau disease. An electron microscopic study. *Arch Pathol Lab Med* 106(5):235, 1982

96. Ichinose H, Hewitt RL, Drapanas T: Minute pulmonary chemodectoma. *Cancer* 28:692, 1971

97. Jacobs JB, Chretien PB, Sugarbaker E et al: Arteriographic discovery of a small contralateral carotid body tumor. *Radiology* 93:837, 1969

98. Jaenisch Rudolf: Mammalian neural crest cells participate in normal embryonic development on microinjection into postimplantation mouse embryos. *Nature* 318:181, 1985

99. Jago R, Smith P, Heath D: Electron microscopy of carotid body hyperplasia. *Arch Pathol Lab Med* 108:717, 1984

100. Johnson TL, Lloyd RV, Shapiro B, Sisson JC, Beierwaltes WH: Cardiac paragangliomas: A clinicopathologic study of four cases. *Lab Invest* 52:31A, 1985

101. Jubb KV, McEntee K: The relationship of ultimobranchial remnants and derivatives to tumor of the thyroid gland in cattle. *Cornell Veterinarian* 49:41, 1959

102. Kahn LB: Vagal body tumor (nonchromaffin paraganglioma, chemodectoma, and carotid body-like tumor) with cervical node metastasis and familial association. *Cancer* 38:2367, 1976

103. Karasov RB, Sheps SG, Carney JA, van Heerden JA, deQuattro V: Paragangliomatosis with numerous catecholamine-producing tumors. *Mayo Clin Proc* 57:590, 1982

104. Kissel P, Andre JM, Jacquier A: The neurocristopathies. p. 262. Masson Publishing, USA, Inc, New York, 1981

105. Kjaergaard J: Anatomy of the carotid glomus and carotid glomus-like bodies (non-chromaffin paraganglia). With electron microscopy and comparison of human foetal carotid, aorticopulmonary, tympanojugular, and vagal glomera. p. 328. FADL's Forlag, Copenhagen, p. 328, 1973

106. Knudson Ag Jr: Mutation and cancer: Statistical study of retinoblastoma. *Proc Nat Acad Sci USA* 68:820, 1971

107. Koufos A, Hansen MF, Copeland NG, Jenkins NA, Lampkin BC, Cavenee WK: Loss of heterozygosity in three embryonal tumours suggests a common pathogenetic mechanism. *Nature* 316:330, 1985

108. Krammer EB: Carotid body chemoreceptor function: Hypothesis based on a new circuit model. *Proc Natl Acad Sci USA* 75:2507, 1978

109. Lack EE: Hyperplasia of vagal and carotid body paraganglia in patients with chronic hypoxemia. *Amer J Pathol* 91:497, 1978

110. Lack EE, Cubilla AL, Woodruff JM: Paragangliomas of the head and neck region. *Human Pathol* 10:191, 1979

111. Lack EE, Cubilla AL, Woodruff JM, Lieberman PH: Extra-adrenal paragangliomas of the retroperitoneum. A clinicopathologic study of 12 tumors. *Amer J Surg Pathol* 4:109, 1980

112. Lack EE, Perez-Atayde AR, Young JB: Carotid body hyperplasia in cystic fibrosis and cyanotic heart disease. A combined morphometric, ultrastructural, and biochemical study. *Am J Pathol* 119:301, 1985

113. Lack EE, Stillinger RA, Colvin DB, Groves RM, Burnette DG: Aortic-pulmonary paraganglioma. Report of a case with ultrastructural study and review of the literature. *Cancer* 43:269, 1979b

114. Larraza-Hernandez O, Albores-Saavedra J, Benavides G, Krause LG, Perez-Merizaldi JC, Ginzo A: Pituitary adenoma, multicentric papillary thyroid carcinoma, bilateral carotid body paraganglioma, parathyroid hyperplasia, gastric leiomyoma, and systemic amyloidosis. *Amer J Clin Pathol* 78:527, 1982

115. Larsson L-I, Goltermann N, Rehfeld JF, Schwartz TW: Somatostatin cell processes as pathways for paracrine secretion. *Science* 205:1393, 1979

116. Lee AK, DeLellis RA, Blount M, Nunnemacher G, Wolfe HJ: Pituitary proliferative lesions in aging male Long-Evans rats. A model of mixed multiple endocrine neoplasia syndrome. *Lab Invest* 47:595, 1982

117. Leestma JE, Price EB Jr: Paraganglioma of the urinary bladder. *Cancer* 28:1063, 1971

118. Le Douarin NM: The neural crest. Cambridge Univ Press, 1982

119. Levit SA, Sheps SG, Espinosa RE et al.: Catecholamine-secreting paraganglioma of glomus-jugulare region resembling pheochromocytoma. *New Engl J Med* 281:805, 1969

120. Lewis RV, Stern AS, Kimura S, Rossier J, Stein S, Udenfriend S: An about 50,000 dalton protein in adrenal medulla: A common precursor of [met] and [leu]-enkephalin. *Science* 200:1450, 1980

121. Lipper S, Decker RE: Paraganglioma of the cauda equina: A histologic, immunohistochemical, and ultrastructural study and review of the literature. *Surg Neurol* 22:415, 1984

122. Llena JF: Paraganglioma in the cerebrospinal axis. *Prog Neuropathol* 5:261, 1983

123. Lloyd RV, Blaivas M, Wilson BS: Distribution of chromogranin and S100 protein in normal and abnormal adrenal medullary tissues. *Arch Pathol Lab Med* 109:633, 1985

124. Lloyd RV, Shapiro B, Sisson JC, Kalff V, Thompson NW, Beierwaltes WA: An immunohistochemical study of pheochromocytomas. *Arch Pathol Lab Med* 108:541, 1984

125. Lloyd RV, Warner TF: pp 127–140 In: *Advances in Immunohistochemistry*. DeLellis RA (Ed), New York: Masson Publishing, Inc, 1984

126. Lynch HT, Lynch PM, Albano WA, Edney J, Organ CH, Lynch JF: Hereditary cancer: Ascertainment and management, pp. 216–232. In: *Cancer – A Journal for Clinicians*, 1979

127. Manning JT, Ordonez NG, Rosenberg HS, Walker WE: Pulmonary endodermal tumor resembling fetal lung. Report of a case with immunohistochemical studies. *Arch Pathol Lab Med* 109:48, 1985

128. Marchevsky AM, Dikman SH: Mediastinal carcinoid with an incomplete Sipple's syndrome. *Cancer* 43:2497, 1979

129. Markel SF, Johnson RM: The clinical features and laboratory diagnosis of functional paragangliomas. *Lab Med* 6(10):39, 65, 1975

130. McCarthy EF, Bonfiglio M, Lawton W: A solitary functioning osseous metastasis from a malignant pheochromocytoma of the organ of Zuckerkandl. *Cancer* 40:3092, 1977

131. Melicow MM: One hundred cases of pheochromocytoma (107 tumors) at the Columbia-Presbyterian Medical Center, 1926–1976. A clinicopathological analysis. *Cancer* 40:1987, 1977

132. Messing A, Chen HY, Palmiter RD, Brinster RL: Peripheral neuropathies, hepatocellular carcinomas and islet cell adenomas in transgenic mice. *Nature* 316:461, 1985

133. Miller TA, Weber TR, Appelman HD: Paraganglioma of the gallbladder. *Arch Surg* 105:637, 1972

134. Morriss TA, Tymms DJ: Oat cell carcinoma, pheochromocytoma and carcinoid tumors – multiple APUD cell neoplasia – a case report. *J Pathol* 313:107, 1980

135. Nathan DM, Daniels GH, Ridgway EC: Gastrinoma and phaeochromocytoma: is there a mixed multiple endocrine adenoma syndrome? *Acta Endocrinol* 93:91, 1980

136. Newsome HH Jr, Weir GC, Daniel TM: Norepinephrine secreting tumor of the organ of Zuckerkandl. *JAMA* 242(b):540, 1979

137. Nicholas G, Orsini MA: Simultaneous ipsilateral carotid body and vagal paraganglioma. Otolaryngol. *Head Neck Surg* 90:246, 1982

138. O'Connor DT, Burton D, Deftos LJ: Chromogranin A: Immunohistology reveals its universal occurrence in normal polypeptide hormone producing endocrine glands. *Life Sciences* 33:1657, 1983

139. Oberg K, Walinder D, Bostrom H, Lundqvist G, Wide L: Peptide hormone markers in screening for endocrine tumors in multiple endocrine adenomatosis type I. *Amer J Med* 73:619, 1982

140. Olson JL, Salyer WR: Mediastinal paragangliomas (aortic body tumor). A report of four cases and a review of the literature. *Cancer* 41:2405, 1978

141. Page DL, DeLellis RA, Hough AJ: Tumors of the adrenal, fascicle 23, Atlas of Tumor Pathology (2nd series), Armed Forces Institute of Pathology, Washington, DC, 1986

142. Parry DM, Pi FP, Strong LC, Carney JA, Schottenfeld D, Reimer RR, Grufferman S: Carotid body tumors in man: Genetics and epidemiology. *J Nat Cancer Inst* 68:573, 1982

143. Payne CM, Nagle RB, Borduin V: Methods in laboratory investigation. An ultrastructural cytochemical stain specific for neuroendocrine neoplasms. *Lab Invest* 51:350, 1984

144. Pearse AGE: The cytochemistry and ultrastructure of polypeptide hormone-producing cells of the APUD series and the embryologic, physiologic and pathologic implications of the concept. *J Histochem Cytochem* 17:303, 1969

145. Pearse AGE: The diffuse neuroendocrine system and the APUD concept. Related "endocrine" peptides in brain, intestine, pituitary, placenta, and anuran cutaneous glands. *Med Biol* 35:115, 1977

146. Pearse AGE, Polak JM: The diffuse neuroendocrine system and the APUD concept. p. 33 in Gut Hormones (SR Bloom, ed) Churchill Livingstone, Edinburgh, 1978

147. Pereira DT, Hunter RD: Familial multicentric non-chromaffin paragangliomas: A case report on a patient with glomus jugulare and bilateral body tumors. *Clin Oncol* 6(3):273, 1980

148. Perrone T, Sibley RK, Rosai J: Duodenal gangliocytic paraganglioma: An immunohistochemical and ultrastructural study and a hypothesis concerning its origin. *Am J Surg Pathol* 9:31, 1985

149. Persson AV, Frusha JD, Dial PF, Jewell ER: Vagal body tumor: Paraganglioma of the head and neck. *CA-A Cancer Journal for Clinicians* 35:232, 1985

150. Pictet RL, Rall LB, Phelps P, Rutter WJ: The neural crest and the origin of insulin-producing and other gastrointestinal hormone-producing cells. *Science* 191, 1976

151. Polak JM, Bloom SR: The diffuse neuroendocrine system. Studies of this newly discovered controlling system in health and disease. *The J Histochem Cytochem* 27:1398, 1979

152. Pollack RS: Carotid body tumors – idiosyncracies. *Oncology* 27:81, 1973

153. Quint LE, Glazer GM, Francis IR, Shapiro B, Chenevert TL: Pheochromocytoma and paraganglioma comparison at MR imaging with CT and I-131 MIBG scintigraphy. *Radiology* 165: 89, 1987

154. Reed JC, Hallet KK, Felgin DS: Neural tumors of the thorax: Subject review from the AFIP. *Radiology* 126:9, 1978

155. Revak CS, Morris SE, Alexander GH: Pheochromocytoma and recurrent chemodectomas. *Radiology* 100:53, 1971

156. Richards MA, Mawdesley-Thomas LE: Aortic body tumors in a boxer dog with a review of the literature. *J Path* 98:283, 1969

157. Robertson DI, Cooney TP: Malignant carotid body paraganglioma: Light and electron microscopic study of the tumor and its metastases. *Cancer* 46:2623, 1980

158. Rosenfeld MG, Amara SG, Birnberg NC, Mermod J-J, Murdock GH, Evans RM: Calcitonin, prolactin and growth hormone gene expression as model systems for the characterization of neuroendocrine regulation. *Recent Prog Horm Res* 39:305, 1983

159. Roth J, LeRoith D, Shiloach J, Rosenzweig JL, Lesniak M, Havrankova J: The evolutionary origins of hormones, neurotransmitters, and other extracellular chemical messengers. *New Engl J Med* 306:523, 1982

160. Ruijs JHJ, van Waes PFGM, deHaas G, Hoekstra A, Mulder PHM, Veldman JE: Screening of a family for chemodectoma. *Radiologia Clin* 47:114, 1978

161. Saito H, Saito S, Sano T, Kagawa N, Hizawa K, Tatara K: Immunoreactive somatostatin in catecholamine-producing extra-adrenal paraganglioma. *Cancer* 50:560, 1982

162. Saldana MJ, Salem LE, Travezan R: High altitude hypoxia and chemodectomas. *Human Path* 4:251, 1973

163. Sano T, Saito H, Inaba H et al: Immunoreactive somatostatin and vasoactive intestinal polypeptide in adrenal pheochromocytoma. *Cancer* 52:282, 1983

164. Sato T, Saito H, Yoshinaga K, Shibota Y, Sasano N: Concurrence of carotid body tumor and pheochromocytoma. *Cancer* 34:1787, 1974

165. Scarpelli DG: Multipotent development capacity of cells in the adult animal. *Lab Invest* 52:331, 1985

166. Schimke RN: The neurocristopathy concept: fact or fiction. p. 344. In: *Advances in Neuroblastoma Research*, Proceedings of the 2nd Symposium on Advances in Neuroblastoma Research held in Philadelphia, 1979. Vol. 12. (Ed.) Evans AE. Progress in Cancer Research and Therapy, 1980

167. Schimke RN: Tumors of the Neural Crest System. In: *Genetics of Human Cancer*, edited by Mulvihill JJ, Miller RW, and Fraumeni JF Jr. Raven Press, New York, 1977

168. Schimke RN, Hartmann WH, Prout TE, Rimoin DL: Syndrome of bilateral pheochromocytoma, medullary thyroid carcinoma and multiple neuromas. A possible regulatory defect in the differentiation of chromaffin tissue. *New Engl J Med* 279:1, 1968

169. Schmale MC, Hensley G, Udey LR: Neurofibromatosis, von Recklinghausen's disease, multiple schwannomas, malignant schwannomas. *Amer J Path* 112:238, 1983

170. Schmechel DE: -Subunit of the glycolytic enzyme enolase: Nonspecific or neuron specific? *Lab Invest* 52:239, 1985

171. Scully RE, Aguirre P, DeLellis RA: Argyrophilia, scrotonin and peptide hormones in the female genital tract and its tumors. *Int J Gynec Path* 3:51, 1984

172. Sibley RK: The intermediate filament profile of neuro- and neuroendocrine neoplasms. *Lab Invest* 52:62A, 1985

173. Sidhu GS: The endodermal origin of digestive and respiratory tract APUD cells: Histopathologic evidence and a review of the literature. *Amer J Pathol* 96:5, 1979

174. Sisson JC, Frager MS, Valk TW, Gross MD, Swanson DP, Wieland DM, Tobes MC, Beierwaltes WH, Thompson NW: Scintigraphic localization of pheochromocytoma. *New Engl J Med* 305:12, 1981

175. Smith DM, Haggitt RC: A comparative study of generic

stains for carcinoid secretory granules. *Amer J Surg Pathol* 7:61, 1983

176. Snyder SH: Brain peptides as neurotransmitters. *Science* 209:976, 1980

177. Soeprono FF, Hodgkin JE: Metastatic chemodectoma with multiple nodular lesions. *CA-A Cancer Journal for Clinicians* 33:98, 1983

178. Spector GJ, Compagno J, Perez CA, Maisel RH, Ogura JH: Glomus jugulare tumors: Effects of radiotherapy. *Cancer* 35:1316, 1975

179. Spector GJ, Sobol S, Thawley SE, Maisel RH, Ogura JH: Glomus jugulare tumors of the temporal bone: Patterns of invasion in the temporal bone. *Laryngoscope* 89:1628, 1979

180. Sponenberg DP, McEntee K: Pheochromocytomas and ultimobranchial (C-cell) neoplasms in the bull: Evidence of autosomal dominant inheritance in the Guernsey breed. *Vet Pathol* 20:396, 1983

181. Stahlman M, Gray ME: Ontogeny of neuroendocrine cells in human fetal lung. I. An electron microscopic study. *Lab Invest* 51:449, 1984

182. Stahlman MT, Kasselberg AG, Orth DN, Gray ME: Ontogeny of neuroendocrine cells in human fetal lung. II. An immunohistochemical study. *Lab Invest* 52:52, 1985

183. Steiner AL, Goodman AD, Powers SR: Study of a kindred with pheochromocytoma, medullary thyroid carcinoma, hyperparathyroidism and Cushing's disease: multiple endocrine neoplasia, type 2^1. *Medicine* 47:371, 1968

184. Stevens RE, Moore GE: Inadequacy of APUD concept in explaining production of peptide hormones by tumours. *Lancet* 1:118, 1983

185. Tannir NM, Cortas N, Allam C: A functioning catecholamine-secreting vagal body tumor. A case report and review of the literature. *Cancer* 52:932, 1983

186. Tateishi R, Ishikawa O: The effect of N-nitrosobis(2-hydroxypropyl)amine on pulmonary neuroepithelial cells in Syrian golden hamsters. *Amer J Pathol* 119:326, 1985

187. Thacker WC, Duckworth JK: Chemodectoma of the orbit. *Cancer* 23:1233, 1969

188. Thomas P, Battifora H, Manderino G: Is neuron-specific enolase specific? An immunohistochemical comparison of a monoclonal and a polyclonal antibody against neuron-specific enolase. *Lab Invest* 54:63A, 1986

189. Tischler AS, Dichter MA, Biales B, Greene LA: Neuroendocrine neoplasms and their cells of origin. *New Engl J Med* 296:919, 1977

190. Tischler AS, DeLellis RA, Perlman RL, Allen JM, Costopoulos D, Lee YC, Nunnemacher G, Wolfe JH, Bloom SR: Spontaneous proliferative lesions of the adrenal medulla in aging Long-Evans rats. *Lab Invest* 53:486, 1985

191. Tischler AS, Lee AK, Nunnemacher G, Said SI, DeLellis RA, Morse GM, Wolfe HJ: Spontaneous neurite outgrowth and vasoactive intestinal peptide-like immunoreactivity of cultures of human paraganglioma cells from the glomus jugulare. *Cell Tissue Res* 219:543, 1981

192. Trojanowski JQ, Lee VM-Y: Expression of neurofilament antigens by normal and neoplastic human adrenal chromaffin cells. *New Engl J Med* 313:101, 1985

193. Van Baars F, Cremers C, van den Brock P, Geerts S, Veldman J: Genetic aspects of nonchromaffin paraganglioma. *Human Genet* 60:305, 1982

194. Van Heerden JA, Kent RB III, Sizemore GW, Grant CS, ReMine WH: Primary hyperparathyroidism in patients with multiple endocrine neoplasia syndromes. Surgical experience. *Arch Surg* 118:533, 1983

195. Van Zwieten MJ, Burek JD, Zurcher C, Hollander CF: Aortic body tumors and hyperplasia in the rat. *J Path* 128:99, 1979

196. Veldman JE, Mulder PHM, Ruijs SHJ, deHaas G, van Waes PFGM, Hockstra A: Early detection of asymptomatic hereditary chemodectoma with radionuclide scintiangiography. A possibility for family screening and surveillance. *Arch Otolaryngol* 106:547, 1980

197. Verhofstad AAJ, Steinbusch HWM, Joosten HWJ, Penke B, Varga J, Goldstein M: Immunocytochemical localization of nonadrenaline, adrenaline and serotonin. In: *Immunocytochemistry. Practical applications in pathology and biology.* Wright PSG. Bristol, p. 143–168, 1983

198. Wasserman K: Recent advances in carotid body physiology. *Fed Proc* 39:2626, 1980

199. Webb TA, Sheps SG, Carney JA: Differences between sporadic pheochromocytoma and pheochromocytoma in multiple endocrine neoplasia, type 2. *Am J Surg Pathol* 4:121, 1980

200. Weber AL, Davis KR, Nadol JB Jr: Chemodectomas (nonchromaffin paragangliomas) of the glomus jugulare, glomus vagale, and carotid body. *Ann Otol Rhinol Laryngol* 91:666, 1982

201. Whang-Peng J, Triche TJ, Knutsen T, Miser J, Douglass EC, Israel MA: Chromosome translocation in peripheral neuroepithelioma. *New Eng Med* 311:584, 1984

202. White MC, Hickson BR: Multiple paragangliomata secreting catecholamines and calcitonin with intermittent hypercalcemia. *J Roy Soc Med* 72(7):532, 1979

203. Wilson BS, Lloyd RV: Detection of chromogranin in neuroendocrine cells with a monoclonal antibody. *Amer J Pathol* 115:458, 1984

204. Wilson H: Carotid body tumors: Familial and bilateral. *Ann Surg* 171:843, 1970

205. Wolfe H, Childers H, Montminy M, Goodman R, Punzak S, Lechan R, DeLellis R, Tischler A: Use of antisense RNA probes for morphologic detection of peptide-producing cells by *in situ* hybridization. *Lab Invest* 52:77A, 1985

206. Wolfe HJ, Melvin KEW, Cervi-Skinner SJ, Saadi AA, Julian JF, Jackson CE, Tashjian AH: C-cell hyperplasia preceding medullary thyroid carcinoma *N Engl J Med* 289:437, 1973

207. Yarrington JT, Capen CC: Fine structural and biochemical investigations of pheochromocytomas in bulls with C-cell (ultimobranchial) neoplasms of the thyroid (UBT). *Proc Electron Microsc Soc Am* 33:438, 1975

208. Young TW, Thrasher TV: Nonchromaffin paraganglioma of the uterus. *Arch Pathol Lab Med* 106:608, 1982

209. Zollinger R, Hedinger C: Pheochromocytoma and sympathetic paraganglioma. 2. Combination with typical associated diseases. Familial occurrence. *Schweiz Med Wochenschr* 113:1086, 1983

7

RARE TYPES OF NEOPLASTIC PROGRESSION

H.E. KAISER

Neoplasms, in general, do not remain unchanged over longer periods of time (exception are dormant neoplastic cells and tissues) but show instead progressive stages of development.

The study of rare neoplasms is of great scientific value because from them we may learn more about basic aspects of neoplastic progression in man. The best information can be gained from a comparative approach.

During their progression, neoplasms exhibit an intimate relation with the host from which they once derived. Tumor and host are two related counterparts in one disease process. This interrelationship plays an important role in the frequent and infrequent types of neoplastic development which can be understood only on this basis. Neoplasms are diseases in their own right characterized by typical speed of growth, wide or rare distribution and high or low metastatic aggressiveness; they have a characteristic pattern regarding age, sex, location, spreading and so on which is species-, strain-, and breed-specific. In Chapter 2/Volume VIII the metastatic pattern of selected human neoplasms has been described. Rare cases of neoplasms may develop at different intervals of neoplastic progression. From the viewpoint of the host, we distinguish among such variations as species, age, sex, racial origin which may vary in frequent and infrequent tumor progression. Regarding the neoplasms, the whole path of progression may be unusual, or only its speed, topographical occurrence, or other aspects. Tumor progression itself can be divided into primary and secondary tumor development.

To avoid confusion, a classification of cases considered "rare neoplasms" is in order. Each arrangement of neoplasms should be done first, according to the sequence of the parent tissues and secondly, according to the facts of intra- and extraspecies comparison.

Amplification of certain oncogenes occurs as a common

Table 1a. Facts serving as basis for an intra-extraspecies comparison.

1. The primary neoplasm(s) (are) is rare in the species
2. The primary neoplasm occurs in a rare region
3. The way of progression of the neoplasm is unusual
4. The local recurrence of the neoplasm is unusual
5. The metastatic occurrence is unusual
6. Secondary neoplasms (also due to therapy) are, until now, rare
7. The neoplasm is rare in this particular age range
8. The neoplasm is rare in the male or female sex
9. The speed of progression is rare

correlation of the progression of some neoplasms on one hand and as a rare sporadic event affecting various oncogenes in different neoplasms on the other. The increase of an amplified oncogene may contribute to the multistep progression of at least some neoplasms (10).

Neoplastic facts which can be compared on an intraspecies and extraspecies level are listed in Table 1a.

Based on these facts, the following chapter is divided into sections as shown in Table 1b.

I. GENERAL ASPECTS

1. Rare speed of neoplastic progression

Epidemiology, statistics and experience have demonstrated that the majority of neoplasms show a characteristic prognosis, which itself depends on the aggressiveness, therefore also the speed, of the neoplastic progression, including local recurrence, metastasis, and systemic and general dissemination. Major variations (shortcuts) occur only rarely, resulting in rare speed of tumor progression. This can happen in different ways: (1) a normally slow-growing tumor may suddenly become aggressive, leading to a grave prognosis; (2) a normally fast-growing, aggressive tumor may

Table 1b. Distinction of various aspects of unusual or rare appearance of neoplasms.

I. *General aspects*
 1. Rare speed of neoplastic progression
 2. Unusual path of neoplastic progression

II. *Specific aspects: primary neoplasms*
 1. Rare neoplasms in particular species
 2. Rare neoplasms in man
  a. Primary neoplasms of uncommon histology (H), in a rare topographical region (L), and at specific site (S)
  b. Rare neoplasms in a particular age
  c. Rare neoplasms of one or the other sex

III. *Specific aspects: secondary neoplastic growth*
 1. Rare neoplastic invasiveness
 2. Uncommon local recurrence
 3. Rare secondary direct spreading
 4. Rare neoplastic seeding
 5. Rare neoplastic circulating cells
 6. Rare metastases; selected aspects: metastases of uncommon primary neoplasms (U) and unusual metastases of common primary neoplasms (C)
 7. Rare neoplastic spontaneous regression

K.W. Brunson (ed) Local invasion and spread of cancer.

Table 2. Rare speed of neoplastic progression: selected cases.

Tissue	Organ	Tumor	Time of revival	Remarks	References
Stratified squamous epithelium	Cervix uteri	Squamous cell ca	After 10 and more years of initial radiation treatment	The long survival is very rare	(290)
Stratified squamous epithelium	Cervix uteri	Squamous cell ca	Local recurrence more than 10 years after initial treatment	This late recurrence is very rare	(234)
Reticular connective tissue	Lymphatic system	Lymphoblastic lymphoma	Initial relapse after 2 years treatment	This late relapse is extremely rare	(222)

unexpectedly turn inactive and indolent; it may even become dormant.

The prognosis for a neoplasm depends widely on the speed of progression and the aggressiveness of the particular tumor. In general, less-differentiated, anaplastic neoplasms exhibit a fast, often fatal, course in contrast to well-differentiated neoplasms which tend to proceed much slower. Of course the way a particular neoplasm develops secondary growth also plays a significant role. Metastasis is more likely from more voluminous neoplasms than small ones. But this also is not always the case if we compare, for example, a breast cancer with an incipient, often still minute, malignant melanoma. The aggressiveness of the melanoma may by far outplay that of the breast cancer, which may be several times larger in size. On certain occasions, neoplasms with a rapid growth, such as oat cell carcinoma of the lung, carcinoma of the exocrine pancreas, carcinoma of the gallbladder or malignant melanoma may show a rarely occurring slow growth whereas neoplasms with a normally slow growth

may suddenly exhibit a rapid course. These changes, even though occurring rarely, are important because we may learn from certain parameters what the causes are for these changes in the speed of growth (Table 2).

2. Unusual paths in neoplastic progression

Neoplastic progression develops generally in a tumor-specific way. Certain neoplasms proceed more often via direct spreading (Chapter 1/Volume III), others by metastasis. Some neoplasms, like the basal cell cancer of the skin, rarely metastasize but invade frequently. Breast cancer in man metastasizes via the lymphatic system; other neoplasms are characterized by blood-borne metastasis. Again, others spread by a combination of paths.

In a 79-year-old woman, a primary liposarcoma of the heart, an extremely rare malignant neoplasm, coexisted with a Brenner tumor. The histologic material of the sarcoma was stained with histochemical methods for lipids; lipid droplets

Table 3. Unusual path of neoplastic progression.

Tissue type	Organ	Tumor	Unusual way of progression	Number of cases known	Remarks	References
Stratified squamous epithelium	Skin	Basal cell carcinoma	Metastases (rarely squamous differentiation), perineural spread. Metastatic spread (lymphogenic and hematogenic) occurs most often to lymph nodes, lungs and bones	170 cases histologically proven (ratio 1 in 1000:35 000)	Male–female ratio 2:1. Age 45. Metastasis after 9 yrs. after onset of primary tumor. Survival with metastasis 8 mos.	von Domarus H, Stevens P, *J Am Acad Dermatol* 10(6):1043, 1984
Stratified columnar epithelium	Mandible	Amelo-blastoma	Very rarely development of metastasis. Case with pulmonary metastasis		Two types of malignant ameloblastomas (1) metastases identical to primary, (2) appearance of undifferentiated carcinoma. No relationship between size of primary, histologic type and course of metastases	Dupuis A et al., *Rev Stomatol Chir Maxillofac* 84(3):154, 1983
Transitional epithelium	Ureter	Ureteral carcinoma	Bilateral primary carcinoma of the ureter	1	Topographically very rare case	Powder JR et al., *J Urol* 132(2):349, 1984
Desmal epithelium	Intra-cranial	Hemangio-pericytoma	Extracranial bone metastasis of this rare intracranial tumor			Marsot-Dupoch K et al., *J Radiol* 65(1):41, 1984
Fibrous connective tiss.	Breast	Cystosarcoma phylloides	Shifting of metastasis to an entirely sarcomatous growth	1	Fatal outcome in 18-year-old woman	Ngala Kenda JF, *Arch Surg* 118(7):871, 1983
Bone	Bones	Osteosarcoma	Skip metastases (rare) to lung and bone	3	Skip metastases indicate grave prognosis. Postoperatively 6, 7 mos. disease-free – extensive dissemination	Malawer MM, Dunham WK, *J Surg Oncol* 22(4):236, 1983

Table 4. Spontaneous neoplasms which are Rare in certain species.

Tissue	Organ	Neoplasm	Domestic animals (general)	Mouse	Rat	Hamster	Dog	Cat	Cattle	Horse	Sheep	Goat	Pig	Exceptions
Epithelia		Tumors											Rare	
Stratified squamous epithelium	Skin	Tumors		Rare		Rare*								*with exception of melanoma in some strains
	Skin	Basal cell & appendage tumors	Rare*											*dog and cat
	Integumentary scent gland	Tumors				Unknown								
	Tongue	Carcinoma					Rare							
	Esophagus	Tumors			Extremely rare									
	Uterine cervix				Unknown (spont. t)									
	Uterine cervix & vagina	Tumors		Extremely rare										
Simple cuboidal/columnar epithelium	Kidney	Clear cell carcinoma	Rare											
	Male genital tract	Tumors				Rare								
	Kidney	Carcinoma				Low incidence								
Simple columnar epithelium	Stomach	Carcinoma	Rare											
	Intestine	Tumors	Relatively rare											
	Alimentary tract	Tumors		Rare										
	Intestine	Tumors			Very seldom									
	Gallbladder	Carcinoma				Unknown								
Pseudostratified columnar epithelium	Upper respiratory tract	Tumors			Unknown									
	Lower respiratory tract	Tumors			Rare									
	Lung	Adenoma	Quite rare											
	Lung	Cancer				Rare								
	Lung	Squamous cell carcinoma					Rare	Rare						
		Anaplastic carcinoma					Rare	Rare						

Organ	Subsite	Tumor type											Note
Transitional epithelium	Urinary tract	Tumors					Very rare						
	Urinary bladder	Tumors		Rare	Very rare			Rare	Rare				
Sebaceous & sweat glands	Auditory sebaceous glands	Tumors			Rare								
Mammary glands		Tumors					Very rare						
		Carcinoma								Extremely rare	Rare	Rare	
Salivary glands		Adenocarcinoma		Very rare	Rare								
Salivary incl. Lacrimal glands		Tumors		Infrequent									
Harderian gl.		Tumors		Low frequency									
Liver		Tumors		Very rare	Very rare								
		Hepatocellular carcinoma		Rare			Very rare						
Exocrine pancreas		Tumors		Rare	Rare			Uncommon					
		Carcinoma	Rare										
Pituitary gland	–	Tumors		Rare									
Parathyroid gland	–	Tumor		Exceedingly rare									
		Cancer	Rare										
Adrenal glands		Tumors		Rare									
Testes		Tumors		Extremely rare									
		Germ cell tumors				Extremely rare							
		Seminoma	Rare*										*Dog: fairly common
Ovary		Tumors		Comparatively rare	Uncommon								
Soft tissues		Mesothelioma		Rare									
		Myxoma		Rare									
		Myxosarcoma		Rare									
Melanogenic system		Melanoma		Rare				Rare*					*Grey and white horses

Table 4. Continued.

Tissue	Organ	Neoplasm	Domestic animals (general)	Mouse	Rat	Hamster	Dog	Cat	Cattle	Horse	Sheep	Goat	Pig	Exceptions
Bone		Tumors				Rare								
		Tumors*	Unknown		Unknown									*Osteosarcoma
		Osteosarcoma	Rare	Rare										
		Primary cancer	Uncommon											
Soft tissues		Tumors			Rare*									*Fibromas, fibrosarcomas, lipomas
Smooth muscle		Tumors	Rare											
Striated muscle		Tumors	Rare											
CNS		Tumors		Rare	Extremely rare	Unreported								
PNS		Tumors		Rare	Extremely rare	Rare								
Teratomas				Rare										

*Topographically Rare melanomas are described in Chapter 19/Volume VIII by Kaiser.

Table 5. Rare and uncommon neoplasms.

Tissue	Organ	Tumor and No. of reported cases	Rare or uncommon location	Type or spreading	Age General	Age Special	Treatment and prognosis	Established	Remarks	Reference
Simple squamous epithelium	Capillary in ovary	Hemangioma first case?	Capillary wall of ovarian cyst	–		35 yrs.	–	G.T. McKee		(241)
Simple/stratified squamous epithelium	Thyroid*	Squamous cell ca 1% of all primary thyroid malignancies		Extremely high local recurrence, also distant metastases	50–60 yrs.		Radical surgery-radioresistant extremely poor prognosis		Metaplastic tumor	(18) pp. 43–44
	Mammary glands	Squamous cell ca (very rare) 0.1% of breast ca, approximately 30 cases known. Sometimes element of sarcomatoid pattern		Distant metastases	54.4 yrs.		Surgery, 3 yrs. survival 30%		More often in left breast	(18) pp. 5–7
	Stomach	Squamous cell ca 0.04–0.7% adenosquamous cell ca		Metastatic			Surgery, 7 mos. survival after diagnosis is characteristic		4 to 1 male preponderance	(18) pp. 8–11
	Colon (squamous nests)	Squamous cell ca approximately 30 cases reported	Increasing rarity: cecum, ascending colon, transverse colon, hepatic flexure, descending c., sigmoid c.		50–70 yrs.		1 to 2 yrs., postoperatively healthy			(18) p. 12
	Prostate	Squamous cell ca (keratinizing) – keratinization, perhaps 30 cases known	Local extension to symphysis pubis, perineum, urinary bladder and rectum, iliac lymph node metastasis as well as to periaortic lymph nodes		65 yrs.		Surgery, radiotherapy, chemotherapy, prognosis poor		Rarest form of prostatic ca, grave prognosis; survival 4 mos. to less than 3 yrs.	(18) p. 13–14
Stratified squamous epithelium	Skin	Primary oat-cell ca, exceedingly rare	Head and neck	Metastases			Surgery			(188)
	Skin	Squamous cell ca, 7 cases	Hand, scalp, groin, lower extremity, penis						Very rare occurrence	(272)
	Skin	Basal cell ca, 109 cases	Skin	Metastasis	40+ yrs.					(307)
	Lip	Basal cell ca basosquamous ca	Lip	Direct spread metastasis			Surgery			(318)
	Oral cavity	Combined nevus	Oral mucosa	None			Benign		Variable histologic appearance	(102)
	Soft palate	Acinic cell ca, 1 case	Soft palate			35 yrs.				(81)

*Squamos cells do not occur in the thyroid, but the tumor known as squamous cell carcinoma of thyroid exists.

Table 5. Continued.

Tissue	Organ	Tumor and No. of reported cases	Rare or uncommon location	Type or spreading	Age General	Age Special	Treatment and prognosis	Established	Remarks	Reference
Stratified squamous epithelium	Skin	Condyloma acuminatum, chronic	Inguinal region bladder, endocervix from pinonidal sinus							(263)
	Skin	Xeroderma pigmentosum; 726 cases	XP is rare itself in each location	Increased no. of tumors	Under 20 or under 40: under 20-yr. old show 2,000-fold increase of basal cell, squamous cell ca, etc. Up to 40, increased brain sarcoma, etc.					(201)
	Skin	Carcinoma adeno/squamous cell 90% – melanomas, sarcomas, unclear histology – 1 case transitional cell ca	Bartholin's gland			50 yrs	Surgery: radical vulvectomy, bilateral lymph adenectomy – 3 to 5 yrs. survival 68% – 55%, respectively			(18) pp. 38-41
Pilonidal sinus		Carcinoma: 21 cases squamous cell ca, 2 basal cell ca, 1 adeno + 2 mixed (squamous and basal cell) ca	Pilonidal sinus	2 cases only had inguinal lymph node metastases; 7 cases developed recurrence; rarely distant metastases		50 yrs.	Surgery		24-25 yrs. predevelopment, 84% male	(18) pp. 15-18
	Vagina	Carcinoma (squamous cell 85-90% – adenoca 6% clear cell ca of cervix belong to latter	Posterior wall of lower vagina	Pelvic lymph node; distant metastasis in lungs (36%); supraclavicular lymph nodes		19.5 yrs 33.4 yrs	Surgery, radiotherapy, chemotherapy			(18) pp. 51-55
	Skin	Burn scar ca 29% of skin ca		Recurrence is often observed; metastases (1/3)	58	18-84 yrs	Surgery, 57% face and neck; 31% lower extremity; 5 yrs. survival	Marjolin 1828	Often a lethal disease growing from the periphery	(18) pp. 19-21
	Skin	Basal cell ca 1 case	Back of shoulder	Metastases	Elderly	22 yrs.			Glucose-6-phosphate dehydrogenase and 6-phosphogluconate dehydrogenase indicate metastasis	(94)
	Skin	Basalioma of	Temporal area	Regional metastases to parotid gland and neck						(93)
	Skin	Merkel cell tumor (trabecular ca)	Unusual skin appendage malignancy	Recurrence						(83)
	Skin	Carcinoma cuniculatum (variant of squamous cell ca), 46 cases		Local invasion extension in bone; rare metastases					Histologically: mature squamous keratinocytes	(178)

Site	Type	Location	Behavior	Age	Survival/Treatment	Author	Comments	Reference
Nail bed	Subunguinal ca	Toes in 20%	Metastasis does not appear, one patient exhibited generalized disease	50; 24–82 yrs.	Surgery: 5 yrs. survival approaches 100%		Amputation results in cure, no lymph node involvement	(18) pp. 22–23
Nasal cavity	Squamous cell ca	Nasal cavity					Uncommon	(29)
Larynx		Rare in larynx					1% of ca in larynx or laryngopharynx	(29)
Ear, nose, throat	Tumors		Very rare cutaneous digital metastasis					(197)
Soft palate, larynx	Squamous cell ca						Sarcomatoid stroma tumors are rare	(80)
Oral cavity, nasal cavity, larynx, genitalia, and peritoneum	Verrucous ca: 4.5% oral ca, oral cavity 73%, larynx 11%, nasal cavity 4%, genitalia and peritoneum 11%	Nasal cavity	Rarely, local recurrence		Larynx: 1–2% of laryngeal ca, surgery – highly curable, perineal location: Burchke-Loewenstein			(18) pp. 140–142
Oral cavity, oropharynx, hypopharynx	Adenoid cystic ca (30% of head and neck tumors with this histology)	Oropharynx only 2%	Metastasis to regional lymph nodes uncommon – local recurrence frequent		Surgery and radiation 70% 5 yrs. survival, 10 yrs. survival 30%			
Hypopharynx	Lymphoepithelial ca	Hypopharynx 1977: 2nd reported case		60-yr-old-man				(100)
Neck	Cystic squamous cell ca, branchial cleft ca, extremely rare, 22 cases			50 average age 40–77 yrs.			Male predominance	(69)
Retromolar trigone	Squamous cell ca acinic cell ca, 1 case		Metastases	63-yr-old man			3 metastatic carcinomas in the neck – 2 deriving from nonsquamous cell occult primaries, first described	(112)
External auditory canal	Adenoid cystic ca (ceruminoma), approximately 30 + cases described		Late distant metastases	44 yrs.	Survival at 15 yrs. 50%			(18) pp. 143–144
Embryologic cloacogenic membrane	2–3% of anorectal neoplasms	Anal canal					Rare but distinct group of anal ca	(36)
Cervix	Adenoid cystic ca of uterine cervix		Lymphatic invasion – 66 metastases to liver, lung, bones, peritoneal cavity- local recurrence	39–89 yrs.	2 yrs. survival	Paolmen and Counsellor 1949		(18) pp. 159–161
Anus	Epidermoid ca	Anus					Relatively rare entity	(243)
Glans penis and prepuce	Balanitis xerotica obliterans		Change to squamous cell ca in rare instances					(244)

Table 5. Continued.

Tissue	Organ	Tumor and No. of reported cases	Rare or uncommon location	Type or spreading	Age (General)	Age (Special)	Treatment and prognosis	Established	Remarks	Reference
Stratified squamous cell epithelium	Vagina, uterine cervix	1–2%		23% of recurrence in 5 yrs.	19.5 yrs.	7–29 yrs.	Surgery and variable types of treatment 2 yrs. survival 87%, 5 yrs. survival in vagina and cervix 91%			(18) pp. 51–55
	Vulva	ca of Bartholin's gland, 90% adenoca or squamous cell ca; 10% melanomas, sarcomas and unclear histology – 1.8% of vulva ca		Metastases, including regional lymph nodes	50 yrs.	Teens to nineties	3 yrs. survival, 68%; 5 yrs. survival, 55%; radical surgery: vulvectomy and bilateral lymphadenectomy	Homan 1897		(18) pp. 38–41
	Anterior male urethra	Primary squamous cell ca; 10 case	Anterior urethra				Surgery: distal lesions have better prognosis			(15)
Simple cuboidal/ columnar epithelium	Kidney	Adenoca							Rare tumors	(291)
	Kidneys	Polycystic renal disease and bilateral hypernephroma	Rare association in this location	Metastasis			Prognosis recently improved	Transfer Kalifat, 1987 from on to the other disease possible		
	Prostate	Cancer; 1 case		Metastasis to an extremity is rare	88-yr. old man					(217)
	Prostate	Carcinoma; 1 reported case, 10 from literature		Epididymal metastasis						(25)
	Prostate	Endometrial ca of prostate, 10 cases		Metastases to skeletal system	61–79 yrs.	68 yrs.	Good prognosis indolent course	Mellicow & Pachter, 1967	Comparable histologically to adenoca of uterus	(18) pp. 59–60
	Seminal vesicles	Papillary adenoca. (soft tissue sarcomas occur too) sarcoma: fibrosarcoma, leiomyosarcoma and pleomorphic		Rather rapid: metastases in regional lymph nodes (66%), lungs (33.3%), and liver (41.6%)	60.7 yrs.		Surgery, radiotherapy, Stilbestrol – death by urinary obstruction and urenia			(18) pp. 46–48
	Endometrium	Clear cell ca. 4.7% of all endometrial ca.		To retroperitoneal lymph nodes, mediastinum, lung and brain, omentum, peritoneum, tumor is more aggressive than typical endometrial adenoca.	68 yrs.		Surgery, pre- and postoperative radiation			(18) pp. 49–50
	Stomach	Cancer, 1 case	Very rare variant of pp(Tja) system						Glycolipids, glycoproteins	(176)

	Site	Tumor / cases	Frequency	Spread / metastasis	Age	Treatment / prognosis	Notes	Ref.
Simple columnar epithelium	Gastro-intestinal tract (APUD system)	Carcinoid tumor of gastrointestinal tract: 2052 cases – stomach: 3.4%		Liver, regional lymph nodes 22% Liver and regional lymph node 22% metastasis	All age groups	Surgery; good 52% (5 yrs. 23%)		(18) pp. 162–172
		– duodenum: 2.3% – jejunum and ileum: 32.2%		Penetration 36% Invasion, metastasis peritoneal cavity, Liver	60–65 yrs.			
		– appendix: 45.5%		1% head metastases,	40 yrs.			
		– rectum: 12%		lymph node metastases and distal spread	20–40 yrs. (9–14)			
		– cecum colon: 2.6%		62% metastases				
		– Meckel's div.: 1.3% (30 cases)		38% metastases in regional lymph nodes	20–40 yrs. (9–14)			
		– gallbladder: 0.5%	Rare					
	Small bowel	Carcinoma, 7 cases	Rare			Curable, when already symptomatic	One patient had 13 separate primary adenocarcinomas in the distal ileum	(143)
	Colon	Carcinoma, 1 case	Extremely rare	Diffusely infiltrating primary colon ca.	45-year-old man			(20)
	GI tract	Carcinoid syndrome	Rare	Involves also respiratory tract, skin and heart		Aggressive surgery		(376)
Carcinoid tumors	Thymus	Carcinoid tumors, approx. 20 cases	–	Recurrence	Male predominance 43 yrs.	Surgery, 5 yrs. Survival 85%	–	(18) pp. 173–174
	Bronchus	Carcinoid tumor 6–10% of all primary lung tumors	–	Local invasion 10–94% (50%) lymph node metastasis: 0–30%, blood-borne metastasis 0–42% sites liver, skeleton, chest wall, brain	45 yrs.	Surgery – radiation, good prognosis, survival 1–21 yrs., survival 95%		(18) pp. 175–178
	Testis	Carcinoid tumors, 15 cases	–		48 yrs.	Excellent prognosis after orchiectomy	–	(18) pp. 179
	Ovary	Carcinoid tumor, (1% of ovarian teratomas, less than 1% of all carcinoids) 50 cases	–	Recurrence (pelvis or abdominal) – liver metastases	55–60 yrs.	Salpingo-oophorectomy, benign cause, 95% survival at 5 yrs., 88% at 10 yrs.	–	(18) pp. 180–181
Simple columnar epithelium/ mesenchyme	Seminal vesicle	Tumors of seminal vesicle	–	Metastases: regional lymph nodes, (66.6%) lungs, 33.3%) and liver, (41.6%)	65 yrs.	Surgery, radiotherapy	Mesenchymal neoplasm less frequent	(18) pp. 46–48

Table 5. Continued.

Tissue	Organ	Tumor and No. of reported cases	Rare or uncommon location	Type or spreading	Age General	Age Special	Treatment and prognosis	Established	Remarks	Reference
Simple columnar cell epithelium	Uterus	Clear cell ca of endometrium	–	Metastasis: retroperitoneal lymph nodes, mediastinum, lung, brain (omentum, peritoneum)	68 yrs.		Surgery, radiation therapy 20.6–55.3% survival			(18) pp. 49–50
	Fallopian tube	Malignant mixed Müllerian tumors, 21 cases approx.	–	Direct extension into pelvis, genital tract, liver, lungs and bones	58 yrs.		Surgery and radiotherapy, survival 15 mos. to more than 4 yrs.			(18) p. 216
	Rectum	Cloacogenic ca of the anorectal junction	–	Metastasis to regional lymph nodes, 34%; inguinal nodes in 50% – 19% of cases, distant metastases to liver, lung, bones, and peritoneum	50–70yrs.	29 yrs.	Surgery – survival well diff. nonkeratinizing 70% 5 yrs. survival less-diff. 40% Klotz: 46.7%	Grinvalsky and Helwig 1956		(18) pp. 377–381
	Cowper's gland	Ca, approx. 15 cases	–	Local growth and extension, local recurrence	17 yrs.		Surgery (locally)			(188) pp. 42–43
	Paranasal sinus	Small cell carcinoma, 4 cases	Paranasal sinus	1 case with bone metastasis					Should be named neuroendocrine ca	(174)
	Nasopharynx	Nasopharyngeal ca		Bone and lung	Very rare in childhood		Extremely poor when metastasizing, irrespective of treatment			(369)
	Nasopharynx	Nasopharyngeal ca and epitheloid granuloma	Rare	Metastasized to cervical lymph nodes	18-year-old woman					(342)
	Nasopharynx	Nasopharyngeal ca	–		12-year-old boy of European origin				Association with Epstein-Barr virus, in Caucasians of this tumor is rare.	(330)
Pseudostratified columnar epithelium	Nose	Adenoid cystic; ca 5% of tumors in this location		Destroys adjacent bone, infiltrates along perineural lymphatics – local recurrence, 75%	40-60 yrs.		Surgery – radiation therapy			(18) pp. 135–139
	Sinuses Nasopharynx						2-19 yrs. 45% 5 yrs.			
	Glottis	Ca (7 tumors)	Primary epidermoid ca of subglottis is extremely rare	15% recurrence, other types of spread are rare	33-77 years		Surgery, radiation therapy		Male preponderance	(49, 67, 323)
	Larynx	Oat cell ca – (anaplastic) few cases		Infiltration of muscle, lymph node metastases	63 yrs.		(Surgery) radiation and chemotherapy, poor – 2.5 yrs. survival is rare			(18) pp. 65–67

Tissue	Organ	Tumor	Metastasis / progression	Age	Therapy / survival	Notes	Reference
	Trachea	Oat cell ca few cases	Metastasis to liver and regional lymph nodes	58 yrs.	Radiotherapy (surgery), prognosis extremely poor		(18) pp. 65–67
Pseudostratified columna epith.	Larynx	Adenoid cystic ca 5%	Rarely cervical lymph node metastases	52%	Total laryngectomy – 3 yrs: 50% rarely up to 16 yrs.	–	(18) pp. 146–147
	Larynx	Oat-cell carcinoma	Larynx		Surgery alone is useless		(284)
	Larynx	Primary neuroendocrine tumors 1 case	Extremely rare in larynx	61-year-old, white	Supraglottic laryngectomy, radical neck dissection	Free of tumor 22 month after operation	(271)
	Larynx	Tumor primary malignant carinoid; 1 case				Endocrine and mucous differentiation	(56)
	Larynx	Clear cell carcinoma – 3 cases	Extremely rare in larynx		Very poor		(279)
	Trachea	Adenoid cystic ca	To tracheal wall, mediastinal structures; metastases to lungs, bone, liver and brain	42–44 yrs below 30–50 yrs.	Surgery, 5 yrs. survival 64%, 10 yrs. 39%, 15 yrs. 17%, also 22–30 yrs. survival		(18) pp. 148–152
	Bronchus	Adenoid cystic ca –	Distal metastasis	45 yrs.	Surgery: survival 4.8 yrs, conservative therapy: survival 2.8 yrs. 5 yrs. surv. 25%	H. Müller 1882	(16) pp. 153–155
	Lung	Blastoma, rarest pulmonary neoplasm, approx. 30 cases	20% of cases hematogenous metastasis to lung, brain, liver, skeleton	?	Surgery – (long survivors in localized disease) longest survivor 15 yrs. with intrathoracic extension up to 1 yr.		(18) pp. 306–308
	Respiratory tract	Mucoepidermoid ca 2–3%	Metastasis to bone (?)	60 yrs., one 32 yr. female	Radiotherapy, chemotherapy, one group with long survival, other group aggressive		(18) pp. 186–187
Simple cuboidal columnar epithelium	Prostate	Transitional cell ca 2.5% of prostatic ca	Local growth – pelvic lymph node metastasis and metastasis to bone, brain and lung	65 yrs. (?)	Surgery, survival 43–160 mos., radiation therapy: 26 mos. survival	Melicow and Hollowell 1952	(18) pp. 61–64
Sebaceous sweat glands	Sweat gland	Carcinoma 0.0011% of skin tumors	Tendency for local recurrence – preference for lymph. dissemination – regional and abdominal lymph node metastases, metastases to skeletal system – hematogenous, also metastasize to lung, pleura, liver, extremity	53 yrs. (24–84 yrs.) most in 6th to 7th decade – youngest 7 yrs.	Surgery, patients w/metastasis lived 10, 20 and 30 yrs. past diagnosis		(18) pp. 24–26

Table 5. Continued.

Tissue	Organ	Tumor and No. of reported cases	Rare or uncommon location	Type or spreading	Age General	Age Special	Treatment and prognosis	Established	Remarks	Reference
	Sebaceous gland	Carcinoma	-	Local recurrence - metastasis	60 yrs.		Surgery, radiotherapy, 5 yrs survival, 70% (Meibomian gland ca)			(18) pp. 27–29
	Parotid gland	Sebaceous cell ca, 2 cases	Parotid gland	Regional lymph nodes	9, 49 years old					(386)
	Eyelid	Meibomian sebaceous gland adenocarcinoma, approximately 200 cases	Eyelid	17–28% regional metastasis			Surgery, radiation therapy; when metastasized, prognosis is poor		Half of the patients where metastasis occurred survived 5 yrs	(236)
Mammary glands	Breast	Adenoid cystic ca, less than 100 cases	Breast gland	Metastases, without involvement of axillary lymph nodes	-		Favorable prognosis		In 79 only 6 well documented cases w/distant metastases were known	(223)
	Breast	Adenoid cystic ca	Breast gland	Nerve infiltration	-		Favorable			(350)
	Breast	Adenoid cystic ca, 0.4% of breast ca		Paucity of lymph node metastasis	50–55 yrs.		Surgery – favorable prognosis		Among 1/6 of tumors with this prognosis	(18) pp. 156–158
	Breast	Rare benign (0.6%; 0.3–9% respectively) rare malignant (6/213 cases)		No invasion, or metastasis	34–68 yrs.		Depending on tumor type		Rare neoplasms of the breast gland may be epithelial, nonepithelial or mixed gland responsible for malignancy	(212, 28)
	Breast	Cystosarcoma phyllodes 0.3–0.5% of all breast tumors		Local recurrence in 1st yr. – metastasis to lung (66%), bone (28%), heart, liver and nearly all organs	5–90 yrs. 58–60 yrs.		Surgery (radiation therapy)			(18) pp. 341–345
	Breast	Secretory ca, 19 cases	Breast	-	Children and adolescents					(349)
	Breast	Rare ductal ca							Normal antigens	(260)
	Breast	Signet ring cell ca		Stomach metastasis	51-yr-old female		Surgery; poor prognosis			(198)
Breast gland	Breast gland	Infiltrating ca with benign multinucleated osteoclast like giant cells – 8 cases	Breast gland	Metastasis			Not particularly favorable			(3)
	Breast gland	Primary carcinoma	Origin in cyst lining	-	-		-	-	-	(200)
	Breast gland	In males	Breast gland	-	Adults, elderly		Unfavorable, due to late diagnosis and detrimental anatomical condition	-	-	(139)
	Breast gland	Subareolar hamartoma	Muscular type							(52)

Site	Sub-site	Tumor	Detail	Metastasis / Recurrence	Age	Prognosis / Treatment	Author	Comments	Ref.
Salivary glands	Salivary glands	Mucoepidermoid ca		30% recurrence following surgical resection – metastasis infrequent	Major glands: 20–30 yrs. age – first to 8th decade, minor salivary glands	Surgery, radiotherapy – low grade tumors have survival of 5 yrs. (94%). high grade tumors, 56%	Stewart et al. 1945		(18) pp. 182-185
	Salivary glands (parotid gland)	Acinic cell ca		Recurrence – hematogenous metastasis to lung	Early teens to late years – mostly fourth and fifth decades	Surgery	Nasse, 1892	Long-time survival, even w/metastasis	(18) pp. 302-305
	Parotid gland	Carcinoma in cystadenolymphomas, 2 cases	Cystadeno-lymphomas			Radiotherapy			(321)
	Parotid gland	Acinic cell ca	In 11 and 12 year-old girls (27 were known in children under 5 years)	High recurrence				3% salivary gland tumors are of this type; 2/3 are females	(9)
	Salivary glands	Acinic cell tumor; 15 cases		Local recurrence, distant metastases	Mean age 41 yrs.	Well-differentiated, good; poorly differentiated, poor prognosis			(62)
Liver		Hepatoblastoma, 1 case	Extremely rare in adults		Adult			Mixed type from epithelial and mesenchymal cells	(287)
	Liver	Cystadenoma w/malignant change	Liver	Widespread metastases: liver, pancreas, spleen and peritoneal carcinomatosis	71-yr.-old male	Poor		Only 2 earlier cases in literature	(194)
	Liver	Primary ca presented as right-sided heart failure and pulmonary hypertension	Liver			Poor		Unique case	(46)
	Liver	Malignant mixed tumor of liver, 1 case	Liver		60-yr.-old male	Poor		Edmonson's grade II hepatocellular ca and chondrosarcoma	(189)
	Liver	Combined hepatocellular-cholangioca; 24 cases							(122)
	Liver	Hepatoblastoma; 2 cases	Liver			Poor to moderate		One patient alive after 2 yrs. and 8 mos; may be the longest survivor	(182)
Exocrine portion of pancreas	Exocrine pancreas	Cystadenoca of pancreas		Late metastases in liver, regional lymph nodes and peritoneum	45 yrs.		Kauffman 1911	76% in females	(18) pp. 338-340 (148)
	Exocrine pancreas	Distinctive solid and papillary epithelia		Metastasis	24-yr.-old ± 24 yrs woman	Mean survival ± 7 yrs.		Only 1 patient died of metastasis	(69)

Table 5. Continued.

Tissue	Organ	Tumor and No. of reported cases	Rare or uncommon location	Type or spreading	Age General	Age Special	Treatment and prognosis	Established	Remarks	Reference
	Exocrine pancreas	Gastrinoma		Recurrence – metastases to lymph nodes and liver (cause of death)	50–70 yrs., but also in those below 20 yrs.		Surgery	Zollinger and Ellison 1955	Familiar inclination	(18) pp. 325–328
	Exocrine pancreas	WDHA syndrome		Metastasis	45 yrs.		Surgery 14 mos survival	Verner and Morrison, 1958		(18) pp. 329–333
	Exocrine pancreas	Pancreatic ca 1 case; ca of pancreas, 1 case	Ureter metastasis		57-yr.-old man 50-yr.-old woman		Surgery poor		Obstruction of the ureter by pancreatic ca is very rare	(339)
	Exocrine pancreas	Tumor containing osteoclast-like cells	Pancreas						Unusual	(355)
Islets of Langerhans	Endocrine pancreas	Insulinoma		Metastases to regional lymph node and liver	42 yrs.		Benign, excellent – surgery if malignant 26 mos.	Wilder et al. 1927		(18) pp. 320–324
	Endocrine pancreas	Pancreatic glucagonoma, approx. 16 patients		Recurrence or metastasis	54 yrs.		Surgery, chemotherapy – long survival (7.13 yrs) due to slow progress of disease	McGavran et al. 1966		(18) pp. 334–337
	Endocrine pancreas	Primary carcinoid cell tumor, 1 case	Pancreatic head		44-yr.-old woman				May have originated from common neuro ectodermal recursor cells	(384)
	Endocrine pancreas	Islet cell ca and carcinoid tumors	Islet cells	Metastasis to liver, lung, bone, brain w/indolent course					Data for therapies are sparse because such malignancies are so rare	(55)
Pineal gland	Pineal gland	Primary pinealoblastoma, with photoreceptor differentiation	Pineal gland			2, 5-year-old boy		Manschot, 1979	First case of this type of tumor	(237, 238)
Pituitary gland										
Thyroid gland	Thyroid gland	Anomalous papillary ca, 1 case	Thyroid gland	Metastasis to thoracic wall, both groins, thigh, lymph nodes	70-year-old woman		9 years after thyroidectomy	Johannesen 1983	1983 the only described case with tetraploid DNS values	(169)
Parathyroid glands	Glomus jugulare	Chemodectoma		Local recurrence (15–20 yrs.) – distant metastasis in 2–4% of cases	Average 48.1 yrs 23–78 yrs.		Surgery diff., radiation therapy	Rosenwasser 1945	Pleural predominance	(18) pp. 291–294
	Glomus intravagale	Chemodectoma		Local invasion, distant metastasis	44–45 yrs.		Surgery	Stout, 1935		(18) pp. 295–296
	Organ of Zuckerkandl	Tumors		Invasion, metastasis	33–38 yrs. (6–81 yrs)		Surgery, palliative radiation therapy			(18) pp. 297–299

Organ	Site	Tumor	Spread / Metastasis	Age / Sex	Treatment	Year	Comments	Reference
	(Lung, prostate, gallbladder, pancreas)	Paragangliomas in bladder, stomach, thyroid, larynx, trachea, orbit	e.g. of duodenum, none metastasized	20 yrs. and over	Surgery		May occur in each organ	(18) pp. 300–301
Parathyroid glands	Parathyroid glands	Carcinoma	Recurrence (70%) metastasis in 30%	44-45 yrs.	Surgery (radiotherapy after recurrence): 5 yrs. survival 50%, 10 yrs. 13% (4 to 5 yrs.)		Death through toxicity of hyperparathyroid state	(18) pp. 30–33
Parathyroid glands	Carotid body	Chemodectoma 500 cases are known	Metastasis: regional lymph nodes, distal viscera, especially lung – vertebrae, ribs	3rd and 4th decades	Surgery			(18) pp. 286–290
	Parathyroid glands	Parathyroid ca					The tumor is a rare cause of hyperparathyroidism	(299)
	Parathyroid glands	Hyperfunctioning parathyroid ca, 12 cases			2-14, and 16-yr. survival after diagnosis and early surgery			(364)
Adrenal glands	Adrenal glands	Primary retroperitoneal tumors					These tumors are rare	(138)
	Adrenal cortex	Adrenal cortical ca, 0.04% of all ca cases	Metastatic to retroperitoneal lymph nodes (68%), lung (71%), liver (42%), bone (26%)	3-74 yrs., median, 53 yrs.	Surgery, survival 3 to 34 yrs. after operation		A second primary ca was found to occur in 20.4% of cases. Breast and lymphoma were most common	(82, 131, 348, 373)
Adrenal medulla	Duodenum	Gangliocytic paraganglioma and duodenal adenocarcinoma – first case? Pheochromocytoma 1 case	Rare association — Metastasis to two regional lymph nodes	71, male			Immunohistochem.	(14)
Adrenal glands	Adrenal medulla	Pheochromocytoma 1 case	Primary in wall of atrium — Metastases	70-yr.-old white female				(370)
	Adrenal medulla	Pheochromocytoma 1 case	Extension into inferior vena cava — Direct		Surgery		Coexistence in this case of a primary bronchoalveolar adenoca was previously unreported	(304)
	Adrenal medulla	Pheochromocytoma	Approximately 100 cases of this t. of the urinary bladder have been reported — Hypogastric lymph nodes	Young to old age w/peak in 4th decade	Pheochromocytosis in the bladder have a more favorable prognosis than those in classical sites	1953	Surgery should include iliohypogastric lymphadenectomy	(76, 103, 242, 289)
Testis	Testis	Polyembryoma, choriocarcinoma are extremely rare						(219, 253)
	Testis	Choriocarcinoma					Distinguished by cyto- and syncytiotrophoblastic cells	(245)

Table 5. Continued.

Tissue	Organ	Tumor and No. of reported cases	Rare or uncommon location	Type or spreading	Age General	Age Special	Treatment and prognosis	Established	Remarks	Reference
Testis	Testis	Malignant chorionic gonadotropin producing germ cell tumor case 1	Anterior mediastinum		36-year-old man				The tumor included components of teratoma, seminoma, and embryonal ca., and produced luteinizing hormone, estrogen, alpha-fetoprotein and lactic dehydrogenase.	(267)
	Breast	Lymph angiosarcoma		Distant metastases are frequent	82 yrs.		Amputation, radiotherapy 19 mos. survival	Stewart and Treves, 1948	See chapter 21/Vol. VI	(18) pp. 241–244
	Nasal region	Angioendotheliomatosis, 1 case 40 reported previously		Systemic dissemination		62-year-old woman				(380)
	Nasopharynx	Hemangioendothelioma	Head and neck region	Benign		52-year-old female	Good		First report in literature	(254)
	Kidney	Hemangioendothelioma	Kidney	Local recurrence, widespread vascular metastases			Very poor prognosis		Hurricane course of or weeks after traditional therapy	(58)
	Spleen	Hemangioma	Spleen	Extensive systemic metastasis	42-year-old man		Poor			(259)
	Femur and tibia	Hemangioendothelioma	Femur and tibia		57-year-old man					(317)
	Vein	Epithelioid hemangioendothelioma	Soft tissue, mediumsized vein	Local recurrences, metastases			Favorable prognosis			(378)
	Soft tissues	Hemangiopericytoma	Soft tissue	High local recurrence						(22)
	Head and neck	Multiple congenital hemangiopericytoma					More benign clinical course			(320)
Testis/ovary	Testis	Gonadoblastoma		Gonadoblastoma does not metastasize but secondary germinomas do	10–38 yrs.		Surgery; gonadoblastoma transformed into embryonal ca, sinus tumors, or chorioca: 18 mos survival	Scully 1953		(18) pp. 369–373
Testis	Testis	Sertoli cell tumor		Recurrence in skin metastasis to lymph nodes, bone	All ages		Inguinal orchiectomy		Stromal tumor	(18) pp. 372–374

Organ	Tumor	Location	Behavior / Metastasis	Age	Treatment / Survival	Author / Year	Notes	Reference
Testis	Interstitial Leydig-cell tumor, 3% of all testicular neoplasms		Metastasis to retroperitoneal nodes, liver, lung, and others, such as skeletal system, abdominal cavity, inguinal, pelvic nodes	Children and in adults only malignant	Radical orchiectomy – 3 yr. survival if malignant form		Stromal tumor	(18) pp. 375–376
Testis	Seminoma, extremely rare in children			Peak at fourth and fifth decade				(203)
Testis	Adenoca of rete testis, approx. 14 cases		Metastasis to local inguinal iliac and periaortic and mediastinal lymph nodes	42 yrs. (30 yr. + up)	Surgery (orchiectomy) – radiotherapy, survival 1 mo. to 4.5 yrs.		One of rarest neoplasms	(18) pp. 44–45
Testis	Germinoma, 9 cases				Rapid response to radiation			(161)
Testis	Feminizing Leydig cell t., 1 case						Questionable if benign or malignant	(75)
Testis, ovary	Germ cell tumors of the pineal and suprasellar region, ?? subtypes		Metastasis to cerebral or spinal subarachnoid species	?	Surgery? radiation	D. Russell 1944		(18) pp. 117–127
Testis, ovary	Germ cell tumors of mediastinum and retroperitoneum		Metastasis to adjacent lymph nodes	27–29 yrs. 15–35 yrs.	Radiotherapy? seminoma: 5 yr. survival, 54%; embryonal ca, no survivors past 2 yrs.; teratorca, 4–5 mos.	Schlumberger 1946		(18) pp. 128–132
Testis	Germ cell tumors	Mediastinum						(298)
Testis	Bilateral seminomas	Testes	Metastasis to chest	51-year-old man	Orchiectomies			(27)
Testis	Primary mediastinal seminoma	Mediastinum	No metastases 6 years after treatment	12-year-old boy	Endoxan and tele-cobalt therapy			(336)
Testis	Primary choriocarcinoma of mediastinum, 1 case	Mediastinum	Death due to massive metastasis on 20th post-operative day	19-year-old male	Surgery			(377)
Ovary	Malignant mixed Müllerian tumors, 1.1% of all malignant primary neoplasms	–	Metastasis to liver and lung	5th to 6th decade	Surgery, postoperative radiotherapy, median survival, 6–8 mos.		Sarcomatous elements predominant in metastasis (histologically)	(18) pp. 214–215
Ovary	Clear cell ca.		Local pelvic metastasis	40–60 yrs.	Surgery – stage I, 57% 5 yrs. survival; stage II, 16% 5 yrs. survival	Schiller 1939		(18) pp. 56–58
Ovary	Granulosa cell tumor		Recurrence along peritoneal spaces; distant metastases extremely rare	50 yrs 3.5 yrs	Surgery 20-yr. survival, 58.3%	von Rokitansky 1855	Thecoma, granulosa cell tumors	(18) pp. 346–351

Table 5. Continued.

Tissue	Organ	Tumor and No. of reported cases	Rare or uncommon location	Type or spreading	Age General	Age Special	Treatment and prognosis	Established	Remarks	Reference
Ovary	Ovary	Granulosa cell tumor, complicated with dermoid cyst		Very rare						(313)
	Ovary	Dysgerminoma, 1–2% all primary ovarian tumors			12–54 yrs.		Surgery, radiation; prognosis good, 5 yrs. 86%	Chenot 1911		(18) pp. 352–356 (211)
	Ovary	Endodermal sinus tumor			1.5–40 yrs.		Surgery, radiotherapy, chemotherapy	Schiller 1939		(18) pp. 357–360
	Ovary	Endodermal sinus tumor, 13 cases	Other location		below 1 yr.		Surgery, chemotherapy, 5 yr. survival less than 10%	Thiele 1971		(18) p. 361
	Ovary	Brenner tumor		Recurrence, metastasis to lung and bone	50 yrs.		Surgery, radiation therapy 5 yrs. surv. 5%	Brenner 1907		(18) pp. 362–364 (226)
	Ovaries	Cystic ovarian tumors and focus of anaplastic carcinoma		Dissemination		50 yrs.	Hysterectomy, bilateral salpingo-oophorectomy; poor prognosis		Refused further therapy; died 12 mos after operation	(136)
	Ovary	Androblastoma, less than 1% of all ovarian neoplasms		Recurrence metastasis ??	10–40 (34) y		Surgery, prognosis poor		Strong stromal; during pregnancy more malignant	(18) pp. 365–68
	Ovary	Malignant struma ovarii – approx. 20 cases reported	Ovaries, bilateral	Multiple metastases					Resembles papillary and follicular ca of thyroid gl. ultrastructure	(273)
Urachus	Urachus	Carcinoma of urachus		Local recurrence, metastases	5th and 6th decade		Surgery, radiation	Campbell, Begg 1931		(18) pp. 34–37
	Ovary	Giant ovarian cyst, endometrial ovarian ca		Peritoneal metastasis	61-year-old woman				The abdomen increased in 10 hours to a waist measure of 188 cm.	(16)
	Ovary	Choriocarcinoma	Two metastases on anterior wall of vagina, several cm behind urethral meatus						Metastases are rare (14–20%), but clinically very distinct.	(71)
	Ovary	Juxtaovarian tumor, 19 cases	Adnexal region	Recurrence, metastases					Low malignant potential	(177)
	Ovary	Teratoma, grade IIb	Ovary	Metastasis			Surgery, 2 mo–1, 4 yr after			(135)
	Ovary	Primary intracranial yolk sac tumor, 3 cases	Pineal location in two cases, suprasellar in one	Metastases restricted to peritoneum						(265)

Category	Organ	Tumor	Location	Metastasis / behavior	Age	Treatment / prognosis	Notes	Ref.
Desmal epithelium	Ovary	Clear cell ca (mesonephroma), 7 patients	Ovary		39–60 years old (average 50 years)		Only one case reported in China by 1955	(99)
	Ovary	Gestational trophoblastic neoplasm	Ovary				Quite rare in Sweden	(341)
	Ovary	Adult teratoma	Ovary		16-year-old girl		With highly differentiated glia	(137)
	Ovary	Mature solid teratoma	Ovary	Gliomatosis peritonei		Prognosis excellent	Treatment of metastasis unnecessary	(95)
	Scalp	Unusual vascular tumor			51-year-old man			(78)
	Heart	Myxoma (most common intracavitary cardiac tumor)		Local recurrence metastasis e.g. to hip	young adult	Surgery	Basically benign tumors	(18) pp. 309–311
	Pericard	Mesothelioma, 100 cases		Direct extension, rarely, metastasis outside thorax	40 yrs.	Chemotherapy		(18) pp. 92–94
	Pericard	Malignant mesothelioma, 1 case		Metastases to lung and regional lymph nodes	54-year-old male		First case from China	(225)
	Omentum	Angiosarcoma		Widespread metastases in viscera and CNS	61-year-old man	Surgery, poor prognosis	Very aggressive tumor	(47)
	Skin	Angiosarcoma of skin and of head and neck		Multicentric extension	12–74 yrs.	Surgery – radiation, survival 1 yr. prognosis: poor 40% 5-yr surviv.		(18) pp. 221–223
	Breast	Angiosarcoma, some 50 cases reported	Breast	Lung metastases	23–24 yrs.	Surgery, prognosis poor		(325)
		Angiosarcoma, 1 case		Hematogenic lung metastasis recurrences	47-year-old woman	Prognosis unfavorable	about first reported occurrence in 2 sisters	(153)
		Angiosarcoma	Breast	Dissemination		5 cases with 5 yrs disease-free survival		(59)
	Bone	Hemangiosarcoma	Very rare primary tumor	No metastases after 4 years, from operation	31 yrs.	Up to 4 years follow up, good	Diagnosis by cytophotometric DNA-measurements	(2)
Mesenchyme		Mesenchymal tumor (desmoid) and malignant lymphoma	Two rare tumors				Caused by exposure to polychlorinated biphenyls	(124)
Desmal ep.	Head and neck	Synovial sarcoma, 80 cases known	Head and neck			Radical surgery with, postoperative radio-therapy and chemo-therapy		(235)

Table 5. Continued.

Tissue	Organ	Tumor and No. of reported cases	Rare or uncommon location	Age (General)	Age (Special)	Type or spreading	Treatment and prognosis	Established	Remarks	Reference
Desmal epithelium	Bone	Angiosarcoma of bone		All ages. 30–35 yrs		Local and distant recurrence	Surgery 5 yrs. 40%	Stout 1943		(18) pp. 224–226
	Liver	Angiosarcoma of liver, 6% of all primary hepatic tumors	–	Infantile and adult form		?	Chemotherapy, radiotherapy, P: poor, survival 3–4 mos.			(18) pp. 227–229
	Spleen	Angiosarcoma of spleen, very rare	–			Early metastasis to liver, lymph nodes, and bones				(18) p. 230
	Heart	Angiosarcoma of heart, 58 cases	–	41 yrs.		Metastasis to lung, liver, lymph nodes, bones	Surgery, radio-chemotherapy, 6 mos. survival			(18) pp. 231–233
	Breast	Angiosarcoma of breast, 48 cases (1976)		Female 2nd and 3rd decades		Blood borne metastasis in skin, bone, lungs, liver, ovaries, and gastro-intestinal tract	Mastectomy, 5 yrs., survival 5%			(18) pp. 234–235
Desmal epithelium		Hemangiopericytoma	–	Teens to octogenarians (41–84 yrs.)		Multiple local recurrence, metastasis, especially to lungs and bones	Surgery, chemotherapy	Stout and Murray 1942	Generally benign course in children	(18) pp. 236–240
		Hemangiopericytoma 3 women	Right sinus, trachea, epiglottis			Frequent metastasis to bones, lungs, and liver			In children rarely malignant	(43)
	Lung	Intravascular bronchioalveolar tumor				Low incidence of metastases, slow clinical course			Related to hemangioendothelioma, endovascular papillary angioendothelioma	(35)
	Serous membranes	Primary tumors							Relatively rare	(125)
Desmal epithelium/synovial origin	Joints? head, neck	Synovial sarcoma of head and neck	–	20–40 yrs.		Few lymph node metastases	Surgery, radiotherapy, chemotherapy, 5 yr. survival 23.5% to (33%) 51%	Smith 1927		(18) pp. 106–109
Desmal epithelium		Epithelioid sarcoma	–	23–29 yrs.		Local recurrence, lymph node, metastasis later	Amputation 60% 5 yr. survival	Enzinger 1970	Male predominance	(18) pp. 259–261
	Tendons, aponeurosis	Clear cell sarcoma of tendons and aponeurosis	–	32 yrs.		Local recurrence and regional lymph node metastasis	Local excision – in case of metastatic type survival for 5 yrs. 292%	Enzinger 1965		(18) pp. 256–258

System	Organ	Tumor	Localization	Metastasis / Dissemination	Age	Prognosis	Comments	Ref
Mesenchyme	Soft tissues	Mesenchymal chondrosarcomas 2 patients	Spinal cord, elbow	Meningeal metastasis, dissemination in lungs, skin, bones and muscles	19 and 27 yrs	Extremely poor	Undifferentiated mesenchymatous cells and mature cartilage are characteristic, typically occurring in young females	(282)
	Heart	Malignant mesenchymoma, 1 case	Left atrium	Metastases to left femur, lung, and hilar lymph nodes	46-year-old woman	Poor	Tumor was composed of mesenchymal elements of fibro-, rhabdo-, chondro- myxo- and liposarcoma	(344)
Reticular connective tissue	Testis	Acute lymphoblastic leukemia	Testis	Testicular metastasis, 11 yrs. after diagnosis of acute lymphoblastic leukemia; pulmonary complications			First time a secondary tumor appeared 9 yrs. after treatment of primary t. and order of pulmonary complications	(133)
	Blood	Pure red cell aplasia					Sometimes associated w/thymomas or solid ca	(387)
	Mediastinum, pelvis, bones, lymph nodes, testes, epidural area, heart	Acute monoblastic leukemia, 4 cases			3 under 6 yrs. of age			(280)
	Blood	Histiocytic lymphoma, cervical ca, 2 cases					Peripheral eosinophilia associated w/malignant disease is a marker of disease progression w/ poor prognosis	(297)
	Blood	Acute megakaryoblastic leukemia, 2 children	Cells in bone marrow	Dissemination			Rare leukemia	(292)
Reticular connective tissue	Various organs	Multicentric reticulohistiocytosis	Subcutis, bone, lung, pericard, larynx, one case				Huge subcut. nodules, bone destruction, pulmonary fibrosis, acute pericarditis, laryngeal compression	(13)
Reticular connective tissue	Lymphatic system	Plasmocytoma	Connected w/hypereosinophilia				Second hypereosinophilia connected w/IgG plasmacytoma	(231)
	Blood	Subacute myelomonocytic leukemia	Dissemination		70-yr-old male	No response to cytostatic treatment		(146)

Table 5. Continued.

Tissue	Organ	Tumor and No. of reported cases	Rare or uncommon location	Type or spreading	Age — General	Age — Special	Treatment and prognosis	Established	Remarks	Reference
Stomach	Stomach	Solitary plasmacytoma, 1 case	Stomach		71-yr-old man		Gastrectomy, splenectomy, radiotherapy; poor prognosis			(360)
		T-lymphomas are rare								(362)
		Hodgkin's disease	Gastrointestinal tract locations are rare							(314)
	Thigh muscle	Lymphoma, 2 cases	Intramuscular				Special techniques			(175)
		Non-Hodgkin's lymphoma, 37 patients	Unusual sites: psoas/iliacus muscle (16 p.), kidney (13 p.), pancreas (5 p.), adrenals (4 p.), skin/subcutaneous tissue (4 p.), abdominal wall musculature (4 p.), peritoneum (4 p.), omentum (3 p.), female reproductive tract (3 p.)						Extranodal involvement was rarely the only site of initial or recurrent lymphoma	(118)
	Lymphatic system	Lymphangioma	mesentery							(363)
CNS		Lymphoma, primary lymphoma; 2% of extranodal non-Hodgkin's lymphomas	Primary CNS lesions				Radiotherapy, surgery median survival 15 mos.			(115, 229)
		Fibrous histiocytoma, 7 personal cases, 63 from literature	Oral and maxillo-facial regions							(352)
	Pelvis, mammary gland	Burkitt-like lymphoma and acute leukemia	Mamma and pelvis		Young female				Renal insufficiency and metabolic acidosis caused death.	(12)
Melanogenic system*										
Adipose tissue	Perineum	Liposarcoma 1 case	Perineum	Invasion			Surgical extirpation		Perineal liposarcoma is extremely rare.	(156)
	Bone	Primary liposarcoma, 1 case	Bone	Large metastasis in left lung	19-year-old white male		Surgery, radiation and chemotherapy; death 10 mos. after diagnosis.			(1)

* For topographically rarely located melanomas see chapter 16/Vol. VIII.

Tissue	Tumor	Location	Metastasis/Clinical	Patient	Treatment	Comment	Ref.
Bone	Primary osteoliposarcoma	Bone		57- and 37-year-old women		More favorable prognosis than osteosarcoma	(73)
Knee	Infiltrating angiolipoma	Knee		19- and 13-year-old white males	Surgery – first patient was disease-free for the last 10 years	Infiltrating angiolipoma is rare	(372)
Lung	Lipoma and liposarcoma, three cases	Endobronchial and pulmonary			Bronchioscopy or lobectomy	The tumors are more rare in the lung than in the bronchi	(84)
Tongue	Lipomas and sarcomas	Mobile tongue				These tumors and other sarcomas are rare in the mobile tongue	(111)
Adipose tissue / Kidneys	Bilateral renal angiomyolipomas with Bourneville's tuberous sclerosis, 1 case			Child			(141)
Kidneys	Bilateral angiolipomas and bilateral hypernephromas of both kidneys with tuberous sclerosis 1 case	Rare combination of kidney tumors					(4)
Reticular connective tissue / Lymphatic system	Nodular, poorly differentiated lymphocytic lymphoma, 1 case	Ruptured cerebral arterial aneurism due to infiltration of lymphoma	Spleen and abdominal lymph nodes	55-yr.-old woman		In contrast to leukemias, cerebral hemorrhage in non-Hodgkin's lymphomas is extremely rare	(294)
Salivary glands	Primary malignant lymphoma	Salivary glands					(221)
Esophagus	Lymphosarcoma, 1 case	Esophagus	Metastasis		Radiotherapy, chemotherapy	Patient alive and free of tumor 6 yrs. after diagnosis	(262)
Esophagus	Malignant lymphoma	Esophagus	Metastasis to local lymph nodes, early infiltrating squamous cell ca	56-yr.-old female	Surgery		(385)
Testis	Reticulum cell sarcoma, 2 cases	Testis		75-and 49-yr.-old men			(233)
	Lymphoepithelioma		Metastasis through anterior vertebral vein	53-yr old man			(347)
	Burkitt's lymphoma	Nerve involvement remote from obvious systemic tumor and brain parenchymal involvement from junction w/nerves					(351)
	Plasmacytoma, 4 patients	Primary intracranial	Dissemination		Surgery		(166)

Table 5. Continued.

Tissue	Organ	Tumor and No. of reported cases	Rare or uncommon location	Type or spreading	Age (General)	Age (Special)	Treatment and prognosis	Established	Remarks	Reference
	Urethra	Extramedullary plasmacytoma	Urethra	Metastasis					First known case, perhaps a late metastasis	(54)
Reticular connective tissue	Nose, nasopharynx, paranasal sinus	Extramedullary plasmacytoma	Skin, CNS, lung, gastrointestinal tract, breast	?	4th and 5th decades		Surgery and radiation		211 patients, male predominance	(18) pp. 110-116
	Nasal cavity and paranasal sinus	Extramedullary plasmacytoma, 7 cases	Nasal cavity and paranasal sinus		37 to 47-yrs		Surgery			(228)
	Thymus	Thymoma, 1 case	2 autoimmune disease, abnormal hypogamma-globulinemia and thymoma	Intrathoracic metastasis	45-yr-old woman		Surgery			(205)
Reticular connective tissue	Thymus	Malignant thymoma (mixed lympho-epithelial), 1 case	Distant metastases	To liver, large peripancreatic and mesenteric lymph nodes, involvement of stomach; micrometastases in myocardium	37-yr-old patient		Surgery poor prognosis			(155)
	Thymus	Thymoma, 1 case	Pleura	Metastasizing					Unusual pleural involvement or metastasizing t.	(134)
	Trachea	Tracheal mass, 1 case	Trachea	No recurrence or metastasis up to 27 mos.	26-yr.-old man		Bronchoscopy			(128)
	Mast cells	Mast cell neoplasias							Mastocytosis lacking primary skin lesions may be aggravated by myeloproliferative disorders and mast cell leukemia. Mast cell sarcoma is extremely rare	(274)
Gelatinous connective tissue	Appendix and ovary	Pseudomyxoma peritonei	Rare complication of mucocele, adenoca of appendix, cystadenoma or cystadenoca of ovary						Precise demonstration possible w/CT	(240)
Gelatinous connective tissue	Shoulder	Myxosarcoma, 1 case	Skin	Metastases very rarely	44-yr-old woman		Surgery			(199)

Tissue	Site	Tumor	Location	Age / demographics	Behavior	Treatment / survival	Comments	Reference
Fibrous connective tissue	Endometrium	Endometrial stromal tumors, 0.2% of all uterine ca	–	42–47 yrs.	Local recurrence metastasis esp. to lung	Surgery, 5 yrs. survival Koss 55%?		(18) pp. 217–220
	Soft tissue	Fibrosarcoma			Metastasizing		Relatively rare	(17)
	Heart	Fibrosarcoma of heart	–	Very young to very old	Metastasis to brain	Surgery		(18) pp. 98–99
		Malignant fibroxanthoma	–		High recurrence (73%) and high metastasis			(18) pp. 266–270
	Head and neck	Fibrosarcoma, less than 50 cases, congenital solitary; unique case of fibrosarcoma in oral cavity		Neonate	Metastasis is rare, local recurrence frequent		1% of head and neck malignancies	(32)
	Bone	Fibrosarcoma, 1 case	Bone	46-yr.-old man	Metastasis to the skin and later to sacrum, rib, and sternoclavicular joint	Surgery		(329)
	Bone	Multifocal fibrosarcoma, 1 case	Left ilium	50-yr.-old woman	Metastasis in liver and lung	Surgery		(160)
	Scapula	Chondromyxoid fibroma	Scapula		No recurrence or metastasis 2½ yrs. after surgery	Surgery, good prognosis		(359)
	Dermis	Dermatofibrosarcoma protuberans, a rare fibrosarcoma	Dermis	64-yr.-old white man	Frequent recurrence, rare metastasis	Surgery	Slow clinically course, 20 yrs in mentioned case	(130, 225)
Fibrous connective tissue	Gingiva	Malignant fibrohistiocytoma	Gingiva				p 21 *ras* oncoprotein	(346)
		Juvenile hyaline fibromatosis one case						(6)
Chorda tissue	Chorda	Chordoma						(18) pp. 278–285
		Cranium (36%)		38 cases (10–39 yrs)				
		Vertebral (15%)						
		Sacrococygeal (49%)		53 cases (50–60 yrs)				
Cartilage	Larynx	Chondrosarcoma; 0.14–0.16% of laryngeal malignancy		5th and 6th decades	Metastases to regional lymph nodes extremely rare – local recurrence – metastatic to lung	Surgery, good prognosis	These chondrosarcomas arise only from hyalin and not from elastic cartilage of the larynx; 70% males	(18)pp. 101–103
	Extraskeletal (soft tissues)	Extraskeletal chondrosarcoma approx. 50 cases		46 yrs.	Recurrence metastases: lymph nodes and lungs	Surgery – 5 yrs. survival 68.4%; Stout and Verner, 1952	Better prognosis of extraskeletal than skeletal chondrosarcoma	(18) pp. 104–105
	Knee	Benign chondroblastoma		18-year-old male				(193)

Table 5. Continued.

Tissue	Organ	Tumor and No. of reported cases	Rare or uncommon location	Type or spreading	Age – General	Age – Special	Treatment and prognosis	Established	Remarks	Reference
	Lower abdomen	Retrovesical chondrosarcoma, 1 patient	Retrovesical region	No local recurrence or metastasis after surgery			Surgery good		First reported case	(195)
		Malignant chondroblastoma			Children		Combined therapy			(114)
	Petrous apex	Benign chondroma			60-year-old woman				Extremely rare	(196)
	Base of skull, convexity of skull	Chondroma 41 and 32 cases respectively in 1975	Skull							
	Trachea	Chondrosarcoma, 1 observed case; 4 in English literature	Trachea				Longest survival is 17 years, prognosis generally poor		Extraordinarily rare tumors	(327)
Bone	Bones	Primary tumors of bone							Rare	(256)
	Hard palate	Primary malignancies							Rare	(63)
	Bone	Benign osteoblastoma, 1% of bone tumors – two fatal cases		Recurrence, and lung metastasis	Males 6 and 19 years					(224)
	Temporal bone	Osteosarcoma	Destroying pyramid and paralyzing facial nerve	Metastases to lung and regional lymph nodes		7-year-old girl				(268)
	Jaws	Osteosarcoma 66 cases	Jaws	Only in 4, metastasis to lung, cervical lymph nodes, spine and brain; most died of uncontrolled local disease	12–79 years, mean 34 years		Chondroblastic osteosarcoma showed best survival		Rare	(65)
	Bone	Osteogenic sarcoma							Rare	(167)
	Knee	Epithelioid osteogenic sarcoma	Left knee	Massive metastasis to the lungs		21-year-old male	Surgery; death after 12 months		Rare variation	(120)
		Multiple osteogenic sarcoma	Many bones	Liver involvement		9-year-old boy			Very rare entity, with widespread osseous destruction	(300)
	Patella	Giant cell tumor, 2 cases	Patella	First patient 7 years after surgery, no metastasis		22-year-old male, 27-year-old female	Surgery		Rare	(193)
	Bone	Ameloblastoma								(113)
Bone	Bone and lung	Osteosarcoma of mandible and lung cancer, 1 case	Rare combination							(266)

Origin	Site	Tumor	Metastatic spread	Age	Treatment / prognosis	Remarks	Ref.
Bone	Long bones, pelvis	Ewing's sarcoma	Lung, skeleton, sometimes nervous system; rapid development of dissemination	10–20 years	Poor	Rare tumor	(285)
Bone	Left orbitonasal region	Extraosseous Ewing's sarcoma	Metastasis to frontal lobe of homolateral cerebral hemisphere	50-year-old woman	Radiotherapy, chemotherapy; no recurrence 6 months after treatment		(366)
Bone	Tibia	Adamantinoma	Late local recurrence and lung metastasis			Rare tumor	(11)
Bone	Finger	Osteofibroma				Very rare	(337)
Smooth muscle	Heart	Leiomyosarcoma of the heart, perhaps 5–10 cases	Widespread metastasis			The existence of this tumor is sometimes questioned	(18) pp. 95–96
	Aorta	Sarcomas (fibrosarcomas, 1 leiomyosarcoma) until 1977, 50 cases in English literature	Metastases, bone, liver, kidneys, and spleen, sometimes without dissemination	50–60 yrs. 56 yrs. 1 infant 3½ mos.	Surgical resection, graft replacement	Male predominance	(18) pp. 312–313
	Pulmonary artery	Sarcomas (leiomyosarcomas, fibrosarcomas, undiff. sarcoma, mesenchymomas) 37 patients	Lung metastasis, sarcomatous metastasis to hilar and mediastinal nodes (16%)	52 yrs.	Surgery, prognosis extremely poor; survival 12 mos. (1–39 mos.)	Male predominance	(18) pp. 314–316
	Superior and inferior vena cava	Leiomyosarcoma 22 cases	Recurrence, late metastatic spreading: liver (17%)	60 yrs.	Surgery 1 and 2 yrs.		(18) pp. 317–319
	Uterus	Benign metastasizing leiomyoma 1 case	Metastasis				(335)
Smooth muscle	Pelvic promontory lymph node	Leiomyomatosis, leiomyomatosis peritonealis disseminata 2 cases	Distribution	50- and 41-year-old women	Prognosis favorable, surgery only		(154)
	Small intestine	Leiomyosarcoma, 0.2% of malignancies of gastrointestinal tract, 28 patients	Lymph node, diffuse			Rare tumor	(60)
	Jejunum	Leiomyoma 73 cases reviewed, 1 original case		55-year-old woman		Rare tumor	(145)
	Cecum	Bizarre leiomyoblastoma, Leser-Trelat syndrome, 1 case		62-year-old man		8 cases of leiomyoblastoma of small intestine (5/8 malignant) reported in Japan.	(163)
	Bladder	Leiomyosarcoma	No metastases	4-year-old girl	Radical cystectomy; 6 years later, free of metastases		(216)

Table 5. Continued.

Tissue	Organ	Tumor and No. of reported cases	Rare or uncommon location	Type or spreading	Age		Treatment and prognosis	Established	Remarks	Reference
					General	Special				
	Colon	Leiomyosarcoma, 1 case	Ascending colon	Extensive metastasis					Leiomyosarcoma of colon, excluding rectum, is exceedingly rare	(295)
	Colon	Leiomyosarcoma, 1 case	Descending colon	Metastases in lungs, left kidney, pancreas, vertebral bodies, peritoneum, mesentery, bone marrow	39-year-old woman		Hysterectomy		Rare	(249)
Smooth musculature	Vein	Leiomyosarcoma, 1 case	Femoral vein	Pulmonary metastases	64-year-old man				Leiomyosarcomas in venous smooth muscle are rare and have a higher mortality rate	(232)
	Vein	Leiomyosarcoma, 1 case	In branch of long saphenous vein	No recurrence or metastasis 3 months after excision	64-year-old man		Excision		Very rare case	(269)
	Vein	Leiomyosarcoma, 1 case reported, 51 cases reviewed	Inferior vena cava		46-year-old man				Rare primary malignant tumor, usually fatal	(276)
	Uterus	Leiomyoma obstructing inferior vena cava and extending into right atrium; 1 case reported, 50 cases reviewed, including 3 of direct extension of pelvic veins into right atrium	Inferior vena cava to right atrium		46-year-old woman		Surgery		Venous extension of uterine leiomyoma is rare.	(353)
	Lung	Leiomyosarcoma, 1 case	Lung	Recurrence, fatal metastasis	14-month-old boy		Surgery, radio- and chemotherapy		These rare tumors may be curable by total excision	(270)
Mesoderm?	Uterus	Sarcomas develop from stromal cells into epithelial and stromal components			63–68 yrs.		Surgery – 5 yr. survival 32% w/homologous variation and 14% heterologous type, 26.7% (41%) carcinosarcoma 16.7%, mixed mesodermal tumor (31%)		In one series of 48 patients obesity was found in (41.7%) hypertension (31.3%) and diabetes (10.4%)	(18) pp. 208–213

Tissue	Tumor	Site	Behavior / metastasis	Age	Treatment / prognosis	Eponym	Notes	Reference
Transverse striated (skeletal) muscle	Malignant granular cell myoblastoma malignant variation 3%	Esophagus	Local recurrence; metastasize lymphatic and hematogenous; very commonly to regional lymph nodes and distant to lung, liver, skeleton and brains	45 yrs.	Surgery; prognosis poor, 5 yr. survival 25%	Abrikossoff 1931	Rare	(16) pp. 251–255
Esophagus	Granular cell myoblastoma	Esophagus		48-year-old man				(358)
Spermatic cord	Embryonal rhabdomyosarcoma	Spermatic cord						(356)
Soft tissue	Rhabdomyosarcoma	Involvement of lymph centers is rare						(57)
Head and neck	Embryonal rhabdomyosarcoma, 3 cases	Palate; ear and mastoid; nasopharynx w/orbital involvement		Children				(96)
Lung	Primary rhabdomyosarcoma, 1 case; 18 reviewed from world literature	Lung	Metastasis in pleura, hilus and mediastinum	22-yr old male	Poor		Very rare disease, not previously reported in China	(220)
Spermatic cord	Rhabdomyosarcoma, 58th case reported in the literature	Spermatic cord	No evidence of recurrence of metastasis one year after surgery	5-year-old boy	Orchiectomy, lymphadenectomy, chemotherapy			(302)
Muscle	Congenital rhabdomyosarcoma, 1 patient	Muscle	Widespread metastases to many locations	Infant, 4 hours old	Death four hours after birth		First case from China, less than 30 cases in the literature	(383)
Urethra, kidney	Fetal rhabdomyoma after nephroblastoma			Child	Nephrectomy, excellent prognosis			(85)
Cardiac muscle	Rhabdomyosarcoma of heart, approx. 45 cases	Heart	Dissemination to lung, liver and mediastinal lymph nodes	45 yrs.	Surgery – radiation therapy, chemotherapy			(18) pp. 96–97
schwannoma (generally, in lower rate); solitary	Alveolar soft part sarcoma		25% local recurrence, metastasis to lung; 50% of patients develop metastasis	Young females, 20 yrs., males 30 yrs.	Surgery? 5 yr. survival 59%	Christopherson, 1952	Young females have better prognosis	(18) pp. 262–265
Transverse striated (skeletal) muscle	Polymorphic rhabdomyosarcoma, rhabdomyosarcoma, rhabdomyoma, and three cases of rhabdomyomasosis	Heart		Children, 2 days to 11 years of age	Surgery, chemotherapy			(117)

Table 5. Continued.

Tissue	Organ	Tumor and No. of reported cases	Rare or uncommon location	Type or spreading	Age — General	Age — Special	Treatment and prognosis	Established	Remarks	Reference
Central nervous system	Head and neck	Neuroblastoma, review of 152 cases	Head and neck	Rapid and widespread metastasis	Children		Surgery, chemotherapy, radiation therapy			(48)
	Olfactory neurons	Olfactory neuroblastoma	Olfactory neurons	Pleural fluid	40-year-old man				Olfactory neuroblastoma (esthesio-neuroblastoma) has better prognosis than more common malignancies of nose	(168)
	CNS	CNS tumors					Therapy favors metastasis by increased survival			(275)
Peripheral nervous system	Adrenal glands	Bilateral adrenal neuroblastoma, 1 case	Adrenal glands, bilateral						Bilateral adrenal neuroblastoma is extremely rare	(202)
Meninges	Lepto-meninges	Primary leptomeningeal gliomatosis (diffuse form), fourth case in the literature	Leptomeninges				Radiotherapy, chemotherapy			(190)
Peripheral glia	Peripheral nerves	Malignant schwannoma (generally, in lower rate), solitary	Retroperitoneum, mediastinum, pelvis,	Recurrence, rare lymph node metastasis	Very young to very old, 5% under 10 yrs., 41–42 yrs., median		Surgery – survival depends on size of neoplasm: 5 cm, 79.3%		Malignant schwannoma appears de novo	(18) pp. 245–250
		Associated with neurofibromatoses		High recurrence	28–30 yrs.		Surgery – 30%, 5 yrs. survival			(18) pp. 245–250
	Oligodendroglia	Oligodendroglioma, 49 cases, 1 primary of spinal cord		Unusual metastases			Good prognosis, if surgery and radical radiation therapy used			(278)
	Peripheral nerve	Schwannoma	Medial plantar branch of posterior tibial nerve of foot		64-year-old man		Amputation or radical excision			(116)
	Peripheral nerve	Schwannoma, malignant		Usually hematogenic metastasis to lungs, liver, bones, or brain; lymphatic metastasis occasionally reported.					Malignant schwannoma is a rare neoplasm of the neural sheath.	(258)

System	Site	Tumor / cases	Location	Clinical features / metastasis	Age	Treatment / survival	Year / Author	Comments	Ref.
Autonomous nervous system	Peripheral nerves	Malignant schwannoma and elephantoid hypertrophy of limb are rare manifestations of von Recklinghausen's neurofibromatosis. 1 case	Limb		17-year-old man			Both rare conditions appeared in the same patient	(375)
	Nasal cavity	Esthesio-neuroblastoma		Extension along meninges – distant metastases, 20–30%, most commonly, cervical lymph nodes and lungs, less commonly bones, thoracic and abdominal lymph nodes		Surgery – 5 yr. survival 50%, average life span 6 yrs.	Berger et al. 1924	Slight male preponderance epithelial component, lacking in esthesioneurocytoma	(18) pp. 273–277
Central glia	Nasal cavity	Esthesioneuroblastoma 31 cases reviewed		Metastases uncommon at diagnosis	10–40 yrs. (young): 66% 7–79 yrs.			This tumor is extremely rare among blacks.	(322)
	CNS							Secondary CNS involvement is rare in the development of sarcoma, with exception of alveolar soft part sarcoma	(50)
	Brain	Glioblastoma, 2 cases		Meningeal and spinal spread				Meningeal spread is considered rare	(368)
	Meninges	Carcinomatosis, 4% of ca patients		Death from systemic disease rare				Not more as rare	(288)
	Spinal cord	Leptomeningeal carcinomatosis, 1 case	Cervical region	Diffuse tumor, infiltration of dura				This type of metastasis was previously unreported	(186)
	Lung	Carcinosarcoma up to 1977, 42 cases		Infiltration to pleura or mediastinum, distant hematogenous metastasis to liver, brain, adrenals, intestine, kidneys, and heart		Surgery – radiation, chemotherapy – central loc. Tumors have better prognosis than peripheral ones: 1 yr. survival, 42%	1908		(18) pp. 197–198
Thyroid	Thyroid	Carcinosarcoma, very rare		Extensive metastasis		Poor prognosis survival less than 1 yr.			(18) p. 199
	Breast	Carcinosarcoma; up to 1974, 16 cases		Metastasis to lung 50%		Surgery (mastectomy)			(18) p. 200

Table 5. Continued.

Tissue	Organ	Tumor and No. of reported cases	Rare or uncommon location	Type or spreading	Age General	Age Special	Treatment and prognosis	Established	Remarks	Reference
	Esophagus	Carcinosarcoma; up to 1973, 28 cases		Extension to mediastinum and bronchi, lymph mode and distant metastasis uncommon	Median, 59 yrs.		Surgery, average survival, 1–5 yrs. (0.5%)	Stout et al. 1949	Male predominance	(18) p. 201
	Stomach	Carcinosarcoma		Extension; distant metastases uncommon					Most common in Japan	(18) p. 203
	Kidney	Carcinosarcoma		Local infiltration and wide metastasis	60 yrs. and older		Surgery (nephrectomy) survival, 6 mos.			(18) p. 204
	Bladder	Carcinosarcoma, approx. 30 cases		Local recurrence, rare metastasis to lung and liver	64 yrs.		Surgery, radiotherapy, 5 yr. survival in 1 case after electrodesiccation		Metastasis of epithelial and mesenchymal components	(18) pp. 205–206
	Prostate	Carcinosarcoma		Metastasis to lung, liver, spine and viscera						(18) p. 207
	Heart	Intermedial teratoma, 5 cases in English literature (3 malignant)		Distant metastasis to lung and spine	Only in children		No special treatment rendered, diagnosis postmortem			(18) p. 100

were also seen by electron microscopy. The liposarcoma was of the pleomorphic type. This case reported by Suzuki and coworkers (340) indicates that rare combinations of tumors may be a part of unusual tumor progression.

There are rare occurrences of neoplastic spreading where an unusual course is taken. It is important to learn why this happens. The following factors may play a role in this rare behavior of neoplasms: topographic site; heterogeneity of tumor cells; immunologic condition of the host; individual specificity. Nutritional influences may also play a role. Table 3 lists a few selected cases.

II. SPECIFIC ASPECTS: PRIMARY NEOPLASMS

1. Rare neoplasms in particular species
Two classes of rarity may be distinguished: (1) Rarity of the neoplasm in a larger taxonomic unit. A typical example is the rare occurrence of epithelial neoplasms (with the exception of ovarian and oviduct neoplasms) in birds. Another example, sarcomas occur at a higher percentage in lower vertebrates, especially fish. (2) Specific tumors are rare in a particular species. We have chosen the domestic and laboratory animals as examples because from these species the most cases are known (Table 4).

2. Rare neoplasms in man
The following section is divided into three aspects: (a) rare topographical region; (b) uncommon histology; (c) specific site. Results are summarized in Table 5. This is followed by a section on rare human neoplasms appearing during a particular age period and, finally, a section on rare neoplasms found either in males or females.

(a) Primary neoplasms in uncommon topographical regions
This section deals with selected neoplasms occurring in unusual body regions. Using examples of a number of tissues, we will show why these neoplasms are rare in specific areas. Development of, topographical, or other influences may play a role.

(b) Primary neoplasms of uncommon histology
The histology of these tumors is unusual for the organ affected. It can be easily seen that the separation of tumors which are rare in certain locations from those which exhibit an uncommon histology or those which are site-specific is not fundamental – there are fluent interchanges. For this reason these different rare tumors are presented in Table 5. Typical examples of tumors with uncommon histology are besides others (98), carcinoid tumors of the bronchus, testes, thymus or the carcinosarcomas, also known as collision tumors, in such organs as lung, esophagus or bladder.

(c) Site specific neoplasms
These tumors are site-specific to smaller organs, such as tumors of the organ of Zuckerkandl, or they appear in specific areas of other organs such as the leiomyomas, tumors of the superior and inferior vena cava.

Rare neoplasms occurring during a particular age period
It is well known that neoplasms may appear at any time during a life span, yet we can distinguish between those which can occur throughout the life of a person and those which occur generally only during a certain time span. The age spectrum of neoplasms was discussed in Chapter 21/ Volume II. In this context, Table 6 lists selected tumors which are uncommon in certain age groups.

The age variation in patients with different types of primary gastric cancer illustrates the variability of various histologically different tumors, as shown in the abstracted article of Katoh (80): "Gastric resection was performed in 632 patients with primary gastric cancer. Infiltration of cancer frequently extended to the whole area of the stomach in the 30's but rarely in the 60's. Histological classification, revealed that papillary adenocarcinoma was rare in the 30's but frequent in the group over 70, and that moderately differentiated tubular adenocarcinoma and signet-ring-cell carcinoma were frequent in the 30's; and according to Lauren's histological classification, the ratio of the intestinal type was low in the 30's and 40's but high in the 60's and over 70 groups; and the ratio of the diffuse type was just the opposite. Metastasis occurred frequently through peritoneal dissemination in younger people, while in the aged it was more frequent through the vein and lymphatic vessel."

As evident from Table 7 a larger number of neoplasms occurs less often in females than in males, a situation which is compensated by the large number of sex-related neoplasms in the female as, for example, breast cancer. There exist neoplasms, of course, which occur equally in both sexes, such as the oligodendroglioma. Experimental evidence and clinical experience indicate that an imbalance of sex hormones may contribute to or cause tumor growth (218). A number of chapters, such as 20/Vol. II, 3/Vol. III, 19/Vol. V, 8/Vol. VI, 13/Vol. VIII, 16/Vol. IV, 12/Vol. VI, 9/Vol. VI, 17/Vol. IV, 20/Vol. IX, deal with the problems of hormonal influence on spontaneous, experimental or treatment-induced changes in tumor growth.

III. SPECIFIC ASPECTS: SECONDARY NEOPLASTIC GROWTH

Some specific neoplasms develop uncommon or rare patterns of secondary tumor. The following aspects must be considered.

1. Rare neoplastic invasiveness
This is seen in such cases as the penetration of arterial walls by neoplastic cells and the continued growth in the lumen. The elastic connective tissue of the arterial wall and the fast movement of arterial blood may be some of the reasons for this rare affection of arteries by neoplasms. Other examples include the neoplastic penetration of fasciae and tendons, e.g., through sarcomas.

2. Uncommon local recurrence
Local recurrence may occur after one type of therapy or another. Examples are regrowth, after surgery, from leftover malignant cells, or from residual cells following chemotherapy against leukemias or lymphomas. Like metastasis, it shows a typical pattern of tumor specificity. For some tumors, metastasis is the preferred type of spread, for others, local recurrence. Sometimes a rare change in some of those patterns is found. Rare cases of recurrence are those neo-

Table 6. Selected aspects of the age spectrum of neoplasms.

Tissue	Neoplasm	Rare age	Common age	Reference
Stratified squamous epithelium	Squamous cell carcinoma of skin	Children or young adults	45 and over	(21) p. 365
Stratified squamous epithelium	Epidermoid carcinoma of vulva	Under 40 yrs	60 to 80 yrs	(21) p. 743
Simple cuboidal/columnar epithelium	Prostate carcinoma	In children	Over 45 increasing max. 60–85 yrs	(21) p. 785
Simple columnar epithelium	Fallopian tube carcinoma	In very young, and old	40 to 60 yrs	(21) p. 738
Simple columnar epithelium	Colon carcinoma	Under 30 yrs.	50 to 70 yrs.	(296)
Pseudostriatified columnar epithelium	Bronchial tumors (carcinoid, mucoepidermoid carcinomas)	Under 12 yrs	50 to 60 yrs.	(213)
Pseudostratified columnar epithelium	Primary bronchial tumors	Under 12 yrs.	50 to 60 yrs.	
Simple columnar epithelium	Carcinoma of gallbladder	Young adults	55 to 75 yrs.	(21) p. 605
Exocrine pancreas	Carcinoma of pancreas	In children	50 to 70 yrs.	(21) p. 612
Fibrous connective tissue	Fibrosarcoma	Infants and children, juvenile fibrosarcoma	50 yrs. and over	(21) p. 23
Adipose tissue	Liposarcoma	Under 30 yrs	Middle and later life	(21) p. 59
Bone marrow	Ewing's tumor		Children in second decade	(361)
Central glia	Ependymoblastoma		2 years	(250)

Table 7. Selected aspects of neoplasms as a function of sex.

Tissue	Neoplasm	Rare, less common sex	Common sex	Reference*
Simple cuboidal, columnar epithelium	Kidney cancer	♀	♂ 2×	(21) p. 801
Simple columnar epithelium	Gallbladder carcinoma	♂	♀	(21) p. 605
Simple columnar epithelium	Carcinoma of colon and rectum	♀	♂ 2×	(21) p. 582
Salivary glands	Parotid gland tumors	♂	♀ preponderance	(21) p. 531
Exocrine pancreas	Pancreas carcinoma	♀	♂ nearly 2×	(21) p. 612
Pineal gland	Pineal gland tumor	♀	♂ more than 3×	(21) p. 497
Pituitary gland	Pituitary chromophobe adenoma	♀ −	♂ +	(21) p. 231
Reticular connective tissue	Hodgkin's disease	♀	♂ 3×	(21) p. 175
Desmal epithelium	Kaposi's sarcoma	♀	♂ predominance	(21) p. 84
Melanogenic system	Malignant melanoma	♂	♀ more than 2×	(21) p. 423
Chordal tissue	Chordoma	♀	♂ more than 2×	(21) p. 141
Cartilage	Chondrosarcoma	♀	♂ 2×	(21) p. 111
Bone	Osteosarcoma	♀	♂ 2×	(21) p. 117
Central glia	Oligodendroglioma	Equal	Equal	(21) p. 451

* The references are summarized by Ashley (21), and used here to save space for reference citations.

Table 8. Metastases and other types of spreading of rare tumors.

Primary tumor with number of cases	Metastases	Comments	Reference
General aspects			
	Metastatic infiltration of scar after laparoscopy	Very rare	(338)
Several types of neoplasms; spindle-cell ca	Metastatic spindle-cell ca of rib		(315)
Uterine carcinosarcoma; 49 patients	Death from local recurrence rather than from distant metastases	Rare and fatal malignancy	(86)
Small cell lung cancer, 134 patients	Isolated brain metatasis was rare		(88)
Nonneuraxial primary tumor, 1 case	M. to arachnoid space		(379)
Stratified squamous cell epithelium			
Merkel's cell ca; 86 patients reviewed, 2 reported	Lymphatic as well as hematogenic metastases		(8)
Adenoca of stomach	Testicular metastasis	Rare, poor prognosis	(101)
Gastric ca	Hematogenous hepatic metastases	These metastases are rare	(308)
Simple columnar epithelium			
Ca of endometrium, 1 case	Lymphonodular metastases to main bronchus and trachea	Rare cause of death	(30)
Endometrial ca, 59-yr.-old woman	M. to femur		(33)
Gastric ca	Osseous m. as first sign		(38)
Gastric ca, 62-yr.-old man	M. to lungs, kidney, adrenal glands	Rare case of malignant acanthosis nigricans	(121)
Gastric ca, 54-yr.-old woman	M. to skin of neck		(129)
Gastric ca, 62-yr.-old man	M. to pancreas and duodenum	Very rare	(159)
Gastric ca, 732 cases	Lymph node m. was rare		(239)
Biliary cystadenoca, 1 case recorded; 59-yr.-old male	Osseous metastases	Very rare	(34)
Neoplasm of kidney; 1 case (clear cell)	M. to parotid		(26)
ca of colon and rectum	Ovarian m. rare	Rare	(144)
Cecal adenoca, 62-yr.-old woman	Umbilical metastasis	Rare	(165)
ca of the colon, 47-yr.-old man	Bilateral testicular metastases		(74)
ca of urogenital tract or lung	Metastases to thyroid	Rare	(106)
Gastric adenoca	Metastases in bone marrow and ovaries	Occurrence of microangiopathic anemia w/o evidence of local occurrence in metastatic nests, is rare	(264)
Squamous cell ca of colorectum; 69 cases reported in Engl. literature	Prognosis depends on visceral m.	One additional case treated successfully by multimodality approach	(127)
Small-cell ca of rectum, 1 case	Death due to widespread m.		(301)
Rectal ca, 63-yr.-old patient; only 29 cases reported previously	Metastasis to a toe	Metastatic lesions of small bones of extremities very rare	(132)
Adenoca of rectum	Rare peritoneal seeding		(123)
Pseudostratified columnar epithelium			
Recurrent respiratory papillomatosis; youngest patient described w/ malignant changes, 6-yr.-old female		Malignant changes usually seen in older patients	(328)
Carcinoid syndrome of right bronchus, 67-yr.-old Japanese male	Large hepatic meatastases	Only 4 reported cases previously in Japan	(345)

Table 8. Continued.

Primary tumor with number of cases	Metastases	Comments	Reference
Transitional epithelium			
Bladder ca	Choroidal metastases	Extremely rare dissemination of bladder ca	(64)
Bladder ca	Adrenal metastases, bilateral	Very rare occasion	(105)
Mammary glands			
Breast ca; 166 patients reviewed	Metastases to endocrine glands (40%) lungs (28%); cardiovascular system (21%); genitourinary system (21%); CNS (14%); bones (10%)		(126)
Breast ca	40–45% ocular metastases	In comparison lung ca 10–29%; ca of digestive system 5% poor prognosis	(171)
ca of breast (adenoca)	Intradural metastasis		(247)
ca of breast	Early metastasis to brain	Brain metastasis occur in 25–50% of cases	(207)
ca of breast, 36-yr.-old woman	M. to pituitary gland	Resulted in chiasmal compression and panhypopituitarism	(72)
ca of breast	Lung metastasis	M. as one solitary round lesion is rare	(306)
ca of breast, 1 case	Endobronchial metastasis	Extremely rare	(77)
ca of breast, 70-yr.-old woman	Esophageal metastasis		(107)
ca of breast, 2 cases	Metastatic disease to cervical esophagus	1982 were no other cases of breast ca metastasis to the cervical esophagus reported	(37)
ca of breast, 5 patients	Uterine metastases	All died of widespread metastases 2–20 mos. later	(261)
ca of breast	Metastases in bones distal to the elbow, knee, and in mandible make about 1% of all metastases	Other bone metastases are much more frequent	(142)
Adeno ca of breast, 56-yr.-old nullipara	Two axillary lymph nodes	Lymph nodes deposits detected first, a rare occasion	(151)
Cystosarcoma phyllodes	Sarcomatous metastasis	Rare, especially infrequent w/benign appearing primary tumor	(23, 40)
Salivary glands			
Minor salivary gland ca of larynx, 18 cases	Distant metastases	ca in minor sal. glands is rare	(68)
Parotid neoplasms	Bone metastases	Very rare	(381)
Mucoepidermoid parotid tumor; perhaps first case described	Metastasizing to stomach	Very rare	(185)
Liver			
Hepatoma, 49-yr.-old woman	Bone metastasis of right orbit	Bone m. of hepatomas very rare; (3–12%), exceptional first t. sign	(152)
Liver tumor, 1 case	Metastasis in heart, growing more than two years	Primary did not recur; metastasis produced jaundice	(367)
Cholangiocellular ca	Pulmonary metastasis	Rare occurrence	(357)
Cystadenoca of liver; 62-yr.-old woman	Metastases are rare	Better prognosis than cholangioca.	(371)
Hepatoma; 42-yr.-old African male	Bone metastases in calvaria	Extremely rare; exceptional first sign of hepatoma	(252)
Hepatoma; 58-yr.-old woman	Pancreatic metastases	Hivet in 1977 found only 27 cases of visceral m. to the pancreas	(147)
Liver ca; 48-yr.-old man	Metastasized to left ilium		(19)

Table 8. Continued.

Primary tumor with number of cases	Metastases	Comments	Reference
Exocrine pancreas			
Adenoca of tail of pancreas	Bilateral temporal bone m.	Bilateral sudden loss of hearing	(158)
ca of head of pancreas, w/penetration of duodenum	Liver metastases	Phlebitis nigrans rare early symptoms of abdominal tumors	(209)
ca of pancreatic head, 70-yr.-old woman	Infiltration into lumen of portal vein; no other metastasis	Chief symptom was abdominal ascites	(326)
Pineal gland			
Pineal germinoma (assumed) in 17-yr.-old boy; 4 previous cases	Metastases to chest		(303)
Pituitary gland			
Hypophyseal tumor	Rare metastasis produced exophthalmos		(310)
Thyroid gland			
Thyroid ca	Ocular and neck metastases	Ocular metastasis of thyroid ca seems to be exceedingly rare	(333)
Thyroid ca combined w/toxic goiter	Metastases very rare		(183)
Follicular ca of thyroid, 75-yr.-old woman	Breast metastasis after 9 yrs.	Also metastasis to lungs	(61)
Thyroid ca	Spinal cord compression	This rare complication is not necessarily preterminal	(119)
Thyroid ca; 2 cases reviewed, 1 described	Renal metastases to kidney after 37 yrs.	Patient donated contralateral kidney to transplantation earlier	(170)
Thyroid ca	Lymphatic metastasis to submental nodes		(179)
Thyroid ca, 64-yr.-old woman	Bone and liver metastases	Endocrine secretion by m.	(251)
Adrenal cortex and medulla			
Pheochromocytoma in a 14-yr.-old girl and 21 cases reviewed	High frequency: regional lymph nodes, bones, lungs are main sites		(192)
Testis			
Germ cell tumors, 154 cases	Rare sites of metastasis: breast, prostate, penis, gallbladder, heart	Chorioca elements metastasize rarely pure	(45)
Germ cell tumors	Leptomeningeal metastases are rare		(316)
Seminoma, 29-yr.-old man	Metastasis to kidney		(70)
Intracranial germinoma, 25-yr.-old black man	Ventriculoperitoneal shunt metastasis	This is the 4th report in the literature	(343)
Germ cell tumor, 35-yr.-old man	Thymoma	This case seems to be the first of leukemia-like infiltration of malignant germ cell tumore	(162)
Testicular teratomas	Consistent pattern to retroperitoneum, mediastinum, lungs, liver	Primaries are rare	(157)
Bilateral sequential testicular ca	Spontaneous regression of metastasis from one tumor		(255)
Ovary			
Placental site trophoblastic tumor	Metastasis to para-aortic lymph nodes and lung		(91)
Small cell ca of ovary; 2nd and 3rd known cases	Metastatic	Patients died 6 mos after diagnosis; it is a ca of the young	(277)
Brenner tumor, 67-yr.-old woman	Local recurrence and metastasis		(230)
Cystadenoca, 78-yr.-old woman	To rectum, 26 yrs. after primary		(42)
Mature solid teratoma	Gliomatosis peritonei		(95)

Table 8. Continued.

Primary tumor with number of cases	Metastases	Comments	Reference
Desmal epithelium			
Angioblastosarcoma in a 16-yr.-old patient	Pulmonary metastases	Rare tumor	(97)
Adenoca in 62-yr.-old	Malignant pleural effusion	Rare complication, only 5 cases in the literature	(208)
Mesenchyme			
Mesenchymal breast sarcoma; 25 cases, 1% of malignant breast tumors	Nodal involvement rare (4%), hematogenous metastases, usual. In 24%, metastases mostly to lung	Local recurrence in 44%	(331)
Mixed mesodermal tumor of uterine body, 61-yr.-old woman	Extensive metastasis		(5)
Maternal sarcomas, 6 women 15 to 39 yrs. of age	Metastasizing to placenta or fetus, rare		(164)
Alveolar soft part sarcoma in a 33-yr.-old man, in 20-yr.-old man, a 25-yr.-old woman, an 8-yr.-old man	First case, metastasis to lung and brain; 2nd case, multiple lung and hepatic metastases; 3rd case, no recurrence or m. after 2 yrs, 4th case, lung m.	First two cases died; 3rd and 4th cases were in good condition 2 yrs. and 15 mos respectively, after surgery	(206)
Reticular connective tissue			
A typical fibroxanthoma of skin on the head	Metastases in region of parotid gland	Most fibroxanthomas exhibit benign behavior	(140)
Chronic myeloid leukemia; 35-yr.-old woman	Mandibular soft tissue and osteo-lytic metastases		(324)
Cutaneous primary lymphomas (excluding mycosis fungoides and Sezary syndrome) 16 cases	Extracutaneous dissemination in lymph nodes and bone marrow		(374)
Bone			
Ewing's sarcoma, reticulosarcoma	Radiation renders local recurrence rare		(305)
Isolated osteolysis after age 40	Almost always a tumor metastasis, because primary neoplasms are rare in this age group		(108)
Mandibular ameloblastoma, 21-year-old man which was resected at age 6	Recurrence at mandible and facial bones with 21, also multiple pulmonary nodules were found		(51)
Giant-cell tumor of bone, 130 cases	Typical, aggressive tumors, rarely metastasized		(53)
Bone metastases occur with carcinomas, lymphomas, leukemias and especially, prostate ca	Metastases are rare in mandibular canal, pulp and periapex; multiple metastatic lesions are also rare.		(90)
Malignant metastasizing ameloblastoma, 26 cases	Lung, lymph nodes, bone, brain kidney, small intestine, liver	Duration 13.1 yrs. after metastasis only 2.6 yrs	(210)
Genitouterine malignancies, 9 cases confirmed histologically	Metastases to bones of feet, most often calcaneus		(109)
Smooth musculature			
Uterine leiomyoma, benign, of 32-year-old woman	Metastatic to para-aortic lymph nodes	3, 5 years after exploratory laparotomy free of symptoms	(79)
Uterine leiomyoma	Pulmonary metastasis, after age 21	Extensive multiple nodules	(286)
Leiomyosarcoma of uterus	Metastases to scalp and back	Exceptionally rare	(7)
Cardiac musculature			
Heart	Malignant tumor involvement is relatively rare		(191)

Table 8. Continued.

Primary tumor with number of cases	Metastases	Comments	Reference
CNS			
282 cases of extraneural metastases of CNS tumors have been reported	These metastases are fatal	They occur especially after craniotomy or diversionary cerebrospinal fluid shunting	(149, 89)
Bilateral retinoblastoma, 35-year-old black man	1 month postoperatively, metastases in mandible, lung, femur and after 21 months, a rare metastatic retinoblastoma		(187)
Medulloblastoma, 7-year-old boy	Skeletal metastases 6–12 months after diagnosis in rigth femur, left ischium and vertebral column, with diffuse bone marrow involvement		(281)
Peripheral nervous system			
Testicular neuroblastoma, young boy	Dissemination started 9 months after orchiectomy	This seems to be the only report of neuroblastoma without disseminated disease at diagnosis	(184)

plasms which do not normally recur but have done so in a few cases.

Chapter 17/Volume VII deals with recurrence. The two examples chosen may illustrate the point: benign pedunculated tumors of the hypopharynx are very rare, but even more rare is the recurrent case of such a fibromatous tumor with malignant change after 20 years (215). Congenital mesoblastic nephroma shows recurrence only rarely (172).

3. Rare secondary direct spreading

The difference between direct spreading and metastatic spreading as forms of tumor distribution is that, in the first case, cells remain connected to the primary tumor, whereas in the second they are freed. Direct spreading cells continue to grow in tissue spaces and other organ channels, such as the interior of veins or at the periphery of veins, and more rarely in or around arteries. (Vasco-neural conduit.) As types of site-specific tumors, neoplasms in the aorta, the pulmonary arteries, the vena cava superior, and the vena cava inferior are rare neoplasms. The tumors in these veins have always originated from smooth musculature and have grown inside the vessel, or penetrated the wall from which they derived towards the outside. It is sometimes a question of judgment whether these tumors can be seen as expansion of the primary tumor or as cases of direct tumor spreading as we know it from common locations in smaller vessels. This will have to be decided from case to case. The following case report serves as an example.

Six years earlier, a 37-year-old woman was operated for thyroid cancer and experienced a few years later a mediastinal metastasis from this tumor. The tumor grew in the left vena brachiocephalica, obstructed this vein completely and was adherent to the left vena jugularis interna only partially; 6 × 3 × 3 cm in size. The tumor exhibited a thin capsule, a smooth and soft consistency, and light yellow color. It was a papillary and follicular metastatic adenocarcinoma (257).

4. Rare neoplastic seeding

Pulmonary tumor embolism resulting from hepatic tumors is rare. A first intraoperative occurrence was reported by Blanloeil (39).

Placement of Broviac catheters for venous access led to metastatic tumor implantation in an adult case with multiple myeloma and in a child with Burkitt's lymphoma. Both patients were in advanced stages of their disease. Tumor implantation is a rare occurrence (334).

5. Rare neoplastic circulating cells

Studies in the rat, using a fibrosarcoma, were intended to investigate the first five minutes of tumor cell lodging. The fibrosarcoma cells were very rigid. The tumor cells became mainly arrested by mechanical trapping in narrow liver sinusoids. Rarely, an arrest of tumor cells by adherence to venular veins was seen. The initial phenomena of tumor cell lodgment seemed not to be influenced by platelets (24).

Intracranial metastases make-up 7–17% of all brain tumors: 5.8–22% in different series. Neoplasms of the lung, breast and melanoma metastasize most often to the brain. Two-thirds of intracranial metastases occur in the brain parenchyma and the remaining third in meningeal envelopes. Leptomeningeal metastases are rare and arise mostly from leukemia, lymphomas and breast carcinoma (41).

An embryonal sarcoma of the liver presented as an intracardiac tumor in a boy 8 years old. Repeated embolization of the tumor led to the death of the patient (110).

A rare case of the combined occurrence of mitral stenosis and left atrial myxoma was reported by Seagle (319).

6. Rare metastases: selected aspects: metastases of uncommon primary neoplasms (U) and unusual metastases of common primary neoplasms (C)

Rare metastases may occur from rare primary tumors or they may present as rare metastases from a common primary tumor. Table 8 exhibits cases for both of these groups.

7. Rare neoplastic spontaneous regression

Tumor regression against a broad comparative background is treated in Chapters 5–9/Volume IV. Only a few remarks added here. A benign osteoblastoma of the mandible regressed spontaneously after biopsy during a 15-year follow-up (92). Duodenal carcinoid tumors are rare and patients may survive over 30 years, even with regional and hepatic metastases. One patient showed a regression of the duodenal primary (66). An adenocarcinoma in the ascending colon of a young woman without predisposing familial or premalignant conditions regressed spontaneously (31). A 37-year-old woman in the second trimester of her pregnancy presented with a supraglottic hemangioma. She had symptoms during her previous pregnancy. This rare tumor regressed postpartum, perhaps due to the effects of estrogen and progesterone (44).

SUMMARY AND CONCLUSION

Neoplasms may be rare from different points of view: in various species or in a single species (interspecies or intraspecies variation). Rare neoplasms not only present with rare morphological aspects of appearance but also with rare behavior, such as speed of growth, unusual path of tumor distribution, age of appearance or progression, sex, and last, not least, tumors interrelationship. The latter especially may be able to open new avenues of research and treatment. This chapter has reviewed these questions, based on an extensive case material.

REFERENCES

1. Addison AK, Payne SR: Primary liposarcoma of bone, case report. *J Bone Joint Surg (AM)* 64(2):301, 1982
2. Adler CP, Reichelt A: Haemangiosarcoma of bone. *Int Orth* 8(4):273, 1985
3. Agnatis NJ, Rosen PP: Mammary carcinoma with osteoclast-like giant cells – a study of eight cases with follow-up. *Pathology* 165(1/2):60, 1979
4. Ahuja S, Loffler W, Wegener OH et al.: Tuberous sclerosis with angiomyolipoma and metastasized hypernephroma. *Urology* 28(5):413, 1986
5. Akashi E, Adachi K, Ohono M, Mizuuchi H, Matsuura M, Kudo R, Kawase N, Hashimoto M: Scanning electron microscopy of mixed mesodermal tumors of the uterine body. *Nippon Sanka Fujinka Gakkai Zasshi* 31(4):459, 1979
6. Aldred MJ, Crawford PJ: Juvenile hyaline fibromatosis. *Oral Surg Oral Med Oral Pathol* 63(1):71, 1987
7. Alessi E, Innocenti M, Sala F: Leiomyosarcoma metastatic to the back and scalp from a primary neoplasm in the uterus. *Am J Dermatopathol* 7(5):471, 1985
8. Alexiou G, Papadopoulou-Alexiou M, Karakousis CP: Primary neuroendocrine carcinoma of the skin (Merkel's cell carcinoma). *J Surg Oncol* 27(1):31, 1984
9. Ali J, Riese KT: Acinic cell cancers of the parotid gland in children: comments based on two affected girls. *Clin Pediatr (Phila)* 14(12):1111, 1975
10. Alitalo K: Amplification of cellular oncogenes in cancer cells. *Med Biol* 621(6):304, 1984
11. Altmannsberger M, Poppe H, Schauer A: An unusual case of adamantinoma of long bones. *J Cancer Res Clin Oncol* 104(3):315, 19??
12. Amadori G, Brigato G, Cordiano V et al.: Pelvic and mammary Burkitt-like lymphoma with simultaneous development of leukemia. *Gynecol Oncol* 26(2):246, 1987
13. Amor B, Kahan A, Laoussadi S et al.: Multicentric reticulo-histiocytosis. A case with unusual clinical, radiologic and ultrastructural aspects. *Rev Rhum Mal Osteoartic* 54(2):113, 1987
14. Anders KH, Glasgow BJ, Lewin KJ: Gangliocytic paragan-

glioma associated with duodenal. *Arch Pathol Lab Med* 111(1):49, 1987
15. Anderson KA, McAninch JW: Primary squamous cell carcinoma of anterior male urethra. *Urology* 23(2):134, 1984
16. Andreasen EE, Hald F: Gigantic ovarian cyst. *Ugeskr Laeger* 142(25):1620, 1980
17. Angervall L: Fibrosarcoma and fibromatosis. XXI Postgraduate Course on Clinical Oncology: Bone and Soft Tissue Tumors. Milan NCI, Bethesda, 1980
18. Antoniades J: Uncommon Malignant Tumors. New York: Masson, 1982
19. Aoki T: A very rare case of primary liver cancer with metastasis to the flat bone. *Jpn J Cancer Clin* 22(1):46, 1976
20. Ashida K, Iwakoshi K, Masamune D, Hirata I, Asada S, Ohshiba S, Kurokawa A: Diffusely infiltrating type of colonic carcinoma: Report of a case. *I To Cho* 17(4):435, 1982
21. Ashley DJB: Evans' Histological Appearances of Tumours. Vols. I and II (3rd edition). Edinburgh–London–New York: Churchill Livingstone, 1978
22. Auguste LJ, Razack MS, Sako K: Hemangiopericytoma. *J Surg Oncol* 20(4):260, 1982
23. Baczako K, Fischer H: Malignant metastasizing cystosarcoma phyllodes of the breast... *Onkologie* 7(6):382, 1984
24. Bagge U, Skolnik G, Ericson LE: The arrest of circulating tumor cells in the liver microcirculation. A vital fluorescence microscopic, electron microscopic and isotope study in the rat. *J Cancer Res Clin Oncol* 105(2):134, 1983
25. Bahnson RR, Snopek, TJ, Grayhack JT: Epididymal metastasis from prostatic carcinoma. *Urology* 26(3):296, 1985
26. Ballanger R, Ballanger P: A rare form of kidney cancer: parotid metastases. *J Urol Nephrol (Paris)* 85(7/8):548, 1979
27. Barbalias GA: Bilateral successive seminomas in scrotal testes. *Del Med J* 46(5):243, 1974
28. Barbanti F, Padovani F: Considerations for diagnosis and therapy of mammary phyllode cystosarcoma. *Radiol Med (Torino)* 67(11):874, 1981
29. Batsakis JG, Rice DH, Solomon AR: The pathology of head and neck tumors: squamous and mucous-gland carcinomas of the nasal cavity, paranasal sinuses, and larynx. Part 6. *Head Neck Surg* 2(6):497, 1980
30. Beckert W: A rare cause of death: pulmonary metastasis of endometrial carcinoma. *Zentralbl Gynaekol* 101(5):354, 1979
31. Beechey RT, Edwards BE, Kelland CH: Adenocarcinoma of the colon: an unusual case. *Med J Aust* 144(4):211, 1986
32. Beeson WH, Singer MI, Lingemann RE: Congenital fibrosarcoma in the oral cavity. First reported case. *Laryngoscope* 90(8, Part 1):1336, 1980
33. Benz G, Brandeis WE, Geiger H, Georgi P: 'Cold' lesion in bone scan of an osteogenic metastasis of Wilms' tumor. *Pediatr Radiol* 6(4):233, 1978
34. Berjian RA, Nime F, Douglass HO, Nava H: Biliary cyst-adenocarcinoma: Report of a case presenting with osseous metastasis and a review of the literature. *J Surg Oncol* 18(3):305, 1980
35. Bhagayan BS, Dorfman HD, Azumi N, Murthy SN, Eggleston J: Intravascular bronchioloalveolar tumor: a low grade sclerosing epithelioid angiosarcoma of lung. *Lab Invest* 46(1):10A, 1982
36. Bhat IK, Gennaro AR: Cloacogenic carcinoma. *Am J Proctol Gastroenterol Colon Rectal Surg* 33(9):6, 22, 1982
37. Biller HF, Diktaban T, Fink W, Lawson W: Breast carcinoma metastasizing to the cervical esophagus. *Laryngoscope* 92(9, Part 1):999, 1982
38. Birla RK, Bowden L: Solitary bony metastasis as the first sign of malignant gastric tumor or of its recurrence. *Ann Surg* 182(1):45, 1975
39. Blanloeil Y, Paineau J, Vissett J, Dixneuf B: Intraoperative pulmonary tumor embolism after hepatectomy for liver carcinoma. *Can Anaesth Soc J* 30(1):69, 1983

40. Blumencranz PW, Gray GF: Cystosarcoma phyllodes. Clinical and pathologic study. *NY State J Med* 78(4):623, 1978

41. Boccardo F, Comelli G, De Menech R, Mina G, Zanardi S: Natural history and staging of brain metastases. *Minerva Med* 75(22–23):1369, 1984

42. Bodin F, Dyan S, Licht H, Conte-Marti J, Crottoggini JJ: Rectal metastasis of an ovarian tumor 26 years after surgery. *Nouv Presse Med*, 1977

43. Bork K, Korting GW, Rumpelt HJ: Diffuse melanosis in malignant melanoma. *Hautarzt* 28(9):463, 1977

44. Brandwein MS, Abramson AL, Shikowitz MJ: Supraglottic hemangioma during pregnancy. *Obstet Gynecol* 69(3 Pt 2):450, 1987

45. Bredael JJ, Vugrin D, Kleinert EL, Whitmore WF: Analysis of treatment failures on 154 patients with testicular cancer coming to autopsy. 75th Annual Meeting, San Francisco, May 18–22, 1980. Amer Urol Association, Inc, 284 pp, 1980

46. Brisbane JU, Howell DA, Bonkowsky HL: Pulmonary hypertension as a presentation of hepatocarcinoma. Report of a case and brief review of the literature. *Am J Med* 68(3):466, 1980

47. Brook IM, Martin BA: Angiosarcoma, metastatic to the mandible and maxilla. *Br J Oral Surg* 18(3):266, 1980

48. Brown RJ, Szymula NJ, Lore JM: Neuroblastoma of the head and neck. *Arch Otolaryngol* 104(7):395, 1978

49. Brugere J, Royer P: Surveillance of a patient treated for cancer of the larynx. *Gaz Med Fr* 88(25):3605, 1981

50. Bryant BM, Wiltshaw E: Central nervous system involvement in sarcoma. A presentation of 12 cases, a review of the literature, and a discussion of possible changing patterns with the use of chemotherapy, placing special emphasis on embryonal tumours. *Eur J Cancer* 16(11):1503, 1980

51. Buff SJ, Chen JT, Ravin CC, Moore JO: Pulmonary metastasis from ameloblastoma of the mandible: Report of case and review of the literature. *J Oral Surg* 38(5):374, 1980

52. Bussolati G, Ghiringhello B, Papotti M: Subareolar muscular hamartoma of the breast. *Appl Pathol* 2(2):92, 1984

53. Campanacci M, Giunti A, Olmi R: Giant-cell tumours of bone: a study of 209 cases with long-term follow-up in 130. *Ital J Orthorp Traumatol* 1(2):249, 1975

54. Campbell CM, Smith JA, Middleton RG: Plasmacytoma of the urethra. *J Urol* 127(5):986, 1982

55. Carter SK, Broder LE: The cytostatic therapy of hormone-secreting tumours of the GI tract. *Clin Gastroenterol* 3(31):733, 1978

56. Cefis F, Cattaneo M, Carnevale Ricci PM, Frigerio B, Usellini L, Capella C: Primary polypeptide hormones and mucin-producing malignant carcinoid of the larynx. *Ultrastruct Pathol* 5(1):45, 1983

57. Cerra R, Masatro AA: Problems in the surgical treatment of soft tissue tumors of the extremities. *Tumori* 67(3, Suppl), 1981

58. Chatterjee D, Powell A: Renal Hemangioendothelioma. *Int Surg* 67(4):373, 1982

59. Chen KT, Kirkegaard DD, Bocian JJ: Angiosarcoma of the breast. *Cancer* 46(2):368, 1980

60. Chiotasso PJ, Fazio VW: Prognostic factors of 28 leiomyosarcomas of the small intestine. *Surg Gynecol Obstet* 155(2):197, 1982

61. Chisholm RC, Chung EB, Tuckson W, Khan T, White JE: Follicular carcinoma of the thyroid with metastasis to the breast. *J Natl Med Assoc* 72(11):1—101, 1980

62. Chomette G, Auriol M, Vaillant JM: Acinic cell tumors of salivary glands. Frequency and morphological study. *J Biol Buccale* 12(2):157, 1984

63. Chung CK, Johns ME, Cantrell RW, Constable WC: Radiotherapy in the management of primary malignancies of the hard palate. *Laryngoscope* 90(4):576, 1980

64. Cieplinski W, Ciesielski TE, Haine C, Nieh P: Choroid metastases from transitional cell carcinoma of the bladder. A case report and a review of the literature. *Cancer* 50(8):1596, 1982

65. Clark JL, Unni KK, Dahlin DC, Devine KD: Osteosarcoma of the jaws. *Am J Clin Pathol* 69(2):212, 1978

66. Clements JL Jr, Roche RR: Carcinoid of the duodenum: a report of six cases. *Gastrointest Radiol* 9(1):17, 1984

67. Cocke EW: Cancer of the larynx. *Surgery CA* 26(4):201, 1976

68. Cohen J, Guillamondegui OM, Batsakis JG, Medina JE: Cancer of the minor salivary glands of the larynx. *Am J Surg* 150(4):513, 1985

69. Compagno J, Oertel JE, Kremzar M: Solid and papillary epithelial neoplasm of the pancreas, probably of small duct origin: a clinicopathologic study of 52 cases. *Lab Invest* 40(2):248, 1979

70. Conrad MR, Ballard J, Epstein R: Renal metastasis from treated seminoma. *J Can Assoc Radiol* 29(3):197, 1978

71. Cornier E, Colau JC, Blum F, Faguer C, Barrat J: Discovery of a post-abortion choriocarcinoma on the occasion of a vaginal metastasis. *J Gynecol Obstet Biol Reprod (Paris)* 7(8):1474, 1978

72. Cox EV: Chiasmal compression from metastatic cancer to the pituitary gland. *Surg Neurol* 11(1):49, 1979

73. Cremer H, Koischwitz D, Tismer R: Primary osteoliposarcoma of bone. *J Cancer Res Clin Oncol* 101(2):203, 1981

74. Cricco RP, Kandzari SJ: Secondary testicular tumors. *J Urol* 118(3):489, 1977

75. Dahl C, Iversen HG, Engelholm SA, Jacobsen M: Leydig cell tumour – a malignant tumour? *Scand J Urol Nephrol* 18(4):337, 1984

76. Das S, Bulusu NV, Lowe P: Primary vesical pheochromocytoma. *Urology* 21(1):20, 1983

77. Daskalakis MK: Endobronchial metastasis from breast carcinoma. *Int Surg* 66(2):165, 1981

78. Dawson J, Mauduit G, Kanitakis J, Euvrard S, Thivolet J: Unusual vascular tumour of the scalp in association with lymphoid aggregates: a variant of angiolymphoid hyperplasia? *J Cutan Pathol* 11(6):506, 1984

79. Deppe G, Clachko M, Deligdisch L, Cohen CJ: Uterine fibroleiomyomata with aortic lymph node metastasis. *Int J Gynaecol Obstet* 18(1):1, 1980

80. Deshotels SJ, Sarma D, Fazio F, Rodriguez F: Squamous cell carcinoma with sarcomatoid stroma. *J Surg Oncol* 19(4):201, 1982

81. Deutsch HL, Millard DR: Acinic cell tumor of the palate. *J Surg Oncol* 9(5):481, 1977

82. Didolkar MS, Bescher RA, Elias EG, Moore RH: Natural history of adrenal cortical carcinoma: a clinicopathologic study of 42 patients. *Cancer* 47(9):2153, 1981

83. Dietz R, Burger L, Merkel K, Schimrigk K: Malignant gliomas–glioblastoma multiforme and astrocytoma III–IV with extracranial metastases. Report of two cases. *Acta Neurochir (Wien)* 57(1/2):99, 1981

84. Dobias J: Endobronchial and intrapulmonary lipomatous tumours. *Cas Lek Cesk* 120(33):980, 1981

85. Dodat H, Paulhac JB, Macabeo V et al.: Benign tumors of the posterior urethra in children. Apropos of an unusual case of rhabdomyoma of fetal type. *J Urol (Paris)* 93(1):43, 1987

86. Doss LL, Llorens AS, Henriquez EM: Carcinosarcoma of the uterus: a 40-year experience from the state of Missouri. *Gynecol Oncol* 18(1):43, 1984

87. Dourov N: The mobile portion of the tongue. Pathologic anatomy. *Acta Otorhinolaryngol Belg* 34 (Suppl 2):55, 1980

88. Doyle TJ: Brain metastases in the natural history of small-cell lung cancer 1972-1979. *Cancer* 50(4):752, 1982

89. Duffner PK, Cohen ME: Extraneural metastases in childhood brain tumors. *Ann Neurol* 10(3):261, 1981

90. Duker J, Otten JE, Schilli W: Differential diagnostic aspects of classification of osseous metastases in x-rays of the jaw.

Dtsch Zahnaerztl Z 36(11):755, 1981

91. Eckstein RP, Russell P, Friedlander ML, Tattersall MM, Bradfield A: Metastasizing placental site trophoblastic tumor: a case study. *Hum Pathol* 16(6):632, 1985

92. Eisenbud L, Kahn LB, Friedman E: Benign osteoblastoma of the mandible; fifteen year follow-up showing spontaneous regression after biopsy. *J Oral Maxillofac Surg* 45(1):53, 1987

93. Eitschberger E, Wangemann HH, Weidner F et al.: Regional metastases or continuous extension in a case of basal cell carcinoma in the temporal area? *HNG* 30(9):346, 1982

94. Elias EA, Elias RA, Bijlsma J, Tazelaar DJ: The enzyme histochemistry of metastasizing basal cell carcinoma of the skin. *J Pathol* 131(3):235, 1980

95. El Shafie M, Furay RW, Chablani LV: Ovarian teratoma with peritoneal and lymph node metastases of mature glial tissue: a benign condition. *J Surg Oncol* 27(1):18, 1984

96. El Shennawy M, Khafagy M, Ishak E: Rhabdomyosarcoma of head and neck in children. *J Laryngol Otol* 94(6):677, 1980

97. Etzel JC, Froehlich C, Hoeffel JC: Radiological appearances of angioblastosarcomas: a report on one case and review of the published literature. *J Radiol Electrol Med Nucl* 61(6/7):411, 1980

98. Faintuch J, Shepard KV, Levin B: Adenocarcinoma and other unusual variants of esophageal cancer. *Semin Oncol* 11(2):196, 1984

99. Fan L, Gao C, Jin F, Hu L, Sun L: Clear cell carcinoma of the ovary – report of seven cases and review of the literature. *Zhonghua Zhongliu Zazhi* 3(4):269, 1981

100. Ferlito A: Primary lymphoepithelial carcinoma of the hypopharynx. *J Laryngol Otol* 91(4):361, 1977

101. Ferlito A: Acinic cell carcinoma of minor salivary glands. *Histopathology* 4(3):331, 1980

102. Ficarra G, Hansen LS, Engebretsen S et al.: Combined nevi of the oral mucosa. *Oral Surg Oral Med Oral Pathol* 63(2):196, 1987

103. Flanigan RV, Wittman RP, Huhn RG: Malignant pheochromocytoma of the bladder. 75th Annual Meeting, San Francisco. Amer Uorological Assoc.

104. Fourcade R, Jardin A, Kuss R: Bladder metastasis from a renal cancer. *J Urol Nephrol (Paris)* 83(7/8):54, 1977

105. Fourcade R, Wechsler B, Garion G, Jardin A: Acute adrenal insufficiency associated with a malignant tumor of the bladder, possibility of bilateral metastases. *Ann Urol (Paris)* 14(5):321, 1980

106. Froidevaux A, Megewand R: Metastases to the thyroid gland: report of two cases. *Helv Chir Acta* 44(1/2):175, 1977

107. Gabrielle R, Schmitz D, Becker JM, Paulignan M: Dysphagia caused by neoplastic metastases following breast cancer. *Rev Fr Gastroenterol* (163):5, 1980

108. Gaillard J, Fournial G, Barthoumieu F: False primary bone and cartilage tumors of the thoracic wall. *Ann Chir Thorac Cardiovasc* 17(1):18, 1978

109. Gall RJ, Sim FH, Pritchard DJ: Metastatic tumors to the bones of the foot. *Cancer* 37(3):1492, 1976

110. Gallivan MV, Lack EE, Chun B, Ishak KG: Undifferentiated ("embryonal") sarcoma of the liver: ultrastructure of a case presenting as a primary intracardiac tumor. *Pediatr Pathol* 1(3):291, 1983

111. Garavaglia J, Guepp DR: Intramuscular (infiltrating) lipoma of the tongue. *Oral Surg Oral Med Oral Pathol* 63(3):348, 1987

112. Gardiner LJ, Pillsbury HC: A case of three synchronous metastatic carcinomas in the neck with two occult primaries. *Otolaryngol Head Neck Surg* 90(5):174, 1982

113. Gardner DG: A pathologist's approach to the treatment of ameloblastoma. *J Oral Maxillofac Surg* 42(3):161, 1984

114. Geschickter CF, Copeland MM: Bone. In: *Management of the Patient with Cancer*, edited by Nealon TF, WB Saunders, Philadelphia, 1976

115. Ghilezan N, Tamburlini S, Marinca F: The involvement of the central nervous system in malignant lymphoma. *Radiobiol Radiother (Berl)* 23(4):375, 1982

116. Giannestras NJ, Bronson JL: Malignant schwannoma of the medial plantar branch of the posterior tibial nerve (unassociated with von Recklinghausen's disease). *J Bone Joint Surg (Am)* 57A(5):701, 1975

117. Gizycka I, Kubicka K, Bieganowska K, Lisicka D, Marcinski A, Karczenski K: Primary cardiac neoplasms in children. *Pol Przegl Chir* 52(9):807, 1980

118. Glazer HS, Lee JK, Balfe DM, Mauro MA, Griffith R, Sagel SS: Non-Hodgkinson's lymphoma: computed tomographic demonstration of unusual extranodal involvement. *Radiology* 149(1):211, 1983

119. Goldberg LD, Ditchek NT: Thyroid carcinoma with spinal cord compression. *JAMA* 245(9):953, 1981

120. Golnik R, Gajewski W: A tumor of the femur resembling aponeurotic sarcoma. *Chir Narzadow Ruchu Ortop Pol* 44(6):115, 1979

121. Gomyoda M, Nishikawa M, Inada Y, Hoshijima E: Marked esophageal changes associated with acanthosis nigricans with scirrhous carcinoma of the stomach – an autopsy case. *I To Cho* 15(3):249, 1980

122. Goodman ZD, Ishak KG, Langloss JM, Sesterhenn IA, Rabin L: Combined hepatocellular-cholangiocarcinoma. A histologic and immunohistochemical study. *Cancer* 55(1):124, 1985

123. Gunderson LL, Sosin H: Areas of failure found at reoperation (second or symptomatic look) following 'curvative surgery' for adenocarinoma of the rectum. Clinicopathologic correlation and implications for adjuvant therapy. *Cancer* 34(4):1278, 1974

124. Gustavsson P, Hogstedt C, Rappe C: Short-term mortality and cancer incidence in capacitor manufacturing workers exposed to polychlorinated biphenyls (PCBs). *Am J Ind Med* 10(4):341, 1986

125. Hackl H: Structural and functional pathologic characteristics in the cytology of body cavities. *Med Welt* 31(34):1197, 1980

126. Hagemeister FB, Buzdar Au, Luna MA, Blumenschein GR: Causes of death in breast cancer. A clinicopathologic study. *Cancer* 46(1):162, 1980

127. Hager J, Riedler L, Eichenauer M: Clinical and pathological aspects of 'rare' metastases of colorectal carcinoma. *Helv Chir Acta* 50(6):757, 1984

128. Hakimi M, Pai RP, Fine G, Favila JC: Fibrous histiocytoma of the trachea. *Chest* 68(3):367, 1975

129. Halama M: A rare case of gastric cancer metastasis to the cervical skin. *Otolaryngol Pol* 32(3):363, 1978

130. Handel N, Rouge D: Dermatofibrosarcoma protuberans: a case report and clinicopathologic review. *Cutis* 26(3):313, 1980

131. Haq MM, Legha SS, Samaan NA, Bodey GP, Burgess MA: Cytotoxic chemotherapy in adrenal cortical carcinoma. *Cancer Treat Rep* 64(8/9):909, 1980

132. Harkonen M, Olin PE: Rectal carcinoma metastasizing to a toe. *Acta Med Scand* 207(3):235, 1980

133. Harousseau JL, Schaison G, Caubarrere I, Tricot G: Acute lymphoblastic leukemia: late testicular recurrence that was associated with lymph node sarcoidosis. *Nouv Presse Med* 9(18):1310, 1980

134. Hartmann CA, Hanke S: Unusual pleural involvement in a metastasizing thymoma. *Pathologe* 5(3):169, 1984

135. Hasumi K, Nagashima K, Yamaguchi K, Sugano H: Clinicopathological study of solid teratoma of the ovary. *Jpn J Cancer Clin* 19(12):1173, 1973

136. Hayman JA, Ostor AG: Ovarian mucinous tumour with a focus of anaplastic carcinoma: a case report. *Pathology* 17(4):591, 1985

137. Heberling D, Rummel HH, Leppien G, Hoffken H: Glioma-

tosis peritonei – a contribution to the biology of metastasizing. *Geburtshilfe Frauenheilkd* 40(8):729, 1980

138. Heckemann R: Ultrasonographic tumor diagnosis in the retroperitoneum. *Therapiewoche* 33(2):123, 127, 133, 137, 1983

139. Heitland Neugebauer Durst: Prognosis of male mammary carcinoma. *Zentralbl Chir* 102(2):125, 1977

140. Helwig EB, May D: Atypical fibroxanthoma of the skin with metastasis. *Cancer* 57(2):368, 1986

141. Hendren WG, Monfort GF: Symptomatic bilateral renal angiomyolipomas in a child. *J Urol* 137(2):256, 1987

142. Herics I, Rado J, Decker A: Certain aspects of bone metastases in breast cancers. 20th Congr of Radiology, Aug 31–Sept 2, 1980, Pecs, Hungary, The Radiology Soc Budapest, 1980

143. Herlinger H, Caroline D, Thompson J, Kressel HY, Laufer I: Detection and differential diagnosis of adenocarcinoma of the small intestine. Scientific Program of the Society of Gastrointestinal Radiologists. Maui, Hawaii, The Society, 1980

144. Herrera LO, Ledesma EJ, Natarajan N, Lopez GE, Tsukada Y, Mittelman A: Metachronous ovarian metastases from adenocarcinoma of the colon and rectum. *Surg Gynecol Obstet* 154(4):531, 1982

145. Higa T, Sakamoto A, Yoshida T, Tanaka K, Shimayama T, Sumiyoshi A: Leiomyoma of the jejunum: a case report and a review of cases in Japanese literature. *I To Cho* 15(10):1097, 1980

146. Hiriart JC, Bodega E, Otero AM, Dighiero G: A rare case of subacute myelomonocytic leukemia. *Rev Med Urug* 2(3):390, 1976

147. Hivet M, Casassus P, Horiot A: Pancreatic metastases. Report of a case of pancreatic metastasis in a liver carcinoma. *Ann Chir* 31(2):163, 1977

148. Hodgkinson DJ, Rettine WH, Weiland LH: A clinicopathologic study of 21 cases of pancreatic cystadenocarcinoma. *Ann Surg* 188(5):679, 1978

149. Hoffman NJ, Duffner PK: Extraneural metastases of central nervous system tumors. *Cancer* 56(7 suppl):1778, 1985

150. Hollins RR, Lydiatt DD, Markin RS et al.: Mesenchymal chondrosarcoma: a case report. *J Oral Maxillofac Surg* 45(1):72, 1987

151. Holt JT, Choi BH: Occult pontine astrocytoma with bony metastases at time or craniotomy: a case report. *Lab Invest* 44(1):28A, 1981

152. Holveck N, Deschler JM, Garnier JP, Voegflin M: Orbital metastasis as a revealer of a primary hepatoma. Arteriographic diagnosis. *J Radiol Electrol Med Nucl* 60(6/7):449, 1979

153. Horcher E, Staffen A, Czech W: Clinical appearance, radiology and therapy of angiosarcomas in the mammary gland. *Chirurg* 48(6):395, 1977

154. Horie A, Ishii N, Matsumoto M, Hashizuma Y, Kawakami M, Sato Y: Leiomyomatosis in the pelvic lymph node and peritoneum. *Acta Pathol Jpn* 34(4):813, 1984

155. Huber O, Megewand R, Baud M: Malignant thymoma and intestinal metastasis; one case and literature review. *Helv Chir Acta* 47(1/2):209, 1980

156. Hulbert JC, Rodriguez PN, Cummings KB: Perineal liposarcoma: diagnosis and management. *J Urol* 131(6):1185, 1984

157. Husband JE, Barrett A, Peckham J: Evaluation of computed tomography in the management of testicular teratoma. *Br J Urol* 53(2):179, 1981

158. Igarashi M, Card GC, Johnson PE, Alford BR: Bilateral sudden hearing loss and metastatic pancreatic adenocarcinoma. *Arch Otolaryngol* 105(4):196, 1979

159. Ikeda M, Kimura M, Niwa H, Sasamoto K, Miki K, Hirayama T, Cho K, Oka H, Oda T, Mhori N: Gastric cancer with peculiar metastatic lesions in the head of the pancreas and the duodenum: report of a case. *Gastroenterol Endosc* 23(12):1832, 1981

160. Imahori SC: Multifocal fibrosarcoma of the bone. *Arch Pathol Lab Med* 104(10):550, 1980

161. Inoue Y, Takeuchi T, Tamakai M, Nin K, Hakuba A, Nishimura S: Sequential CT observations of irradiated intracranial germinomas. *Am J Roentgenol* 132(3):361, 1979

162. Irie J, Kawai K, Ueno Y, Kumagai K, Matsuo K, Tsuchiyama H: (1985). Malignant germ cell tumor of the anterior mediastinum with leukemia-like infiltration. *Acta Pathol Jpn* 35(6):1561, 1985

163. Ishihara K, Horitani K, Kinochi J, Kano S, Hoshika K, Hiamoto N, Fushimi A, Uchida J, Kihara T: A case of bizarre leiomyoblastoma of the ileum associated with Leser-Trelat syndrome. *I To Cho* 16(10):1091, 1981

164. Jafari K, Lash AF, Webster A: Pregnancy and sarcoma. *Acta Obstet Gynecol Scand* 57(3):265, 1978

165. Jager RM, Max MH: Umbilical metastasis as the presenting symptom of cecal carcinoma. *J Surg Oncol* 12(1):41, 1979

166. Jakubowski J, Kendall BE, Symon L: Primary plasmocytomas of the cranial vault. *Acta Neurochir (Wien)* 55(1/2):117, 1980

167. Jaulerry C, Bataini J, Brunin F, Pouillart P, Mazabraud A: Osteosarcomas. *Rev Prat* 32(55/56):3497, 3501, 3507, 3513, 1982

168. Jobst SB, Ljung BM, Gilkey FW, Rosenthal DL: Cytologic diagnosis of olfactory neuroblastoma: a case report with multiple diagnostic parameters. *Lab Invest* 46(1):42A, 1982

169. Johannessen JV, Sobrinho-Simoes M et al.: Anomalous papillary carcinoma of the thyroid. *Cancer* 51(8):1462, 1983

170. Johnson MW, Morettin LB, Sarles HE, Zaharoppoulos P: Follicular carcinoma of the thyroid metastatic to the kidney 37 years after resection of the primary tumor. *J Urol* 127(1):114, 1982

171. Jones WL: Intraocular metastatic disease to the eye. *J Am Optom Assoc* 52(9):741, 1981

172. Joshi VV, Banerjee AK, Yadav K, Pathak IC: Cystic partially differentiated nephroblastoma. A clinicopathologic entity in the spectrum of infantile renal neoplasia. *Cancer* 40(2):789, 1977

173. Kalifat R, Sellami F: Polycystic renal disease and bilateral renal cancer. *Ann Urol (Paris)* 21(1):3, 1987

174. Kameya T, Shimosato Y, Adachi I, Abe K, Ebihara S, Ono I: Neuroendocrine carcinoma of the paranasal sinus. A morphological and endocrinological study. *Cancer* 45(2):330, 1980

175. Kandel RA, Bedard YC, Pritzker KP, Luk SC: Lymphoma. Presenting as an intramuscular small cell malignant tumor. *Cancer* 53(7):1586, 1984

176. Kannagi R, Levine P, Watanabe K, Hakomori SI: Recent studies of glycolipid and glycoprotein profiles and characterization of the major glycolipid antigen in gastric cancer of a patient of blood group genotype pp TJA – first studied in 1951. *Cancer Res* 42(13):5249, 1982

177. Kao GF, Norris HJ: Juxtaovarian adnexal tumor – clinical and pathologic study of 19 cases. *Lab Invest* 38(3):350, 1978

178. Kao GF, Graham JH, Helwig EB: Carcinoma cuniculatum (verrucous carcinoma of the skin). A clinicopathologic study of 46 cases with ultrastructural observations. *Cancer* 49(11):2395, 1982

179. Kasai N, Uchida M, Sakamoto A, Hosoya T, Watanuki T: Clinical studies on metastatic patterns of carcinoma of the thyroid. *J Jpn Soc Cancer Ther* 13(5):537, 1978

180. Katoh M, Minami M, Inoue K, Boku S, Murayama Y et al.: A clinicopathological study of gastric cancer: its characteristics in relation to the age of the patients. *Nippon Shokaki Geka Gakkai Zasshi* 12(11):832, 1979

181. Kawamura K: A case of adenoid cystic carcinoma of the trachea treated with circumferential segmental resection of the trachea. *Nippon Kyoba Seka Gakkai Zasschi* 28(12):1908, 1980

182. Kawarada Y, Uehara S, Noda M, Yatani R, Mizumoto R:

Nonhepatocytic malignant mixed tumor primary in the liver. Report of two cases. *Cancer* 55(8):1790, 1985

183. Kazeev KN, Bazarova EN, Babin AV, Bronshtein ME, Iureva NP: Thyrotoxicosis and thyroid cancer. *Sov Med* (9):46, 1980

184. Kellie SJ, Waters KD: Testicular neuroblastoma. *J Surg Oncol* 29(3):201, 1985

185. Kibsgaard K: Gastric metastases from muco-epidermoid parotid tumor. Endoscopic diagnosis. *Gastrointest Endosc* 25(3):106, 1979

186. Kim KS, Weinberg PE, Hemmati M: Spinal pachymeningeal carcinomatosis: myelographic features. *Am J Neuroradiol* 1(2):199, 1980

187. Kimball JC, Cangir A: Occurrence of testicular metastasis in a child with bilateral retinoblastoma. *Cancer Treat Rep* 63(5):803, 1979

188. Kimmelman CP, Haller DG: Unusual oat cell carcinomas of the head and neck. *Otolaryngol Head Neck Surg* 89 (5, section 2):192, 1981

189. Kishimoto Y, Hijiya S, Nagasako R: Malignant mixed tumor of the liver in adults. *Am J Gastroenterol* 79(3):229, 1984

190. Kitahara M, Katakura R, Wada T, Nawiki T, Suzuki J: Diffuse form of primary leptomeningeal gliomatosis. Case report. *J Neurosurg* 63(2):283, 1984

191. Kline IK: Malignancy metastatic to the heart: its incidence and significance. *Am J Clin Pathol* 69(2):214, 1978

192. Knoepfle G, Foedisch HJ, Evers KG, Juergens H: Malignant pheochromocytoma in childhood and adolescence-clinical case and review of the literature. *Klin Pediatr* 196(3):156, 1984

193. Kochhar VL, Srivastava KK: Unusual lesions of the patella. *Int Surg* 61(1):37, 1976

194. Kohnoe K, Nomura H, Tokumitsu S, Takeuchi T: An autopsy case of cystadenocarcinoma arising from cystadenoma of the liver. Proc Jap Cancer Assoc, Japanese Cancer Association, Tokyo, Japan, 1977

195. Kohri K, Nagai N, Matsuura T, Kaneko S, Iguchi M, Minami K, Akiyama T, Yachiku S, Kurita T: Retrovesical chondrosarcoma. *J Urol* 123(5):768, 1980

196. Komisar A, Som PM, Shugar JM, Sacher M, Parisier SC: Benign chondroma of the petrous apex. *J Computer Assit Tomography* 5(1):116, 1981

197. Komminoth J, Florange W, Staehling V: Cutaneous digital metastasis of a cancer of the buccal floor. *Ann Otolaryngol Chir Cervicofac* 94(1/2):53, 1977

198. Kondo Y, Akita T, Sugano I, Isono K: Signet ring cell carcinoma of the breast. *Acta Pathol Jpn* 34(4):875, 1984

199. Kopf AW, Bart RS: Tumor conference number 7. Tumor on shoulder arising after excision of a cyst. *J Dermatol Surg* 2(3):196, 1976

200. Koss LG: The breast and nipple. Diagnostic Cytology and its Histopathologic Bases, edited by Koss LG, Philadelphia: Lippincott. Vol 2, 1979

201. Kraemer KH, Lee MM, Scotto J: DNA repair protects against cutaneous and internal neoplasia: evidence from xeroderma pigmentosus. *Carcinogenesis* 5(4):511, 1984

202. Kramer SA, Bradford WD, Anderson EE: Bilateral adrenal neuroblastoma. *Cancer* 45(8):2208, 1980

203. Krane RJ: Seminoma. Invitational Assembly for Advanced Urology: Urologic Malignancies Pinehurst, North Carolina Duke University, Medical Center, 1982

204. Krayenbuehl H, Yasargii MG: Chondromas. *Prog Neurol Surg* 6:435, 1975

205. Krieger G, Wuchter J: Aplastic amenia, Sjögren-syndrome and hypogammaglobulinemia associated with thymoma. *Therapiewoche* 31(6):718, 1981

206. Kroon BB, Albus-Lutter ChE, Van Dongen JA: The alveolar soft part sarcoma. *Med Tijdschr Geneeskd* 125(3):87, 1981

207. Krutchik AN, Buzdsar AU, Tashima CK, Blumenschein

208. Kumar UN, Varkey B: Subcutaneous metastasis. Rare complication of drainage of malignant pleural fluid. *Postgrad Med* 60(5):253, 1976

209. Kuntz HD, May B: Phlebitis migrans with pancreas carcinoma. *MMW* 122(41):53, 1980

210. Kunze E, Donath K, Luhr HG, Engelhardt W, De Vivie R: Biology of metastasizing ameloblastoma. *Pathol Res Pract* 180(5):526, 1985

211. Kurman RJ, Norris HJ: Germ cell tumors of the ovary. *Pathol Annu* 13(1):291, 1978

212. Kurschwitz S, Schubel HW: Histological diagnosis and therapy of rare breast tumors. *Zentralbl Gynaekol* 97(9):552, 1975

213. Lack EE, Harris GB, Eraklis AJ, Vawter GF: Primary bronchial tumors in childhood. A clinicopathologic study of six cases. *Cancer* 51(3):492, 1983

214. Lafreniere R, Ketcham AS: Primary squamous carcinoma of the rectum. Report of a case and review of the literature. *Dis Colon Rectum* 281:2967, 1985

215. Laurent C, Lindholm CE, Nordlinder H: Benign pedunculated tumours of the hypopharynx. 3 case reports, 1 with late malignant transformation. *ORL Otorhinolaryngol Relat Spec* 47(1):17, 1985

216. Laurenti C, De Dominicis C, Dal Forno S, Bologna G: Leiomyosarcoma of the bladder in a girl. *Eur Urol* 8(3):185, 1982

217. Lee JR, Zubrod CG: Osteolytic metastasis of the humerus: primary source. *JAMA* 239(9):870, 1978

218. Lee YT: Better prognosis of many cancers in female: a phenomenon not explained by study of steroid receptors. *J Surg Oncol* 25(4):255, 1984

219. Le Guillou M, Perrin P: Tumours of the testis. *J Urol (Paris)* 87(6):331, 1981

220. Lei Z, Du C, Song D: Primary rhabdomyosarcoma of the lung: a review of literature and a case report. *Zhonghua Jiehe He Huxixi Jibing Zazhi* 4(2):84, 1981

221. Lennert K, Schmid U: Immunosialadenitis (Sjögren syndrome) – a model of lymphomagenesis. Modern Trends in Human Leukemia V, June 21–23, 1982, Wilsede, W Germany Deutsche Gesellschaft für Hämatologie und Onchologie, New York, Springer Verlag, 1982

222. Levine PL, Berberich FR, Burke JS, Mott MG, Wilbur JR: Lymphoblastic lymphoma: late relapse in childhood. *Med Pediatr Oncol* 11(1):33, 1983

223. Lim SK, Kovi Y, Warner OG: Adenoid cystic carcinoma of breast with metastasis: a case report and review of the literature. *J Natl Med Assoc* 71(4):329, 1979

224. Ling L: Fatality of 'benign osteoblastoma'. Proposal of a new nomenclature. *Zhonghua Guke Zazhi* 1(1):55, 1981

225. Liu F: Diagnosis and prognosis of dermatofibrosarcoma protuberans. *Zhonghua Pifuke Zazhi* 14(2):92, 1981

226. Liu S, Kang Y, Wang C, Mao L: Analysis of treatment results in ovarian epithelial carcinoma using surgery as the primary treatment. *Zhonghua Fuchanke Zazhi* 17(1):53, 1982

227. Liu Y, Deng X: A case of malignant mesothelioma of the pericardium. *Zhonghua Zhongliu Zazhi* 3(1):74, 1981

228. Liu Z, Meng Y, Ma S: Extramedullary plasmacytoma of the nasal cavity and paranasal sinuses: a comprehensive report of 7 cases. *Zhonghua Er Bi Yanhouke Zazhi* 15(3):185, 1980

229. Loeffler JS, Ervin TJ, Mauch P, Skarin A, Weinstein HJ, Canellos G, Cassady JR: Primary lymphomas of the central nervous system: patterns of failure and factors that influence survival. *J Clin Oncol* 8(4):490, 1985

230. Lotze W, Richter P: Malignant Brenner tumor of the ovary. *Zentralbl Gynakol* 107(17):1085, 1985

231. Lovisetto O, Manachino D, Biarese V, Marchi L, Andrione P: Blood hypereosinophilias. IV. Symptomatic hypereo-

sinophilias: connective tissue diseases, neoplasms, blood diseases, various causes. *Minerva Med* 76(25):1181, 1985

232. Luper WE, Klima T: Leiomyosarcoma of the femoral vein. *Bull Tex Heart Inst* 1(5):428, 1975

233. Macnicol MF, Rebello G, Kirkpatrick JR et al.: Reticulum cell sarcoma of the testis. *J R Coll Surg Edinb* 19(2):116, 1974

234. Maehara Y, Sakurai T, Hareyama M, Nishio M, Saito A, Kagami Y, Kanemoto T: Late local recurrence of cervical cancer after initial treatment. *Gan No Rinsho* 29(12):1441, 1983

235. Mamelle G, Richard J, Luboinski B et al.: Synovial sarcoma of the head and neck: an account of four cases and review of the literature. *Eur J Surg Oncol* 12(4):347, 1986

236. Maniglia AJ: Meibomian gland adenocarcinoma of the eyelid with neck metastasis. *Laryngoscope* 88(9, part 1):1421, 1978

237. Manschot WA, van Strik R: Choroid melanoma: Analysis of published therapeutic results. *Fortschr Ophthalmol* 84(2):183, 1987

238. Manschot WA, Stefanko SZ: Pinealoblastoma with photoreceptor differentiation. *Ophthalmologica* 178(1/2):94, 1979

239. Matsusaka T, Miyazaki M, Soejima K, Kodama Y, Yoshimura K, Inokuchi K: Clinico-pathological analysis of macroscopically early, but microscopically advanced gastric cancer. *Gan No Rinsho* 24(14):1197, 1978

240. Mayes GB, Chuang VP, Fisher RG: CT of pseudomyxoma peritonei. *AJR* 136(4):807, 1981

241. McKee GT, Fletcher CD, McKee PH: Visceral intravascular capillary hemangioma. *Arch Pathol Lab Med* 111(4):390, 1987

242. Meyer JJ, Sane SM, Drake RM: Malignant paraganglioma (pheochromocytoma) of the urinary bladder: report of a case and review of the literature. *Pediatrics* 63(6):879, 1979

243. Michaelson RA, Magill GB, Quan SH, Leaming RH, Nikrui M, Stearns NW: Preoperative chemotherapy and radiation therapy in the management of anal epidermoid carcinoma. *Cancer* 51(3):390, 1983

244. Mikhail GR: Cancers, precancers, and pseudocancers on the male genitalia. A review of clinical appearances, histopathology, and management. *Dermatol Surg Oncol* 6(12):1027, 1980

245. Miller A, Seljelid R: Histopathologic classification and natural history of malignant testis tumors in Norway, 1959–1963. *Cancer* 28(4):1054, 1971

246. Miller RW: Prenatal origins of cancer in man: epidemiological evidence. *IARC Sci Publ* (4):175, 1973

246a. Miller RW, Watanabe S, Fraumeni JF Jr, Sugimura T, Takayama S, Sugano H (eds): Unusual Occurrences as Clues to Cancer Etiology. Tokyo, Japan Scientific Societies Press; London – Philadelphia, Taylor & Francis Ltd., 1988

247. Mohlen K, Brandt M: Compression of the spinal cord secondary to an intradural metastasis from a primary carcinoma of the breast. *Geburtshilfe Frauenheilkd* 38(8):648, 1978

248. Montesinos M: Metastasis in the rectum from ovarian mesonephroma up to 10 years after removal of the tumor. *Takoginecol Pract* 33(40):405, 1974

249. Morioka M, Uehata Y, Koyama M, Sakurada K, Shiraishi T, Miyasaka M, Suzuki K, Nojima T, Fujioka Y: An autopsy case of primary leiomyosarcoma of the descending colon. *Gan No Rinsho* 26(3):301, 1980

250. Mørk SJ, Rubinstein LJ: Ependymoblastoma. A reappraisal of a rare embryonal tumor. *Cancer* 55(7):1536, 1985

251. Mornex R, Pousset G, Briere J, Daumont M, Paffoy JC: Hyperthyroidism by autonomous metastasis of thyroid carcinoma. *Am Endocrinol (Paris)* 37(2):113, 1976

252. Morvan G, Marsault C, Brault B: Observation of one case of primary hepatoma metastasis in the calvaria. *J Radiol Electrol Med Nucl* 57(2):167, 1976

253. Mostofi FK: Classification of tumors of testis. *Ann Clin Lab Sci* 9(6):455, 1979

254. Motomura M: Benign hemangioendothelioma of the nasopharynx – report of a case. *Jibi Inkoka* 54(2):149, 1982

255. Mueh JR, Greco CM, Green MR: Spontaneous regression of metastatic testicular carcinoma in a patient with bilateral sequential testicular tumor. *Cancer* 45(11):2908, 1980

256. Murray RD: Lesions resembling malignant tumours of bone. *J Belge Radiol* 62(1):1, 1979

257. Muta N, Wada J, Kusajima K, Muroya K: A metastasis grown in the vein, from cancer of the thyroid. *Nippon Acta Radiol* 38(1):14, 1978

258. Nagel K, Ghussen F: The malignant schwannoma. *Med Klin* 77(2):45, 1982

259. Nakazawa M, Hanada T, Nakamura H, Nagasawa T, Yoda Y, Abe T, Kikuchi M, Kojima M: A case of splenic hemangiosarcoma complicated by disseminated intravascular coagulation. *Rinsho Ketsueki* 22(10):1558, 1981

260. Natali PG, Giacomini P, Bigotti G, Nicotra MR, Bellocci M, De Martino: Heterogeneous distribution of actin, myosin, fibronectin and basement membrane antigens in primary and metastatic human breast cancer. *Virchows Arch (A)* 405(1):69, 1984

261. Newman J, Fortune MJ: Metastasis of breast carcinoma to the uterus. *R Coll Surg Edinb* 24(1):42, 1979

262. Nissan S, Bar-Moar JA, Levy E: Lymphosarcoma of the esophagus: a case report. *Cancer* 34(4):1321, 1974

263. Norris CS: Giant condyloma acuminatum (Buschke-Loewenstein tumor) involving a pilonidal sinus: a case report and review of the literature. *J. Surg Oncol* 22(1):47, 1983

264. Obana M, Mita S, Harada K, Irimajiri S, Fujimori I, Fukuda J: An autopsy case of gastric cancer associated with microangiopathic hemolytic anemia without local relapse 6 years after gastrectomy. *Rinsho Ketsueki* 21(9):1395, 1980

265. O'Brien M: Primary intracranial yolk tumors. *Childs Brain* 5(6):570, 1979

266. Ohya T, Takeda Y, Yoshida H et al.: A rare case of simultaneous malignant tumors: osteosarcoma of the mandible and lung cancer. *J Oral Maxillofac Surg* 45(3):261, 1987

267. Ono J, Kawate N, Matsushima Y, Sawa H, Kato H, Kawamura I, Hayata Y, Hayakawa K, Takahashi M: A case of HCG-producing malignant germinal cell tumor originating in the anterior mediastinum. *Kyobu Geka* 33(9):657, 1980

268. Opric M, Cvetkovic S, Planovic Z, Todorovic P, Popovic B: Osteosarcoma of the temporal bone. *Libri Oncol* 8(2/3):187, 1979

269. Ostergaard Laursen S, Beck HI: Leiomyosarcomas of veins. *Ugeskr Laeger* 142(38):2484, 1980

270. Ownby D, Lyon G, Spock A: Primary leiomyosarcoma of the lung in childhood. *Am J Dis Child* 130(10):1132, 1976

271. Paladugu RR, Nathwani BN, Goodstein J, Dari LE, Memoli VE, Gould VE: Carcinoma of the larynx with mucosubstance production and neuroendocrine differentiation: an ultrastructural and immunohistochemical study. *Cancer* 49(2):343, 1982

272. Paletta FX: Squamous cell carcinoma of the skin. *Clin Plast Surg* 7(3):313, 1980

273. Pardo-Mindan FJ, Vazquez JJ: Malignant struma ovarii. Light and electron microscopic study. *Cancer* 51(2):337, 1983

274. Parwaresch MR, Horny HP, Lennert K: Tissue mast cells in health and disease. *Pathol Res Pract* 179(4–5):439, 1985

275. Pasquier B, Pasquier D, Lachard A et al.: Extraneural metastasis of central nervous system tumors. *Bu-l Cancer (Paris)* 66(1):25, 1979

276. Patel JK, Englander LS: Leiomyosarcoma of the inferior vena cava. *J Surg Oncol* 21(4):238, 1982

277. Patsner B, Piver MS, Lele SB, Tsukada Y, Bielat K, Castillo

NB: Small cell carcinoma of the ovary: a rapidly lethal tumor occurring in the young. *Gynecol Oncol* 22(2):233, 1985

278. Payne DG, Simpson WJ: Oligodendroglioma: surgery and radiation in 49 cases. Twenty-fourth Ann Meeting of the Amer Soc of Ther Radiologists October 25–29, Orlando, Florida. Amer Society of Therapeutic Radiologists, 1982

279. Pesavento G, Ferlito A, Recher G: Primary clear cell carcinoma of the larynx. *J Clin Pathol* 33(12):1160, 1980

280. Peterson L, Dehner LP, Brunning RD: Acute monoblastic leukemia in patients presenting with extramedullary masses. *Lab Invest* 42(1):142, 1980

281. Pfister-Goedeke L, Pluss HJ, Isler W: Skeletal metastasis in medulloblastomas. 18th Congr European Soc of Pediatr Radiol, Oslo, May 20–23, 1981. The Society, pp AB 1981, 1981

282. Pialat J, Bejui-Thivolet F, Perrin G et al.: Mesenchyma chondrosarcoma: two cases. *Lyons Med* 243(10):621, 1980

283. Pizzarello RA, Goldberg SM, Goldman MA, Gottesman R, Fetten JV, Brown N, Kahn EI, Stein HL: Tumor of the heart diagnosed by magnetic resonance imaging. *J Am Coll Cardiol* 5(4):989, 1985

284. Pizzi GB, Sotti G, Zorat PL, Tomio L, Calzawara F, Poliodoro F, Ferlito A: Chemo-radiotherapy regimen in the treatment of the oat cell carcinoma of the larynx. UICC Conf on Clinical Oncology, October, 1981, Lausanne/Switzerland. IUAC, 131 pp, 1981

285. Plager C: Ewing's sarcoma. *Cancer Bull* 31(7):208, 1979

286. Pocock E, Craig JR, Bullock WK: Metastatic uterine leiomyomata. *Cancer* 38(5):2096, 1976

287. Popper H: Bidermal hepatoblastoma in an adult. *Zentralbl Allg Pathol* 124(5):403, 1980

288. Posner JB, Shapiro WR: Brain tumor: current status of treatment and its complications. *Arch Neurol* 32(12):781, 1975

289. Potts IF: Phaeochromocytoma of the bladder. *Br J Uroli* 49(3):240, 1977

290. Prempree T, Amornmann R, Villasanta U, Kwon T, Scott RM: Retreatment of very late recurrent invasive squamous cell carcinoma of the cervix with irradiation. II. Criteria for patients' selection to achieve the success. *Cancer* 54(9):1950, 1984

291. Probst W, Joss R, Triller J, Schoenenberger A, Greiner R, Brunner KW: Adenocarcinoma of the kidney (hypernephroma). *Schweiz Med Wochenschr* 114(41):1406, 1984

292. Pui CH, Rivera G, Mirro J, Stass S, Peiper S, Murphy SB: Acute megakaryoblastic leukemia. Blast cell aggregates simulating metastatic taumor. *Arch Pathol Lab Med* 109(11):1033, 1985

293. Quan SH: Anal and para-anal tumors. *Surg Clin North Am* 58(3):591, 1978

294. Rahko PS, Nollet DJ, Blomberg DJ: Infiltration of a cerebral artery aneurysm by malignant lymphoma cells with acute rupture: report of a case. *Hum Pathol* 11(4):396, 1980

295. Rao BK, Kapur MM, Roy S: Leiomyosarcoma of the colon: a case report and review of literature. *Dis Colon Rectum* 23(3):184, 1980

296. Rao BN, Pratt CB, Fleming ID, Dilawari RA, Green AA, Austin BA: Colon carcinoma in children and adolescents. A review of 30 cases. *Cancer* 55(6):1322, 1985

297. Reddy SS, Hyland RH, Alison RE, Sturgeon JF, Hutcheon MA: Tumor-associated peripheral eosinophilia: two unusual cases. *J Clin Oncol* 2(10):1165, 1984

298. Redman HC: CT tumors of the retroperitoneal tissues. *Exerpta Med Int Congr Ser* (463):251, 1979

299. Reynolds LR, Flueck JA: Evaluation of the hypercalcemic patient. *Am Fam Physician* 23(4):105, 1981

300. Riebel T: So-called "multiple" osteogenic sarcoma of childhood. 18th Congress of European Society of Pediatric Radiology, Oslo, Norway, May 20–23, The Society, pp A10, 1981

301. Robidoux A, Monte M, Heppell J, Schurch W: Small-cell carcinoma of the rectum. *Dis Colon Rectum* 28(8):594, 1985

302. Rosi P, Trippitelli A, Turini D, Carini M: Rhabdomyosarcoma of the spermatic cord. *Minerva Urol* 34(4):291, 1982

303. Rubery ED, Wheeler TK: Metastases outside the central nervous system from a presumed pineal germinoma. *J Neurosurg* 53(4):562, 1980

304. Russinovich NA, Recio MG, Tishler JM et al.: Intracaval extension of pheochromocytoma ultrasonographic demonstration. *J Can Assoc Radiol* 33(1):53, 1982

305. Sack H: Radiotherapy of malignant bone tumors. 99 Kongr Deutsche Ges Chirurgie, Apr 14–17, Munich, pp A72, 1982

306. Saegesser F: Surigcal treatment of round pulmonary foci in a man and six women with breast cancer. Solitary metastases? A second primary pulmonary cancer? A round benign foci? *Helv Chir Acta* 44(5/6):647, 1978

307. Safai B, Good RA: Basal cell carcinoma with metastasis: review of literature. *Arch Pathol* 101:327, 1977

308. Saiga H, Nagao K, Matsuzaki O et al.: Clinicopathological analysis of vascular invasion in early gastric cancer. *Gan No Rinsho* 25(10):1046, 1979

309. Saito R, Nakajima T, Shingaki S, Yokobayashi T: Primary intraosseous epidermoid carcinoma of the mandible. *J Oral Maxillofac Surg* 49(1):41, 1982

310. Sammartino A, Bonavolonta G, Pettinato G, Loffredo A: Exophthalmos caused by an invasive pituitary adenoma in a child. *Ophthalmologica* 179(2):83, 1979

311. Sasaki K, Tani S, Nagamine Y, Takahashi M: Pseudosarcomatous carcinoma of the esophagus – reference to its histogenesis. *Acta Pathol Jpn* 28(5):779, 1978

312. Sato S, Fitzpatrick TB: Ultrastructural studies of melanosis cutis secondary to metastatic malignant melanoma. XIth Internat'l Pigment Cell Conf Sendai, Japan, Tohoku University, 1980

313. Sato Y, Ueda G, Yamasaki M, Yoshinare S, Okudaira Y, Hayakawa K: Clinical histochemical and ultrastructural studies of ovarian granulosa cell tumors. Gann; Pp 177 in Gan Proc Jpn Cancer Sssoc, 33rd Ann Meeting, 1974

314. Sauvegrain J, Kalifa G, Kalifa C: Abdominal presentation of malignant lymphomas in childhood. *J Belge Radiol* 63(1):13, 1980

315. Schantz HD, Ramzy Y, Tio FO, Buhaug J: Metastatic spindle-cell carcinoma. Cytologic features and differential diagnosis. *Acta Cytol (Baltimore)* 29(3):435, 1985

316. Schold SC, Vurgrin D, Golbey RB, Posner JB: Central nervous system metastases from germ cell carcinoma of testis. *Semin Oncol* 6(1):102, 1979

317. Schuhl JF, Paillot JM, Trillat A, Bied JC, Patricot LM: Concerning an observation of hemangioendothelioma of the bone. *Lyon Med* 240(14):79, 1978

318. Schuller DE, Berg JW, Sherman G, Krause CJ: Cutaneous basosquamous carcinoma of the head and neck: a comparative analysis. *Otolaryngol Head Neck Surg* 87(4, Set 1):420, 1979

319. Seagle RL, Nomeir AM, Watts LE: Left atrial myxoma associated with rheumatic mitral stenosis. *Clin Cardiol* 7(6):370, 1984

320. Seibert JJ, Seibert RW, Weisenburger DS, Allsbrook W: Multiple congenital hemangiopericytomas of the head and neck. *Laryngoscope* 88(6):1006, 1978

321. Seifert G, Bull HG, Donath K: Histologic subclassification of the cystadenolymphoma of the parotid gland. Analysis of 275 cases. *Virchows Arch (Pathol Anat)* 388(1):13, 1980

322. Shah JP, Feghali J: Esthesioneuroblastoma. *Am J Surg* 142(4):456, 1981

323. Shaha AR, Shah JP: Carcinoma of the subglottic larynx. *Am J Surg* 144(4):456, 1982

324. Sharma SC, Patel FD, Gupta SK, Ayyagari S, Dutta TK, Gupta BD: Soft tissue and bone lesions in chronic myeloid

leukaemia – a case report. *Indian J Cancer* 17(3):188, 1980

325. Shi H, Gao W: Angiosarcoma of the breast in 2 sisters. *Zhonghua Zhongliu Zazhi* 2(4):314, 1980
326. Shishido M, Hiwada K, Ueda E, Kokubu K, Yoshida H, Fukunishi R: An autopsy case of pancreatic head cancer with proliferation and infiltration only of the portal vein. *Nippon Rinsho* 38(2):452, 1980
327. Slasky BS, Hardesty RL, Wilson S: Tracheal chondrosarcoma with an overview of other tumors of the trachea. *J Comput Tomogr* 9(3):225, 1985
328. Solomon D, Smith RR, Kashima HK, Leventhal BG: Malignant transformation in non-irradiated recurrent respiratory papillomatosis. *Laryngoscope* 95(8):900, 1985
329. Sonobe H, Fujioka I, Nakatoh S, Miyake K, Taguchi K, Motoi M, Ogawa K: Central fibrosarcoma of the bone. Report of a case. *Acta Pathol Jpn* 29(3):479, 1979
330. Souillet G, Maisonneuve J, Lenoir G, Gilly J, Brunat-Mentigny M, Duc H, Hermier M: Undifferentiated carcinoma of the nasopharynx associated with Epstein–Barr virus. Diagnostic value of serological studies of the Epstein–Barr virus. *Pedaitrie* 35(6):541, 1980
331. Spielmann M, Toussaint C, Malcoste G, LeChevalier T et al.: Mesenchymal breast sarcomas. Apropos of 25 cases. *Bull Cancer (Paris)* 72(3):202, 1985
332. Sridhar KS, Rap RK, Kunhardt B: Skeletal muscle metastases from lung cancer. *Cancer* 59(8):1530, 1987
333. Stangl R: Choroid membrane metastases of a papillary thyroid gland carcinoma in a 9-year-old girl. *Ophthalmologica* 175(3):175, 1977
333a. Stefanko SZ, Manschot WA: Pinealoblastoma with retinoblastomatour differentiation. *Brain* 102(2):321, 1979
334. Stellato TA, Gauderer MW, Kazura J: Tumor metastastis from multiple myeloma and Burkitt's lymphoma in Broviac catheter tracts. *Cancer* 55(11):2715, 1985
335. Stephenson CA, Henley FT, Goldstein AR: Benign metastasizing leiomyoma. *Ala J Med Sci* 21(1):78, 1984
336. Stoba C, Gross R: Primary mediastinal seminoma in a boy. *Pediatr Pol* 56(6):683, 1981
337. Stock HJ: Two rare bone tumors of the band. *Zentralbl Chir* 102(7):420, 1977
338. Stockdale AD, Pocock TJ: Abdominal wall metastasis following laparoscopy: a case report. *Eur J Surg Oncol* 11(4):373, 1985
339. Stosch M, Steinhoff H: Carcinoma of the pancreas presenting with urological symptoms. Report of two cases. *Urologe (A)* 20(6):394, 1981
340. Suzuki T, Hirota M, Hoshino H, Yamasaku F, Terada I: An extremely rare autopsy case of cardiac liposarcoma and Brenner tumor. *Gan No Rinsho* 31(4):434, 1985
341. Szabolcs A, Borell U, Lundstrom V: Management of gestational throphoblastic neoplasma during a thirteen years period. Third World Conf of Human Reproduction, Berlin, FRG, Internat'l Acad of Reproductive Med, 1981
342. Takimoto T, Furukawa M, Morishita K, Yoshida K, Morishita Y, Umeda R: Nasopharyngeal carcinoma associated with tuberculoid granuloma – case report. *Nippon Jibiinkoka Gakkai Kaiho* 85(1):33, 1982
343. Talamo TS, Mendelow H: Primary intracranial germinoma with massive ventriculoperitoneal shunt metastases. *J Surg Oncol* 28(1):39, 1985
344. Tanaka T, Bunai Y, Nishikawa A, Kawai T, Mori H, Takahashi M: Malignant mesenchymoma of the heart. *Acta Pathol Jpn* 32(5):851, 1982
345. Tanaka M, Matsubara O, Takemura T, Watanabe S, Suzuki K, Okano T, Unn Kawaoi A, Kasuga T: Cardiovascular lesion of carcinoid syndrome. An autopsy case of bronchial carcinoid. *Acta Pathol Jpn* 34(1):201, 1984
346. Tanaka T, Slamon DJ, Battifora H et al.: Expression of p21 ras oncoproteins in human cancers. *Cancer Res* 46(3):1465, 1986

347. Tatsuno I, Michigishi K, Watanabe K: A case of so-called lymphoepithelioma. *Jpn J Clin Radiol* 22(1):161, 1977
348. Tattersall MH, Lander H, Bain B, Stocks AE, Woods RL, Fox RM, Burne E, Trotten JR, Roos I: Cis-platinum treatment of metastatic adrenal carcinoma. *Med J Aust* 1(9):419, 1980
349. Tavassoli FA, Norris HJ: Secretory carcinoma of the breast. *Cancer* 45(9):2404, 1980
350. Taylor HB: Histologic patterns of breast cancer with special significance. In: *Early Breast Cancer: Detection and Treatment*, edited by Gallagher HS, New York: Wiley & Sons, 1975
351. Templeton AC: Nerve involvement in malignant lymphoma. *Lab Invest* 46(7):82A, 1982
352. Thompson SH, Shear M: Fibrous histiocytomas of the oral and maxillofacial regions. *J Oral Pathol* 13(3):282, 1984
353. Timmis AD, Smallpiece C, Davies AC, Macarthur AM, Gishen P, Jackson G: Intracardiac spread of intravenous leiomyomatosis with successful surgical excision. *New Engl J Med* 303(18):1043, 1980
354. Tomeno B, Feuilhade de Chauvin P: Chondrosarcomas. *Rev Prat* 32(55/56):3523, 3527, 1982
355. Trepeta RW, Mathur B, Lagin S, LiVolsi VA: Giant cell tumor ('osteoclastoma') of the pancreas: A tumor of epithelial origin. *Cancer* 48(9):2022, 1981
356. Trippitelli A, Rosi P, Selli C, Carini M, Turini D: Rhabdomyosarcoma of spermatic cord in adult. *Urology* 19(5):533, 1982
357. Tsai GL, Liu JD, Siauw CP, Chen PH: Thoracic roentgenologic manifestations in primary carcinoma of the liver. *Chest* 86(3):430, 1984
358. Tune JM, Bowles MH, Grunow WA, Patel GK, Texter EC: Granular cell myoblastoma of the esophagus. Report of two cases. *Am J Gastroenterol* 75(6):426, 1981
359. Uematsu A, Coy JT, Hodges SO, Goodman RP, Brower TS: Malignant chondromyxoid fibroma of the scapula. Case report. *South Med J* 70(12):1469, 71.
360. Ulfohn A, Raju M, Sweiss K, Gruss L: Gastric plasmocytoma. *Md State Med J* 31(3):65, 1982
361. Unni KK: Ewing's sarcoma-systemic or metastatic disease. XXI Postgraduate Course on Clinical Oncology: Bone and Soft Tissue Tumors, June 23–27, Milan, NCI, Bethesda, Maryland, 1980
362. Van den Heule B, Hupin J, Capel P, Bron D, Andry G: Contribution of immunologic surface markers to the differential anatomo-pathological diagnosis of malignant lymphomas. *Ann Pathol* 1(3):233, 1981
363. Van der Zee DC, van Elk PJ: Lymphangioma of the mesentery: an uncommon cause of abdominal discomfort. *Neth J Surg* 36(2):61, 1984
364. van Heerden JA, Weiland LN, Rettine WH, Walls JT, Purnell DC: Cancer of the parathyroid glands. *Arch Surg* 114(4):475, 1977
365. Vichard P, Tropet Y, Pinon P, Watelet F, Carbillet JP: Chondrosarcoma of the extraskeletal soft tissues of the hand. *Ann Chir* 34(9):743, 1980
366. Vigano W, Colombo A, Brenna A, Tagliabue M, Buratti C: A case of extraosseous Ewing's sarcoma of rare orbitonasal localization. *Minerva Otorinolaringol* 32(4):381, 1982
367. Villett WT, Burger EG, Bezuidenhout DJ: Metastatic hepatocellular carcinoma of the heart. *S Afr Med J* 53(25):1036, 1978
368. Vincent FM: Spinal leptomeningeal invasion from intracranial glioblastoma multiforme. *Arch Phys Med Rehabil* 64(1):34, 1983
369. Vita HC, Shaw DL, Someren A, Mendiondo DA, Jelden G, Rene JB, Whitehead T: Carcinoma of the nasopharynx in the second decade of life. RNSA Scientific Program, 66th Annual Meeting, Dallas, 1980, The Radiological Society of North America, Inc, 313 pp, 1980

370. Voci V, Olson H, Beilin L: A malignant primary cardiac pheochromocytoma. *Surg Rounds* 5(9):88, 1982
371. Voigt JJ, Fretigny E, Cassigneul J, Marty C, Monrozies X: Primary liver cystadenocarcinoma associated with cystadenoma. *Gastroenterol Clin Biol* 6(3):279, 1982
372. Watkins FB, White AA: Infiltrating angiolipoma. *Bull Hosp Joint Dis* 4:105, 1981
373. Weatherby RP, Carney JA: Childhood adrenocortical tumors: pathologic features and prognosis. *Lab Invest* 46(1):17P, 1982
374. Wechsler J, Caillaud JM, Clerici T, Ghozali F, Micheau C, Pinaudeau Y: Primary malignant cutaneous lymphomas excluding mycosis fungoides. Anatomoclinical study of 16 cases. *Ann Pathol* 4(4):273, 1984
375. Wehbe MA, Mickelson MR: Malignant schwannoma in neurofibromatous elephantiasis of the upper extremity. *Clin Orthop* (167):164, 1982
376. Weidner PA, Ziter FM: Carcinoid tumors of the gastrointestinal tract. *JAMA* 245(11):1153, 1981
377. Weiss AM, Frey N, Andreassian B, Potet F: Primary choriocarcinoma of the mediastinum in a male. *Sem Hop Paris* 52(20):1235, 1976
378. Weiss SW, Enzinger FM: Epithelioid hemangioendothelioma. A vascular tumor often mistaken for a carcinoma. *Cancer* 50(5):970, 1982
379. West CG: Spinal subarachnoid metastatic spread from non-neuraxial primary neoplasms. Case report. *J Neurosurg* 51(2):251, 1979
380. Wick MR, Banks PM, McDonald TJ: Angioendotheliomatosis of the nose with fatal systemic dissemination. *Cancer* 48(11):2510, 1981
381. Wilms G, Baert AL, Van Damme B: Osteoblastic metastasis of parotid carcinoma with sun-ray periosteal reaction. *J Belge Radiol* 62(1):87, 1979
382. Woolfson JM, Dulisch ML, Tams TR: Intrathoracic lipoma in a dog. *J Am Vet Med Assoc* 185(9):1007, 1984
383. Wu P, Fing L: Congenital rhabdomyosarcoma – autopsy report of one case. *Zhonghua Zhongliu Zazhi* 2(4):308, 1980
384. Yamaoka H, Oku T, Matsumoto T, Okuda S, Isiglo K, Takahashi M: A case of carcinoid-islet cell tumor of the pancreas. *Gan No Rinsho* 26(11):12847, 1980
385. Yang K, Wang Z, Zhang X, Ma J: A case of primary malignant lymphoma associated with early infiltrating carcinoma of esophagus. *Zhonghua Zhongliu Zazhi* 3(1):8, 1981
386. Yi G: Sebaceous cell carcinoma of the parotid gland. *Zhanghua Kouqiangke Zazhi* 16(3):191, 1981
387. Zucker S: Anemia in cancer. *Cancer Invest* 3(3):249, 1985

8

THE OCCULT PRIMARY MALIGNANCY: CONCEPTS OF SPREAD AND SCHEME FOR EVALUATION

JOHN A. ARCADI and HARVEY A. GILBERT

Metastases may occur only if the extracellular matrix of the tumor and the extracellular matrix (including basement membrane) of a vascular or lymphatic channel become confluent. The extracellular matrix is composed of the fibrous connective tissue and the amorphous "ground substance." We conceive this matrix to be in a gelatinous state of variable and varying density or degree of aggregation.

The density of this gel is under the control of steroid hormones that are secreted or transmitted to the gel by the fibroblasts in the matrix. The varying density of this gel has been recognized since the turn of the century (10). (See discussion by Maximow). The role of the amorphous matrix in the growth and control of the epithelial cells was noted in the prostate of man in 1954–55 (1, 2).

Tumor cells must invade the matrix as it separates from the main tumor mass and must penetrate a similar matrix that surrounds a vascular channel to enter the transport system for metastases-lymph and venous channels. When the tumor embolus reaches a tissue that is conductive for further cell growth, the endothelial cells and the contiguous connective tissue with its extracellular matrix are penetrated.

The metastatic or migratory capacity of a cell may be related to its nuclear roundness, and this may relate to its vibratory capacity. Coffey (per com.) believes that this roundness factor is controlled by the nuclear matrix which is formed on a DNA framework. The least round a cell nucleus is the higher the degree of malignancy of the cell in growth activity and, therefore, in metastatic potential.

The brilliant work of Liotta and his associates have clearly shown that tumor cells can secrete a collagenase that will cause degradation of basement membrane collagen (19). This type IV collagenase is secreted in increasing amounts from cells of increasing malignancy or metastatic potential.

Of considerable importance in the metastatic process is the observation of Biswas that human tumor cells secrete a factor which stimulates human fibroblasts to produce a collagenase(s) (4). Since collagenase and collagenase-like substances are at the tumor cell-extracellular matrix junction where the dissolution of the matrix occurs and malignant cells have a propensity for movement, metastases occur from this site. From the growing front of invading malignant cells, long irregular pseudopodia extend into the matrix which shows focal dissolution in the immediate area around the pseudopodia (9). It is probably from these pseudopodia that the proteases, such as collagenase IV, are secreted.

The ease with which tumor cells penetrate the gel of the extracellular matrix depends not only on the concentration of the collagenase but also on the density of the gel. The softer or less dense the extracellular matrix is, the easier it is for tumor cells to penetrate.

Some years ago we presented evidence clearly indicating that "... connective tissue glycoprotein (extracellular matrix component) of untreated prostatic cancer is quite different in histological appearance than that of estrogen – or castration – treated prostatic cancer ... The ground substance of untreated prostatic cancer was found, histochemically, to be soluble in a buffer solution at pH 7.0. It was much less soluble when the tumor had previously been treated by estrogen administration or by castration. This study suggested that the serum glycoproteins might be elevated in untreated prostatic cancer, and that they might be decreased after treatment" (3).

This hypothesis, as presented in 1958, was found to be correct. The serum glycoproteins in untreated prostatic cancer ranged from 23.3 to 86.0 mg percent with an average of 49 mg percent. In treated prostatic cancer, the serum glycoproteins fell to below 20 mg percent. (Normal serum glycoproteins averaged 13.2 mg percent.)

This study, again, shows the intimate relationship between a growing cancer cell and its adjacent extracellular matrix.

Since the tumor cell emboli do not carry stroma with them, there are no metastatic macrophages or fibroblasts to produce an organ-specific collagenase. We believe the innate organization of the tumor cell (a nuclear matrix function) determines the site for metastatic deposition of tumor cell emboli. This concept is reinforced by the work of Cerra and Natale (5), who demonstrated that tumor cell lines which have high specificity for lungs will have a much less affinity for kidneys and liver matrix than for lung matrix. The cells in their study seem to have a recognition for lung matrix. A collagenase is secreted by the tumor cell. This collagenase not only breaks down the endothelial membrane of the vascular channel but also stimulates the endothelial cell to produce a collagenase. Both sources of Type IV collagenase allow the tumor cell mass to enter the ECM.

From the data we have presented it seems apparent that the process of metastasis is complex on the one hand but, on the other hand, relatively simple. The complexity rests in the enzymatic kinetics involved in the secretion of collagenases/proteases from tumor cells, fibroblasts and macrophages, and related factors to stimulate these secretions. In its simplest form, metastasis is a function of the integrity of the extracellular matrix, a gelatinous substance whose rigidity is controlled by fibroblast-secreted substances.

In the most basic context, metastases of tumors is directly

K.W. Brunson (ed) Local invasion and spread of cancer.

related to the organization and modification of the extracellular matrix or ground substance.

Several excellent reviews of the clinical aspects of the OPM have been recently published (17, 18, 20, 21, 23). These reviews have pointed out both semantic problems facing the reviewer of the literature as well as the diverse clinical entities that compromise the OPM. Therefore, in attempting to understand the problem, we need to recognize the wastebasket nature of this diagnosis and attempt to bring some order to the inherent chaos of the field.

Somewhere between 1 and 7% of all cancer patients present findings that are cause for inclusion into the category of OPM. For all practical purposes, we would like to define this entity in the following manner: The patient with an occult primary malignancy (OPM) will have the disease discovered by finding a dominant mass in a site that is typically metastatic and with a histological appearance that usually does not arise primarily in that site. In addition, a "reasonable" work-up to eliminate sites of other obvious primary malignancies is performed and is negative. Important aspects of the history to emphasize are smoking, pain (especially abdominal), changing bowel habits, alteration in voiding pattern, abnormal bleeding, pelvic discomfort or history of previous biopsy or surgery. The extent of the initial work-up usually includes a chest x-ray, physical exam, stool for occult blood, CBC, UA, automated chemistry panel (e.g. SMA 20) and any test that is directed by the anatomic and histologic nuances of the particular metastatic site where the OPM was found. Some OPM sites require a more detailed histologic and geographical locational analysis. For example upper neck nodes usually represent spread from a supraclavicular primary and lower neck nodes usually arise from an infraclavicular primary site (7). It can be generally stated that a random search for a primary cancer site in every case of an OPM is wasteful and, more often than not, misleading. In fact, it has been shown that a positive radiologic finding can most often be attributed to an additional metastasis and not the primary site of origin (6, 15, 16).

Table 1 will give some insight into the anatomic and histologic patterns found that indicate the primary site of an OPM.

As illustrated in the preceding Table 1, there are some hints as to how a presenting anatomic site and histologic type can influence the investigation for the primary site of tumor origin. When nodes appear in the upper neck, it can usually be accepted that the primary arose from head and neck sites (oral cavity and Waldyers's ring in the majority, with a few cases arising from larynx, sinus and esophagus). Another example is when an axillary node is discovered as the initial metastatic site and the histologic study reveals an adenocarcinoma with positive estrogen receptors. In this situation there is a high degree of probability that the primary arose in the breast. This is true even when the clinical examination and mammograms are negative.

An additional aspect of our attempt toward making the search for an OPM more logical and more directed is the use of tumor markers. After obtaining tissue, a variety of special stains, and in some circumstances electron microscopy are extremely helpful. Also several serologic tests are useful. Some of these tissue and serologic tumor markers are listed in Table 2, and they are correlated with the primary tumor that gives rise to them (11, 12, 13).

The tumors that have a significant chance of responding to a palliative or curative therapy are listed in Table 3a and Table 3b.

In summary, the evaluation of a patient with an OPM should be logical and based on all anatomic, histologic, serologic and treatability criteria that we can avail ourselves of.

These include the following factors:

(1) The anatomic patterns listed in Table 1.
(2) The histologic subtype listed in Table 1.
(3) The tumor markers listed in Table 2.
(4) The chance that discovery of the primary will eventually lead one to selecting effective therapy as listed in Table 3a and Table 3b.

Table 1. Anatomic and histologic patterns of primary sites.

Site discovered	Typical history	Typical primary site
Neck – upper	Squamous carcinoma	Head and neck
– lower	Adenocarcinoma	Lung, GI
Lung	Squamous	Lung
	Adenocarcinoma	Lung, breast gastrointestinal, kidney
Inguinal nodes	Squamous	Anal, vulva
	Adenocarcinoma	Prostate, ovary
	Other	Testicle
Axillary nodes	Adenocarcinoma	Breast, lung
	Squamous	Lung
Skin	Melanoma	Skin
	Adenocarcinoma	Breast, kidney, ovary
Liver	Adenocarcinoma	Gastrointestinal, pancreas, lung, breast
Bone	Adenocarcinoma	Kidney, breast, ovary gastrointestinal carcinoid
Brain	Large cell (Adenoma) oat cell CA	Lung
	Adenocarcinoma	Breast, prostate, pancreas, melanoma
Epidural cord compress	Multiple histologic	Lung, breast
		Lymphoma, prostate
Pleural effusions	Adenocarcinoma	Lung (also squamous) breast, ovary, GI pancreas
Ascites	Adenocarcinoma	Ovary, pancreas colon
Umbilical mass	Adenocarcinoma	Stomach, other GI

Table 2. Serologic and tissue tumor markers.

Test marker	Usual primary site
I. Enzymatic markers	
Diastase resistant PAS & Mucicarmine	Adenocarcinoma
Acid phosphatase	Prostate
Muramidase	Histiocytic lymphoma
	Multiple tumor types
	Medullary CA of thyroid
Alkaline phosphatase	
Calcitonin	
II. Hormones	
Thyroglobulin	Thyroid CA
Pancreatic hormone	Pancreatic cell tumor
HCG	Gonadal or placental tumor
Testosterone	Stromal-gonadal or adrenal
Estradiol	Stromal-gonadal tumor
III. Oncofetal antigens	
Alpha fetoprotein	Germ cell and liver CA
CEA	Multiple enteral tumors
IV. Serum proteins	
Immunoglobulins	Lymphoma
Alpha-I-antitrypsin	Liver or germinal tumors
V. Other products	
Alpha lactalbumin	Breast CA
Myoglobin	Skeletal muscle
Actin-Myosin	Smooth and skeletal muscle
Factor VIII antigen	Endothelial tumor
Mesothelial antigen	Mesothelioma
Glial fibrillary acid protein	Glioma
Keratin	Epithelial malignancy
S-100 antigen	Melanoma and sarcoma
CA-125	Ovary
Estrogen receptors	Breast, ovary, melanoma
Electron microscopic markers	Squamous, adeno, lymphoma, sarcoma and melanoma

The numbers of patients who have an unknown primary will significantly decrease as the number of cell specific antigens are developed. A valuable approach to the problem will be more profitable than a shotgun approach.

TREATMENT

The emphasis of this chapter is on the mechanisms of metastasis and the evaluation of the patient with a clinical OPM, and not treatment; but a short note about treatment is indicated.

Of course, in those patients whose initial OPM is identified and is listed in Table 3a and Table 3b, the treatment is obvious and will be directed by the treatment philosophy of the individual physician. For those patients whose OPM remains clinically occult, the critical distinction is to separate the local regional metastasis from the distant metastasis. For the latter group, treatment is only marginally effective. The use of an Adriamycin based treatment regimen is the most useful of the many proposed regimens, when treatment has been elected (8, 14).

Table 3a. Tumors that have excellent response and benefit from systematic therapy with prolongation of survival.

(1) Serum cell tumors
(2) Hodgkins disease
(3) Non-Hodgkins disease
(4) Trophoblastic tumor
(5) Breast cancer
(6) Ovarian cancer
(7) Oat cell cancer of the lung
(8) Head and neck cancer
(9) Adrenal cancer
(10) Prostate cancer
(11) Osteosarcoma

Table 3b. Tumor types displaying a response rate of more than 20%, but no survival prolongation.

(1) Stomach
(2) Pancreas
(3) Colon
(4) Kidney
(5) Undifferentiated sarcoma
(6) Melanoma

For patients who have their OPM as a manifestation of local regional disease, treatment should be directed at the potential primary sites and the presenting metastasis (upper cervical neck nodes). This might include irradiation of the Waldeyer's area and hypopharynx as well as the neck. The treatment morbidity is high and the benefits are limited. An alternate proposal that has similar survival benefits, is to treat the metastatic neck nodes and to just observe the upper aerodigestive tract for the later appearance of a primary site. When treated at a later date, the newly discovered primary can at times be salvaged by irradiation or surgery. We favor the later approach.

REFERENCES

1. Arcadi JA: Role of the ground substance in atrophy of normal and malignant prostatic tissue following estrogen administration and orchiectomy. *Journal of Clinical Endocrinology and Metabolism* 14:1113, 1954
2. Arcadi JA: The influence of hormones upon some constituents of connective tissue in prostatic cancer. *Texas Reports on Biology and Medicine* 13:591, 1955
3. Arcadi JA: Serum mucoproteins in prostatic carcinoma. *J Urology* 80:192, 1958
4. Biswas C: Collagenase stimulation in cocultures of human fibroblasts and human tumor cells. *J Cell Biology* 99:87a (329), 1984
5. Cerra FR, Natale RB: Selective adhesion of tumor cells to organ specific matrix. *J Cell Biology* 101:214a (811), 1985
6. Fer MF, Greco FA, Oldham RK: Poorly differentiated neoplasms and tumors of unknown origin: Introduction: *Semen Oncol* 9:393, 1982
7. Fred MP, Diehl Wm Jr, Brownson RJ, et al: Cervical metastasis from an unknown primary site. *Awn Otol Laryngol* 85:152, 1975
8. Indupalli SR, Bedikian AY, Bodey GP: Adenocarcinoma of unknown primary origin; Impact of chemotherapy on survival. *South Med J* 74:1431, 1981
9. Kramer RH, Bensch KG, Rezaee M, Wong J: Invasion of

reconstituted basement membrane matrix by fibrosarcoma cells. *J Cell Biology* 101:214a (813), 1985

10. Maximow A: Bindegewebe und blutbildende Gewebe. Amorphe Grundsubstanz, pp 247–250. In: *Die Gewebe, Handbuch der Mikroskopischen Anatomie des Menschen* 2:247, 1927

11. MacKay B, Ordonez NG: The role of the pathologist in the evaluation of poorly differentiated tumors. *Semen Oncol* 9:416, 1982

12. Neel HB, GR, Weiland LH et al.: Immunologic detection of occult primary cancer of the head and neck. *Otolaryngol Head and Neck Surg* 89:230, 1981

13. Neel HB, Pearson GR, Weiland LH et al.: Immunologic detection of occult primary cancer of the head and neck. *Otolaryngol Head and Neck Surg* 89:230, 1981

14. Nelson RB: Chemotherapy of metastatic adenocarcinoma of unknown origin. *N Engl J Med* 303:1478, 1980

15. Neumann KH, Nystrom JS: Metastatic cancer of unknown origin: Nonsquamous cell type. *Semen Oncol* 9:427, 1982

16. Nystrom JS, Weiner JM, Heffelfinger-Juttner J et al.: Metastatic and histologic presentations in unknown primary cancer. *Semen Oncol* 4:53, 1977

17. Osteen RT, Koph G, Wilson RE: In pursuit of the unknown primary. *AMJ Surg* 135:494, 1978

18. Richardson RG, Parker RG: Metastasis from undetected primary cancers – Clinical experience at a radiation oncology center (Medical Information). *West J Med* 123:337, 1975

19. Salo T, Liotta LA, Tryggvason K: Purification and characterization of a murine basement membrane collagen-degrading enzyme secreted by metastatic tumor cells. *J Biol Chem* 258:3058, 1983

20. Smith PE, Krementz ET, Chapman W: Metastatic cancer without a detectable primary site. *J Surgery* 133:633, 1967

21. Stewart JF, Tattersall MHN, Woods RL, et al.: Unknown primary adenocarcinoma; Incidence of overinvestigation and natural history. *British Journal of Medicine* Vol. I:1530, 1533, 1979

22. Turpeenniemi-Hujanen T, Thorgeirsson UP, Hart IR, Grant SS, Liotta LA: Expression of collagenase IV (Basement Membrane Collagenase) activity in murine tumor cell hybrids that differ in metastatic potential. *J National Cancer Institute* 75:99, 1985

23. Ultmann JE, Phillips TL: Chapter 49, 1843–1853, Cancer of unknown primary site. In: Cancer, Principles and Practice of Oncology, edited by DeVita V, Hellman S, Rosenberg S, Lippincott JP, Philadelphia, 1985

POSTSCRIPT

A rise in serum calcitonin can be used in the diagnosis of occult medullary carcinoma of the thyroid in children with multiple endocrine neoplasia syndrome (2). Occult testicular tumors which are not eliminated by chemotherapy due to the presence of a blood-testicular barrier may lead to late recurrences in long-term survivors of germ cell neoplasms (1).

POSTSCRIPT REFERENCES

1. DeLeo MJ, Greco FA, Hainsworth JD, Johnson DH: Late recurrences in long-term survivors of germ cell neoplasms. *Cancer* 62(5):985–8, 1988

2. Graham SM, Genel M, Toulooukian RJ et al.: Provocative testing for occult medullary carcinoma of the thyroid: findings in seven children with multiple endocrine neoplasia type IIa. *J Pediatr Surg* 22(6):501–3, 1987

NEOPLASMS OF THE IMMUNE SYSTEM WITH INVOLVEMENT OF LYMPHORETICULAR STRUCTURES

H.E. KAISER and J. SUTHERLAND

NEOPLASMS OF THE IMMUNE SYSTEM

Leukemias and lymphosarcomas are a group of important neoplastic diseases, also regarded as systemic neoplastic diseases in contrast with the so-called solid tumors. The classification of neoplasms (including leukemias) of hematopoietic and lymphoreticular tissues has undergone revision, based especially on immunological aspects. It is still somewhat vague with respect to man; no wonder, then, that even more confusion exists when we consider the diseases of other animal groups such as feline, bovine and avian leukoses, lymphoreticular and hematopoietic diseases in reptiles, amphibians and fishes and, finally, in the invertebrates of which those found in insects and mollusks are best known.

In our classification we have used and revised the WHO system. This introductory chapter is intended as a review of the intra- and interspecies comparisons of the diseases concerned. Such a comparative approach may shed new light on their development. The process of metastasis or, in the case of the leukemias, of dissemination produces heterogenous pictures because of the different cells becoming malignant and because of cellular heterogeneity in the various malignant cell lines themselves. Thus, even an intraspecies comparison based on the conditions in man is difficult because of diversity and becomes even more complicated when an interspecies comparison is attempted. The distribution of the tissues involved with various body fluids throughout the animal phyla was reviewed by Kaiser (8). The knowledge of leukemias and related diseases in the various phyla is not limited, but a comparison of this diversified group of diseases with each other needs an exact base and this is still lacking.

Table 1 offers a review of reticular, hematopoietic and free connective tissue cells of the organisms in the various animal phyla.

Table 2 is a review of human leukemias, lymphomas and related disease. At present, evaluation and classification of the neoplasms deriving from the reticular connective tissues are in a state of flux (6). Although names and nomenclature based on anatomic appearance are of importance, of greater interest is the fact that the systemic diseases of this group, the leukemias, are now seen more as neoplasms of various components of the immune system with distinct biochemical abnormalities, making the function of these components and the biochemical deficiencies resulting from their perturbation much more understandable. Failure of maturation may be the real cause for the mass production of the different types of immature leukemia cells as well as the

functional deficiency of these malignant cells. Leukemias represent not only of certain groups of immature cells or immature versions of the free cells of the reticular connective tissues, but there is also a change in internal host functions. The study of these interrelationships leads to a better understanding of these changes in the importance of a comparative evaluation of human disease and diseases in different species. Therefore, the value of an interspecies comparison of these malignancies cannot be overestimated. The present distinction and arrangement of the diseases set forth in this chapter, however, should be considered as tentative.

COMPARABLE DISEASES IN INVERTEBRATES

In invertebrates, what tissues are diseased depends on the phylogenetic background of the host. Mesodermal tissues, connective tissue cells, circulatory systems, lymphatic and immune systems in the different animal phyla exhibit great variability. The normal conditions have been summarized (8).

Some hematopoietic neoplasms are known in bivalve mollusks and insects (*Drosophila* sp.), but our knowledge or evaluation of these diseases is limited and their comparative value is small. The progressive stages of this disease group are well known only in a few species. Chapters 5/Volume V (Leucosis in invertebrates) and (7/Volume V. Selected aspects of neoplastic growth in arthropods) deal with some details.

COMPARABLE DISEASES IN NON-HUMAN VERTEBRATES

Fishes show a more pronounced occurrence of sarcomas than the higher vertebrates. Leukoses in amphibians were reviewed by Kaiser in 1981. A section on amphibians is contained in NCI Monograph 32 (1968) by Clyde Dawe in his paper about leukoses in poikilothermic animals. Kaiser (1981) lists several pertinent leukoses in Chapter 47(9) and a case occurring in an axolotl is mentioned by Anver in Chapter 9/Volume V.

In birds, epithelial neoplasms are rather rare but leukoses and lymphoma are the most significant and widely distributed neoplasms (see Chapter 12/Volume V by Fredrickson, 13/Volume V by Purchase, 14/Volume V by Sharma and 15/Volume V by Moriguchi). In mammals, with the special development of the lymphatic system and the development of the mammary glands, we find a special situation (see

K.W. Brunson (ed) Local invasion and spread of cancer.

Table 1. Cells of the reticular, free connective and hematopoietic tissues of various phyla and the systemic and associated neoplasms to which they may give rise.

Cells	Neoplasms
I. Connective tissues of man	
A. Mast cells	Malignant mastocytosis
B. Histiocytes-macrophages	Malignant histiocytosis
	Histiocytosis X
	Eosinophilic granuloma
	Hand Schüller Christian disease
	Letterer Siwe disease
II. Hematopoietic tissues of man	
A. Lymphoid or lymphatic tissue	Acute lymphocytic leukemia
	Chronic lymphocytic leukemia
	Nodular and diffuse lymphomas
	(see Table 2)
	Primary macroglobulinemia of Waldenström
	Mycosis fungoides
	Sezary's syndrome
	Plasmacytoma
	Multiple myeloma
	Plasma cell leukemia
	Hairy cell leukemia
B. Myeloid tissue	
a. Neutrophilic, eosinophilic and basophilic myelocytes and their precursors	Acute myelocytic leukemia
	Chronic myelocytic leukemia
	Progranulocytic leukemia
	Chronic eosinophilic leukemia
	Acute monocytic leukemia
	Chronic monocytic leukemia
	Acute myelomonocytic leukemia
b. Cells of the erythrocytic series	Polycythemia vera
	Acute erythraemia (Di Guglielmo)
	Erythroleukemia
	Chronic erythraemia (Heilmeyer-Schoen)
c. Megakaryocytes-thrombocytes	Megakaryocytic leukemia?
	Idiopathic thrombocythaemia
	Polycythaemia vera (see above)
	Myelosclerosis with myeloid metaplasia
III. Connective and hematopoietic tissues of non-mammalian vertebrates	
A. Fish	
a. Myeloid tissue	Acute granulocytic leukemia in chinook salmon, *Oncorhynchustshawytscha*
	(29 species of bony fish have been reported with hemic neoplasms – see Harshbarger (4))
b. Lymphatic tissue	Approximately two dozen lymphomas in various trout species – see Harshbarger (4)
	Undifferentiated lymphomas in northern pike, *Esox lucius* (retroviral-related)
	Malignant lymphomas in muskellunge, *Esox masquinongy*
	Lymphosarcoma in *Conger conger*, *Oncorhynchus keta* and others
c. Connective tissue	Reticulum cell sarcoma in sandbar sharks, *Carcharhinus plumbeus*
B. Amphibians	
a. Myelocytic tissue	Granulocytic leukemia in African clawed frogs, *Xenopus laevis*
b. Lymphatic tissue	Lymphosarcoma in frogs, *Xenopus Laevis laevis*, *Xenopus fraseri* and *Rana pipiens*
	Lymphosarcoma in urodeles, *Cynops pyrrhogaster* and *Ambystoma mexicanum*

Table 1. Continued.

Cells	Neoplasms
C. Reptiles	
a. Lymphatic tissue	Lymphoblastic leukemia in *Varanus bengalensis*
	Lymphosarcoma in California king snakes, *Lampropeltis getulis californiae* and in *Eunectes murinus* and *Naja naja*
	Lymphomas in *Testudo hermanii* and *Lacerta sica*
D. Birds	
a. Myeloid tissue	Erythroblastosis, myeloblastosis, myelocytomatosis (retrovirus-related)
b. Lymphoid tissue	Marek's disease (herpes virus-related)
	Lymphoproliferative disease of turkeys and lymphoid leukosis in other species (retroviral-related)
c. Connective tissues	Acute reticulum cell neoplasia (reticuloendotheliosis virus-related)
c. Connective tissue	Mast cell neoplasms in axolotls, *Ambystoma mexicanum*
IV. Connective and hematopoietic-related tissues of invertebrates	
A. Mollusks*	
a. Leukoses	Chemically-related hemic neoplasms in the blue mussel, *Mytilus edulis*, freshwater clams, *Unio pictorum* and the American oyster, *Crassostrea virginicae*
	Viral-related hemic neoplasm in the soft-shelled clam, *Mya arenaria*
B. Arthropods	
a. Leukoses	Plasmacytic neoplasms in *Drosophila melanogaster* (viral-related)
	Hematopoietic neoplasms in *Heptagenia lateralis* and *Tipula paludosa*
	Lymphoma-like condition leading to fatal type of leukemia in mayflies, *Ecdyonurus lateralis* and *Rhitrogena semicolorata* when both are parasitized by the wasp *Symbiocladius rhithrogenae*

*See also chapter 4, Volume V: Selected Aspects of Neoplastic Progression in Mollusks by CA Farley

Chapter 16/Volume V by Kaiser). The species specificity of this disease group in the mammal is remarkable, but too little knowledge exist regarding the various mammalian species (see also Chapter 20/Volume V by Sass and Chapter 26/Volume V by Williams and Thorne). Table 3 lists the chapters dealing with leukemias and lymphomas in the various groups of organisms discussed in this book.

SUMMARY AND CONCLUSIONS

Phylogenetic development and species diversity of hematopoietic and lymphoreticular neoplasms and related diseases is far from established, but their study may result in a better understanding of this group of diseases.

Table 2. Systemic and related neoplasms of man and other phyla and their phenotypic expression.

I. Leukemias and lymphomas in mammalian vertebrates, especially man

Neoplasm	Phenotypic cellular expression
A. *Acute leukemias and related diseases*	
Acute lymphocytic leukemia	Lymphoblasts
Acute myelocytic leukemia	Myeloblasta and promyelocytes
Acute monocytic leukemia	Immature monocytes
Erythroleukemia (Di Guglielmo)	Immature erythroid and granuloid cells
Megakaryocytic leukemia	Immature megakaryocytes
Acute panmyelosis	All bone marrow cells
Acute leukemia, unclassified	Unclassified cells
B. *Chronic lymphoid leukemia and other lymphoproliferative disorders*	
Chronic lymphocytic leukemia	Small lymphocytes
Primary macroglobulinemia of Waldenström	Plasmacytoid lymphocytes
Myeloma	Immature plasma cells
Plasma cell leukemia	Immature plasma cells and plasmablasts
Heavy chain disease	Plasmacytoid lymphocytes in the bone marrow
Mycosis fungoides	T lymphocytes
Sezary's syndrome	T lymphocytes
Chronic lymphoproliferative disease, unclassified	Unclassified lymphocytes
C. *Chronic myeloid leukemia and other myeloproliferative diseases*	
Chronic myelocytic leukemia	Mature and immature granulocytes
Variants of chronic myelocytic leukemia	
a. neutrophilic leukemia	neutrophilic granulocytes
b. eosinophilic leukemia	eosinophilic granulocytes
c. basophilic leukemia	basophilic granulocytes
Chronic erythraemia (Heilmeyer-Schoener)	Immature erythrocytes
Polycythemia vera (Vaquez-Osler)	Erythrocytosis, granulocytosis, and thrombocytosis
Idiopathic thrombocythemia	Megakaryocytes and thrombocytes
Myelosclerosis with myeloid metaplasia	Myeloid cells and megakaryocytes
Chronic myeloproliferative diseases, unclassified	Unclassified myelocytic cells
D. *Chronic monocytoid leukemia and systemic histiocytoid diseases*	
Chronic monocytic leukemia	Monocytes
Histiocytosis X	Histiocytes
Malignant histiocytosis	Malignant histiocytes
Hodgkin's disease	Interdigitaling reticulum cells
E. *Unclassified leukemias*	
Hairy cell leukemia	*Lymphoid-appearing cells* with hair-like projections
F. *Others*	
Malignant mastocytosis	Tissue mast cells
G. *Lymphomas*	
Low grade (clinical prognosis)	
malignant lymphoma, small cell lymphocytic	small lymphocytes
malignant lymphoma, follicular	small cleaved lymphocytes
malignant lymphoma, follicular, mixed	small cleaved and large lymphocytes
Intermediate grade	
malignant lymphoma, follicular, predominantly large cell	large lymphocytes
malignant lymphoma, diffuse, predominantly small cell	small cleaved lymphocytes
malignant lymphoma, diffuse, mixed small and large cell	small cleaved and large lymphocytes
malignant lymphoma, diffuse, large cell	large lymphocytes
High grade	
malignant lymphoma, large cell, immunoblastic	large immunoblastic lymphocytes
malignant lymphoma, lymphoblastic	lymphoblasts
malignant lymphoma, small noncleaved cell (Burkitt's)	small, noncleaved lymphocytes

Table 2. Continued.

I. Leukemias and lymphomas in mammalian vertebrates, especially man	
Neoplasm	*Phenotypic cellular expression*
Miscellaneous	
histiocytic lymphoma	malignant histiocytes
mycosis fungoides	T lymphocytes
extramedullary plasmacytoma	immature plasma cells
unclassifiable	unclassifiable cells

II. Leukemias and lymphomas in non-mammalian vertebrates	
Neoplasm	*Phenotypic cellular expression*
A. *Fish*	
Acute granulocytic leukemia in chinook salmon, *Oncorhynchustshawytscha* (29 species of bony fish with hemic neoplasms have been reported – see Harshbarger(4))	Immature granulocytes
Undifferentiated lymphomas in northern pike, *Esox lucius* (retrovirus-related)	Undifferentiated lymphocytic cells
Malignant lymphomas in muskellunge *Esox masquinongy* retrovirus related	Immature lymphocytes
Lymphosarcoma in *Conger conger*, *Oncorhynhus keta* and others	Immature lymphocytes
Reticulum cell sarcoma in sandbar sharks *Carcharhinus plumbeus* (approximately 24 lymphomas in various trout species – see Harshbarger	Reticulum cells
	Lymphocytes
B. *Amphibians*	
Granulocytic leukemia in African clawed frogs, *Xenopus laevis*	Immature granulocytes
Lymphosarcoma in frogs, *Xenopus laevis laevis*, *Xenopus fraseri*, and *Rana pipiens*	Immature lymphocytes
Lymphosarcoma in urodeles, *Cynops pyrrhogaster* and *Ambystoma mexicanum*	Immature lymphocytes
Mast cell neoplasms in axolotls, *Ambystoma mexicanum*	Mast cells
C. *Reptiles*	
Lymphoblastic leukemia in *Varanus bengalensis*	Lymphoblasts
Lymphosarcoma in California king snakes, *Lampropeltis getulis californiae* and in *Eunectes murinus* and *Naja naja*	Immature lymphocytes
Lymphomas in *Testudo hermanii* and *Lacerta sica*	Immature lymphocytes
D. *Birds*	
Erythroblastosis (retrovirus-related)	Erythroblasts
Myeloblastosis (retrovirus-related)	Myeloblasts
Myelocytomatosis (retrovirus-related)	Myelocytes
Marek's disease (herpes virus-related)	Lymphocytes
Lymphoproliferative (retrovirus-related) disease of turkeys	Lymphocytes
Lymphoid leukoses (retrovirus-related)	Lymphocytes
Acute reticulum cell (reticulo-endotheliosis virus-related) neoplasia	Lymphocytes or reticulo-endothelial cells

III. Connective and hematopoietic-related tissues of invertebrates	
Neoplasm	*Phenotypic cellular expression*
A. *Mollusks*	
Chemically-related hemic neoplasms in the blue mussel, *Mytilus edulis*, freshwater clams, *Unio pictorum* and the *American oyster, Crassostrea virginica*	Atypical hemocytes
Viral-related hemic neoplasms in the soft-shelled clam, *Mya arenaria*	Atypical hemocytes
B. *Arthropods*	
Plasmatocytic neoplasms in mutant larvae of *Drosophila melanogaster* (viral-related)	Plasmatocytes

Table 2. Continued.

I. Leukemias and lymphomas in mammalian vertebrates, especially man Neoplasm	Phenotypic cellular expression
Hematopoietic neoplasms in *Heptagenia lateralis* and *Tipula paludosa*	
Lymphoma-like, leading to fatal type of leukemia in mayfly naiads, *Ecdyonurus lateralis* and *Rhitrogena semicolorata* when both are parasitized by the wasp *Symbiocladium rhithrogenae*	Hemocyte, probably

Table 3. Review of chapters dealing with leukemias and lymphomas (leucoses) in various species.

1. *General*
   7/Vol. I   The Influence of the Body Structure on Tumor Development
               HE Kaiser
   22/Vol. II Extremely Low Frequency Electromagnetic fields as Promoters of Carcinogenesis
               N. Wertheimer
   23/Vol. II Medical Geography and Neoplasms
               JA Fulton
   13/Vol. VI Urbanization Parameters as Moderators of the Background Radiation – Leukemia Connection: Comparison with Single Variable and Multifactor Models
               HW Wendt and KA Birdsey

2. *Man (Homo sapiens)*
   16/Vol. X   Bone Marrow Transplantation
               D Kirkpatrick and L Delmonte
   18/Vol. X   The sphygmochron for chronobiologic blood pressure and heart rate assessmnent in cancer patients. J Halberg, G. Cornelissen, Franz Halberg, Francine Halberg, E. Halberg
   10/Vol. VII Progression of Neoplastic and Related Diseases Deriving From Hematopoietic Tissues – A Review
               ES Groves and D Longo
   11/Vol. VII Neoplastic Progression of the Myeloid Leukemias
               A Raza and HD Preisler
   12/Vol. VI Systemic Mastocytosis
               WR Henderson and EY Chi
   13/Vol. VI Histiocytic Tumors: Immunological Classification
               S Watanabe
   14/Vol. VI Eosinophilic Granuloma
               WR Henderson and EY Chi
   15/Vol. VI Malignant Lymphoma: Immunological Aspects
               S Watanabe
   15/Vol. IV Hematological Complications of Cancer From the Species-specific Point of View
               JR Cotelingam, D Patrick and HR Schumacher

3. *Other vertebrates*
   A.   *Mammals*:
   26/Vol. V   Spontaneous Tumors of Free-ranging Terrestrial Mammals of North America
               E Williams and ET Thorne
   12/Vol. I   Comparative Importance of the Lymphatic System During Neoplastic Progression
               HE Kaiser
   24/Vol. V   Bovine Lymphoma – Epidemiology, Diagnosis, Transmission, Pathology
               B Sass
   B.   *Birds*
   12/Vol. V   Review of Tumor Progression in Typical Bird Neoplasms (Neoplasms Metastasis in Birds)
               T Fredrickson
   14/Vol. V   Progression of Avian Lymphoid Leucosis
               HG Purchase
   15/Vol. V   Selected Immunological Aspects of Neoplastic Progression in Marek's Disease
               HM Sharma
   15/Vol. V   Feather Pulp Lesions During the Course of Marek's Disease Virus Induced Lymphoma Formation in Chickens
               R Moriguchi
   C.   *Reptiles*
   11/Vol. V   Lymphatic Neoplasms in Reptiles and Fish
               SV Machotka
   D.   *Amphibians*
   9/Vol. V   Metastases in Amphibians
               M Anver
   E.   *Fishes*
   11/Vol. V   Lymphatic Neoplasms in Reptiles and Fish
               SV Machotka

4. *Invertebrates*
   5/Vol. V   Leucoses in Invertebrates
               HE Kaiser
   6/Vol. V   Metastases of Invertebrate Neoplasms
               KR Cooper
   7/Vol. V   Selected Aspects of Neoplastic Growth in Arthropods
               HE Kaiser

REFERENCES

1. Ashley DJB: *Evans' Histological Appearances of Tumours.* Vol 1, pp 161–220. Edinburgh-London-New York: Churchill Livingstone, 1978
2. Cohen WD (ed) *Blood Cells of Marine Invertebrates: Experimental Systems in Cell Biology and Comparative Physiology.* New York: Alan R. Liss, Inc, 1985
3. Couch JA, Harshbarger JC: Effects of carcinogenic agents on aquatic animals: an environmental and experimental overview. *Environ Carcinogenesis Revs* 3(1):63, 1985
4. Dawe CJ: Phylogeny and Oncogeny. In: *Neoplasms and Related Disorders of Invertebrate and Lower Vertebrate Animals.* Monograph 31. Bethesda, Maryland: U.S. Department of Health, Education, and Welfare, National Cancer Institute, 1969
5. Harshbarger JC: Epizootiology of leukemia and lymphoma in poikilotherms. In: *Advances in Comparative Leukemia Re-*

search, edited by John DS and Blakeslee JR, Elsevier North Holland, pp 39–46, 1982

6. Jaffe ES, Green I: Neoplasms of the immune system. In: *Mechanisms of Tumor Immunity*, edited by Green I, Cohen S, McCluskey RT, New York: John Wiley & Sons, Inc, 1977

7. Kaiser HE: *Species-specific Potential of Invertebrates for Toxicological Research*. Baltimore: University Park Press, 1980

8. Kaiser HE: Distribution of true (real) tissues in organisms: A preliminary condition of neoplastic growth. In: *Neoplasms – Comparative Pathology of Growth in Animals, Plants, and Man*, edited by Kaiser HE, Baltimore: Williams & Wilkins, pp 43–88, 1981

9. Kaiser HE: The species-specific spectrum of neoplasms. In: *Neoplasms – Comparative Pathology of Growth in Animals, Plants, and Man*, edited by Kaiser HE, Baltimore: Williams & Wilkins, pp 649–721, 1981

10. Kaiser HE: Animal neoplasms – A systematic review. In: *Neoplasms – Comparative Pathology of Growth in Animals, Plants, and Man*, edited by Kaiser HE, Baltimore: Williams & Wilkins, pp 747–812, 1981

11. Mathe G, Rappaport H, in collaboration with O'Conor GT, Torloni H: Histological and cytological typing of neoplastic diseases of hematopoietic and lymphoid tissues. WHO Internat'l Histological Classification of Tumours No. 14, Geneva, 1976

12. Mix MC: Cancerous diseases in aquatic animals and their association with environmental pollutants: a critical literature review. Mar Environ Res vol. 20 (1 and 2):141 pp, ATh Heath (ed), Elsevier Appl Science, Crownhouse, New York, 1986

13. National Cancer Institute Sponsored Study of Classifications of non-Hodgkin's Lymphomas. *Cancer* 49:2110, 1982

PROGRESSION OF LYMPHOPROLIFERATIVE DISORDERS AND HEMATOLOGIC MALIGNANCIES

ERIC S. GROVES and DAN L. LONGO

I. INTRODUCTION

Figures 1–3 show the differentiation pathways, markers, and associated malignancies for hematopoietic cells, B lymphocytes, and T lymphocytes, respectively. As can be seen from the figures, distinct malignancies have been shown to have surface antigen characteristics similar to cells at virtually every identified differentiation step.

Normal hematopoietic and lymphoid cells are required to migrate throughout the body during the course of normal differentiation or function and therefore, differ from cells of other histogeneses. Hence, the patterns of tissue involvement by hematopoietic and lymphoid neoplasms reflect not only the usual metastatic processes but may also reflect the specific patterns of migration of normal hematopoietic and lymphoid cells. In order to clarify the influence of trafficking

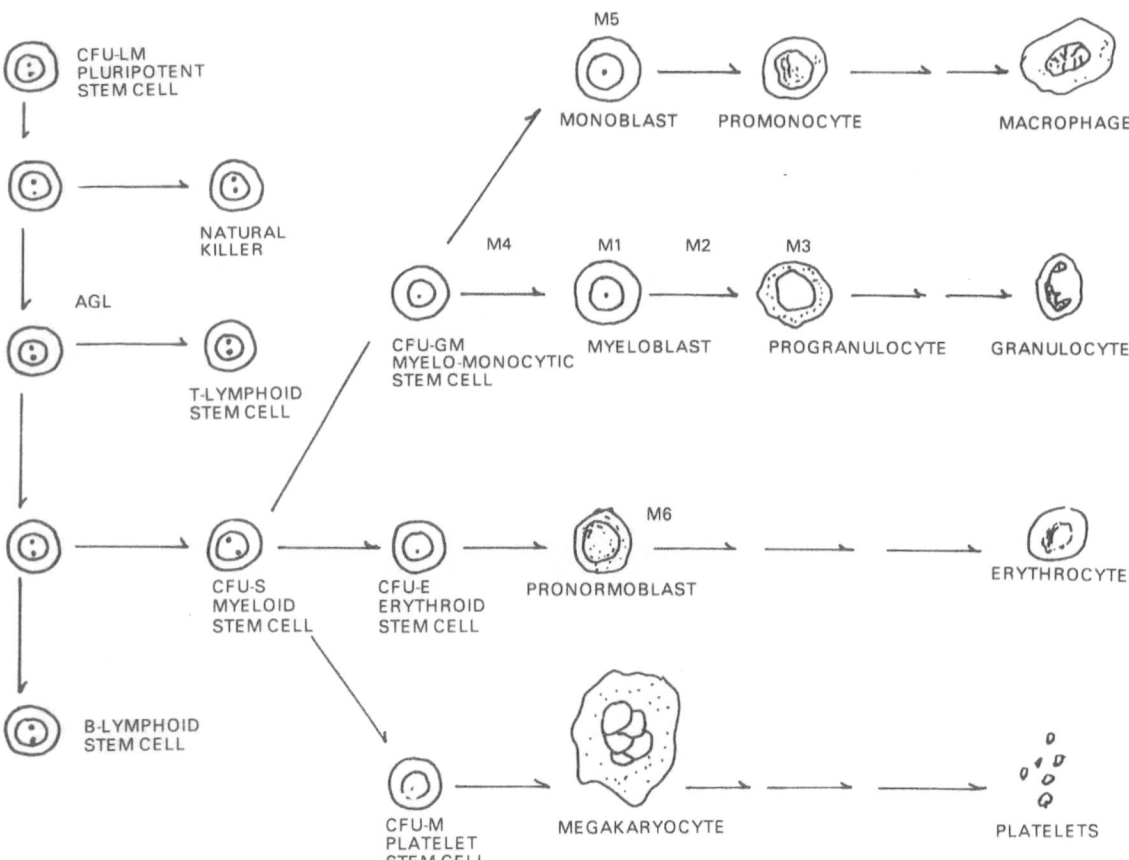

Figure 1. Scheme of myeloid differentiation showing normal cell phenotypes and their relationship to the French–American–British (FAB) subgroups of acute granulocytic leukemia (AGL). M1, undifferentiated myeloid; M2, myeloid; M3, progranulocyte; M4, myelomonocytic; M5, monocytic; M6, erythroleukemia. Differentiation stages as assayed by standard colony forming cell assays are indicated: CFU-LM, colony forming unit- lymphocytic-myelocytic; CFU-S, colony forming unit- splenic; CFU-GM, colony forming unit-granulocytic-monocytic; CFU-E, colony forming unit- erythrocytic; CFU-M, colony forming unit- megakaryocytic.

K.W. Brunson (ed) Local invasion and spread of cancer.
© 1989, Kluwer Academic Publishers, Dordrecht.

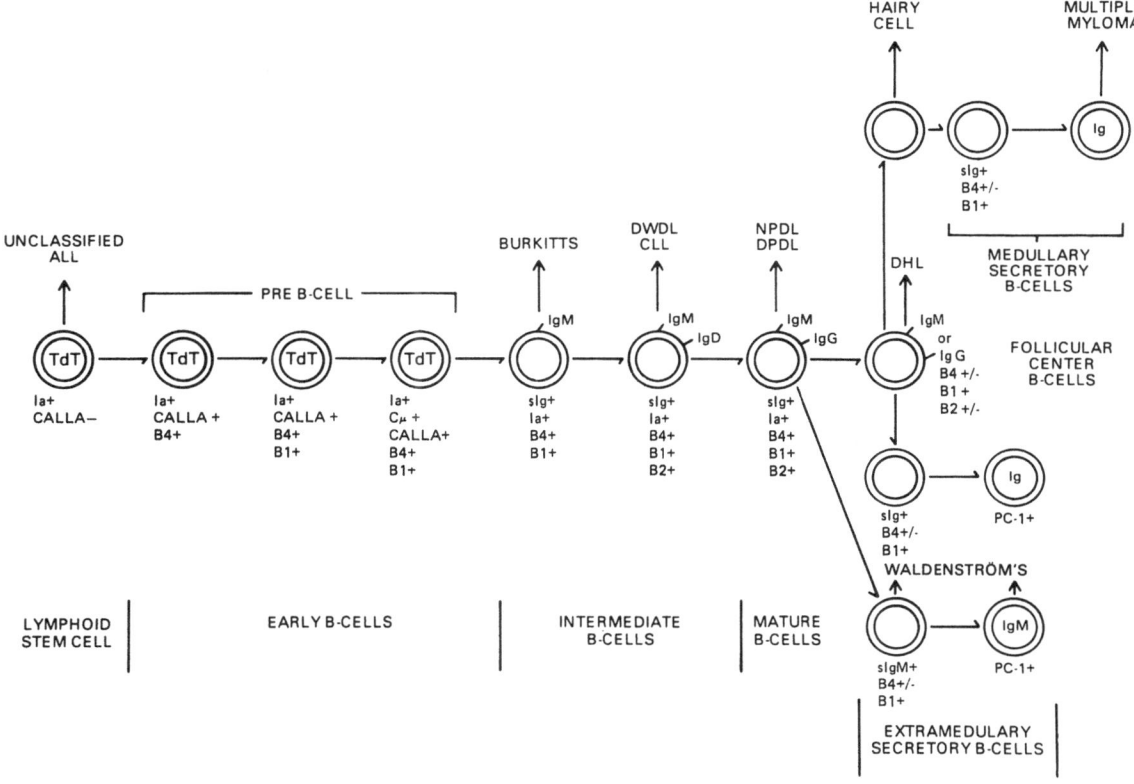

Figure 2. Scheme of B-lymphocyte differentiation showing cell phenotypes and their relationship to the lymphoproliferative disorders. ALL, acute lymphoblastic leukemia; CALLA, common anti-lymphoblastic leukemia antigen; DWDL, diffuse well-differentiated lymphocytic lymphoma; CLL, chronic lymphocytic leukemia; NPDL + DPDL, nodular and diffuse poorly differentiated lymphocytic lymphoma; DHL, diffuse histiocytic lymphoma; hairy cell, hairy cell leukemia; Cμ, cytoplasmic μ heavy chain; sIg, surface membrane immunoglobulin; TdT, terminal deoxynucleotidyl transferase. B1, B2, B4, Ia, PC-1 are cell surface antigens recognized by antibodies.

mechanisms we will briefly review what is known about these migration and traffic patterns.

II. DETERMINANTS OF NORMAL AND NEOPLASTIC CELL DISTRIBUTION

A. Differentiation and migration patterns of hematopoietic stem cells

The hematologic stem cells have been identified in various cell colony forming (CFU) assays and are designated CFU-XX, where the XX designates the specific assay. Thus far these cells have poorly defined cell surface marker phenotypes. The apparent differentiation sequence is depicted in Figures 1–3. The majority of data describing the ontogeny and differentiation of hematopoietic and lymphoid cells comes from studies performed using mice and rats. In what follows we will indicate what has been learned and attempt to extrapolate to the human system.

In the murine embryo, the CFU-LH cells appear to originate in the yolk-sac, migrate to the fetal liver then to the bone marrow (4). Some of these cells may differentiate to CFU-S, prior to reaching the marrow and thus supply early lymphoid progenitors. In adult mice, CFU-S are localized almost exclusively in the marrow (~ 98%), spleen (2%) and blood (> 1%). Hypoxia, anemia, or injection of antigens or endotoxin lead to decreased marrow and increased blood and spleen concentrations, suggesting migration of CFU-S from the marrow to the spleen (2, 5–8). Studies in lethally irradiated mice with one limb shielded have demonstrated that stem cell migration from the protected to irradiated sites does occur (1, 3). Hence stem cells (presumably CFU-LH as well as CFU-S) retain the capacity to migrate and "home" to the marrow.

Each of these colony forming stem cells retains the ability to replicate or self-replace, a capacity which appears more extensive in cells located earlier in the differentiation chain. However, even for the earliest committed stem cells there is an absolute limit, as demonstrated by the eventual decline of self-renewal and repopulation in serially transplanted marrows (9).

B. Differentiation and migration patterns of maturing non-lymphoid cells

As seen in Fig. 1, granulocytes and monocyte-macrophages are believed to share a common progenitor. Neutrophils apparently differentiate from the CSF-GM within the mar-

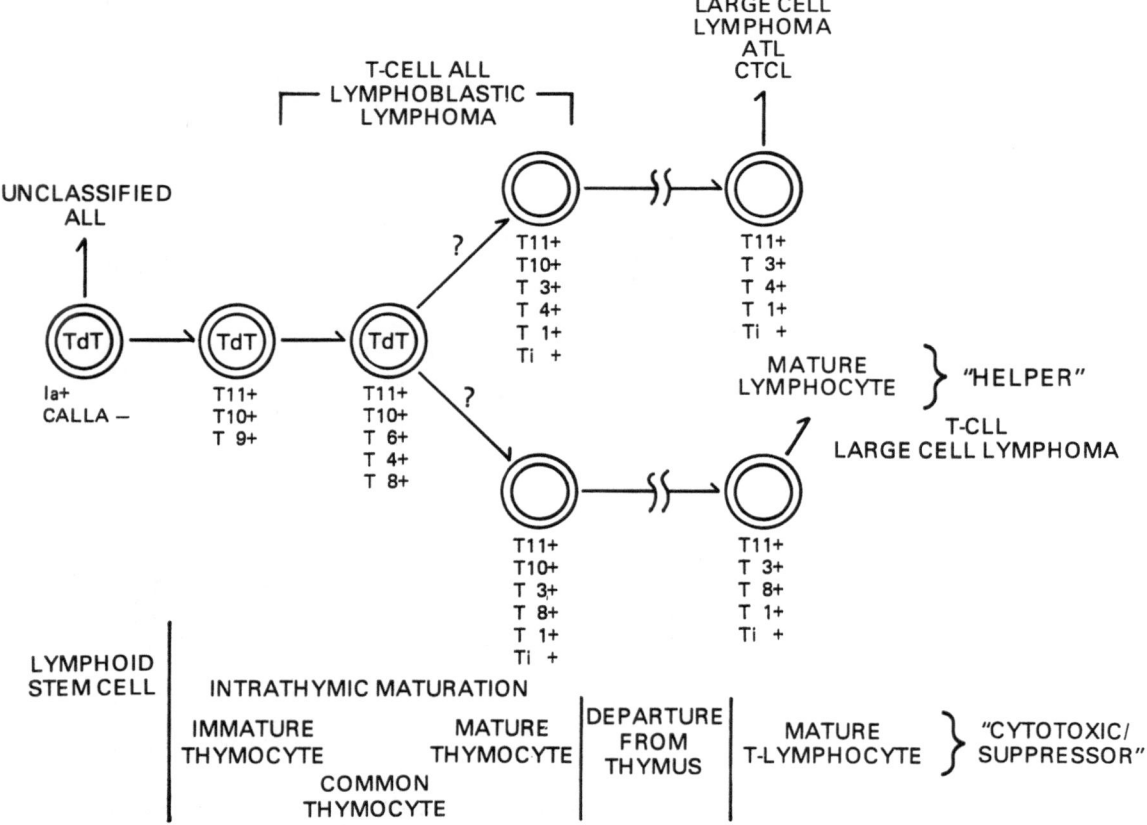

Figure 3. Scheme of T-lymphocyte differentiation showing cell phenotypes and their relationship to the lymphoproliferative disorders. ALL, acute lymphoblastic leukemia; CLL, chronic lymphoblastic leukemia; ATL, adult T-cell leukemia/lymphoma; TdT, terminal deoxynucleotidyl transferase. T1, T3, T4, T6, T8, T9 and T10 are cell surface membrane antigens recognized by antibodies.

row, are stored for an interval, and then are discharged into the blood. Shortly thereafter they transfer to tissues. Their lifetime in tissues is believed to be on the order of a few days. The monocyte/macrophage migration pattern appears similar, however, the tissue life time of these cells may be quite long. Megakaryocytic and erythrocytic differentiation appear to be confined solely to the marrow, except in the instance of myelofibrosis where myeloid metaplasia of the liver and spleen may be seen.

Feedback circuits exist which relay the demand for mature cells to their progenitors, influencing cells at least as early as CFU-LH, as evidenced by the cycling behavior of mature populations seen in humans with cyclic neutropenia (10).

C. Differentiation and migration patterns of maturing lymphocytes

Lymphocytes are subdivided into B, T and natural killer cell lineages. B cells mature into antibody producing plasma cells and T cells mature into helper, cytotoxic, and regulatory cells. The differentiation of lymphocytes proceeds in two stages. The first stage occurs during fetal and early neonatal development and lays a framework for lymphocytes in various stages of differentiation situated throughout the body. The second stage is an ongoing process of replacement of finite-lived mature cells by the progeny of cells placed earlier in the differentiation pathways (11, 12, 15, 16).

Prenatal B cell ontogeny
B cell genesis in the mouse occurs in a single wave evolving during the 20-day murine gestation period. B precursor cells appear sequentially in the blood (day 10), liver (day 12), spleen (day 15) and bone marrow (day 17). Cells in all sites mature simultaneously, producing increasing numbers of surface IgM positive (sIgM$^+$) cells just before birth (20 days). At birth most sIgM$^+$ spleen cells lack sIgD, Ia antigens and complement receptors. These first appear by neonatal day 10 and the proportion of sIgM$^+$ cells displaying sIgD rises progressively thereafter. Neonatal sIgM$^+$ cells are still immature in both receptor expression and function and may be rendered unresponsive rather than activated by antigen exposure (i.e. may be tolerized to antigen). The wave of B cell genesis in the mouse liver ends by neonatal week 2 and in the spleen by neonatal week 3. Thereafter, the production of committed B cell progenitors occurs only in the bone marrow.

Postnatal B cell differentiation
Postnatally, pre-B cells reside predominantly in the bone marrow and produce progeny at a rate which appears to permit the whole repertoire of antigenic specificities to be generated anew every few days (12, 15). Maturation proceeds through rather discrete stages beginning with large dividing pre-B cells (cytoplasmic μ^+ ($c\mu^+$)), followed by small postmitotic pre-B cells ($c\mu^+$, $s\mu^-$) (the most numerous population of marrow pre-B cells), $sIgM^+$ B cells, and then finally as $sIgM^+$, $sIgD^+$ cells which are exported to extramedullary sites. There is significant cell death at the stage which is $sIgM^+$, $sIgD^-$. This fact and observations with anti-IgM treated neonatal mice have been used to argue that tolerance induction (or elimination of self-reactive clones) occurs at this stage. The surface marker pattern of differentiating B cells is shown in Fig. 2. This pattern permits identification of the normal phenotype which corresponds to the malignant cells in many cases.

T cell prenatal differentiation
Again the best data describing the process in mammals derive from murine studies. In mice, shortly after the earliest appearance of the thymus, Thy^+ cells derived from precursors in the yolk sac and para-aortic mesoderm enter the thymus. T cells first entering the thymus do not express their antigen receptor (Ti) and do not have the receptor alpha and beta chain genes rearranged. During subsequent development, first the β chain of the Ti receptor and then the α chain are rearranged to form the expressed genes defining the Ti receptors displayed by mature T cells. In human similar intrathymic populations differentiate first into a subgroup in which the Ti genes remain unrearranged, and then develop into mature "helper" ($OKT4^+$, Ti^+, $T3^+$ (10%)), mature "suppressor/cytotoxic" ($OKT8^+$, Ti^+, $T3^+$ (10%)) or non-functional "double positive" cells ($OKT4^+$–$OKT8^+$, Ti^-, $T3^+$ (80%). It is likely that the double positive population gives rise to the mature populations. (The exact details of this final developmental sequence still are controversial but are depicted in Fig. 3). In the mouse, just prior to birth, mature cells begin to migrate from the thymus to extra-thymic sites. The intrathymic progenitor subset has been demonstrated to contain cells capable of homing to the thymus and repopulating it. Evidence has been presented suggesting an extrathymic pathway of T cell maturation for a small fraction of cells. However, probably all T cells undergo their receptor gene rearrangements intrathymically.

Postnatal T cell differentiation
The initial developmental sequence occurs in a wave, requiring the entry into the thymus of relatively small numbers of $Thy\ 1^+$ precursors. Postnatally, the release of T cells from the thymus has a periodicity which suggests that the numbers of progeny produced by each entering $Thy\ 1^+$ precursor are relatively fixed and that reinitiation of the cycle requires the entrance of a new group of $Thy\ 1^+$ precursors (13). The time required to regenerate a set of T cells exhibiting the complete receptor repertoire is on order of seven to twelve weeks in mice. Postnatally, prethymic T cell precursors are present in the bone marrow, as demonstrated by the success of T cell reconstitution after bone marrow transplantation, but they are also present in reduced numbers in such sites as the spleen and perhaps in even the peripheral blood.

Extra-thymic populations
Mature T cells exiting the thymus and $sIgM^+$, $sIgD^+$ B cells leaving the bone marrow appear to enter the bloodstream and migrate to the lymphoid organs, the spleen, lymph nodes and Peyers's patches. This migration marks their entrance into a recirculating pool of lymphocytes which traffic between blood and lymph nodes or between blood and spleen. The majority of these newly released lymphocytes appear to have a relatively short life span. Radioautographic studies suggest a mean life span of 5–7 weeks for recirculating B cells and 16 weeks for T cells (18). However, in functional studies with radiation induced chromosome abnormalities, evidence exists for longer lived subsets which are believed to have been recruited by antigenic stimulation and which apparently form the cellular basis of immunologic memory (12, 15). With increasing age, these longer lived subsets appear to form a larger fraction of the extra-thymic, extra-bone marrow population. This causes a reduction in the entry of new cells into the population. Thus, with time the thymus undergoes involution and the fraction of nucleated marrow cells that are pre-B cells declines.

Natural killer circulation
Precursors for the natural killer lymphocyte population are ill defined, however, evidence (14) suggests that the mature population has a relatively short life span (several days) in the spleen and other lymphoid organs and that its immediate precursors are located in the bone marrow.

Lymph node organization and cellular traffic
Cells appear to enter lymph nodes from the blood at the site of the high endothelial post-capillary venules (HEV). There is evidence that this endothelial surface has characteristics (or antigens) which permit lymphocytes to distinguish Peyer's patches from mesenteric lymph nodes or peripheral lymph nodes. Mouse cells bound with an antibody (Mel-14)

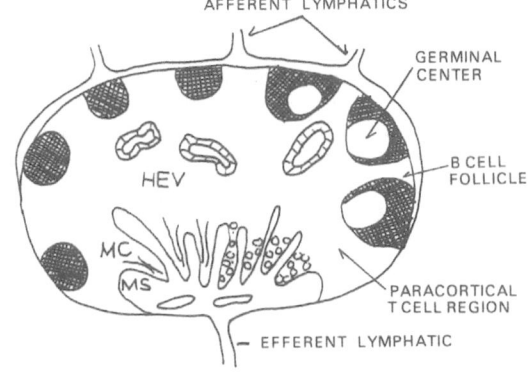

Figure 4a. Schematic of lymph node architecture showing resting (or unimmunized) architecture on the left half of drawing and activated (immunized) architecture on the right. The paracortical area is indicated in white, the medullary cords by MC, the medullary sinuses by MS and the B cell follicles by the black hatching. Two histologically prominent features of immunized lymph nodes are illustrated on the right half: (a) germinal centers (white parafollicular circles), clusters of dividing and differentiating B cell blasts responding to the immunization and (b) distension of the medullary cords with plasma cells.

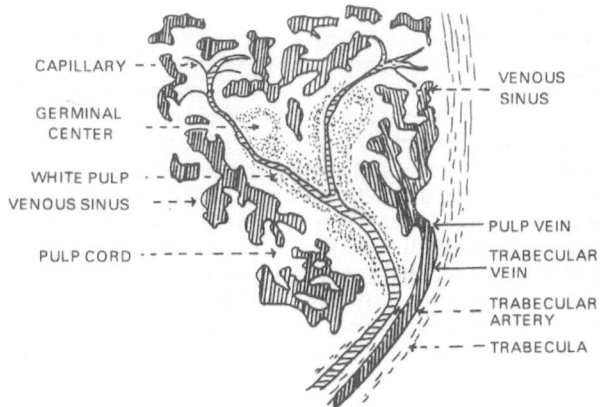

CAPILLARY

GERMINAL
CENTER

WHITE PULP
VENOUS SINUS

PULP CORD

VENOUS
SINUS

PULP VEIN

TRABECULAR
VEIN

TRABECULAR
ARTERY

TRABECULA

Figure 4b. Schematic of splenic architecture showing a subunit organized around an afferent trabecular artery and an efferent trabecular vein. The details of the vascular connection between capillaries and venous sinuses remains controversial, and whether or not a direct connection exists between the two is unclear.

to one set of HEV receptors fail to show the characteristic binding to HEV endothelium *in vitro* and acutely alter their traffic pattern *in vivo* (17). This ability to "home" established substreams of traffic, one apparently recirculating mainly through the peripheral nodes and another through gut-related lymphoid tissues. Access to the spleen apparently does not require the HEV receptor.

All the lymph nodes of the body demonstrate a similar structural organization as shown in Fig. 4a. Afferent lymph, containing some lymphocytes, macrophages and occasionally antigen drains into the subcapsular space, percolates through the paracortical area (white) and the medullary cords (MC) to the medullary sinuses (MS) and leaves via the efferent lymphocyte vessels. B and T lymphocytes enter the node predominantly from the blood via the walls of the HEV.

Within the lymph node, B and T cells appear to linger initially in the deep cortex for a period of 3–6 hrs after which B cells move to the follicles of the superficial cortex, where they remain for about 30 hrs prior to exiting the lymph node. The T cells remain in the deep cortex a further 10 hrs before exiting. This segregation results in the characteristic zones of B and T cell concentration with B cells dominantly in the follicules and T cells in the paracortex. Scattered cells of both types exist within the zones of the other, presumably permitting antigen presentation and helper and suppressor function to occur (17).

Similar architectural subdivisions occur within the spleen. It is organized into anatomic subunits by its vasculature; a functional subunit is indicated in Fig. 4b. The pariarterial sheath (PAS) regions (white pulp) contain the majority of splenic B and T cells and appear to provide a lymphocyte environment and immunologic function is similar to that of the lymph node cortex. The venous regions (red pulp) are filled primarily with blood elements (e.g. red cells and platelets) but also with macrophages and a few plasma cells. The red pulp is the site of the splenic extramedullary hematopoiesis seen in certain disease states. At the interface of the white and red pulp is the marginal zone. This is the site of entry for most lymphocytes to the PAS (from blood as the spleen has virtually no lymphatics).

Antigenic stimulation leads to an increase in antigen specific lymphocytes within the lymph nodes or spleen. This occurs both through arrest of lymphocyte exit and through local proliferation. This proliferation takes place at the boundaries of the follicle and T cell regions. The sites of this proliferation from the morphologically distinct germinal centers is indicated in Fig. 4a. In a primary antigen response, B cells which are sIgM$^+$, sIgD$^+$, are the primary proliferating population, although nearby T cells also proliferate. After secondary or repeated immunizations, cells within the germinal centers express predominantly sIgG in lymph nodes or sIgA in Peyer's patches (17), suggesting that the germinal center is the site of immunoglobulin heavy chain class switching. IgA is a secretory immunoglobulin and is the dominant product of the gut-associated lymphatic tissue.

With primary antigenic stimulation some B cells appear to rapidly differentiate to mature IgM producing plasma cells while others go on to form the B cells of the germinal center (whether this set of IgM secreting plasma cells derive from the germinal center cells or differentiate from pre-germinal center B cells is not yet clear). With secondary stimulation some B cells again go on to differentiate into antibody secreting plasma cells within the lymph node or spleen. (It has been postulated that the germinal center is the origin of these cells.) However, some apparently arrest their differentiation prior to antibody secretion and migrate to the bone marrow. This migration results in the observed shift in the dominant site of antibody producton from the peripheral lymphoid tissues to the bone marrow after the first week of a secondary response. It also explains why approximately 90% of circulating antibodies have been produced by cells within the bone marrow. Individual plasma cells appear to have a life span of a few days.

D. Metastatic behavior

Dispersion of cells from the site at which the first tumor cell arises, is the result of a cascade of interdependent and competing processes. Metastasizing cells differ from normal migrating cells which "home" to various sites with good survivability, in that only a small fraction survive this cascade to flourish at another anatomic site. Experimental investigation suggests that the principle determinants which define sites at which major metastatic groups of cells (i.e. 10^8–10^9 cells) will occur are: (1) anatomic site of initial tumor; (2) surface properties of the tumor cells (e.g. laminin receptors); (3) routes and potential mechanisms of cellular access to the metastatic sites; (4) growth environment provided by the metastatic site; (5) growth requirements of the tumor cells, and (6) host anti-tumor responses (e.g. immunologic reactions).

In addition to these general determinants, it has been found experimentally that tumors exhibit a heterogenous metastatic potential. For example Poste *et al.* (20) found that murine B-16 melanoma cells clonally selected for high metastatic potential gradually developed subpopulations distinguishable for high, medium and low metastatic potential themselves.

Finally, the phenotype of a malignancy may change with time. This can occur as a consequence of the well documented genetic instability of malignancies, either through the activation of new oncogenes (19), through clonal selection, or as the result of therapy. Both chemotherapy (22) and radiation (21) have been demonstrated to alter the metastatic distribution of tumors, presumably through effects on host tissue or on the malignancy or on both. The sum of all of the above influences will be referred to in what follows by the phrase "usual metastatic processes".

The determinants of disease progression in the lymphocytic and hematopoietic malignancies are even more complicated since the normal cells in these systems are, in general, not sessile. They are free to move about, and, in fact, must do so to accomplish their physiological role. Thus, for hematologic and lymphoid malignancies, the additional complications of cell trafficking and differentiation must be added to all of the aforementioned determinants of metastatic behavior. Malignancies composed of trafficking cells have an ill-defined primary anatomic site in most instances (although one might see the tumors confined to a characteristic circulation route). Since the overwhelming majority of hematologic and lymphoid malignancies are clonal in origin, and the tumors seem to be malignant transformations of cells with cell surface phenotypes corresponding to a stage of normal differentiation, it is reasonable to assume that the tumors originate in the anatomic site of the normal counterpart of the malignant cell. However, with rare exception, this notion is not helpful because by the time the tumor is clinically detectable the cells are usually found in remote sites. The rules of spread that are applicable to other tumors (e.g. first spread to draining lymph nodes, then to organs containing the first capillary bed distal to the primary organ site, then widespread hematogenous spread) simply do not apply.

Furthermore, features of normal lymphoid and hematopoietic cells that determine their trafficking are poorly understood. Therefore, there is little science in the chronicling of disease progression in these tumors. Yet there are some strikingly predictable patterns of spread specific for particular tumor types, and such patterns make it likely that further study will reveal the underlying mechanisms.

For example, Hodgkin's disease quite commonly originates in the left supraclavicular node group, a fact based on the observation that when only one site is involved, it is usually the left supraclavicular node group. And when Hodgkin's disease spreads, it tends to go to contiguous lymph node groups rarely skipping anatomic sites. Thus, one might conclude that the origin of the Sternberg-Reed cell (the malignant cell of Hodgkin's disease) has something to do with the interaction of the lymphatic system with the thoracic duct, since these systems come together in the left neck. And one might suggest that the malignant cell does not circulate widely, but may migrate from one lymph node to the adjacent nodes in a predictably stepwise fashion. Finally, one can conclude that for Hodgkin's disease, much like malignancies in other organ systems, an anatomically based staging system might provide reasonable prognostic information; and in fact, it does. Thus, without knowing very much at all about the normal counterpart of the malignant cell and its pattern of migration and trafficking, observation of patients has taught us a great deal.

This is not the case with a large number of lymphoid and hematopoietic tumors. We do not understand why the ma-

lignant cells of myelomonocytic leukemia have a predilection for the gingivae. We do not understand the striking splenic tropism of hairy cell leukemia which is not only a disease that primarily affects the spleen, but also seems to be dependent on the presence of the spleen or some splenic factors for tumor cell proliferation. We do not understand why patients with gamma heavy chain disease have palatal edema. We do not understand the connection between Waldeyer's ring and gastrointestinal involvement with malignant lymphomas of intermediate grade. We do not understand the basis of the predilection of mature T-cell malignancies for the skin. However, it is likely that we will one day be able to relate these findings to the normal trafficking or physiology of the nonmalignant counterpart.

Already some of the observations on patterns of disease origin and spread made by clinicians have resulted in successful prophylaxis and a reduction in morbidity and mortality. For example, it was observed by Burkitt that the lymphoma that bears his name often presented as a rapidly enlarging jaw tumor. Furthermore, it has been felt that in a large fraction of patients with African Burkitt's lymphoma, malignant transformation of a B cell by Epstein-Barr virus is the etiology. Epstein-Barr virus is readily obtainable from the saliva of the vast majority of people. Because of the mandibular primaries that were found in Africa, it proposed that a B cell in the mandible became infected and transformed by EBV that gained access to the mandibular marrow through severely carious teeth. Thus, it is hoped that the institution of a thorough dental prophylaxis system in high risk populations might decrease the incidence of the disease.

Another area in which the observation of patterns of disease involvement has resulted in successful prophylactic measures is the involvement of the central nervous system in patients with intermediate and high grade lymphomas. CNS involvement with lymphoma occurs in about 5% of all cases, and its occurrence is virtually always in patients with diffuse large cell or undifferentiated histology. In fact, if a patient with an indolent histologic subtype of lymphoma develops signs and symptoms of CNS disease, nearly all of those patients will have found to have undergone histologic progression to diffuse lymphoma. Except for the rare primary CNS lymphomas, which nearly always occur in the setting of primary or secondary immunosuppression, patients developing CNS lymphoma almost always have bone marrow involvement with lymphoma. It is felt that the lymphoma spreads to the meninges via Batson's veins. Because of this association, patients with diffuse lymphoma and bone or bone marrow involvement now routinely receive CNS prophylaxis upon achieving a complete remission. As a result, secondary spread of diffuse lymphoma to the CNS occurs in less than 1% of cases. Similar success of prophylaxis has been shown in the childhood lymphoblastic leukemias.

Despite the complexity of the lymphoid and hematopoietic systems, careful observation may result in clinical advances. It is hoped that further scientific study of normal and malignant cell trafficking may lead to new therapies designed to limit the spread of these tumors.

In what follows we will describe for the major hematologic and lymphoid malignancies the known patterns of presentation and progression, followed by what is known regarding the phenotype of the malignant cells and finally, where there is sufficient knowledge will relate this phenotype to clinical behavior of the malignancy.

III. STEM CELL DISORDERS

E. Chronic granulocytic leukemia (CGL) and polycythemia vera (PV)

CGL is a hematopoietic stem cell disorder associated initially with excessive production of mature granulocytic elements apparently derived from an abnormal myeloid stem cell. In its terminal stage, it is characterized by progression to a less well-differentiated or "blastic" phase resembling acute leukemia. The disease is usually detected by routine blood counts. Patients in the initial or chronic phase may present asymptomatically ($\sim 20\%$) or with mild systemic symptoms (e.g. fatigue, malaise, fever) or with symptoms associated with increased myeloid mass (e.g. bone pain), splenomegaly (e.g. abdominal discomfort), or thrombocytosis (e.g. hemorrhage) (29). About 20% of acute leukemias over actually blast transformation of CGL in which the chronic phase was asymptomatic.

Initially, the granulocytes appear to function normally but, later in the disease course subtle abnormalities appear suggesting increasing dysfunction (24). Granulocyte intravascular lifetime also appears to be prolonged. Platelet function is abnormal but hemorrhagic problems are rare (24). The bone pain is felt to be secondary to marrow expansion (29). This disease may cause truly massive splenomegaly. The splenomegaly and the later hepatomegaly are secondary to initiation of extramedullary hematopoiesis at these sites (29) (presumably reflecting the capacity of the malignant stem cell to migrate to these sites). The appearance of lymphadenopathy usually heralds impending blastic transformation.

By cytogenetic analysis, approximately 95% of the leukemic cells have the characteristic Philadelphia chromosome (Ph^1) abnormality associated with a t(9; 22) translocation (although other translocations with chromosome 22 are seen less frequently). The Ph^1 marker as well as glucose 6-phosphate dehydrogenase (G6PD) heterozygosity have been used to demonstrate CGL clonal involvement of granulocytes, monocytes, erythrocytes, platelets, and their precursors. Subsequent studies have shown involvement of B lymphocytes. T cell involvement remains controversial (summarized in (25)), although at least one example of pH^1 involvement of T cells has been observed (28).

Blastic transformation seems to occur with the advent of a subclone, bearing the phenotype of any one of these precursors (including fibroblasts as seen in Ph^{1+} myelofibrosis), which has an unrestrained or leukemic growth pattern. Consistent with this model of subclone appearance, $\sim 1/3$ of Ph^{1+} ALL will remit after therapy to an evolving Ph^1 positive chronic phase which may last several years before developing a myeloid blast phase (26). Blast transformation leukemias most frequently have myeloid morphology (60%), followed by B lymphoid (30%), erythroid (5%), megakaryoblastoid (5%) and T lymphoid (> 1%) morphologies.

The clinical spread of these blast transformation leukemias appears to conform to the patterns characteristic of their morphology, except for the important clinical difference that the response of these leukemias to therapy is usually poorer than Ph^1 negative leukemias not associated with anticedent CGL.

In summary, during the chronic phase of CGL the progeny of the abnormal stem cell clone appears to differentiate normally, function nearly normally and migrate normally; upon blast transformation they behave like therapeutically resistant manifestations of their respective acute leukemias.

Polycythemia vera (or Rubra vera) is another myeloproliferative stem cell disorder. Cells of the erythroid series form the predominate proliferating group although lesser relative elevations of granulocytes and platelets are also seen. Initial presentation is usually the result of sysmptoms or signs associated with the hypervolemia and hyperviscosity associated with the increased red cell mass. Modest splenomegally develops in 75%, with hepatomegaly in 40%. Pruritus (50%) and urticaria (10%) can also be prominent. The usual course is protracted, with the phase of persistent erythrocytosis lasting 5 to 25 years. Eventually, patients enter a "burned out phase" with reduced normal or subnormal erythrocyte production; however, the thrombocytosis and leukocytosis usually persists. During this latter phase, myeloid metaplasia in the spleen, liver, lymph nodes and kidneys may appear.

From the phenotypes of the progeny of the involved stem cell, it appears to be a cell prior to the irreversible separation of lymphocytes from the granulocyte, erythrocyte, megakaryocyte differentiation pathway. The progeny of this abnormal stem cell appear to function normally and traffic normally; hence the morbidity of the disease results from overproduction of apparently normal progeny.

IV. IMMATURE LYMPHOID AND NON-LYMPHOID NEOPLASIA

F. Acute lymphoblastic leukemia (ALL)

ALL predominantly affects children. The course is usually acute with histories measured in days or weeks. Table 1 indicates clinical findings and symptoms at presentation. Two major classifications exist: Table 2 shows the immunologic classification, Table 3 the morphologic classification. L-3, Burkitt's or B-cell ALL is clearly a clinically distinct entity under both schemes and it has been suggested that it represents the leukemic phase of Burkitt's lymphoma

Table 1. Presenting characteristics of 1,024 patients with acute leukemia (1948–1971) in the Southwest Oncology Group.

Characteristic	Percent
Liver enlarged	79
Spleen enlarged	69
Cervical nodes enlarged	62
Inguinal nodes enlarged	54
Axillary nodes enlarged	47
CNS Involvement	2

Modified from Sutow WW, Vietti TJ, Fernbach DL, Clinical Pediatric Oncology, 3rd ed. C.V. Mosby, St. Louis, 1980.

Table 2. Immunologic classification on acute lymphoblastic leukemia.

	"Common"	Null-cell	T-cell	B-cell Burkitt's	Non-Burkitt's
Frequency (%)	58	20	20	2	
E-C rosettes	−	−	+	−	−
Mitotic Rate	Low	?	High	High	?
Surface Ig	−	−	−	+	+
Thy antigen	−	−	+	−	−
ALL antigen(s)	+	−	−	?	+
WBC	Low	High	High	High	High or Low
Sex	M = F	?	M > F	M = F	?
Origin	Marrow	?	Thymus	Nasopharynx	?
Remission	Long	Long	Short	Shortest	?

(see the section on Burkitt's lymphoma for further discussion). The remaining immunotypes are scattered fairly evenly between the L-1 and L-2 morphologic classifications. T cell ALL probably behaves as a clinically distinct entity, however, historically data have not always segregated presentations by T cell markers, hence the frequency with which non-T cell ALL presents with the mediastinal mass "characteristic" of T cell ALL is not known. Patients usually present with a relatively large malignant cell mass. Leukemic infiltration of virtually every organ has been reported and, although difficult to assess, has been estimated to be as high as 50% for extramedullary sites (35, 38) at presentation. Clinically, the two most important extramedullary sites are the CNS and the testes. Clinical involvement of these sites during the course of disease is more frequent in T cell ALL, but the etiology of this predilection remains unclear and does not reflect a known normal T cell tropism. As is noted in Table 1, overt CNS involvement is infrequent at presentation. However, the frequency of relapse from untreated CNS sites is high and has made CNS therapy a component of all treatment regimens. Access to the CNS is proposed to proceed stepwise from diseased bone marrow, through the leptomeningeal veins to the meninges (see e.g. (31). The frequency of this involvement has ap-

parently increased in the chemotherapeutic era; whether this reflects that the CNS is a sanctuary site unavailable to chemotherapy permitting subsequent leukemia outgrowth or whether the chemotherapy facilitates leukemic access to the CNS is unclear.

With relapse from the CNS or the testis, the bone marrow rapidly becomes involved. Studies with testicular relapses suggest that this repopulation proceeds through metastatic mechanisms rather than direct homing to the marrow, i.e. retroperitoneal lymph nodes are involved first (31), then presumably the blood and marrow.

As is noted in Table 2, all ALL appears to be of either B or T cells origin. Present clinical data are consistent with a rapid, neoplastic proliferation of marrow-bound B cell progenitors or thymus-bound T cell progenitors spreading via the usual metastatic processes to other sites with minimal contribution to this spread from lymphocyte migration. This picture has been made more complex by the finding that at least some T cell ALL's can be made to switch to myeloid morphology with treatment by deoxycoformycin, an adenosine deaminase inhibitor (34, 36), suggesting that the malignant cell may actually be a "stem" cell whose differentiation stage precedes the irreversible separation into the lymphoid or myeloid pathway.

Table 3. French–American–British classification of "lymphoblastic" leukemias.

Cytologic features	L1	L2	L3
Cell size	Small cells predominate	Large heterogeneous in size	Large and homogeneous
Nuclear chromatin	Homogeneous in any one case	Variable-heterogeneous in any one case	Finely stippled and homogeneous
Nuclear shape	Regular, occasional clefting or indentation	Irregular, clefting and indentation common	Regular-oval to round
Nucleoli	Not visible or small and inconspicuous	One or more present, of ten large	Prominent; one or more vesicular
Amount of cytoplasm	Scanty	Variable, often moderately abundant	Moderately abundant
Basophilia cytoplasm	Slight or moderate, rarely intense	Variable, deep in some	Very deep
Cytoplasmic vacuolation	Variable	Variable	Often prominent

Bennett JM, Catovsky D, Daniel MT, et al. Proposals for the classification of the acute leukemias. *Br J Haematol* 33:451, 1976

Table 4. Classification of acute non-lymphocytic leukemias.

Subtype	Morphology	Incidence in adults %	Cell size	Characteristics of immature cells				Comments
				Cytoplasm-nucleus ratio	Nucleoli	Cytoplasmic granules	Auer rods	
M1	Myeloblastic leukemia without maturation	35	Small to large	About equal	Distinct	Scarce	Occasional	Easily confused with L2 without special studied
M2	Myeloblastic leukemia with maturation		Large	About equal	Distinct	Present	Occasional	Predominant cells are blasts and early promyelocytes
M3	Hypergranular promyelocytic leukemia	10	Large	Increased	Distinct	Large, abundant, and atypical	Common, often multiple and branched	Associated with a high incidence of DIC
M4	Myelomonocytic leukemia	45	Large with monocytoid features	Increased	Distinct	Present	Occasional	Monocytic component may be more prominent in the blood than in the marrow
M5	Monocytic leukemia; (M5a); well differentiated (M5b)	7	Large with convoluted nuclei; often bizarre	About equal	Large	Present	Rare	Confirmation of diagnosis is necessary using fluoride-inhibited esterase reactions
M6	Erythroleukemia (usually progresses to M1, M2, or M4)	3	–	–	–	–		Prodrome of anemia, florid megaloblastoid erythroid hyperplasia, and bizarre multinucleated erythroblasts

Table 5. Symptoms and findings in patients with ANLL (39, 40).

		% of patients	Characteristic of subtype
Symptoms:	None	$\sim 10\%$	
	Fatigue	Most	
	Infection	$\sim 30\%$	
	Purpura	Most	
	Overt bleeding		Many M_3
Tissue involvement:	Lymphadenopathy	Unusual	
	Splenomegaly with or without hepatomegaly	$\sim 25\%$	
	Gingival hypertrophy		$\sim 50\%$ $M_{4,5}$
	Rectal lesions (e.g. fissures)		$\sim 10\%$ $M_{4,5}$
	Skin nodules	$\sim 5\%$	More frequent $M_{4,5}$
	Granulocytic sarcoma (chloroma) (of skin bone, GI tract, ovary, breast, lung)	Rare	
	Lung leukostasis		End stage $M_{4,5}$
	Retinal infiltration	Rare	
	CNS	Rare at presentation, high relapse rate if untreated $M_{4,5} > M_{1-3,6}$	

G. Acute non-lymphocytic leukemia (ANLL)

ANLL is a set of diseases predominantly affecting a population older than that affected by ALL. These diseases are reviewed elsewhere in this volume. Table 4 lists a current classification scheme. Patients usually present with a very short history of days to weeks and present with findings consistent with a high mass of disease. Table 5 describes the clinical and laboratory findings at presentation and indicates important subtype specific clinical findings (39, 40). The $M_{4,5}$ propensity for involvement of extramedullary sites (e.g. gingiva) is poorly understood but does not clearly reflect a well-established, normal, mature cell migratory pattern. As in ALL, subclinical involvement or therapy facilitated involvement (or both) of the CNS sanctuary site has been used to justify prophylactic therapy to prevent relapse at this site.

This set of diseases appears to represent neoplastic proliferation of marrow-bound cells. Their spread to sites outside of the marrow apparently reflects usual metastatic processes rather than normal migratory patterns.

V. LYMPHOMAS OF UNCERTAIN CELLULAR ORIGIN

H. Hodgkin's disease (HD)

HD is a disease which is among those best characterized but least understood. The pattern of clinical spread has been very well defined yet why the disease remains so confined to this pattern remains obscure.

The majority of these patients at presentation are found to have peripheral adenopathy. With workup, $\sim 50\%$ are found to have mediastinal node involvement. The disease tends to spread from a primary site to contiguous nodes and exhibits limited nodal skipping. A formal staging procedure, the Ann Arbor Staging Scheme (Table 6) (41), has been developed to characterize the degree of spread and facilitate

Table 6. The Ann Arbor staging classification.

Stage I
Involvement of a single lymph node region (I) or localized involvement of a single extranodal organ/site (I_E).

Stage II
Involvement of more than one lymph node region on the same side of the diaphragm (II) or of one or more lymph node regions and localized involvement of an extralymphatic organ/site (II_E) on the same side of the diaphragm.

Stage III
Involvement of lymph node regions on both sides of the diaphragm (III), which may be accompanied by involvement of the spleen (III_S) or by localized involvement of an extralymphatic organ/site (III_E) or both (III_{SE}).

Stage IV
Diffuse or disseminated involvement of one or more extralymphatic organ/site with or without lymph node involvement.

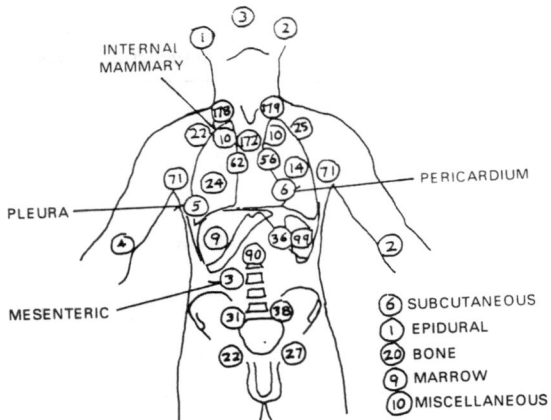

INTERNAL
MAMMARY

PERICARDIUM

PLEURA

MESENTERIC

Ⓢ SUBCUTANEOUS
Ⓔ EPIDURAL
㉒ BONE
Ⓜ MARROW
⑩ MISCELLANEOUS

Figure 5. Hodgkin's disease distribution showing a schematic of the anatomic sites of involvement in 285 consecutive, unselected, previously untreated cases. (Adapted from Kaplan HS, Dorfman RF, Nelson TS *et al.*: Staging laparotomy and splenectomy in 285 consecutive, unselected patients. *Natl Cancer Inst Monogr* 36:291, 1973).

therapeutic decisions. This system is used to characterize the extent of both HD's and the non-Hodgkin's lymphomas (though it is poorly applicable to the latter). Figure 5 shows the results of 285 unselected staging evaluations at Stanford (46). Typically, ~ 15% of patients are Stage I, ~ 35% Stage II, ~ 10% Stage IV. The frequency of "B" symptoms increases with stage. As can be seen from Fig. 5, the distribution of lymphoid tissue involvement is not at all uniform.

Certain tissues frequently involved in non-Hodgkin's lymphomas are spared by HD. These include the tonsils, Waldeyer's ring, and the mesenteric lymph nodes. HD virtually never involves epitrochlear or popliteal nodes. Extranodal primaries occur in HD but are rare, and extranodal involvement is usually an expression of very advanced disease or advanced local extension. Skin, bone, bone marrow and CNS involvement are usually associated with advanced or advancing disease.

The preference of the disease for lymphoid tissue remains unexplained. The surface markers of the malignant Sternberg-Reed (SR) cell suggest it is derived from interdigitating reticulum (IR) cells (45, 46). These cells usually are T200$^+$, HLA-DR$^+$, Leu10$^+$, A1G3$^+$, Tac$^+$, OKT9$^+$, LeuM1$^+$. They are negative for the usual B and T cell markers and are negative for the markers of monocyte (OKM1$^-$, Mo-2$^-$, G3D-3$^-$), follicular dendritic cells (DRC-1$^-$) and natural killer cells (Leu 7$^-$, Leu 11a$^-$, B73.1$^-$). A HD cell line has been used to stimulate an allogenic MLR (42) consistent with the antigen presenting activity supposedly possessed by IR cells. While little is known regarding the traffic of such IR cells, it is presumed that it is limited. Recently antibodies have been made to the SR cell line (43). Stein *et al.* (47) have used this marker as a basis for proposing that SR cells are of activated lymphoid origin instead of being IR cells, but their findings are controversial.

Since little information exists about the behavior of either IR cells or activated lymphoid' cells, the relationship of these cells to HD has thus far contributed little new understanding to HD behavior. Thus, the characteristic spread of HD from lymph node to contiguous lymph node with liver involvement only following splenic involvement and

Table 7. Comparison of the classification schemes for non-Hodgkin's lymphomas.

Rappaport	Working formulation	Lukes-Collins	Kiel
	Malignant lymphoma:		
DWDL/CLL	Small lymphocytic	Small lymphocytic and plasmacytoid lymphocytic	Lymphocytic, CLL lymphoplasmacytic/lymphoplasmacytoid
NPDL	Follicular, small cleaved cell	Small cleaved follicular center cell (FCC) follicular or follicular diffuse	Centroblastic-centrocytic (small) follicular
NML	Follicular, mixed small cleaved and large cell	Small cleaved FCC, follicular also large cleaved FCC, follicular	Centroblastic-centrocytic (small) follicular
NHL	Follicular, predominantly large cell	Large cleaved and/or non-cleaved FCC, follicular	Centroblastic-centrocytic (large) follicular
DPDL	Diffuse, small cleaved cell	Small cleaved FCC, diffuse	Centrocytic, small
DML	Diffuse, mixed small and large cell	Small cleaved, large cleaved or large non-cleaved FCC, diffuse	Centroblastic-centrocytic, diffuse and lymphoplasmacytoid polymorphic
DHL	Diffuse, large cell	Large cleaved or large non-cleaved FCC, diffuse	Centroblastic-centrocytic (large) diffuse; centrocytic (large), and centroblastic, diffuse
DHL	Large cell, immunoblastic	Immunoblastic sarcoma, T- or B-cell type	Immunoblastic and T-zone lymphoma
Lymphoblastic convoluted/non-convoluted	Lymphoblastic	Convoluted T cell	Lymphoblastic, convoluted or unclassified
Diffuse undifferentiated, Burkitt's, & non-Burkitt's	Small non-cleaved cell	Small non-cleaved FCC	Lymphoblastic, Burkitt's type and other B-lymphoblastic

involvement of extranodal sites seen only later remains unexplained.

VI. B CELL NEOPLASIA OF INTERMEDIATE MATURITY

These are the B-cell non-Hodgkin's lymphomas. Table 7 shows the current non-Hodgkin's lymphoma classification schemes. Table 8 subdivides them into good and poor prognosis disease. As will be made clear, the morphologic classification scheme of Table 7 does not subdivide malignancies into those of B or T cell origin, however, certain morphologies are predominantly one phenotype or the other.

Table 8. Histologic classification and prognosis.

Good prognosis*	Poor prognosis*
Nodular poorly differentiated lymphocytic (NPDL)	Nodular histiocytic (NH)
Nodular mixed lymphocytic-histiocytic (NM)	Diffuse histiocytic (DH)
Diffuse well differentiated lymphocytic (DWDL)	Diffuse mixed lymphocytic-histiocytic (DM)
Diffuse poorly differentiated lymphocytic (DPDL)	Pleomorphic or stem cell
	Lymphoblastic

* Good prognosis connotes an expectation of greater than 1-year median survival with palliative radiotherapy or single-agent chemotherapy. Poor prognosis implies a median survival of less than 1 year if complete remission is not achieved by aggressive therapy.

I. B-cell chronic lymphocytic leukemia (B cell CLL)

B-cell CLL is a proliferation of small, well-differentiated B cells. Patients usually present with bone marrow, blood, and lymph node involvement. With progression, patients develop hepatic involvement and may develop pulmonary leukemic infiltrates, renal involvement and skin involvement. The Rai staging classification (Table 9) correlates with prognosis and essentially is a measure of tumor cell mass.

Table 9. Rai classification.

Stage	Extent of disease	Survival
0	Lymphocytosis of bone marrow (> 40% lymphocytes) and blood (< 15,000/mm³)	> 12 years
I	Stage 0 plus lymphadenopathy	~ 10 years
II	Stage 0 or I plus splenomegaly and/or hepatomegaly	~ 7 years
III	Stage 0, I, or II plus anemia (hemoglobin < 11.0 gm/dl)	~ 1.5 years
IV	Stage 0, I, or II plus thrombocytopenia (platelets < 100,000/mm³)	~ 1.5 years

The majority ($\sim 50\%$) of cells bear both sIgM and sIgD (49), thus corresponding in phenotype to B cells, preantigen activation. Their normal B cell counterparts would have undergone light chain and heavy chain variable region rearrangements in the bone marrow and then produced a burst of cells which differentiated in the marrow to express sIgM and sIgD. These cells would then be released to circulate through the blood and lymphoid organs. Finally, if not antigen activated within a short time, they would have died. For the B-cell CLL subgroup, bearing sIgM and sIgD, the clinical pattern of early disease corresponds to the normal migration pattern for cells with this phenotype.

A smaller fraction of cells ($\sim 20\%$) is $sIgM^+$ only. Whether these cells (which are not known to exhibit a different clinical behavior) correspond to cells prematurely released from the marrow at an earlier developmental stage or whether they represent a subset which is postantigen-activation and destined to serve as recirculating IgM memory cells, is as yet unclear.

Nearly all CLL cells, regardless of surface immunoglobulin phenotype (including the rare sIgG + only, which are almost certainly post antigenactivation) may be differentiated to antibody secretion with suitable agents e.g. phorbol esters (48), suggesting that the accumulation of these cells is not secondary to an intrinsic differentiation block but rather is caused by uncontrolled clonal overproduction followed by the absence of the antigen necessary to stimulate further differentiation.

Hence for low mass disease, the pattern of involvement appears to conform to the normal migration pattern. The progression to involve sites such as the skin or kidney presumably proceeds through metastatic rather than "normal" migration. It is not known whether the immunologic or chromosomal phenotype of the cells infiltrating these other sites is the same as that seen in lower stages of disease.

We have labelled CLL cells obtained at leukapheresis with [111]Indium-tagged monoclonal antibody (T101) and reinjected the labelled cells into the patient. The striking finding was that within 6 hours, label was readily detectable in involved lymph nodes suggesting rapid exchange with the circulating pool.

When the clinical picture is dominated by lymphadenopathy rather than increased circulating cells, the disease is called diffuse well-differentiated lymphocytic lymphoma (DWDL). The cells of DWDL have the exact cell surface phenotype of B cell CLL cells, but it is obvious that they must lack a receptor that gets them out of lymph nodes, since we know that both CLL and DWDL cells can get into nodes.

Progression to a lymph node based neoplasm with the histologic characteristics of a large cell or diffuse histocytic lymphoma is seen in $\sim 5\%$ these patients; this phenomenon has been termed Richter's syndrome. This event has been taken as suggestive of a chemotherapy or drug induced differentiation to a lymph node bound B-cell type which behaves as an aggressive lymphoma (51). However, the well-known tendency of B-cell lymphomas to undergo histologic evolution casts doubt on this theory.

Blastic leukemic transformation is an extremely rare terminal event, occurring in 2 of 340 in one series (50), suggesting that rarely, if ever, is the malignant cell a progenitor earlier in differentiation than the clinically dominant cell.

J Burkitt's lymphoma

Burkitt's lymphoma is a malignant proliferation of small B cells predominantly involving extranodal sites. The disease presents in two patterns: "American" and "African", characterized by different epidemiologies and a differing association with Epstein-Barr virus (EBV).

Patients with the "American" disease usually present with massive abdominal disease occasionally combined with CNS or bone marrow involvement. Those with the "African" disease typically present with maxilla or mandible tumors with or without orbital involvement; this latter pattern is almost never seen in "American" disease. "African" disease is associated with EBV in the malignant cells; "American" is not. Table 10 shows experience with clinically involved sites at presentation for a series of 224 "African" and 86 "American" patients (56).

For "African" patients, most of whom are children, the initial site of involvement has not been identified. The site is not clearly lymphoid tissue or a site involving an active immune response. Typically, there is involvement of unerupted molar or premolar teeth. When the "African" variant involves the abdomen, the disease is usually confined to the retroperitoneum, mesentery and omentum, seldom involving the bowel itself. The "American" variant with abdomi-

nal presentation appears to have as the primary site the bowel itself, (Peyer's patch?), (~ 20% of the NIH series presented with involvement at the ilial-colonic junction or the appendix) hence clinical presentation with intussusceptibility, perforation or intestinal obstruction occurs in about 20% of these patients.

CNS prophylaxis is usually required to avoid a high frequency of CNS relapses. This suggests that occult seeding has occurred prior to or during therapy.

Efforts to correlate the pattern of presentation with immunologic phenotype have thus far not been rewarding. The surface markers of Burkitt's cells (see Fig. 2) are those of marrow pre-B cells, post immunoglobulin gene rearrangement but prior to expression of sIgD and release from the marrow to the preantigen-activation cell pool. This phenotype corresponds to that which may be tolerized and eliminated by antigen binding to its sIgM. However, as noted above, this is a tumour which apparently occupies the marrow as a late or advanced effect. Hence it has been argued that the cell of origin is a post-primary-antigen-activation, peripheral B cell, whose immature phenotype corresponds to that of either a small, nonmarrow subpopulation or reflects a neoplastic change induced regression. In support of this second position is the apparent preferential occupation of germinal center sites seen in a few cases (57). More research will be required to understand the correlation between immunologic phenotype and presentation.

Approximately 90% of Burkitt's neoplasms are found to have a t(8;14)(q24; q23) chromosomal abnormality. A smaller number exhibit t(8;22)(24;q11) or t(2;8)(p12;q24) abnormalities. Chromosome 8 is the site of the c-*myc* oncogene and the result of the (8;14) translocation is to place the c-*myc* gene within the heavy chain enhancer region (53–55) on chromosome 14. Presumably this translocation occurs at the differentiation step during which the heavy chain is first being rearranged, a step which occurs in the bone marrow.

Experiments in which the c-*myc* gene prefaced by the heavy chain enhancer gene have been introduced into transgenic mice show that most (but not all) of these animals develop aggressive lymphomas (52). This failure of all mice to develop lymphoma added to the observation that these lymphomas are monoclonal, suggests that a further triggering event may be required in addition to simple heavy chain expression. Finally, the cells of some of these lymphomas have been observed to differentiate along the pathway towards plasma cells. Thus, the appearance of cells of the Burkitt's morphology and the characteristic t(8;14) abnormality both as a leukemia (in B cell ALL) and as a lymphoma may reflect the details of the triggering event.

In summary, the clinical pattern of tumor spread is one of a nonmigratory cell type which grows aggressively and spreads rapidly from its primary site apparently through the usual metastatic processes. Because of its aggressive character patients usually present with relatively high mass disease. Whether the entity of L-3 or Burkitt's leukemia is distinct from the lymphoma or whether it is merely a reflection of increased tumor mass at presentation is not known. The primary site predilection exhibited by the "African" and "American" types are similarly unexplained, however, as noted above, these differences reflect the site of the triggering event.

Table 10. Comparison of disease sites at presentation in 'African' and 'American' Burkitt's lymphoma patients (56).

Site[a]	African		American	
	No.	%	No.	%[b]
Abdomen (all)	130	58	78	91
Ascites	–		19	(39)
Hepatosplenomegaly	25	11	15	(31)
Right iliac fossa mass	–		8	(17)
Bowel	–		26	(54)
Stomach	–		4	(8)
Ovary	–		7	(15)
Kidney	–		7	(15)
Retroperitonenum	–		8	(17)
Pelvis	–		13	(15)
Unspecified	–		30	(38)
Pleural effusion	7	3	16	19
Bone marrow	16	7	17	20
Peripheral nodes	9	4	11	13
Bone	18	8	8	9
Cerebrospinal fluid/central nervous system	43	19	12	14
Paraspinal	38	17	2	2
Testis	4	2	5	6
Pharynx	0	0	9	10
Jaw	136	58	6	7
Mediastinum	1	0.5	3	3
Orbit	25	11	1	1
Other[c]	38	17	7	15
Total patients	224		86	

[a] Many patients had multiple sites of disease.
[b] Percentage of those with abdominal involvement is indicated in parentheses.
[c] Includes thyroid, breast, skin, shoulder, and thigh.

K. Follicular lymphomas

This group includes the indolent histologies of NPDL and NML as well as the more aggressive NHL. Data describing the clinical pattern of these entities were collected during a period predating the present classification schemes. Therefore the clinical presentation and evolution of many subtypes cannot be distinguished.

The usual history is one of an indolent course prior to diagnosis, with the patient having noted enlarged lymph nodes whose size may have waxed and waned over several years. In the study by Spiro *et al.* (64), patients, particularly those younger than 40, displayed extensive and often massive enlargement of discrete nonadherent lymph nodes. Involved sites included those that are rarely involved in diffuse lymphoma such as: preauricular, mastoid, occipital, epitrochlear, infraclavicular or supra- and infrascapular lymph nodes. Lymphangiography frequently discloses involvement of the iliac and para-aortic nodes. Cells bearing the immunoglobulin idiotype of the lymphoma are often found in the blood of patients with advanced disease. Similarly extranodal and skin involvement as well as "B" symptoms may be found in advanced disease.

Most patients present with advanced stage disease (59, 62). In the first study (59, 61) 58% had involvement of lower cervical/supraclavicular nodes, 18% mediastinal/hilar nodes and 54% the upper para-aortic nodes. In a staging study (60), 72% had abdominal involvement and 28% marrow involvement. In a study confined to 118 laparotomy-staged, stage I and II patients (62), 45% had supradiaphragmatic and 54%, subdiaphragmatic disease; 13% had extranodal lesions, usually GI or skin, and 6% had "B" symptoms.

As noted in Fig. 1, these malignancies appear to be tumors of germinal center cells. The usual surface marker expression is sIgM$^+$ and sIgD$^+$ sIgG$^+$ alone (58). Data have been advanced suggesting that malignancies expressing a C3 receptor and/or sIgD in addition to sIgM have a more indolent course (63).

In the model of lymphocyte differentiation described earlier, cells with a germinal center location and the above surface phenotypes are the progeny of cells which have undergone primary-activation and are now undergoing heavy chain class switching and "memory" cell generation. This model would predict that the malignant cells would be largely lymph node bound, shedding a few cells for memory generation. Spread would be through metastatic rather than traffic/migration processes. The relative reluctance of the cells to grow in extranodal or non-bone-marrow sites suggests a continued dependence upon the environment provided by nodal or marrow sites. An alternative model of dissemination would distinguish between the lymph node bound phenotype described above, making stage I, II lymphomas entirely this type, and a phenotype involving production of more "memory" cells, which would therefore present with early spleen, liver and bone marrow involvement (i.e. stage III, IV). Present data do not distinguish these

Table 11. Distinguishing features of diffuse, aggressive non-Hodgkin's lymphomas (61).

	Mixed small and large cell	Large cell	Large cell immunoblastic	Lymphoblastic	Small noncleaved Burkitt's	Non-Burkitt's
Median age	58 years	57 years	51 years	17 years	8 years	34 years
Sites	Lymph nodes, skin lung	Lymph nodes, G.I. tract, gonads, other extranodal sites	Lymph nodes, lungs, skin, other extranodal sites	Lymph nodes, mediastinum, bone	G.I. tract, gonads, jaws	Lymph nodes and extranodal sites
Histologic localization (when focal)	Variable	Variable	Variable	Paracortex (T-cell zone)	Germinal center (B-cell zone)	Variable
Nuclei	Mixture of small and large; follicular center cell or other	Large follicular center cell (cleaved or non-cleaved), single nuclei, 2–3 nucleoli	Large single or multinuclear; prominent nucleoli	Small, fine chromatin; small nucleoli	Uniform, round to oval, small (similar diameter as admixed macrophages); 2–5 nucleoli	Heterogeneous shape and size but similar to macrophages; sometimes multiple; may have large nucleoli
Cytoplasm	Moderate; may be clear in large cells	Moderate	Abundant; amphophilic or clear	Scant	Scant but distinct	Sometimes abundant
Immunologic phenotype (%)						
B	10	95	25	20 (per-B)	100	85
T	80	5	70	70	0	15
Null	10	0	2	10 (common)	0	0
Histiocytic	0	0	2	0	0	0
Tdt	–	–	–	+	–	–

models. However, since the cells are usually readily detectable in the peripheral blood, even at small tumor burdens, it seems likely that the cells possess receptors for nodal egress.

L. Intermediate and aggressive B cell lymphomas

These are the NHL, DPDL, DML, and DHL of the Rappaport classification. The majority of DML's and immuno-

blastic lymphomas appear to be of mature T cell origin (68) and are discussed under the section on peripheral post-thymic T cell lymphoma (see Table 11). Clinical experience suggests that the pattern of spread of DML and immunoblastic B cell lymphomas are not sufficiently unique to be distinguished from DHL. Both DPDL and NHL appear to have a high frequency of progression to the DHL morphology (74). The NIH experience with the infrequent morphology NHL is reviewed in (71). Further, NHL is a rare entity and DPDL and DML are infrequent, hence case experience

Table 12. Relationship between histologic subtype and pathologic stage (65).

	Pathologic stage			
Histologic type	I	II	III	IV
Nodular				
NPDL	3 (3.4%)	5 (5.7%)	29 (33.0%)	51 (58.0%)
NML	6 (8.1%)	11 (14.9%)	29 (39.2%)	28 (37.8%)
NHL	2 (12.5%)	1 (6.3%)	4 (25.0%)	9 (56.3%)
All nodular patients	11 (6.2%)	17 (9.6%)	62 (34.8%)	88 (49.4%)
Diffuse				
DWDL	0	2 (5.1%)	9 (23.1%)	28 (71.8%)
DPDL	6 (9.4%)	8 (12.5%)	11 (17.2%)	39 (60.9%)
DML	4 (12.1%)	7 (21.2%)	7 (21.2%)	15 (45.5%)
DHL	7 (7.7%)	20 (22.0%)	16 (17.6%)	48 (52.7%)
DUL	3 (11.5%)	8 (30.8%)	6 (23.1%)	9 (34.6%)
Burkitt's	2 (5.3%)	8 (21.1%)	3 (7.9%)	25 (65.8%)
All diffuse patients	22 (7.6%)	53 (18.2%)	52 (17.9%)	164 (56.3%)
Total	33 (7.0%)	70 (14.9%)	114 (24.3%)	252 (53.7%)

* Percentages indicate proportion of patients within a specific Rappaport histologic subtype.

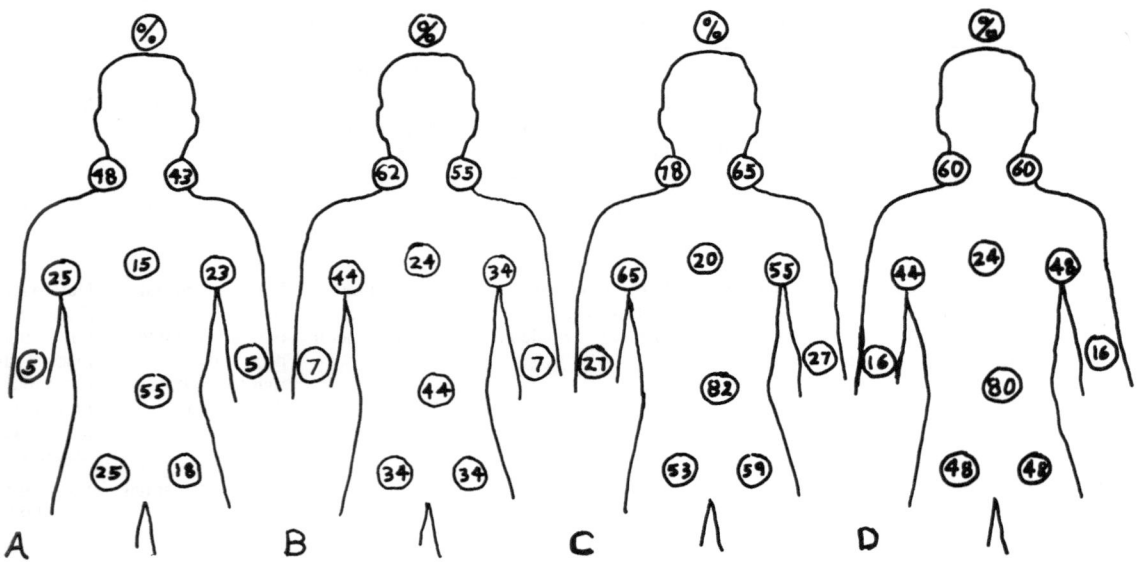

Figure 6. Schematic body diagrams showing the percentage of patients with lymph node involvement in each of the major lymph-node-bearing areas, including epitrochlear, axillary, cervical and supraclavicular, mediastinal or hilar, para-aortic, and inguinal. Nodal involvement was determined by clinical examination, chest X-ray, and lymphangiogram and does not include results of surgical staging.
A: 40 patients with diffuse histiocytic lymphoma.
B: 29 patients with diffuse poorly differentiated lymphocytic lymphoma.
C: 49 patients with nodular poorly differentiated lymphocytic lymphoma.
D: 25 patients with nodular mixed lymphocytic-histiocytic lymphomas.
Chabner BA, Johnson RE *et al.*: Sequential nonsurgical and surgical staging of non-Hodgkin's lymphoma. *Ann Int Med* 85:149, 1976

with the more aggressive lymphomas is dominated by the behavior of DHL.

These lymphomas appear to arise within lymph nodes as well as arising extranodally. Table 12 (65) shows the NIH experience with patient presentation by pathologic stage. Experience indicates that the frequency of "B" symptoms increases with stage. Figure 6 shows the distribution of positive sites for a subset of the NIH series (67). Extranodal involvement is frequent and in the Stanford series was 52% (73). As can be seen from Table 12, the majority of patients present with advanced stage and a clear primary site is not identifiable. Table 13 (73) shows the sites of involvement among the subset of 111 stage IE patients in which these are presumed to be the primary sites and indicates the diversity of primary sites. Table 14 (66) shows the frequency of bone marrow involvement. As can be seen from Table 13, the GI tract is the most frequent site of extranodal involvement. Table 15 shows the GI sites, stages and histologies.

Several correlations between sites of involvement have been demonstrated. Jones *et al.* noted that spread appeared

to be to contiguous sites primarily, and the success of treating stage I disease with wide local therapy supports this observation. However, other patterns are also seen. Two of significance are: (1) the association of abdominal involvement, either at presentation or subsequently, seen in patients presenting with Waldeyer's ring involvement (66); and (2) the association of bone marrow involvement with subsequent CNS relapse (69, 76). This latter association motivates the use of prophylactic CNS treatment in these patients. In contrast to ALL, a high frequency of testicular relapse has as yet not been noted.

By morphology these lymphomas are of follicular origin and most bear sIg, although in variable amounts (70, 72, 74). The clinical pattern of spread primarily to contiguous sites, correlates with the nonmigratory behavior of the corresponding normal cells. However, the frequent involvement of extranodal sites suggests that the malignant transformation of these cells has rendered them relatively independent of the factors and signals supplied by a nodal environment. The pattern of spread is one of a solid tumor, of a nonmi-

Table 13. Extralymphatic sites of 111 patients with diffuse lymphoma (73).

Site	No. of patients	5-year survival (%)	5-year FFR (%)
Gastrointestinal tract	47	40	54
Head and neck	13	38	44
Lung	10	54	50
Skin	7	42	36
Thyroid	7	86	72
Testis	5	40	40
Bone	5	30	40

Note: Sites not listed include brain (three patients), epidural space (three patients), soft tissue (three patients), pericardium (three patients), cervix (two patients), peritoneum (two patients), and breast (one patient).

Table 14. Non-Hodgkin's lymphoma relative frequency of bone marrow involvement vs. histopathologic type (59)*.

Nodular no. positive		Diffuse no. positive	
Type	No. evaluated (%)	Type	No. evaluated (%)
NH	3/27 (11)	DH	8/94 (9)
NM	9/70 (13)	DM	6/40 (15)
NLPD	23/64 (36)	DLPD	11/38 (29)
NLWD	2/5 (40)	DLWD	3/7 (43)
		DU	0/11 (0)
Total nodular	37/166 (22)	Total diffuse	28/190 (15)

* Number of patients with bone marrow involvement at presentation total number evaluated, and percent.

Table 15. Non-Hodgkin's lymphomas sites and stages for patients with initial gastrointestinal involvement (59).

		Sites				Diagnosis confirmed by	
	Stage	Stomach	Small intestine	Colon	Multiple	Laparotomy	X-ray examinations
Diffuse lymphomas	I_E(1) II_E(15)	7	7	3[a]	0	13	3
	III_E(1) IV	12	11	6	5	26	8
	Total 51 cases	19	18	9	5	39	11
Nodular lymphomas	I_E(1) II_E(1)	1[b]	1	0	0	2	0
	III_E(1) IV	3	5	2	1	8	3
	Total 13 cases	4	6	2	1	10	3

[a] Stage I_EA: rectal mucosa only involved by DH lymphoma
[b] State I_EA: stomach only involved by NLWD lymphoma

gratory cell type, whose site specific growth requirements are minimal and which spreads rapidly via usual metastatic processes.

M. Hairy cell leukemia

This is a rare B cell disease usually characterized by pancytopenia, thrombocytopenia and splenomegaly in which marrow, spleen and blood are found to contain "hairy" cells which are sIg$^+$ and contain (tartrate-resistance acid phosphatase) (TRAP). Table 16 shows the presenting physical findings of a group of 102 patients (78) and a set of autopsy findings of 14 patients. With disease progression, patients have been observed to develop increased lymphadenopathy, and rarely CNS (meningeal) infiltration and skin infiltration. The marrow dysfunction and immunologic dysfunction induced by the disease, coupled with its slow growth rate, usually result in patients succumbing to infection or complications of marrow dysfunction rather than problems associated with extramedullary masses.

The characteristic "hairy cells" are found to usually be sIgM$^-$, sIgG$^+$, suggesting that their stage in differentiation is that of a B cell postprimary activation but prior to secondary-activation (i.e. post heavy chain class switch). As was noted, some B cells at this stage of differentiation migrate from peripheral lymph nodes to spleen and marrow or from spleen to marrow, adding weight to the suggestion that these cells might be such a population. "Normal" circulating sIgG$^+$, sIgM$^-$ cells frequently exhibit the cytoplasmic projections of "hairy cells" (77).

Prior to the use of interferon, splenectomy was the therapy of choice. The favorable results with splenectomy seem to largely be secondary to a reduction in splenic sequestration and potentially some debulking, rather than removal of the prime favorable growth site for these cells, as the degree of marrow involvement appears uninfluenced by splenectomy.

A subset of atypical patients, whose abnormal cells are confined to the marrow has been identified (79). Whether these represent early cases of very low mass disease and therefore suggest that the migration pattern is the reverse of that described above or whether they represent patients whose cells have differentiated one step further is unknown.

In summary, in this disease the distribution of the malignant "hairy cell", except for its appearance in the liver, appears to conform to the pattern of post-heavy-chain-class-switch B cells, migrating from lymph node to spleen and marrow or from spleen to marrow.

Table 16. Hairy cell leukemia (77).

Presenting physical signs (102)		Autopsy cases (14)	
CNS involvement	1	Bone marrow involvement	14
Splenomegaly	93	Spleen (sinusoids)	14
Hepatomegaly	38	Liver	14
Lymphadenopathy	22	Peripheral lymph nodes (T cell region)	3
		Blood	14

VII. B CELL NEOPLASIA OF MATURE CELLS

N. Waldenström's macroglobulinemia

This is a disease in which the malignant cells secrete IgM. At presentation, clinically involved sites are the lymph nodes, spleen and liver. Abnormal cells may be found in the blood and marrow. The distribution of involved sites is consistent with that observed for nonmalignant B cells which have differentiated through the point of primary antigen-activation to plasma cell secretion. In the model discussed earlier, such cells are confined to the lymph nodes and spleen and do not migrate to the marrow.

Initially clinical problems relate to hepato-splenomegaly and the hyperviscosity induced complications of IgM overproduction. Late in the disease course, some patients develop an immunoblastic sarcoma. This latter event is consistent with the possibility that in a certain number of patients, the true 'malignant' cell is a presecretory cell which during the chronic phase of the disease is able to differentiate into the IgM secretory cell. With the development of the more acute phase this differentiation is blocked, or occurs at low frequency.

O. Alpha-heavy chain disease

This is a disease in which patients have lymphoplasmacytic infiltrates of mucosa or adjacent lymphoid tissue (80–82). Patients have been reported from the Netherlands and the USA with the respiratory tract as the primary site and from the Mediterranean Basin, Asia and South America with an enteric form. In the enteric form, patients have retroperitoneal and mesenteric lymph node as well as intestinal mucosal infiltration. In late disease, infiltrates are found in the spleen, liver and blood. The anatomic distribution is consistent with a malignant conversion of that set of B cells involved in GI or respiratory traffic which have undergone primary-activation and made the heavy chain class switch to the alpha chain. The failure to secrete complete IgA molecules presumably is secondary to the malignant change as the apparent stage of differentiation is post light-chain-rearrangement. This is in contradistinction to the circumstances in myeloma in which nearly always light chains are secreted in excess of heavy chains.

P. Multiple myeloma (MM)

Multiple myeloma is a disease of malignant plasma cells. In the majority of cases the clonal plasma cells diffusely involve the marrow and are apparently confined to this site. However, approximately 5% are found at presentation to exhibit either lymphadenopathy or splenomegaly suggesting involvement of these sites and more advanced disease. The majority of myelomas secrete IgG (53%), followed by IgA (25%), IgD (1%) and 20% will have light chains only in the serum and urine (85).

Late in the disease course, the tumor growth rate appears to increase and the responsiveness of the tumor to chemotherapy decreases. At this time plasma cell infiltrates may be found in virtually any organ including skin, liver,

Table 17. Criteria for staging plasma cell myeloma patients.

Stage	Criteria	Myeloma cell mass (cells $\times 10^{12}/M^2$)

I	All of the following
	1. Hemoglobin > 100 g/liter
	2. Normal serum calcium
	3. Normal bone structure, or
	    bone plasmacytoma
	4. Low M-protein production rates:
	    a. IgG < 50 g/liter
	    b. IgA < 30 g/liter
	    c. Urinary k or < 4 g/24 hr
		< 0.6
		(low)

II	Fitting neither Stage I nor III	0.6–1.2 (Intermediate)

III	One or more of the following:
	1. Hemoglobin < 85 g/liter
	2. Serum calcium > 12.0 mg/dl
	3. More than 3 lytic bone lesions
	4. High M-protein production rates:
	    a. IgG > 70 g/liter
	    b. IgA > 50 g/liter
	    c. Urinary k or > 12.0 g/24 hr
		> 1.2
		(high)

Subclassification
A. BUN < 10.8 mmol/liter, creatinine < 176 mmol/liter
B. BUN > 30 mg/dl, creatinine > 2.0 mg/dl

Adapted from Durie, BGM, Salmon, SE: A clinical staging system for multiple myeloma. Correlation of measured myeloma cell mass with presenting clinical features, response to treatment and survival. *Cancer* 36:842, 1975

meninges, and brain. Table 17 indicates the present staging procedure which is based on the clinical experience that prognosis is dependent upon total myeloma cell mass.

The distribution and circulation of MM cells appear to correspond to that of normal cells bearing this phenotype. The usual bone marrow presentation is consistent with the idea that these are tumors of transformed B cells, whose progenitors have undergone primary-activation followed by heavy-chain-class-switching (most likely in the spleen or lymph nodes) and then have made their way to the bone marrow. Although antibody secreting cells can be grown and cloned from at least some myeloma patients, two pieces of data suggest that for at least some patients the malignant cell may be the progenitor cell. The first piece of data is that in many patients, nonsecreting marrow cells may be found which bear an immunoglobulin idiotype identical to their nonidiotype bearing progeny, the idiotype secreting plasma cells (84). The second, somewhat weaker information, is that in late stage myeloma, the dominant cell type frequently becomes an "immature" plasma cell suggesting a maturation block of the earlier malignant progenitor cell.

Table 18. Plasma cell tumors originating in skeletal (multiple and solitary) or extramedullary sites.

	No.	%
Plasma cell tumors of bone		
multiple	856	93.2
solitary	26	2.8
Extramedullary plasma cell tumors	37	4.0
Total	919	100.0

As can be seen in Table 18, the disease presents about 7% of the time, as a solitary plasmacytoma of the bone or of an extramedullary site. Table 19 lists the frequency sites of extramedullary involvement. A priori these patients might be taken as examples of low mass disease but the evidence for this view is mixed. Solitary plasmacytomas are distinguished from MM by their epidemiology; thus, as can be seen in Table 20, prognosis, male dominance and urinary M protein quantity all differ. Further heterogeneity is exhibited by the response of plasmacytomas to local therapy (chiefly radiotherapy). Disease of extramedullary sites exhibits limited recurrence, with apparent cures, while that involving bony sites recurs at a predictable rate, and apparently is incurable (83).

The differing response to local therapy of extramedullary and bony plasmacytomas is consistent with the notion that

Table 19. Sites of extramedullary plasma cell tumors (83).

	No.	%

Upper air passages
    (tonsil, palate, nasal sinuses,
    nasopharynx, nose, orbit)
	248	76

Lymph nodes and spleen	18	6
Bronchi and lung	13	4
Skin and subcutaneous	12	3.5
Gastrointestinal tract	10	3
Thyroid	9	3
Testes	3	1
Other	12	3.5
Total	325	100

Table 20. Comparison of plasma cell tumors originating in skeletal (multiple and solitary) and extramedullary sites (83).

	Solitary bone plasmacytoma	Multiple myeloma	Extramedullary plasmacytomas
Number	114	290	325
Age (years)			
medium	53	64	62
range	14–72	29–93	10–87
Percent males	72	55	73
M protein in serum or urine	10/38	–	8/29
M protein/tested	26%	98%	28%
Median survival (months)	114	30	192

the latter cases represent early MM, while the former are derived from cells at a slightly different stage of differentiation. As was noted in the discussion on B cell migration, early in an antibody response, post heavy-chain-class-switch, there are a subset of plasma cells which secrete antibody within lymph nodes (or presumably other lymphoid tissue). These cells may correspond in phenotype to that of extramedullary plasmacytomas.

In summary, myeloma is usually a disease of marrow bound plasma cells (or their progenitors) which only late in the disease (when the tumor mass is large) are found in other sites. Access to sites outside of the bone marrow, blood or lymphoid tissue presumably proceeds via usual metastatic processes, as these sites are not involved in the usual migration circuit of the plasma cells (or their progenitors).

VIII. T CELL NEOPLASIA OF INTERMEDIATE MATURITY

Q. Lymphoblastic lymphoma (LL)

LL is a rare T cell lymphoma (about 3%) seen primarily in adolescents and young adults, and characterized by an acute course and mediastinal involvement. A fraction of cases present without the mediastinal disease but these are those confined to the older age groups (88). The malignant cell of

LL is morphologically and phenotypically indistinguishable from that of T cell ALL. LL and T cell ALL probably have a relationship similar to CLL and DWDL. LL and T cell ALL have a similar natural history, but LL may be somewhat more refractory to treatment. T cell ALL appears to present in the marrow and to secondarily involve the mediastinum. LL usually presents in the mediastinum and secondly involves the marrow. Table 21 is a compilation of the sites of presentation of LL reported by Nathwani *et al.* (88) and the NCI experience summarized by Magrath (87). Frequent late development of CNS and gonadal involvement has prompted the incorporation of prophylactic CNS therapy as part of treatment programs.

As may be seen, the majority of patients present with stage III or IV high mass disease and even with low mass disease, the primary site may be obscure. Hence matching the pattern of spread with the immunologic phenotype of the cell is different. However, histologic findings of abnormal cells in "T" cell regions of partially involved nodes suggests "homing" behavior consistent with the T cell surface markers (86). T_{11} positivity suggests a thymocyte phenotype. LL cells may coexpress OKT4 and OKT8 consistent with a cortical thymocyte origin or may express either OKT4 or OKT8 (and not both) indicating a more mature medullary phenotype. Some tumors express the cortical thymocyte marker OKT6. However, the persistence of TDT$^+$ and the failure of the cells to express OKT3 (associated with the T-cell receptor) would be compatible with aberrant differentiation of an earlier progenitor. Assignment of cortical or medullary thymocyte phenotype is compatible with the pattern of apparent primary mediastinal involvement, with nearby nodes as the sites of early metastatic involvement.

In summary, this disease is an aggressive neoplasm of a thymus bound cell type having minimal site-specific growth requirements and capable of rapid metastasis.

IX. POST-THYMIC T CELL NEOPLASIA

Table 22 lists a classification scheme for peripheral or mature T cell malignancies. As has been noted, the morphologic classifications of the Working Formulation result in most

Table 21. Findings at presentation for patients with lymphoblastic lymphoma.

Nathwani (88)	LL	Magrath (87)	LL
Mediastinum/thymus	40/95 (42%)	Mediastinal mass	50–80%
Generalized adenopathy	44/95 (46%)	Dyspnea/dysphagia of SVC	Frequent
Splenomegaly	–	Pleural effusion	~ 50%
Bone marrow (BM) only	18/81 (22%)	Pericardial effusion	Not uncommon
Blood only	–	Neck/cervical/axillary adenopathy	Common
Both BM and Blood	8/81 (11%)	Hepatosplenomegaly	Uncommon
'B' Symptoms	45/79 (57%)	Renal involvement	Uncommon
Leukemic conversion over t ≥ 12 months	28/53 (53%)	GI	Rare
Progression to BM only	5/53 (9%)	Para-aortic adenopathy	Uncommon
Late development of involvement of		Skin	< 10%
CNS	8/46 (17%)	Bone lesions	Uncommon
Gonadal	2/46 (4%)	CNS	Uncommon
Stage at presentation:			
I or II	8/92 (9%)		
III or IV	84/92 (91%)		

Table 22. Classification of post-thymic T-cell malignancies.

I. T-cell chronic lymphocytic leukemia
   Helper
   Suppressor
   Prolymphocytic
II. Mycosis fungoides/Sezary syndrome
III. Peripheral T-cell lymphomas
   Subtypes and/or related terms:
      Node-based T-cell lymphoma
      T-zone lymphoma
      AILD-like T-cell lymphoma
      Lymphoepitheloid cell (Lennert's) lymphoma
      Multilobated T-cell lymphoma
IV. Adult T-cell leukemia/lymphoma
   (HTLV-I-associated disease)
V. Angiocentric immunoproliferative lesions
   (Lymphomatoid granulomatosis)
   (Polymorphic reticulosis)
   Angiocentric lymphomas

subtypes being comprised of B cell and T cell derived malignancies. Further, the lack of established differentiation steps similar to immunoglobulin heavy chain class switching or plasma cell formation make the relationship of the established T-cell malignancies to their stage of differentiation obscure (89, 90).

R. T-cell chronic lymphocytic leukemia (T cell CLL)

T cell CLL is a disease clinically similar to B cell CLL and comprises 1.5–5% of all CLL cases. Table 23 shows the experience of Pandolfi *et al.* (93). Similar experience was obtained by Brouet *et al.* (91). Patients present with bone marrow and blood involvement (although the lymphocyte count may only be moderately elevated), minimal to no adenopathy and minimal to massive splenomegaly. Skin involvement occurs in more advanced disease and consists of dermal infiltrates without the epidermal infiltration seen in cutaneous T cell lymphomas (CTCL). The course is usually protracted, however, in some cases disease may progress rapidly with a Richter-like transformation to an aggressive lymphoma.

Morphologically the malignant cells are small and mature. The usual surface phenotype is E^+, Fc^-, $OKT3^+$, $OKT1^{+/-}$, $OKT8^+$, $OKT4^-$, $HLA-Dr^{+/-}$. Some patients are $OKT4^+$, $OKT8^-$. (In the first series (93), those patients whose cells were $OKT4^+$, $3A1^-$ (the phenotype of CTCL) had skin involvement). ADCC and suppressor function have been demonstrated in these cells and instances of $OKT8^+$ cells being associated with neutropenia, pure red cell aplasia and hypogammaglobulinemia have been observed. The distribution of involved sites does not correspond to that of a known T cell subtype.

This disease is a relatively rare entity and its clinical description may be obscured by inclusion of indolent cases of HTLV-I, or HTLV-II disease as well as cases in which the increased cell size, cytoplasmic basophilia, hepatosplenomegaly, markedly elevated white blood cell counts and acute course fit the description of acute prolymphocytic leukemia of Galton *et al.* (92).

S. Cutaneous T cell lymphoma (CTCL)

CTLL consists of the mycosis fungoides and Sezary syndromes (95). Tables 24 and 25 describe the staging schema. The mycosis fungoides form is characterized initially by skin changes which worsen from nonspecific erythematous findings to plaque and tumors. Associated with these skin changes is a progressive infiltration of nonlymphoid organs in late stage disease. The Sezary syndrome consists of pruritis, generalized exfoliative erythroderma and abnormal hyperchromatic, hyperconvoluted mononuclear cells in the peripheral blood and is now recognized as an advanced form of CTCL. CTCL is not caused by HTLV-I but the "d'emblee" presentation of CTCL, which consists of the appearance of skin tumors without preceding skin lesions, may be confused with HTLV-I associated adult T cell leukemia/lymphoma (94).

The initial skin manifestations of the disease mimic a variety of dermatoses and may lead to multiple misdiagnoses over a number of years prior to proper diagnosis. Biopsy (often several are required) shows a histologic picture of polymorphic lymphoid infiltration. The form is characteristically "epidermotrophic" with exocytosis of single cells or clusters of mycosis/Sezary cells. Epidermal clusters are termed Pautriers's microabscesses. The infiltrate is usually in the upper dermis in close proximity to the epidermis. With advancing stage, abnormal cells may pene-

Table 23. Significant clinical and laboratory data in seven T-CLL cases at diagnosis and survival time (93).

| | Name | Sex | Age | Enlargement of | | | Mediastinal mass | Skin lesions | Rai stage | WBC ($\times 10^3$/cu mm) | Percent lymphocytes | | Survival time* (mo) |
				Spleen	Liver	Peripheral nodes					PB	BM	
1.	PT	M	83	−	−	−	−	−	0	18.0	98	70	31
2.	EM	F	70	+	−	+	−	−	2	15.0	96	70	> 18
3.	GG	F	46	−	−	−	−	−	0	20.0	94	45	> 20
4.	EDF	M	70	−	+ +	+	−	−	2	15.5	68	64	> 10
5.	AV	M	67	−	−	−	−	−	3	33.0	87	90	> 14
6.	EO	M	55	−	+	+ +	−	+	2	62.0	91	71	> 36
7.	NC	F	78	+	+	−	−	+ +	2	45.2	86	65	11

PB, peripheral blood; BM, bone marrow; (−) absent; (+) slight, (+ +) moderate; (+ + +) massive.
* Calculated from date of diagnosis.

Table 24. TMN classification of CTCL (95).

Classification	Description
T: Skin[a]	
T_0	Clinically and/or histopathologically suspicious lesions
T_1	Limited plaques, papules, or eczematous patches covering 10% or more of the skin surface
T_2	Generalized plaques, papules, or erythematous patches covering 10% or more of the skin surface
T_3	Tumors, one or more
T_4	Generalized erythroderma
N: Lymph nodes[b]	
N	No clinically or palpably abnormal peripheral lymph nodes, pathology negative for CTCL
N_1	Clinically abnormal peripheral lymph nodes, pathology negative for CTCL
N_2	No clinically abnormal peripheral lymph nodes, pathology positive for CTCL
N_3	Clinically abnormal peripheral lymph nodes, pathology positive for CTCL
B: Peripheral blood	
B_0	Atypical circulating cells not present or < 5%
B_1	Atypical circulating cells present in 5% or more; total white blood count, total lymphocyte counts, and number of atypical cell/100 lymphocytes recorded.
M: Visceral organs	
M_0	No involvement of visceral organs
M_1	Visceral involvement (must have confirmation of pathology, and organ involved should be specific)

[a] Pathology T_{1-4} is diagnostic of a CTCL. When characteristics of more than one T exist, both are recorded and the highest is used for staging, e.g. $T_{4(3)}$.
[b] The number of sites of abnormal nodes are recorded, e.g., cervical (left + right), axillary (left + right), inguinal (left + right), epitrochlear, submandibular, etc.

trate further into the dermis. The centering on the upper papillary dermis and epidermis distinguishes the infiltrates from those seen with other T cell malignancies where the maximal concentration of cells is in the mid to lower dermis.

Initial infiltration of lymph nodes is occult although in-

Table 25. Staging classification of CTCL (95).

Stage	Classification		
	T	N	M
IA	1	0	0
IB	2	0	0
IIA	1–2	1	0
IIB	3	0–1	0
III	4	0–1	0
IVA	1–4	2–3	0
IVB	1–4	0–3	1

Table 26. Frequency, at presentation, and survival expectation with respect to skin stage in CTCL (95).

Skin stage	Patients		Mean survival (years)	5-year survival (%)
	No.	%		
Limited plaque (T_1)	306	38	9	90
Generalized plaque (T_2)	225	28	7	67
Cutaneous tumor (T_3)	137	17	2.5	35
Generalized erythroderma (T_4)	137	17	3.5	40

Table 27. Frequency of extracutaneous disease determined by conventional staging studies in patients with CTCL (95).

Study*	Percent positive	
	of all patients	of erythrodermic patients
Lymphadenopathy	47	83
Lymphography	40	66
Lymph node histology	36	81
Peripheral blood	20	90
Bone marrow biopsy	2	5
Liver biopsy	16	39

* Note: Determined by physical examination. X-rays, and review of tissues of conventional microscopy.

stances of nodes showing the early changes of "dermatopathic lymphadenitis" containing malignant cells identified by their Ti β chain have been observed. The peripheral adenopathy of low stage disease may be more strongly influenced by skin breakdown than cellular infiltration (so called dermatopathic adenopathy). Tables 26 and 27 show the disease extent at presentation. With progression of disease, atypical cells are seen in the T cell paracortical areas and with further progression effacement of nodal architecture is observed. Finally, extensive organ involvement develops and involvement of virtually every organ has been described. Table 28 shows the sites of involvement at autopsy.

Phenotypically these cells appear to be of the helper/inducer subtype i.e. E^+, $OKT11^+$, $OKT1^+$, $OKT3^+$, $OKT4^+$, $3A1^-$, $OKT8^-$, $OKT6^-$. Circulating cells are usually $HLA-DR^-$, but cutaneous tumor cells are frequently $HLA-DR^+$ and $3A^+$ (96). In keeping with the $OKT4^4$, $OKT8^-$ markers, when the cells manifest an immune function, they appear to be able to function as helpers for *in vitro* immunoglobulin secretion. The skin focusing displayed by these apparently mature cells, has been used to suggest that normal helper T cells follow a migration circuit involving the lymphoid organs and the skin. None has thus far been demonstrated.

T. Peripheral post-thymic T-cell lymphomas

Peripheral T-cell lymphomas may appear as DML, Lennert's and immunoblastic lymphomas. As was noted before (sections K and L), differing percentages of each of the Working Formulation morphologic subtypes are T cell derived. Table 29 shows an estimate of these percentages.

Table 28. Sites of extracutaneous involvement by cutaneous T-cell lymphoma at autopsy (95).

Reference	Lymph nodes	Spleen	Liver	Lungs	Bone marrow	GI tract	Kidneys	Heart	CNS
Rappaport and Thomas	24/32	19/32	17/32	21/32	12/31	–	14/32	12/32	4/28
Long and Mihm	15/15	12/15	13/15	8/15	7/15	6/15	2/15	1/15	–
Epstein *et al.*	51/86	43/86	35/86	37/86	23/86	30/86	23/86	15/85	17/86
Cyr *et al.*	4/23	6/23	5/23	4/23	–	2/23	5/23	2/23	–
Farber *et al.*	4/7	6/7	6/7	–	0/7	2/7	2/7	2/7	–
Crawley	7/10	4/10	2/10	2/10	5/10	–	2/10	4/10	–
Total	105/173	90/173	78/173	72/166	47/149	40/131	48/173	36/173	21/114
%	61	52	42	43	32	31	28	21	18

Table 29. Analysis of peripheral T-cell lymphoma by the Rappaport classification* (90).

Classification	% of cases
Well-differentiated lymphocytic (WDL)	2
Poorly differentiated lymphocytic (PDL)	16
Mixed cell type (MCT)	40
'Histiocytic' (large cell) (LC)	42

* Based on an analysis of cases diagnosed and immunotyped at the National Cancer Institute, Bethesda, MD.

Table 30. Sites of involvement in peripheral T-cell lymphoma* (90).

Site	% of cases
Lymph nodes	85
Skin and/or mucosa	50
Liver	50
Peripheral blood	30
Peripheral blood with positive skin	60
Bone marrow	30
Lung and/or pleura	20

* Approximate figures based on a series of cases studied and immunotyped at the National Cancer Institute, Bethesda, MD.

Most patients in the NIH series (Table 30) (90) presented with stage IV disease, by virtue of involvement of the skin, liver, peripheral blood, lungs and/or pleura. Additionally, patients usually exhibited generalized lymphadenopathy. The skin involvement, when present, was dermal, sparing the epidermis, thus distinguishing it from that seen with CTCL. Of interest is that no patient had peripheral blood involvement without skin involvement. Additionally, the majority of the patients had 'B' symptoms. Evidence of immune dysfunction preceding the development of lym-

phoma occurred in 15% of the patients and included gluten-sensitive enteropathy, Hashimoto's thyroiditis and Sjögren's syndrome (90).

Surface markers are those of mature T cells. The majority of cases typed are Leu M1$^-$, PNA$^-$, OKT4$^+$, OKT8$^-$ however, some are OKT4$^-$, OKT8$^+$. The majority are able to form E rosettes and are frequently 3A1$^-$. Spread of the tumor appears to be from a primary site via metastatic processes, rather than T-cell migration processes. Response to therapy or relapse pattern has not thus far separated them from the other aggressive B-cell tumors (97).

U. Adult T cell leukemia/lymphoma (ATL)

ATL is a recently recognized disorder in which the viral causative agent has been isolated (100). Aggressive manifestations and more indolent ones have been observed; the latter usually being grouped with the T cell CLL patients. Table 31 shows the histopathology of a series of these patients demonstrating the diversity of the morphology. The patients with the acute syndrome present with stage IV disease. Table 32 (99) shows the sites of involvement at presentation for 13 patients in the United States. Associated with the extensive organ involvement observed at presentation is a paraneoplastic syndrome involving clinically significant hypercalcemia and associated bone resorption. Patients displaying skin manifestations may have the histopathology of cutaneous T-cell lymphoma on biopsy or may have sparing of the overlaying epidermis.

Surface markers are those of mature T helper cells i.e. E rosette$^+$, TDT$^-$, OKT4$^+$, OKT8$^-$, OKT6$^-$. Most are OKT1$^+$, OkT3$^+$, OKT10$^+$, OKT11$^+$, and TAC$^+$ (102). Studies (102) indicate suppressor rather than helper function. All ATL cells express the TAC (or interleukin-2 receptor) yet they do not proliferate in response to IL-2. The virus

Table 31. Histopathology of adult T-cell leukemia/lymphoma (90).

Lymphoma study group	Rappaport	Working formulation	Hamaoka (98) (95 cases)	Jaffe (99) (13 cases)
Small cell	Well-differentiated lymphocytic	Small cell	2%	0%
Medium-sized cell	Poorly differentiated lymphocytic	Unclassifiable	35%	15%
Mixed cell	Mixed cell	Mixed small and large cell	8%	38%
Large cell	Histiocytic/Undifferentiated	Large cell	8%	8%
Pleomorphic	Histiocytic/Mixed cell	Large cell, immunoblastic	42%	38%
Other	Other	Other	3%	0%

Table 32. Clinical manifestations of HTLV associated leukemia/lymphoma.

Manifestation	At presentation (%)	During course (%)
Leukemia	69	100
Hypercalcemia	75	83
Lytic bone lesions	38	–*
Lymphoadenopathy	77	85
Hepatosplenomegaly	61	–
Skin lesions	61	–
Bone marrow positive	58	–
Stage IV	100	–

*: Unchanged during clinical course.

virus integration site in the genome is apparently not crucial (101). But each tumor is monoclonal and the size of the restriction fragment containing the provirus is an excellent tumor marker. ATL cells appear to have no limitations on their sites of spread. The origin of their invasive properties is not clear.

ACKNOWLEDGEMENT

The authors wish to thank Ms Ruth Morsillo, Ms Louise Pastuck and Ms Jackie Owen for preparation of the manuscript and to thank Michael A Bookman, M.D. and Walter Urba, M.D., Ph.D. for helpful discussions.

REFERENCES

A. Differentiation and migration patterns of hematopoietic cells

1. Hanks GE: *In vitro* migration of colony forming units from shielded bone marrow in the irradiated mouse. *Nature* 203:1393, 1964
2. Hanks GE, Ainsworth EJ: Endotoxin protection and colony-forming units. *Radia Res* 32:367, 1964
3. Maloney MA, Patt HM: Migration of cells from shielded to irradiated marrow. *Blood* 39:804, 1972
4. Moore MAS, Metcalf D: Ontogeny of haemopoietic system: Yolk sac origin of *in vivo* and *in vitro* colony forming cells in the developing mouse embryo. *Br J Haematol* 18:279, 1970
5. Quesenberry PJ, Morley A, Ryan M, Howard D, Stohlman F, Jr: The effect of endotoxin on murine stem cells. *J Cell Physiol* 82:239, 1973
6. Quesenberry PJ, Levin J, Zuckerman K, Rencricca N, Sullivan R, Tyler W: Stem cell migration induced by erythropoietin or haemolytic anemia: The effects of actinomycin and endotoxin contamination of erythropoietin preparation. *Br J Haematol* 41:253, 1979
7. Rencricca NJ, Rizzoli V, Howard D, Stohlman F, Jr: Stem cell migration and proliferation during severe anemia. *Blood* 36:764, 1970
8. Rickard KA, Rencricca NJ, Shadduck RK, Monette, FC, Howard DE, Garrity Mand Stohlman F, Jr: Myeloid stem cell kinetics during erythropoietic stress. *Br J Haematl* 20:537, 1971
9. Siminovitch L, Till JE, McCulloch EA: Detective in colony-

forming ability of marrow cells subjected to serial transplantation into irradiated mice. *J Cell Comp Physiol* 64:23, 1964

B. Differentiation and migration patterns of maturing non-lymphoid cells

10. Guerry D, Dale DC, Omine M, Pensy S, Wolff SM: Periodic hematopoiesis in human cyclic neutropenia. *J Clin Invest* 52:3220, 1973

C. Differentiation and migration patterns of maturing lymphocytes

11. Cooper MD, Velardi A, Calvert JE, Gathings WE, Kubagawa H: Generation of B-cell clones during ontogeny. In: *Progress in Immunology V*, edited by Yamamura Y, Tada T, Academic Press, New York, 603, 1983
12. Everett NB, Tyler (Caffery) RW Lymphopoiesis in the thymus and other tissues: Functional implications. *Int Rev Cytol* 22:205, 1967
13. LeDouarin N, Dieterlen-Lieve F, Oliver PD: Ontogeny of primary lymphoid organs and lymphoid stem cells. *Am J Anat* 170:261, 1984
14. Miller SC: Production and renewal of murine natural killer cells in the spleen and bone marrow. *J Immunol* 129:2282, 1982
15. Osmond DG: The origins, life spans and circulation of lymphocytes. In: *Sixth Annual Leucocyte Culture Conference*, edited by Schwartz MR, Academic Press, New York, 3, 1972
16. Owen JJT, Jordan RK, Robinson JH, Singh Y, Willcox HNA: *In vitro* studies on the generation of lymphocyte diversity. *Cold Spring Harbor Symp Quant Biol* 41:129, 1977
17. Rouse RV, Reichert RA, Gallatin WM, Weissmann IL, Butcher EC: Localization of lymphocyte subpopulation in peripheral lymphoid organs: Directed lymphocyte migration and segregation into specific environments. *Am J Anat* 170:391, 1984
18. Sprent J: Recirculating lymphocytes. In: *The lymphocyte: Structure and function. Vol. 5*, edited by Marchalonis JJ, Marcel Dekker, New York. 43, 1977

D. Metastatic behavior

19. Greig RG, Koestler TP, Trainer DL, Corwin SP, Miles L, Kline T, Sweet R, Yokoyama S, Poste G: Tumorigenic and metastatic properties of 'normal' and *ras*-trnsfected NIH/3T3 cells. *Proc Natl Acad Sci USA* 82:3698, 1985
20. Poste G, Doll J, Fidler IJ: Interactions among clonal subpopulations affect stability of the metastatic phenotype in polyclonal populations of B-16 melanoma cells. *Proc Natl Acad Sci USA* 78:6226, 1981
21. Sugarbaker EU: Patterns of metastasis in human malignancies. *Cancer Biol Rev* 2:235, 1981
22. Van Patten LM, Kram LKJ, Van Dierendonck HHC, et al.: Enhancement by drugs of metastatic lung nodule formation after intravenous tumor cell injection. *Int J Cancer* 15:588, 1975

E. Chronic granulocytic leukemia and polycythemia vera

23. Bartram CR: *bcr* rearrangement without juxtaposition of *c-abl* in chronic myelocytic leukemia. *J Exp Med* 162:2175, 1985

24. Canellos GP: Chronic leukemias: In: *Principles and Practice of Oncology* DeVita VT, Jr, Hellman S, Rosenbey S, eds Philadelphia Lippincott, 1739–1752, 1985
25. Canellos GP, Griffin JD: Chronic granulocytic leukemia: The heterogeneity of stem cell differentiation within a single disease entity. *Semin Oncol* 12:281, 1985
26. Catovsky D: Ph¹-positive acute leukemia and chronic granulocytic leukemia: one of the two diseases? (Annotation). *Br J Haematol* 42:493, 1979
27. Groffen J, Stephenson JR, Heisterkamp N, deKlein A, Bartram CR, Grosveld G: Philadelphia chromosomal breakpoints are clustered within a limited region – bcr – chromosome 22. *Cell* 36:93, 1984
28. Nitta M, Kato Y, Strife A, Wachter M, Fried J, Perez A, Jhanwar S, Duigou-Oserndorf R, Chaganti RSK, Clarkson B: Incidence of involvement of the band T lymphocyte lineage in chronic myelogenous leukemia. *Blood* 66:1053, 1985
29. Skassin AT: Pathology and morphology of chronic leukemias and related disorders. In: *Neoplastic Diseases of the Blood*, edited by Wiernick PH, Canellos, GP, Kyle RA, Schiffer CA, Edinburgh Churchill Livingstone, 19–49, 1985

F. Acute lymphoblastic leukemia

30. Azzarelli B, Mirkin LD, Goheen M, Muller J, Crockett C: The lepto-meningeal vein: A site of re-entry of leukemic cells into the systemic circulation. *Cancer* 54:133, 1984
31. Baum E, Nesbit M, Tilford D, Heyn R, Krivit W: Extent of disease in pediatric patients with acute lymphocyte leukemia experiencing an apparent isolated testicular relapse. *Proc Am Soc Clin Oncol* 20:435, 1979
32. Fernbach DJ: Natural history of acute leukemia. In: *Clinical Pediatric Oncology*, edited by Sutow WW, Fernbach DJ, Vietti TJ, St. Louis, Mosby, 1980
33. Freeman A, Brecher ML: Diagnosis and treatment of childhood acute lymphocytic leukemia. In: *Neoplastic Diseases of the Blood*, edited by Wiernik PH, Canellos GP, Kyle RA, Schifter CA, Edinburgh Churchill Livingstone, 267, 1985
34. Herschfield MS, Kuntsberg J, Harden E, Moore JO, Whang-Peng J, Haynes BF: Conversion of a stem cell leukemia from a T-lymphoid to a myeloid phenotype induced by the adenosine deaminase inhibitor 2¹-deoxycoformycin. *Proc Natl Acad Sci USA* 81:253, 1984
35. Mathe G, Schwarzenberg L, Mery AM, et al: Extensive histological and cytological survey of patients with acute leukemia in "complete remission." *Br Med J* 1:640, 1966
36. Murphy SB, Stass S, Kalwinsky D, Rivera G: Phenotypic conversion of acute leukemia from T-lymphoblastic to myeloblastic induced by therapy with 2₁-deoxycoformycin. *Brit J Haemat* 55:285, 1983
37. Nocheles TF: *The acute leukemias* New York, Stratton, 1979
38. Simone JJ, Holland E, Johnston W: Fatalities during remission of childhood leukemia. *Blood* 39:759, 1972

G. Acute non-lymphocytic leukemia

39. Necheles TF: *The Acute Leukemias*, Stratton, 71, 1979
40. Wiernik PH: Diagnosis and treatment of acute nonlymphocytic leukemia. In: *Neoplastic Diseases of the Blood*, edited by Wiernik PH, Canellos GP, Kyle RA, Schiffer CA, Churchill Livingstone, 335, 1985

H. Hodgkin's disease

41. DeVita VT, Jr, Jaffe ES, Hellman S: Hodgkin's disease and the non-Hodgkin's lymphomas. In: *Cancer: Principles and Practice of Oncology*, edited by DeVita VT, Jr, Hellman S, Rosenberg SS, Philadelphia Lippincott, 1623, 1985
42. Fisher RI, Bates SE, Bostick-Bruton F, Tuteja N, Diehl V: Neoplastic cells obtained from Hodgkin's disease function as accessory cells for mitogen-induced human T cell proliferative responses. *J Immunol* 132:2672, 1984
43. Hecht TT, Longo DL, Cossman J, Bolen JB, Hsu S, Israel M, Fisher RI: Production and characterization of a monoclonal antibody that binds Reed-Sternberg cells. *J Immunol* 134:4231, 1985
44. Hsu S, Yang K, Jaffe ES: Phenotypic expression of Hodgkin's and Reed-Sternberg cells in Hodgkin's disease. *Am J Pathol* 118:209, 1985
45. Kadin ME: Possible origin of the Reed-Sternberg cell form an interdigitating reticulum cell. *Cancer Treat Rep* 66:601, 1982
46. Kaplan HS, Dorfman RF, Nelson TS, et al.: Staging laparotomy and splenectomy in Hodgkin's disease: Analysis of indications and patterns of involvement in 285 consecutive, unselected patients. *Natl Cancer Inst Monogr* 36:291, 1973
47. Stein H, Mason DY, O'Connor N, Wainscoat J, Pallesen G, Gatter K, Falini B, Delsol G, Lemke H, Schwarting R, Lennert K: The expression of the Hodgkin's disease associated antigen Ki-1 in reactive and neoplastic lymphoid tissue: Evidence that Reed-Sternberg cells and histiocytic malignancies are derived from activated lymphoid tissue. *Blood* 66;848, 1985

I. B cell CLL

48. Degan M, Maeda K: Differentiation of chronic lymphocytic leukemia cells after *in vitro* treatments with Epstein-Barr virus or phorbol esters. I. Immunologic and morphologic studies *Am J Hematol* 17:335, 1984
49. Dillman RO, Beauregard JC, Lea JW, Green MR, Sobol RE, Royston I: Chronic lymphocytic leukemia and other chronic lymphoid proliferations: Surface marker phenotypes and clinical correlations. *J Clin Oncology* 1(3):190, 1983
50. McPhedran P, Heath CW, Jr: Acute leukemia occurring during chronic lymphocytic leukemia. *J Hamatol* 35:7, 1970
51. Trump DL, Mann RB, Phelps R et al.: Richter's syndrome: Diffuse histiocytic lymphoma in patients with chronic lymphocytic leukemia. A report of five cases and a review of the literature. *Am J Med* 68:539, 1980

J. Burkitt's lymphoma

52. Adams JM, Harris AW, Pinkert CA, Corcoran LM, Alexander WS, Cory S, Palmiter RD, Brinster RL: The c-myc oncogene driven by immunoglobulin enhancers induces lymphoid malignancy in transgenic mice. *Nature* 318:537, 1985
53. Cory S: Activation of cellular oncogenes in hemopoietic cells by chromosomal translocation. *Adv Cancer Res* 47:189–234, 1986
54. Klein G, Klein E: *Immunol Today* 6:208, 1985
55. Leder P: Translocations among antibody genes in human cancer. *Science* 222:765, 1983
56. Magrath J: Burkitt's lymphoma: Clinical aspects and treatment. In: *Diseases of the Lymphatic System, Diagnosis and Therapy*, edited by Molander DW, Springer-Verlag, 103, 1983
57. Mann RB, Jaffe ES, Braylan RB et al.: Nonendemic Burkitt's lymphoma: B cell tumor related to germinal centers. *N Engl J Med* 295:685, 1976

K. Follicular lymphomas

58. Cossman J, Neckers LM, Hsu S, Longo D, Jaffee ES: Low grade lymphomas: Expression of developmentally regulated B-cell antigens. *Am J Pathol* 115(1):117, 1984
59. Jones SE, Fuks Z, Bull M, Kadin ME, Dorfman RF, Kaplan HS, Rosenberg SA, Kim H: Non-Hodgkin's lymphoma. IV. Clinicopathologic correlation in 405 cases. *Cancer* 31:806, 1973
60. Kim H, Dorfman RF: Morphological studies of 84 untreated patients subjected to laparotomy for the staging of non-Hodgkin's lymphomas. *Cancer* 33: 657, 1974
61. Lennert K, Mohri N: Histopathology and diagnosis of non-Hodgkin's lymphomas. In: *Malignant Lymphomas*, edited by Lennert K, Heidelberg Springer-Verlag, 111, 1978
62. Paryani SB, Hoppe RT, Cox RS, Colby TV, Rosenberg SA, Kaplan HS: Analysis of non-Hodgkin's lymphomas with nodular and favorable histologies, stages I and II. *Cancer* 52:2300, 1983
63. Rudders RA, Ahl ET, Jr, Delellis RA, Bernstein S, Begg CB: Surface marker identification of small cleaved follicular cancer cell lymphomas with a highly favorable prognosis. *Cancer Res* 42:349, 1982
64. Spiro S, Galton DAG, Wilthshaw E, Lohmann RC: Follicular lymphoma: A survey of 75 cases with special reference to the syndrome resembling chronic lymphocytic leukemia. *Brit J Cancer* 31, Suppl. II, 60, 1975

L. Intermediate and aggressive B cell lymphomas

65. Anderson T, Chabner BA, Young RC, Bernard CW, Garvin AJ, Simon RM, DeVita V, Jr: Malignant lymphoma. I. The histology and staging of 473 patients at the National Cancer Institute. *Cancer* 50:2699, 1982
66. Bunn PA, Jr, Schein PS, Banks PM, DeVita VT, Jr: Central nervous system complications in patients with diffuse histiocytic and undifferentiated lymphoma: Leukemia revisited. *Blood* 47:3, 1976
67. Chabner BA, Johnson RE, Young RC, Canellow GP, Hubbard SP, Johnson SK, DeVita VT, Jr: Sequential nonsurgical and surgical staging of non-Hodgkin's lymphoma. *Ann Int Med* 85:149, 1976
68. Cossman J: Diffuse aggressive non-Hodgkin's lymphoma. In: *Surgical Pathology of the Lymph Nodes and Related Organs.* edited by Jaffe ES, Philadelphia Saunders, 1985
69. Cossman J, Jaffe ES, Fisher RI: Immunologic phenotypes of diffuse, aggressive non-Hodgkin's lymphomas. *Cancer* 54:1310, 1984
70. Horning SJ, Doggett RS, Warnke RA, Dorfman RF, Cox RS, Levy R: Clinical relevance of immunologic phenotype in diffuse large cell lymphoma. *Blood* 63(5):1209, 1984
71. Jones R, Hubbard SM, Osborne C, Merrill J, Garvin J, Young R, DeVita Vt, Jr: Histologic conversions in non-Hodgkin's lymphoma. *Proc Am Fed Clin Res* 26:437A, 1978
72. Osborne CK, Young RC, Garvin AJ, Simon RM, Bernard CW, Hubbard CW, DeVita VT, Jr: Nodular histiocytic lymphoma: An aggressive nodular lymphoma with potential for prolonged disease-free survival. *Blood* 56:98, 1980
73. Paryani S, Hoppe RT, Burket JS, Dawley D, Cox RS, Rosenberg SA, Kaplan JS: Ectalymphatic involvement in diffuse non-Hodgkin's lymphoma. *J Clin Oncol* 1:682, 1983
74. Rudders RA, Delellis RA, Ahl ET, Jr, Bernstein S, Begg C: Adult non-Hodgkin's lymphoma: Correlation of cell surface marker phenotype with prognosis, the new working formulation, and the Rappaport and Lukes-Collins histomorphologic schemes. *Cancer* 52:2289, 1983
75. Soul SH, Kapadia SB: Primary lymphoma of Waldeyenn's ring. *Cancer* 56:157, 1985
76. Young RC, Howser DM, Anderson T, Fisher RI, Jaffe E,

DeVita VT, Jr; Central nervous system complications of non-Hodgkin's lymphoma. *Am J Med* 66:435, 1979

M. Hairy cell leukemia

77. Machii T, Kitani T: Similarities between IgG-bearing lymphocytes and hairy cells: cytologic and cytochemical studies. *Blood* 64:166, 1984
78. Turner A, Kjeldsberg CR: Hairy cell leukemia: A review. *Medicine* 57:477, 1978
79. Westbrook CA, Groopman JE, Golde DW: Hairy cell leukemia: Disease pattern and prognosis. *Cancer* 54:500, 1984

O. Alpha-heavy chain disease

80. Galian A, Lecestre MJ, Scotio J, et al.: Pathological study of alpha-chain disease, with special emphasis on evolution. *Cancer* 39:2081, 1977
81. Stoop JW, Bullieux RE, Higmens W, et al.: Alpha-chain disease with involvement of the respiratory tract in a Dutch child. *Clin Exp Immunol.* 9:625, 1971
82. Tabban S, Tabbane F, Cammoun M, et al.: Mediterranean lymphomas with alpha-heavy chain monoclonal gammapathy. *Cancer* 38:1989, 1976

P. Multiple myeloma

83. Bergsagel DE, Rider WD: Plasma cell neoplasms. In: *Cancer: Principles and Practice of Oncology,* edited by DeVita VT, Jr, Hellman S, Rosenberg SA, Philadelphia Lippincott, 1753, 1985
84. Kubagawa H, Voglen LB, Lowton AR, Cooper MD: The extent of clonal involvement in multiple myeloma. In: *Progress in Myeloma* edited by Potter M, Amsterdam Elsevier, North-Holland, 195, 1980
85. Longo DL, Broder S: Plasma cell disorders. *Harrison's Textbook of Medicine,* edited by Braunwald E, McGraw Hill, 1396, 1987.

Q. Lymphoblastic lymphoma

86. Cossman J, Chused TM, Fisher RI, Magrath I, Bollum F, Jaffe ES: Diversity of immunological phenotypes of lymphoblastic lymphoma. *Cancer Res,* 43:4486, 1983
87. Magrath I: Malignant lymphomas. In: *Cancer in the Young.* edited by Levine AS, Masson Pub., 473, 1982
88. Nathwani BN, Diamond LW, Winberg CD, Kim H, Bearman RM, Glick JH, Jones SE, Gams RA, Nissen NI, Rappaport H: Lymphoblastic lymphoma: A clinical pathologic study of 95 patients. *Cancer* 48:2347, 1981

IX. Post-thymic T cell neoplasia

89. Catovsky D, Linch DC, Beverley PC: T cell disorders in haematological diseases. *Clin Haematol.* 11(3):661, 1982
90. Jaffe ES: Post-thymic lymphoid neoplasia. In: *Surgical Pathology of the Lymph Nodes and Related Organs.* edited by Jaffe ES, Philadelphia Saunders 218, 1985

R. T cell CLL

91. Brouet JC, Seligmann M: T-derived chronic lymphocytic leukemia. *Path Research and Pract.* 171:262, 1981

92. Galton DAG, Goldman JM, Wiltshaw E, Catovsky D, Henry K, Goldberg GJ: Prolymphocytic leukemia. *Br J Haematol.* 27:7, 1974

93. Pandolfo F, DeRossi G, Semenzato G, Quinti I, Ranucci A, De Sanctis G, Lopez M, Gasparotto G, Aiuti F: Immunologic evaluatiion of T chronic lymphocytic leukemia cells: Correlations among phenotype, functional activities and morphology. *Blood* 59(4):688, 1982

S. Cutaneous T cell lymphoma

94. Poiesz BJ, Ruscetti FW, Gazdar AF, Bunn PA, Minna JD, Gallo RC: Detection and isolation of type C retrovirus particles from fresh and cultured lymphocytes of a patient with cutaneous T-cell lymphoma. *Proc Ntl Acad Sci USA* 77:7415, 1980

95. Winkler CF, Bunn PA, Jr: Cutaneous T-cell lymphoma: A review. *CRC Crit. Rev. Onc/Hema.* 1(1):49, 1983

96. Wood GS, Deneau DG, Miller RA, Levy R, Hoppe R, Warnke RA: Subtypes of cutaneous T-cell lymphoma defined by expression of Leu-1 and Ia. *Blood* 59(5):876, 1982

T. Peripheral Post-thymic T-cell lymphomas

97. Jaffe ES, Cossman J, Fisher RI: Immunologic, pathologic and clinical analysis of peripheral T-cell lymphomas. *Blood* 58 (Suppl. 1): 160a, 1981

U. Adult T cell leukemia/lymphoma

98. Hamaoka M: Progress in adult T-cell leukemia research. *Acta Pathol. Jpn.* 32 (Suppl. 1):171, 1982

99. Jaffe ES, Blattner WA, Blayney DW, Bunn PA, Cossman J, Robert-Guroff M, Gallo RC: The pathologic spectrum of adult T cell leukemia/lymphoma in the United States. *Am J Surg Pathol* 8:263, 1984

100. Poiesz BJ, Ruscetti FW, Gazdar AF, Bunn PA, Jr, Minna JD, Gallo RC: Detection and isolation of type-C retrovirus particles form from fresh cultured lymphocytes of a patient with cutaneous T-cell lymphoma. *Proc Natl Acad Sci.* USA 77:7415, 1980

101. Seiki M, Eddy R, Shrows TB, Yoshida M: Non-specific integration of the HTLV provirus genome into adult T-cell leukemia cells. *Nature* 309:640, 1984

102. Takatsuki K, Uchiyama T, Ueshima Y, Itattori T, Toibana T, Tsudo M, Wano R, Yodoi J: Adult T cell leukemia; Proposal as a new disease and cytogenetic, phenotypic and functional studies of leukemic cells. In: *Adult T cell leukemia and related diseases.* Japan Sci. Soc. Press/Plenum edited by Hamaoka M, Takatsuki K, Shimoyama M, 13, 1982

103. Urba WJ, Longo DL: Clinical spectrum of human retroviral-induced diseases. *Cancer Res.* 45:4637s, 1985

11

NEOPLASTIC PROGRESSION OF THE MYELOID LEUKEMIAS

H.D. PREISLER and A. RAZA

The expression, neoplastic progression, refers to the evolution of neoplastic cells from a less to a more malignant state. This evolutionary process is associated with increasing refractoriness to therapy, increasing metastatic potential, and usually a decrease in the level of differentiation of the neoplasm. Karyotypic evolution is often recognized during this process. The key(s) to understanding neoplastic diseases and hence the key to their control, probably is to be found within this process. We have been studying neoplastic progression in the myeloid leukemias and what follows is a discussion of our concepts of this process.

CHRONIC MYELOCYTIC LEUKEMIA (CML)

General clinical characteristics

The natural history of CML has been well defined by the Japanese investigators who monitored the aftermath of the atomic bombing of Hiroshima and Nagasaki (30). Initially immature elements appear in the peripheral blood, the white blood cell count rises, and splenomegaly appears. The patient becomes symptomatic when the white blood cell count reaches 40,000–50,000/μl. After a variable period of time (ranging from 1–12 years, median 3.5 years) the disease enters an acute phase following which survival is limited to only a few months. While patients may be found to have CML at any point in this evolutionary process, CML is usually diagnosed during the chronic phase of the disease.

The chronic phase of the illness is easily controlled by the administration of one or more agents which lower the WBC to the normal range (25, 32). When the blastic phase appears the patients develop constitutional symptoms, the white blood cell count becomes difficult to control, immature cells predominate in the blood and marrow and what is essentially an acute leukemia is present. Any cell in the myeloid series may predominate during the blastic phase including B lymphocytes and if megakaryocytic transformation occurs the marrow may become fibrotic.

Hence, CML provides an excellent example of tumor progression since it consists of a benign chronic phase of variable duration and a rapidly progressive acute phase.

Clinical characteristics of neoplastic progression in CML

Does neoplastic progression in CML occur gradually or in discrete steps? It has been reported that when CML patients were treated with intermittent busulfan therapy each successive unmaintained remission was shorter than the previous one until finally blastic crisis occurred. These observations were interpreted as indicating that neoplastic progression occurred gradually in CML until finally blastic crisis was present (17, 64). These conclusions were based on observations which involved less than 10 patients. Recent studies in our unit suggest that successive remissions do not necessarily become progressively shorter. Hence, evidence for the gradual progression of this disease from a benign to a malignant form is weak.

Nevertheless, the clinical transition from the chronic phase to the acute phase may be explosive or the disease may go through an 'accelerated' phase where blastic crisis and the chronic phase may appear to coexist for a variable period of time. The variety of transitions to the chronic phase are probably not reflections of chronic phase cells gradually acquiring the properties of blastic phase cells but rather they simply represent the different ways in which a newly appeared clone of cells can replace a clone which is responsible for ongoing hematopoiesis. This process may be gradual or rapid with the rate depending upon the relative proliferative rates of the chronic phase and blastic phase clones and on the degree of survival advantage of the blastic cells over the chronic phase cells. Additionally, the fact that hematopoiesis during the chronic phase of CML occurs in the liver, spleen, lymph nodes and bone marrow means that blastic crisis can begin in any one of these sites (66) and that the large chronic phase tumor load present in many areas of the body must be replaced by the blastic clones before the clinical definition of blastic crisis is fulfilled. Hence, while the clinical transition from chronic phase to blastic phase disease may be gradual, the reasons for this need not be based on a gradual alteration in the properties of individual cells.

Cytogenetic evidence for a discrete event as being the ultimate cause of blastic crisis

The chronic phase of CML is marked by the presence of the Ph[1] chromosome. While cases of so called "Ph[1] negative CML" are reported in the literature (13, 39) it should be remembered that CML was originally defined as a clinical syndrome long before cytogenetic techniques were introduced and hence the Ph[1] negative syndrome is an entity which is not identical to Ph[1] positive CML. In the majority of cases of Ph[1] positive CML essentially all myeloid metaphases bear this chromosomal marker. Several pieces of evidence point to the preexistence of a Ph[1] negative state. Reports that the identical twins of patients with Ph[1] positive CML are Ph[1] negative (18, 29) are consistent with preexistence of a Ph[1] negative state before CML appeared. Second-

148

K.W. Brunson (ed) Local invasion and spread of cancer.
© 1989, Kluwer Academic Publishers, Dordrecht.

ly, both Ph[1] negative and Ph[1] positive metaphases can be detected in the bone marrow and peripheral blood of some patients at the time of diagnosis but with longer follow-up the Ph[1] negative cells become undetectable (3, 7, 54). Patients presenting with this cytogenetic mosaic pattern tend to have longer survivals than patients in whom all detectable metaphases at the time of diagnosis are Ph[1] positive. Hence, the data suggest that the mosaic state is characteristic of an early stage in the illness.

Finally, recent reports of the persistence of Ph[1] negative cells in the bone marrows of CML patients (8) are compatible with a preexistent Ph[1] negative state as are the reports that aggressive chemotherapy can at times result in the reappearance of Ph[1] negative cells and non-monoclonal hematopoiesis (9, 56, 58, 59).

At the time of blastic crisis new chromosomal abnormalities are detected in 80% of the cases. These involve the appearance of one of 3 specific abnormalities: a second Ph[1] chromosome, an isochromosome 17 or a trisomy 8 (40, 44, 61). If the patient lives long enough all of these abnormalities may be present in the same cell (63) suggesting that each may convey a distinct and perhaps different biological advantage to the cell. Perhaps prophase banding techniques (69) will demonstrate new abnormalities in the 20% of cases in whom conventional banding methodologies fail to detect new abnormalities at the time of blastic crisis. The intimate association between the clinical appearance of blastic crisis and the appearance of these new discrete well defined cytogenetic abnormalities demonstrates that clonal evolution underlies blastic crisis and that if the patient survives long enough clonal evolution is detectable during the blastic phase as well.

The process of clonal evolution

The survival of patients with CML is represented by a curve which has an initial shoulder representing the fact that few patients enter blastic crisis during the first year after diagnosis. The shoulder is followed by an exponential decline towards zero, with the base line being crossed at approximately 12 years (60). The exponential portion of this curve, which represents the occurrence of blastic crisis, has been felt to be indicative of a random event which produces blastic crisis, i.e. a mutation. This view, as we have already seen, is probably correct in that the appearance of new cytogenetically marked clone is intimately associated with the onset of blastic crisis. Given that these changes occur in virtually every patient with CML, one must conclude that the Ph[1] clone is genetically unstable and therefore that the chronic phase of CML is similar to the genetic instability syndromes (55) and that in both situations mutations occur much more frequently than under normal conditions and that such mutations are at times causally related to the appearance of a neoplastic process. Hence, it is likely that during the chronic phase new cytogenetically distinct clones are evolving continuously from the genetically unstable Ph[1] clone and that only those clones associated with the distinctive cytogenetic abnormalities described above are better adapted to the environment than the Ph[1] chronic phase clones and therefore are able to replace these clones. Consistent with this possibility is the fact that if one characterizes several hundred metaphases at the time of initial diagnosis many cytogenetically distinct clones are recognizable, clones which may never become clinically relevant and which are represented so infrequently that if one characterizes 25 metaphases they are virtually undetectable (61).

There is suggestive evidence that the state of genetic instability may in fact precede the appearance of even the Ph[1] chromosome. Fialkow and colleagues (14) established B lymphocyte tissue culture cell lines from a chronic phase patient who was heterozygous for glucose-6-phosphate dehydrogenase (G6PD). In this patient peripheral blood cells containing the Ph[1] chromosome had only the type B enzyme while cultured skin fibroblasts contained both the B and A types of the enzyme in a 1:1 ratio. Seventy-four B lymphocyte cell lines were established, 9 of which were Ph[1] positive and 65 Ph[1] negative. Eighteen of these Ph[1] negative cell lines contained the A type enzyme, 45 the B type enzyme, and 2 clones had both enzymes. Hence, a statistically significantly higher proportion of cell lines contained the type B enzyme than would have been expected by chance. Eight of the 33 cytogenetically evaluable cell lines contained chromosome abnormalities while this was true for none of the 14 cell lines with type A enzyme (p > 0.05). The G6PD data suggest that at least some of the B cell lines were derived from the leukemic clone and also that such clones may be Ph[1] negative and genetically unstable. Hence, the suggestion was made that the Ph[1] negative cells in CML patients may be abnormal in that they have unstable genomes and may be members of the CML clone even though they lack the Ph[1] chromosomes.

We interpret these data somewhat differently. The development and evolution of CML may in fact occur in 3 stages. Our hypothesis is that the initial event is the appearance of a clone of genetically unstable hematopoietic cells. These genetically unstable cells acquire a Ph[1] chromosome and as a result become less responsive to normal regulators of growth but their responsiveness to inducers of differentiation is unaltered. These Ph[1] positive cells are also genetically unstable. The third stage occurs when the Ph[1] positive cells undergo further genetic changes which result in a loss in their ability to differentiate and perhaps their responsiveness to regulators of proliferation is further reduced as well. Our model (see below) differs from that of Fialkow in that we believe that the Ph[1] negative genetically unstable clone is not part of CML per se but rather may be a common state which proceeds the development of many leukemias.

Genetic instability itself could be the final common pathway of one or more processes. For example, genetic stability could result from a mutation which results in a reduction of a cell's ability to repair damaged DNA, with abnormalities being possible in one or more different DNA repair genes (53). On the other hand, genetic instability could occur in cells which have normal DNA repair processes but which are exposed to inordinately high levels of DNA damaging agents. These high levels could result directly from environmental exposures to carcinogens or would occur in a practical sense if a cell's ability to activate carcinogens were greater than normal. The possible relationship between any or all of these possibilities and the time to blastic crisis has never been explored.

The concept that differences in the genomic stability of the CML cells of different patients may account for the differences in time to blastic crisis is attractive since if correct and if one could assess the genomic stability of different patients then one could distinguish between patients at high or low risk to enter blastic crisis. This would permit rational decisions regarding the use of high risk therapies during the chronic phase of the illness.

ACUTE NONLYMPHOCYTIC LEUKEMIA (ANLL)

The strongest evidence for neoplastic progression in the majority of patients with ANLL is the development of resistance to chemotherapy. When any of the currently available aggressive remission induction regimens are administered more than 50% of patients will enter a state of complete remission (CR) with leukemic cell drug resistance being an uncommon cause of treatment failure (47, 48). On the other hand, the CR rate falls with each relapse with persistence of leukemia being associated with treatment failure in an increasing proportion of patients (49). In most reports these data are not presented in a clear cut manner since remission induction failures are often not classified as to type. However, in the Intergroup Leukemia Study of high dose cytosine arabinoside therapy the proportion of treatment failures ascribable to drug resistance increased from 30% in previously untreated patients to 47% in first relapsed patients and 52% in 2nd relapsed patients, with the 1st two patient groups receiving high dose araC therapy only and the latter group receiving the same high dose araC therapy together with mAMSA. These data are paralleled by studies *in vitro* of araC sensitivity in that the leukemic cells of previously untreated patients were essentially sensitive to the drug while with multiple relapses drug resistance became increasingly apparent and became an increasingly common cause of treatment failure (50).

It is of interest that despite repeated exposures of normal marrow to chemotherapeutic agents, the normal cells do not become drug resistant. Clearly these cells are less adaptable than leukemic cells to their environment. As will be discussed below the same phenomenon of genetic instability present in CML may also exist in ANLL and may account for the ability of ANLL cells to develop resistance to chemotherapeutic agents. This hypothesis also suggests that the normal cells which characterizes the remission state of these individuals are indeed normal or else they also might be expected to become drug resistant when exposed to repeated courses of consolidation or maintenance therapy.

The development of drug resistance is likely to be a genetic phenomenon since it appears to be stable in time during the course of the illness (although in truth this has not been rigorously tested since patients whose leukemia has been proven to be resistant to an agent(s) are rarely retreated with these agents). Interestingly, resistance seems to develop towards groups of agents simultaneously as evidenced by the fact that agents which are effective in early stage disease may be ineffective in late stage disease even though the patients with advanced disease have never been treated with the agents.

Cytogenetic studies in ANLL

The cytogenetics of ANLL are more complicated than that of CML. Abnormalities are detectable by conventional banding techniques in 50–60% of patients (19) but this may be an underestimate of the proportion of patients with chromosomal abnormalities (63). While there are no cytogenetic abnormalities which are absolutely characteristic of ANLL, some are more common than others including the presence of a trisomy 8 and the abnormalities of the 5th and 7th chromosome associated with secondary leukemias (52). Despite claims to the contrary, cytogenetic evidence points to the coexistence of normal and leukemic clones with the latter returning when remissions are induced and being suppressed once again at the time of relapse (15, 21, 23, 24, 35, 67, 71).

Demonstrable cytogenetic evolution is less uncommon in ANLL than in CML. With respect to spontaneous ANLL, as noted above, when cytogenetic abnormalities are detected at the time of diagnosis, they usually disappear when a remission is induced and reappear at the time of relapse (15, 21, 23, 24, 35, 67, 71). We would locate reports of serial cytogenetic studies in 164 patients with acute leukemia. In these patients there was evidence of clonal evolution in 39 (24%). This may be an underestimate since conventional banding techniques were used and some of the patients being followed were still in remission at the time of the reports. The most extensive study of this phenomena (67) included 60 of the 164 patients referred to above and reported that when clonal evolution occurred the most frequent change was the gain of one or more chromosomes (in 12 of 17 patients) and that 10 of the 12 patients acquired an extra chromosome 8 while 6 had an extra chromosome 18.

Among the 10 patients who presented at the time of diagnosis with an abnormal clone and in whom chromosomal evolution occurred, all but 1 occurred in the original abnormal clone. In a study of 71 patients with acute leukemia in whom cytogenetic studies were performed after a minimal remission time of 6 months, new clones appeared in 11 patients while the original clone was detected at relapse in 60 patients (71). In 7 of the 11 the original karyotype was normal so all 7 might represent clonal evolution of the original cytogenetically normal clone while in 4 patients the original karyotype was abnormal and at relapse was normal. In the authors' opinion this did not represent a new disease but rather represented the outgrowth of karyotypically normal leukemic cells which were initially present but undetected. Hence the occurrence of detectable new clones in acute leukemia at relapse appears to be less common than in CML.

A problem in interpreting these data relates to the mathematics of cytogenetic studies. Most involve the characterization of 20–25 metaphases, and not all by banding methodology. If one characterizes 25 metaphases and finds only a single clone, a 2nd clone may represent as many as 5% of the cells present and yet be undetected (28). If one characterized 50 metaphases a 2nd clone may represent as many as 1% of the metaphases and still be undetected. Hence, substantial numbers of cytogenetically marked leukemic cells may go undetected. Three additional factors make recognition of the appearance of new clones even more difficult. Firstly, the agreed to definition of a clonal abnormality requires the presence of either two identical hyperdiploid or 3 identical hypodiploid cells. The statistics referred to above regarding the detectability of 2nd clones in the presence of a dominant clone are inoperative when this definition is used but using these criteria, the detection and recognition of a 2nd clone would be even more unlikely than described above. The second factor which complicates the problem is that for a clone to be detected its cells must be able to undergo cell division under the *in vitro* conditions employed in the cytogenetic study. Different clones may have different growth requirements with some being able to undergo mitosis only under specific conditions (6, 37). These clones could theoretically be the dominant clone *in vivo* and yet go undetected. Finally, since the mitotic index, even under ideal conditions, is determined not only by the proportion of cells in mitosis but also by the percentage of the entire cell cycle time which is metaphase, the karyotypes of a dominant clone may go undetected if the generation time of this clone is significantly longer than that of a minor clone.

A small subset of patients with ANLL pass through a clinically recognizable preleukemic state before florid leukemia is diagnosed. This may or may not have developed subsequent to exposure to known marrow toxins (36). 'Preleukemia' however represents a wastebasket of hematologic abnormalities only some of which are probably part of the evolutionary pathway to ANLL (11). Patients in whom cytogenetic abnormalities are detected during the preleukemic state appear to be more likely to evolve into true leukemia (45). Clonal evolution has been demonstrable in several preleukemic patients whose illness evolved into florid ANLL. The preleukemic state in that patients with successfully treated ANLL may revert back to the preleukemic state rather than back to normal hematopoiesis as patients treated in the blastic phase of CML may revert to the chronic phase of the illness.

In summary, neoplastic progression occurs in ANLL. It has been demonstrated both clinically and cytogenetically. The question as to whether a preleukemic state characterized by genetic instability is present in all patients prior to the appearance of leukemia per se will be discussed below.

THE PATHOGENESIS OF THE MYELOID LEUKEMIAS

Chronic myelocytic leukemia
Given the evidence that CML cells are genetically unstable, and that Ph^1 negative cells in Ph^1 patients may also be unstable, the 1st event in the development of CML might be a mutation in a gene related to cellular DNA repair functions (53). This 1st step in the development of CML might be in fact a common step in the development of all myeloid leukemias and preleukemias in that this step would predispose to further genetic changes and these latter changes could determine the nature of the subsequent illness.

For CML, the next step would be the appearance of the Ph^1 chromosome. As already noted, this genetic abnormality would produce the clinical syndrome of chronic phase CML which represents a loss or a reduction in responsiveness to regulators of cellular proliferation. In the usual case of CML the development of the Ph^1 chromosome is the result of a reciprocal translocation between chromosomes 9 and 22 (1, 10, 20, 27). The chromosomal material involved includes a transfer of the cellular homologue of the simian sarcoma virus (*sis* oncogene) from chromosome 22 to 9 and the transfer of the cellular homologue of the Abelson leukemia virus (*abl*) from chromosome 9 to 22. These studies have

demonstrated a further difference between Ph^1 positive and Ph^1 negative CML in that the *abl* oncogene is not translocated in the latter syndrome (1).

While the function of the oncogene product of the *abl* oncogene is not known, the *sis* gene product is platelet derived growth factor (PDGF) (12, 42, 68). PDGF stimulates the proliferation of fibroblasts (31) and it should be remembered that marrow fibrosis is common in CML. PDGF may stimulate the proliferation myeloid stem cells as well (16). Hence altered and/or increased expression of the *sis* oncogene may be an integral part of the syndrome of CML. The possible greater relevance of the *sis* oncogene as opposed to the *abl* oncogene is also suggested by the fact that while the Ph^1 chromosome is always present in CML, the 9th chromosome is not always involved (26). Nevertheless, even when the translocation involves the number 22 and a chromosome other than chromosome 9, the course of *Cml* is unaltered. Demonstration that the *sis* oncogene is or is not translocated under these conditions would be useful.

The actual mechanism by which the *sis* oncogene product gives rise to the chronic phase of CML could be its ability to stimulate expression of the *myc* oncogene since this gene appears to be related to cellular proliferation and the transition of cells from the G_0 to the G_1 state (31). Increased expression of this oncogene or expression not responsive to normal feedback could account for the clinical phenomena associated with the chronic phase of CML.

The final step in the evolution of CML is the development of blastic crisis. This event involves alterations in or the acquisition of additional chromosomes which are known to be the site of oncogenes. Trisomy 8 is common in blastic crisis and this chromosome contains 2 oncogenes – *myc* and *mos* (41), chromosome 17 carries the *erb* b oncogene, and the Ph^1 chromosome has already been discussed. Hence, the evolution of CML to blastic crisis may be due to the further alterations of oncogene expression associated with karyotypic evolution. This stepwise evolution is compatible with what is known about carcinogenesis per se and has been elegantly demonstrated in the neoplastic conversion of rat embryo fibroblasts *in vitro* (34). Thus the genesis and evolution of CML may be explainable on the basis of genetic instability with stepwise chromosomal rearrangements which alter oncogene expression and which confer upon the newly appearing cells an increased advantage over their forebearers.

Acute nonlymphocytic leukemia
As already described above, neoplastic progression is also a characteristic of ANLL and there is also evidence of genetic instability in the leukemic clones. As with CML, there is increasing recognition that the cytogenetic abnormalities associated with this illness are also those involving sites of oncogenes. For example, the most common chromosomal abnormality in ANLL is trisomy 8, which is also a common abnormality in the blastic crisis of CML. A unique chromosomal translocation between chromosome 8 and 21 which is present in many patients with FAB M_2 has been shown to involve the *mos* oncogene (51) while the *fes* oncogene may be involved in FAB M_3 ANLL (57). Additionally, the *erb* a oncogene has been located on chromosome 7

and, as noted earlier, abnormalities in this chromosome are frequently seen in secondary ANLL.

In some cases of ANLL a process involving at least 2 steps has been demonstrated (46). The recognition of a pre-leukemic syndrome which develops into florid ANLL is becoming increasingly common. This is especially so because of the widespread use of alkylating agents and radiation therapy in the treatment of neoplastic and nonneoplastic diseases (4, 33, 43, 70). Hematologic and cytogenetic abnormalities often appear in these patients prior to the appearance of florid ANLL and progression to ANLL may be accompanied by further karyotypic evolution. This process is probably akin to that described above for CML and might be initiated by damage to DNA repair genes produced by the initial exposure to carcinogens. In ANLL and in blastic crisis of CML the level of cellular differentiation at which the cytogenetic evolution occurs will determine the cellular nature of the leukemia.

While chromosomal rearrangement of normal cellular genes may result in neoplasms, undoubtedly in some cases a direct alteration in the oncogene itself without translocation may alter its expression sufficiently to result in neoplastic transformation (65). The number of cases of ANLL and CML where this is the direct cause of the neoplastic transformation is unknown.

SUMMARY

We have tried to summarize relevant biological information regarding both CML and ANLL and derive testable hypothesis regarding the nature of these illnesses. Clearly, understanding of the processes described above are essential if we are to be able to move from the era of cytotoxic therapy and killing of the "last leukemic cell" to rational therapy which is a more humane and effective form of therapy.

REFERENCES

1. Bartram CR, deKlein A, Hagemeijer A, van Agthoven T et al.: Localization of the c-*abl* oncogene adjacent to a translocation break point in chronic myelocytic leukemia. *Nature* 306:239, 1983
2. Bernstein R, Morcom G, Pinto MR, Mendelow B et al.: Cytogenetic finding in chronic myeloid leukemia; Evaluation of karyotype blast morphology, and survival in the acute phase. *Cancer Genet and Cytogenet* 6(1):23, 1980
3. Brandt L, Mitelman F, Panani A, Lenner HC: Extremely long duration of chronic myeloid leukemia with Ph¹ negative and Ph¹ positive bone marrow cells. *Scand J Haematol* 16:321, 1976
4. Cadman EC, Capizzi RL, Bertino JR: Acute nonlymphocytic leukemia. A delayed complication of Hodgkin's disease therapy: Analysis of 109 cases. *Cancer* 44:1930, 1979, 1977
5. Cantrell ET, Warr GA, Busbee PL et al.: Induction of aryl hydrocarbon hydroxylase in human pulmonary alveolar macrophages by cigarette smoking. *J Clin Invest* 52:188, 1973
6. Carbonell F, Grilli G, Fliedner TM: Cytogenetic evidence for a clonal selection of leukemic cells in culture. *Leuk Res* 5:395, 1981
7. Carbonell F, Benitez J, Prieto F, Budra L et al.: Chromosome banding patterns with chronic myelocytic leukemia. *Cancer Genet and Cytogenet* 7:287, 1982
8. Coulombel L, Kalousek DK, Eaves CJ, Gupta CM et al.: Long-term marrow culture reveals chromosomally normal hematopoietic progenitor cells in patients with Philadelphia chromosome-positive chronic myelogenous leukemia. *N Engl J Med* 308:1493, 1983
9. Cunningham I, Gee T, Dowling M, Chaganti R et al.: Results of treatment of Ph¹+ chronic myelogenous leukemia with an intensive treatment regimen (L-5 protocol). *Blood* 53:375, 1979
10. deKlein A, van Kessel AG, Grosveld G, Bartram CR et al.: A cellular oncogene is translocated to the Philadelphia chromosome in chronic myelocytic leukemia. *Nature* 300:765, 1982
11. Dreyfus B: Preleukemic states. I Definition and classification II refractory anemia with an excess of myeloblasts in the bone marrow. *Blood Cells* 1:163, 1976
12. Doolittle RF, Hunkapillen MW, Hood LE, Aaronson SA et al.: Simian sarcoma virus *onc* gene, v-*sis*, is derived from the gene (or genes) encoding a platelet-derived growth factor. *Science* 22(1):275, 1983
13. Ezdinli EZ, Sokal JE, Crosswhite L, Sandberg AA: Philadelphia-chromosome-positive and negative chronic myelocytic leukemia. *Ann Int Med* 72:175, 1970
14. Fialkow PJ, Martin PJ, Najfeld V, Penfold GK et al.: Evidence for a multistep pathogenesis of chronic myelogenous leukemia. *Blood* 58:158, 1982
15. Fitzgerald PH, Crossen PE, Hammer JW: Abnormal karyotypic clones in human acute leukemia: Their nature and clinical significance. *Cancer* 31:1069, 1973
16. Francis GE, Michalevicz R, Wickremasinghe RG: Chronic myeloid leukaemia and the Philadelphia translocation: Do the c-*sis* oncogene and platelet-derived growth factor provide the link? *Leuk Res* 7:817, 1983
17. Galton DAG: Treatment of chronic leukemias. *Brit Med Bull* 15:78, 1959
18. Gob K, Swisher SN, Herman EC: Chronic myelocytic leukemia and identical twins. Additional evidence of the Philadelphia chromosome as postzygotic abnormality. *Arch Int Med* 120:214, 1967
19. Golomb HM, Vardiman JW, Rowley JD, Testa JM et al.: Correlation of clinical findings with quinacrine banded chromosomes in 90 adults with acute nonlymphocytic leukemia. An eight year study. *N Eng J Med* 299:613, 1978
20. Groffen J, Heisterkamp N, Stephenson JR, van Kessel AG et al.: C-*sis* is translocated from chromosome 22 to chromosome 9 in chronic myelocytic leukemia. *J Exp Med* 158:9, 1983
21. Gunz FW, Bach BI, Crossen PE, Mellor JEL et al.: Relevance of the cytogenetic status in acute leukemia in adults. *J Natl Cancer Inst* 50:55, 1973
22. Hagemeijer A, Smit EME, Lowenberg B, Abels J: Chronic myeloid leukemia with permanent disappearance of the Ph¹ chromosome and development of new clonal subpopulations. *Blood* 53:1, 1979
23. Hagemeijer A, Hahlen K, Abels J: Cytogenetic follow-up of patients with nonlymphocytic leukemia II Acute nonlymphocytic leukemia. *Cancer Genet Cytogenet* 3:109, 1981
24. Hart JS, Trujillo JM, Freireich EJ, George SL et al: Cytogenetic studies and their clinical correlates in adults with acute leukemia. *Ann Int Med* 75:353, 1971
25. Haut A, Abbott WS, Wintrobe MM, Cartwright GE: Busulfan in the treatment of chronic myelocytic leukemia. The effect of long term intermittent therapy. *Blood* 27:1, 1961
26. Hayata I, Sakurai, M, Kakati S, Sandberg AA: Chromosomes and causation of human cancer and leukemia. XVI Banding studies of chronic myelocytic leukemia, including five unusual Ph¹ translocations. *Cancer* 36:1177, 1975
27. Heistenkamp N, Stephenson JR, Groffen J, Hansen PF et al.: Localization of the c-*abl* oncogene adjacent to a translocation break point in chronic myelocytic leukemia. *Nature* 306:239, 1983
28. Hook E: Exclusion of chromosomal mosaicism: Table of 90%,

95% and 99% confidence limits and comments on use. *Am J Hum Genet* 29:94, 1979

29. Jacobs EM, Luce JK, Caillean R: Chromosome abnormalities in human cancer. Report of a patient with chronic myelocytic leukemia and his nonleukemic monozygotic twin. *Cancer* 19:869, 1966

30. Kamada N, Urchino H: Chronologic sequence in appearance of clinical and laboratory findings characteristic of chronic myelocytic leukemia. *Blood* 51:843, 1978

31. Kelly K, Cochran BH, Stikes CD, Leder P: Cell-specific regulation of the c-*myc* gene by lymphocyte mitogens and platelet-derived growth factor. *Cell* 35:603, 1983

32. Kennedy BJ: Hydroxyurea therapy in chronic myelogenous leukemia. *Cancer* 29:1052, 1972

33. Kyle RA: Second malignancies associated with chemotherapeutic agents. *Semin Oncol* 9:131, 1982

34. Land H, Parada LF. and Weinberg RA: Tumorigenic conversion of primary embryo fibroblasts require at least two cooperating oncogenes. *Nature* 304:596, 1983

35. Lawler SD, Summersgill B, Clink HM. and McElwain TJ: Cytogenetic follow-up study of acute nonlymphocytic leukaemia. *Br J Haem* 44:395, 1980

36. Linman, JW. and Bagby GC: The preleukemic syndrome: Clinical and laboratory features, natural course, and management. *Blood Cells* 2:11, 1976

37. Lowenberg B, Hagemeijer A, and Swart K: Karyotypically distinct subpopulation in acute leukemia with specific growth requirements. *Blood* 59:641, 1982

38. McCulloch EA: Stem cells in normal and leukemic hemopoiesis. *Blood* 47:705, 1976

39. Mintz U, Vardiman J, Golomb HM. and Rowley JD: Evolution of karyotypes in philadelphia chromosome-negative chronic myelogenous leukemia. *Cancer* 43:411, 1979

40. Mitelman F, Levan G, Nilsson PG. and Brandt L: Non-random karyotypic evolution in chronic myeloid leukemia. *Int J Cancer* 18:24, 1976

41. Neel BG, Jhanwar SC, Chaganti RSK, and Hayward WS: Two human c-*onc* genes are located on the long arm of chromosome 8. *Proc Nat Acad Sci* 79:7842, 1982

42. Niman HL: Antisera to a synthetic peptide of the *sis* viral oncogene product recognize human platelet-derived growth factor. *Nature* 303:180, 1984

43. O'Donnell JF, Brereton HD, Greco FA, Gralnick HR, et al.: Acute nonlymphocytic leukemia and acute myeloproliferative syndrome following radiation therapy for non-Hodgkin's lymphoma and chronic lymphocytic leukemia: Clinical studies. *Cancer* 44:1930, 1979

44. Pedersen B: Clonal evolution and progression in chronic myeloid leukemia. *Blood Cells* 1:227, 1975

45. Pierre RV: Cytogenetic studies in preleukemia: Studies before and after transition to acute leukemia in 17 subjects. *Blood Cells* 2:33, 1975

46. Preisler HD.and Lyman GH: Acute myelogenous leukemia subsequent to therapy for a different neoplasm: Clinical features and response to therapy. *Am J Hematol* 3:209, 1977

47. Preisler HD: Failure of remission induction in acute myelocytic leukemia. *Med Pediatr Oncol* 4:275–276, 1978

48. Preisler HD and Rustum YM: Prediction of therapeutic response in acute myelocytic leukemia. *Hamatol Bluttransfus* 23:93–98, 1979

49. Preisler, HD: Treatment failure in AML. *Blood Cells* 8:585–602, 1982

50. Preisler HD, Epstein J, Raza A, Browman G, et al.: Inhibition of DNA synthesis by cytosine arabinoside: Response of ANLL to remission induction therapy to stage of the disease. *Eur J Cancer Clin Oncol* 20(8):1061–1068, 1984

51. Rowley JD: Identification of a translocation with quinacrine fluorescence in a patient with acute leukemia. *Ann Genet* 16:109, 1973

52. Rowley JD, Golomb HM. and Vardiman J: Non-random chromosomal abnormalities in acute nonlymphocytic leukemia in patients treated for Hodgkin's disease and non-Hodgkin's lymphoma. *Blood* 47:705, 1976

53. Rubin JS, Joyner AL, Bernstein A, and Whitmore GF: Molecular identification of a human DNA repair gene following DNA-mediated gene transfer. *Nature* 306:206, 1983

54. Sakurai M, Hayata I, and Sandberg AA: Prognostic value of chromosomal findings in Ph[1] positive chronic myelocytic leukemia. *Cancer Res* 36:313, 1976

55. Schroeder TM: Genetically determined chromosome instability syndromes. *Cytogenet Cell Genet* 33:119, 1982

56. Sharp JC, Wayne AW, Crofts M, McArthur, G et al.: Karyotypic conversion in Ph[1]−positive chronic myeloid leukemia with combination chemotherapy. *Lancet* 1:1370, 1979

57. Sheer D, Hiorns LR, Stanley KF, Goodfellow PN, et al.: Genetic analysis of the 15:17 chromosome translocation associated with acute promyelocytic leukemia. *Proc Nat Acad Sci* 80:6036, 1983

58. Singer JW, Arlin Z, Nejveld V, Adamson JW, et al.: Restoration of non-clonal, presumably normal hematopoiesis accompanying a chemotherapeutic conversion of Ph[1] positive chronic myelogenous leukemia to Ph[1] negative. *Blood* 54(1):176a (abstr 459), 1979

59. Smalley RV, Vogel Huguley CM. and Miller D: Chronic granulocytic leukemia: Cytogenetic conversion of the bone marrow with cycle-specific chemotherapy. *Blood* 50:107, 1977

60. Sokal JE: Evaluation of survival data for chronic myelocytic leukemia. *Am J Hematol* 1:493, 1976

61. Sonta S. and Sandberg AA: Chromosomes and causation of human cancer and leukemia: XVIII. Value of detailed chromosome studies on large numbers of cells in CML. *Am J Hematol* 3:121, 1977

62. Sonta S. and Sandberg AA: Chromosomes and causation of human cancer and leukemia. XXIX. Further studies on karyotypic progression in CML. *Cancer* 41:153, 1979

63. Stoll C. and Oberling F: Non-random clonal evolution in 45 cases of chronic myeloid leukemia. *Leuk Res* 3:61, 1979

64. Stryckmans PA: Current concepts in chronic myelocytic leukemia. *Semin Hemat* 11:101, 1974

65. Sukamar S, Notario V, Martin-Zanca D, and Barbaud M: Induction of mammary carcinomas in rats by nitroso-methylurea involves malignant activation of H-*ras*-1 locus by single point mutations. *Nature* 306:658, 1983

66. Swolin B, Weinfeld A, Waldenstrom J, and Westin J: Cytogenetic studies of bone marrow and extramedullary tissues and clinical course during metamorphosis of chronic myelocytic leukemia. *Cancer Genet Cytogenet* 9(3):197, 1983

67. Testa JR, Mintz U, Rowley JD, Vardiman JW, et al.: Evolution of karyotypes in acute nonlymphocytic leukemia. *Can Res* 39:3619, 1979

68. Waterfield MD, Scrace GT, Whittle N, Stroobant P, et al.: Platelet derived growth factor is structurally related to the putative transforming protein p28[sis] of simian sarcoma virus. *Nature* 304:35, 1983

69. Yunis JJ, Bloomfield CL.D. and Ensrud K: All patients with acute nonlymphocytic leukemia may have a chomosomal defect. *N Engl J Med* 305:135, 1981

70. Zarrabi MH. and Rosner F: Acute myeloblastic leukemia following treatment for non-hematopoietic cancers: Report of 19 cases and review of the literature. *Am J Hematol* 7:357, 1979

71. Zuelzer WW, Inone S, Thompson RI. and Ottenbreit MJ: Long term cytogenetic studies in acute leukemia of children: The nature of relapse. *Am J Hematol* 1:143, 1976

SYSTEMIC MASTOCYTOSIS

WILLIAM R. HENDERSON and EMIL Y. CHI

STRUCTURE AND FUNCTION OF MAST CELLS

Mastocytosis is the condition of unknown etiology characterized by an abnormal accumulation of mast cells occurring in various tissue sites. Mast cells are normally located throughout the body in loose connective tissue with particularly high numbers found in the lungs, skin and gastrointestinal tract. In the lungs, mast cells are associated with large blood vessels and are located in the submucosa of the bronchi and bronchioles (10). In contrast, mast cells in the skin are associated with small blood vessels and also in close proximity to glandular ducts and nerves (28, 58). Mast cells in the gastrointestinal tract occur generally throughout the lamina propria in a random pattern (61). Other sites where mast cells and mast cell precursors are noted in high numbers are in the peritoneal cavity, the thymic capsule and in lymph nodes (50). The origin of mast cells is unclear. Although their presence in the connective tissue has suggested a relationship to fibroblasts, some experiments have suggested their derivation from T lymphocytes (33, 34, 45). These findings are not supported, however, by the presence of typical numbers of mast cells in athymic mice (nu/nu strain) which lack T lymphocytes (49). Other investigators have shown by bone marrow transplantation studies using Chediak-Higashi syndrome mice which have distinctive giant granules that mast cells can be derived from a marrow stem cell precursor (51). The relationship of mast cells to the bone marrow-derived and peripherally circulating basophilic leukocyte is also unknown. Both mast cells and basophils have Fc receptors for IgE on their surface (5, 57) and their granules contain histamine and stain metachromatically when treated with certain dyes such as toluidine blue. Mast cells are characterized by their content of large membrane-bound granules which contain a variety of chemical agents (eg histamine, heparin) which are important mediators of the immediate hypersensitivity reaction.

Mast cells from rats (Fig. 1) and mice contain many large uniformly electron-dense cytoplasmic granules which are membrane-bound (53). The mast cell nucleus is round and in a central location. Cytoplasmic organelles such as mitochondria, Golgi apparatus and endoplasmic reticulum are present and many intermediate filaments are noted. The cell membrane contains numerous, small surface projections which are evenly distributed. Human mast cells also are characterized by their many membrane-bound granules (Fig. 2A, B). Their cytoplasmic granules, unlike those from rodents, however, have a varied appearance. Human mast cell granules have predominant crystalline contents (Fig. 2B) that appear in various patterns including whorls or scrolls and lattices (12, 53) which differ from the appearance of rat leukemia basophil (RBL) cells (Fig. 3) and human basophils (Fig. 4).

Allergic reactions are typically initiated by antigen interaction with IgE antibodies on the surface of mast cells leading to degranulation and mediator release (3). Mast cell degranulation may also be initiated by a variety of secretagogues including the anaphylatoxins C_{3a} and C_{5a} generated by complement activation (47), by cationic polypeptides from polymorphonuclear leukocyte granules (46) and by eosinophil and neutrophil peroxidase oxidative systems (40). Activation of membrane phospholipid metabolism and generation of lipoxygenase products of arachidonic acid metabolism are thought to play an important role in the initiation of secretion in mast cells and highly purified preparations of phospholipase A_2 can initiate mast cell degranulation (15).

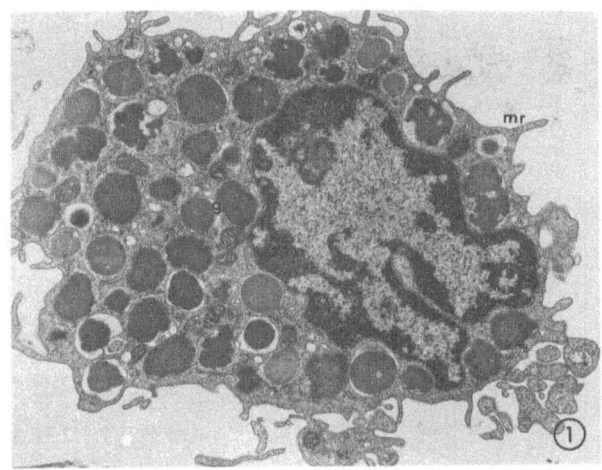

Figure 1. Rat peritoneal mast cell. An unstimulated mast cell was studied by transmission electron microscopy ($\times 1,200$) and is characterized by its many electron-dense membrane-bound granules (g). The nucleus is ovoid and Golgi vesicles and other organelles are present. Numerous microridges (mr) extend from the cell surface.

Supported in part by National Institutes of Health grant AI17758 William R. Henderson is the recipient of Allergic Diseases Academic Award AI00487 from the National Institute of Allergy and Infectious Diseases.

K.W. Brunson (ed) Local invasion and spread of cancer.

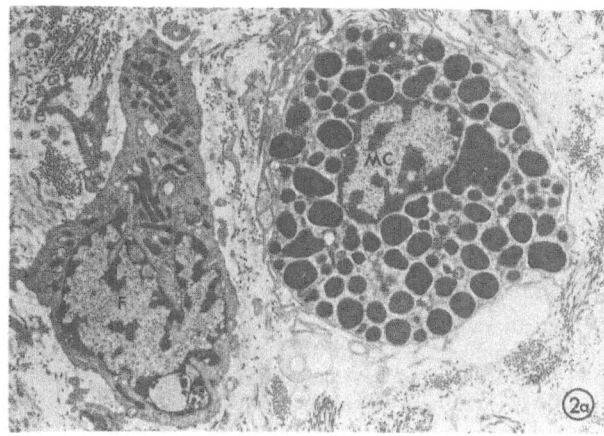

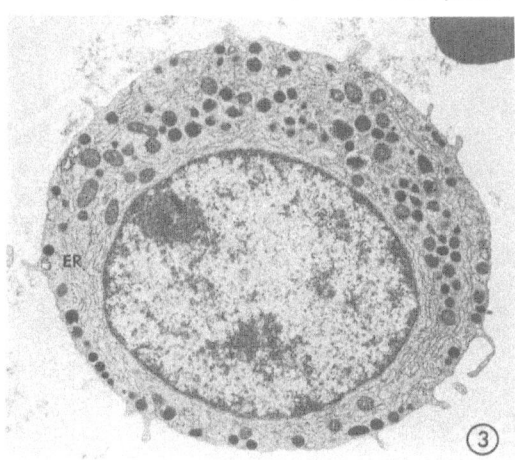

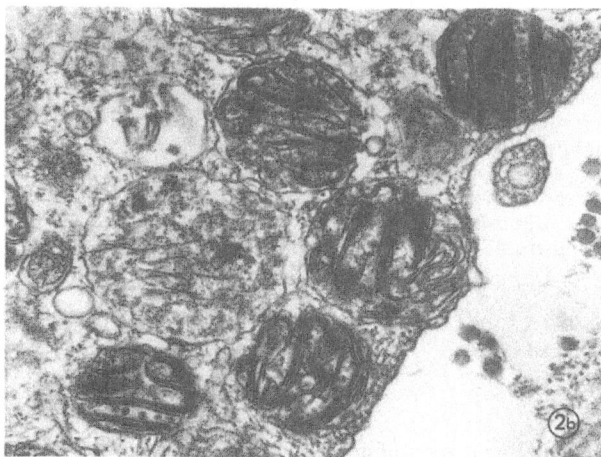

Figure 3. Rat leukemia basophil (RBL) cell. Transmission electron microscopy (× 12,000) This malignant cell contains abundant endoplasmic reticulum (ER). The granules are smaller than seen in mast cells.

serotonin which are easily eluted from the granules and released extracellularly with mast cell secretion. A second class of molecules form the granular matrix such as heparin, chymotrypsin, galactosidase, arylsulfatase, superoxide dismutase and peroxidase. These molecules are also preformed but are poorly solubilized in extracellular fluids. A third group of potent compounds are newly generated by mast cells as a consequence of the secretory process including the arachidonic acid metabolites such as prostaglandins, thromboxanes and leukotrienes. This review will focus on several molecules from each of these groups which may be relevant in the mast cell response to neoplasia and which also may account for the symptoms of systemic mast cell disorders.

Figure 2. Human mast cell. The mast cell (MC) embedded in the connective tissue of a nasal polyp was examined for transmission electron microscopy (a; × 8,000, b; × 60,000). Many adjacent collagen fibers are noted as is a nearby fibroblast (F). Mast cells are often seen closely associated with nerves and blood vessels. As seen in (a), the nucleus is ovoid in shape and the cytoplasm contains both round and irregularly shaped, electron-dense granules. At higher magnification (b), the lamellar structure of the granules is evident.

Mast cell degranulation is characterized initially by the fusion of the membranes of adjacent granules in the peripheral cytoplasm (Fig. 5A). When granules fuse, they become swollen and less electron-dense as their contents are released into cytoplasmic channels. Fusion of perigranular and plasma membranes produces surface pores in the cell membrane (Fig. 5B). Mast cell granule contents can then be discharged through these pores with release of biologically potent mediators such as histamine extracellularly. As a consequence of degranulation, mast cells become swollen with a diminution of surface membrane projections.

Mast cell degranulation produces three distinct groups of biologically potent material. The first group of molecules consists of low molecular weight compounds that are preformed, granule-associated molecules such as histamine, eosinophil chemotactic factor of anaphylaxis (ECF-A) and

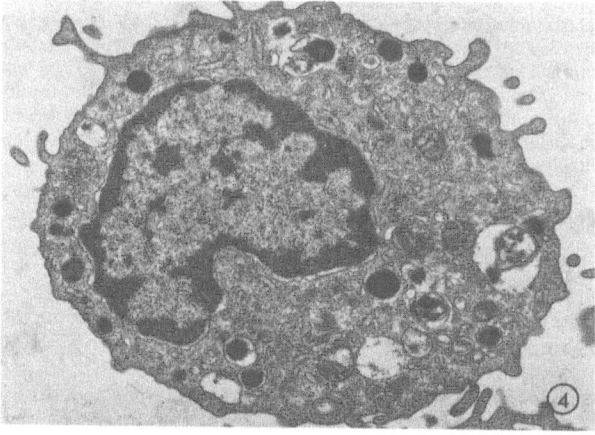

Figure 4. Human peripheral blood basophil. Transmission electron microscopy (× 16,000). The characteristic multilobed nucleus and fewer cytoplasmic granules differentiate this cell from a human mast cell. The basophil granules also do not exhibit the lamellar structure of human mast cell granules when examined at higher magnification.

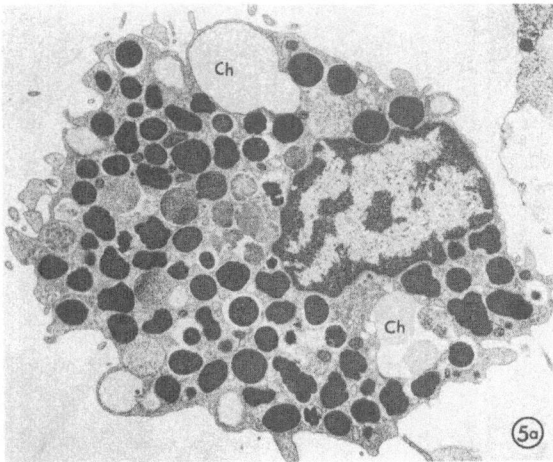

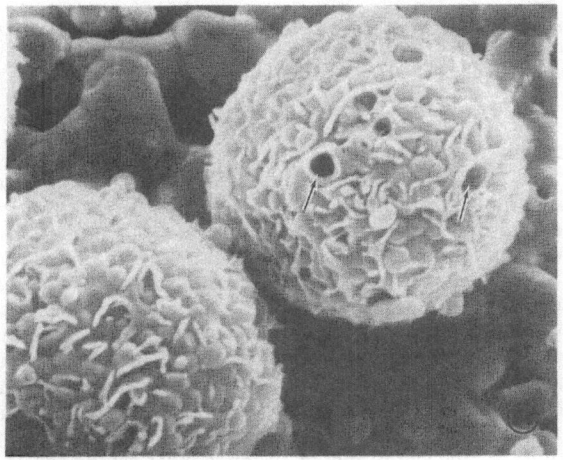

Figure 5. Rat peritoneal mast cell degranulation. Mast cells were incubated with the calcium ionophore A23187 (1 μM, final concentration) for 15 minutes at 37°C and examined for transmission electron microscopy (a; × 10,000) or scanning electron microscopy (b; × 8,000). Typical changes of degranulation are seen in (a); many granules are swollen and of decreased electron density. These altered granules are present in intracellular channels (CH) not found in unstimulated cells as seen in Fig. 1. Pores (arrows) are noted in the surface membrane (b) where intracellular channels open to the outside of the cells.

GRANULE-ASSOCIATED SOLUBLE MEDIATORS

Histamine

Mast cells are the principle tissue source of histamine in mammals (66). Histamine which is B-imidazolylethylamine is synthesized by mast cells from L-histidine by histidine decarboxylase (4). Histamine is stored in the mast cell granule and binds non-covalently to carboxyl groups of the protein-heparin core (52, 76). Upon exposure of the granular matrix to extracellular fluids during degranulation, cations in the extracellular fluid readily displace histamine which is then soluble and fully functional. Histamine reacts with two types of receptors (H_1, H_2) in tissues (4). Histamine causes precapillary smooth muscles to relax (H_1 and H_2

effect) causing vasodilation of small vessels; increased permeability of capillaries occurs by its contractile effect on endothelial cells which opens gaps between cells leading to extravasation of fluid (55). Through H_1 effects, histamine causes contraction of smooth muscles (eg bronchi, intestines, uterus). A specific H_2 effect of histamine is to increase gastric acid secretion. Classical antihistamines such as diphenhydramine block only H_1 actions and thus the more recently synthesized group of H_2 receptor antagonists such as cimetidine must be added to H_1 antihistamines to block local edema formation. Histamine release may also be important in inflammatory reactions by its effects on eosinophil recruitment to the inflammatory site (1, 16). At low histamine concentrations (10^{-8}–10^{-6} M) histamine promotes eosinophil chemotaxis whereas at high concentrations (10^{-5} M) it inhibits eosinophil chemotaxis; these effects of histamine on eosinophil movement are not mediated by either H_1 or H_2 receptors. Histamine is rapidly metabolized by two different pathways: methylation oxidation and deamination by histaminase (4). Histaminase has been found in both neutrophils and eosinophils (83, 84).

Serotonin and ECF-A which constitute a group of low molecular weight tetrapeptides are also preformed in mast cell granules and released in the same fashion as histamine. They selectively attract eosinophils.

Serotonin is found in rat and mouse mast cell granules (7) but is not normally demonstrated in human cells; it has been demonstrated in a human mastocytoma, however (59).

GRANULE MATRIX, POORLY SOLUBILIZED MEDIATORS

Heparin

The metachromatic staining of mast cells is the characteristic identifying feature of these cells by light microscopy. This metachromasia is secondary to their large granule content of heparin. Rat mast cell heparin is a proteoglycan macromolecule of approximately 750,000 molecular weight, composed of glycosaminoglycans covalently linked to a protein core (44, 80). The glycosaminoglycan side chains are composed of highly sulfated disaccharide subunits (which account for the unique staining reaction of heparin with metachromatic dyes) and the protein core consists of a copolymer of repeating and glycine subunits. Although heparin is secreted immunologically from mast cells, it is not readily displaced from the secreted granules (76, 81) Heparin and other granule components such as chymotrypsin are firmly bound to or intrinsic to the relatively insoluble granule matrix and require very high, non-physiological salt concentrations for release. The anticoagulant and antithrombin activity of heparin (and the proteolytic activity of chymotrypsin) are almost totally masked in the discharged mast cell granule (3) whereas its anticomplementary activity (inhibition of the alternate complement pathway) is completely functional (78). Rat heparin as a component of mast cell granules is highly resistant to degradation by proteolytic enzymes but is phagocytosed and degraded by macrophages and fibroblasts. Phagocyte production of oxygen radicals including hydroxyl radicals may be an important mechanism of heparin degradation in tissues (56). A characteristic difference of basophils is that they lack heparin and contain chondroitin sulfate instead.

Peroxidase

Rat peritoneal mast cells contain peroxidase as a granule constituent as demonstrated both histochemically and enzymatically (39). Rat and human mast cells from heart, thyroid gland, skin and connective tissue have all been demonstrated to contain peroxidase. Peroxidases when combined with hydrogen peroxide and a halide are toxic to a variety of target cells including tumor cells by generation of potent oxygen radicals such as hypochlorous acid (HOC1) (17).

NEWLY GENERATED MAST CELL MEDIATORS

Superoxide

Appropriate stimulation of various inflammatory cells (eg neutrophils, eosinophils, macrophages) is associated with activation of the hexose monophosphate shunt pathway and a respiratory burst in which oxygen consumption is greatly increased. Much if not all of the added oxygen consumed is initially reduced to superoxide (O_2^-) which forms hydrogen peroxide (H_2O_2) by spontaneous or superoxide dismutase-catalyzed dismutation as follows: $O_2^- + O_2^- + 2H^+ \rightarrow O_2 + H_2O_2$. Human lung mast cells and human leukemic basophils have been demonstrated to newly generate O_2^- after both immunologic and non-immunologic stimulation (38). O_2^- and its byproducts (hydroxyl radicals and singlet oxygen) have potent microbicidal and cytotoxic activity. Secretory granules from both basophils and mast cells have superoxide dismutase as a preformed component of their matrix (38). Both O_2^- and superoxide dismutase could be involved in host defenses involved in immediate hypersensitivity reactions.

CYCLOOXYGENASE AND LIPOXYGENASE PRODUCTS OF ARACHIDONIC ACID

Arachidonic acid is released from the membrane phospholipids of inflammatory cells after appropriate stimulation of membrane phospholipases. Two oxidative pathways, the cyclooxygenase and lipoxygenase enzyme pathways, are present in polymorphonuclear and mononuclear leucocytes which can oxidatively metabolize arachidonic acid.

Mast cells are capable of metabolizing arachidonic acid by both pathways to form biologically potent mediators. The primary cyclooxygenase products produced by rat mast cells are prostaglandin D_2 (PGD_2), prostaglandin I_2 (PGI_2) and thromboxane A_2 (TXA_2) (67). PGD_2 has chemokinetic activity for neutrophils and is also a potent bronchoconstrictor. PGI_2 has impressive vasodilator activity whereas TXA_2 contracts smooth muscles. Stimulated human lung and mouse mast cells also generate leukotrienes which are a group of compounds with three conjugated double bonds formed by the oxidation of arachidonic acid by the lipoxygenase pathway. The sulfidopeptide leukotrienes C_4 and D_4 which are produced by both human lung and mouse bone marrow derived mast cells (54, 65) constitute the slow reacting substance of anaphylaxis (SRS-A). These sulfidopeptide leukotrienes have potent bronchiolar smooth muscle contracting activity, increase vascular permeability and are thought to play an important role in the pathogenesis of immediate hypersensitivity reactions.

ROLE OF MAST CELLS IN INFLAMMATION

Thus mast cells can release an impressive array of biologically potent mediators which may play an important role in the pathogenesis of allergic disease. Allergic asthma is thought to result from IgE-mediated mast cell degranulation with release of mediators such as leukotrienes C_4 and D_4 and histamine. Alternatively mast cells may function in host defense reactions against parasites and tumor cells. Mast cell numbers greatly increase in the small intestine of animals after nematode and cestode infection and the mast cells are thought to play a critical role in the expulsion of these gastrointestinal parasites and in the host resistance to reinfection (69). Depletion of mast cells by treatment with reserpine or compound 48/80 can abrogate cutaneous inflammatory responses and immunologic rejection of *Schistosoma mansoni* in mice (2, 72). *In vitro*, mast cells adhere to schistosomula through a C_3 receptor (72) but their exact role in the protection of the host against parasites is unknown. Mast cells may also augment the host defense against certain neoplasms. Mast cells have been seen in increased numbers near carcinoma *in situ* of the uterine cervix (35), in the stroma and parenchyma of skin tumors in humans (13) and in both spontaneous tumors and those induced by carcinogenic agents in animals (19). *In vitro* studies have demonstrated that rat mast cells, when supplemented with hydrogen peroxide and iodide, are cytotoxic to mammalian tumor cells (41); this toxicity is mediated by the peroxidase contained in mast cell granules (Fig. 6).

When mast cells proliferate and accumulate for unknown reasons in various tissue sites, clinical disorders termed mastocytosis occur.

MASTOCYTOSIS CLASSIFICATION

In the limited form of mastocytosis, called urticaria pigmentosa, only cutaneous sites are involved, and lesions are present as reddish-brown macules and papules which are widely dispersed (26, 60) or as a solitary collection of mast cells which is described as a mastocytoma (36). These cutaneous lesions are characterized by their urtication after mechanical stimulation (ie Darier's sign) (21) and are also often associated with dermatographism. In one study at St. Batholomew's Hospital, London, England, urticaria pigmentosa composed one in every 2,500 attendances to the dermatology division (37).

In the systemic form called systemic mastocytosis, there is widespread mast cell infiltration of the skin, liver, spleen, gastrointestinal tract, bones and lymph nodes. Hepatosplenomegaly and lymph node enlargement is thought to be secondary to both proliferation of mast cells and fibrosis (27, 77).

Both osteoporotic and osteosclerotic bone involvement is seen in systemic mastocytosis (71). Myelofibrosis may also occur with resulting anemia and thrombocytopenia. Eosino-

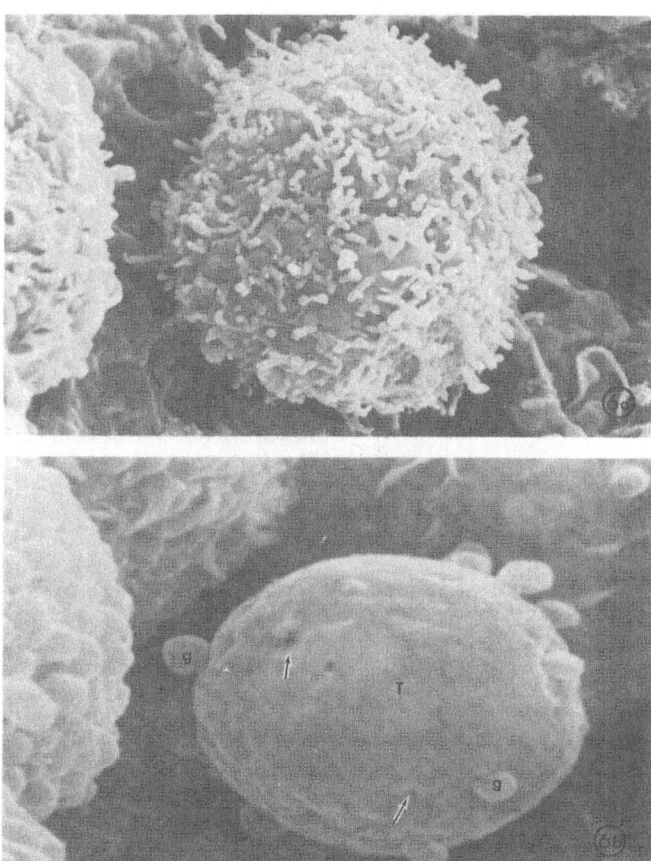

Figure 6. Mast cell induced tumor cell cytotoxicity. Scanning electron microscopy. Maloney virus-induced ascites lymphoma cells (designated as LSTRA) were incubated in buffer alone (a; × 8,000) or with rat peritoneal mast cells in the presence of hydrogen peroxide (10^{-4} M) and iodide (10^{-4} M) (b; × 12,000). In (a), the control LSTRA tumor cell has numerous microvillous projections evenly distributed on the cell surface. In (b), the addition of hydrogen peroxide and iodide induced non-cytotoxic release of peroxidase containing mast cell granules (g). The extracellularly released granules adhered tightly to the surface of the tumor cells (T) causing cytotoxic tumor cell damage. Holes (arrows) formed in the tumor cell surface accompanied by an alteration of cell shape and loss of normal surface projections of the tumor cells as a consequence of the MCG peroxidase system is observed.

philia is noted in 12% of patients with mastocytosis and one patient has been described with both mastocytosis and eosinophilic granuloma (71). Progression of systemic mastocytosis to mast cell leukemia occurs as a rare event with widespread mast cell invasion of the bone marrow, lymph nodes and visceral organs. Mast cell leukemia has been characterized by peripheral white blood cell counts of 50,000 to 100,000 with greater than 50% mast cells in some cases (25, 30).

Mastocytosis is thought to occur as a primary disorder but occasionally can be acquired secondarily or concomitantly to a carcinoma (18) or leukemia (31). Mast cell neoplasms have been described in a variety of animals including dogs (8, 9) and mice (24, 32) with the murine P-815 mastocytoma cell line used extensively in investigations of the biology of this neoplasm (Fig. 7).

neoplasms have been described in a variety of animals including dogs (8, 9) and mice (24, 32) with the murine P-815 mastocytoma cell line used extensively in investigations of the biology of this neoplasm (Fig. 7).

Clinical symptoms of systemic mastocytosis include pruritus, urticaria, flushing, diarrhea and abdominal pain and are thought to result from the chemical mediators produced by mast cells. The majority of patients with systemic mastocytosis have greatly augmented levels of histamine in their skin lesions compared to adjacent normal skin (74, 82), histaminuria (22, 62, 74) and some patients have elevated blood or plasma histamine levels (73). Clinical symptoms are secondary to stimulation of H_1 and H_2 histamine receptors. H_1 stimulation causes smooth muscle constriction, increased vascular permeability and pruritus whereas H_2 stimulation induces gastric acid secretion and mucous secretion. Vasodilation (hypotension), flushing and headache are the effect of both H_1 and H_2 receptor activation. Thus in normal human volunteers given intravenous

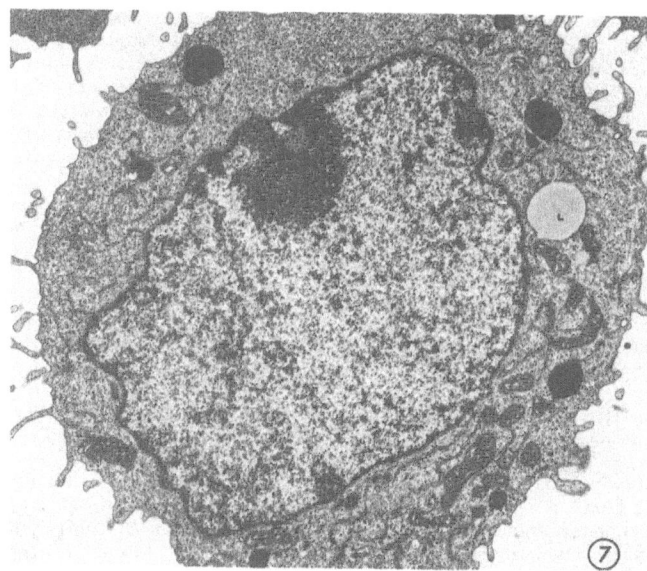

Figure 7. Murine P-815 mastocytoma cell. Transmission electron microscopy ($\times$ 17,000). This cell resembles in some aspects an immature mast cell because of its abundant endoplasmic reticulum (ER), large nuclear to cytoplasmic ratio and few cytoplasmic granules. These mastocytoma cells can bind IgE on their cell surface and contain small amounts of histamine in their granules. Lipid (L) collections are often noted in the murine mastocytoma cells but are rarely observed in normal mast cells.

infusions of histamine, pretreatment with H_1 antihistamines prevented lung mechanics changes and tachycardia whereas both H_1 and H_2 antihistamine premediation was required to prevent headache, flushing and pulse pressure changes (48). In mastocytosis patients, H_1 and H_2 antihistamines have been used to decrease flushing, pruritis and whealing episodes and H_2 antihistamines have been particularly useful in decreasing gastric acid secretion and peptic ulcer formation (29).

The fact that H_1 and H_2 antihistamine blockade does not prevent hypotension, flushing and tachycardia in some patients has suggested that other mast cell mediators are involved in the pathophysiology of this disorder.

Two mastocytosis patients with periodic attacks of flushing, accompanied by hypotension and tachycardia have been reported to overproduce prostaglandin D_2. One of these patients had a major reduction in symptoms by the use of aspirin inhibition of prostaglandin biosynthesis in conjunction with combined blockage of H_1 and H_2 histamine receptors (68).

Elevated plasma levels of thromboxane B_2, another cyclooxygenase product of arachidonic acid metabolism, have been demonstrated in patients with systemic mastocytosis (63).

Other mast cell mediators have been implicated in the pathophysiology of attacks in this syndrome. A child with urticaria pigmentosa was shown to have an increased plasma heparin level during a period of widespread urtication and gastrointestinal bleeding (11). An infant with flushing and apnea post irradiation of a cutaneous mastocytoma had high levels of vasoactive intestinal peptide (VIP) in both the draining venous bed and in the tumor itself (79). VIP has also been shown to be released concomitantly with histamine from stimulated rat mast cells (20).

Treatment of systemic mastocytosis consists initially of the aforementioned use of H_1 and H_2 antihistamines (and aspirin in patients with prostaglandin D_2 overproduction). Since symptoms are not usually totally controlled by antihistamines (43), other drugs have been used in treatment. Oral disodium cromoglycate ingestion has been associated with improvement of such clinical manifestations as diarrhea (23, 74) and cognitive function disorders (74) in patients with systemic mastocytosis.

REFERENCES

1. Archer RK: The eosinophil response in the horse to intramedullary and intradermal injections of histamine, ACTH and cortisone. *J Pathol* 72:87, 1956
2. Askenase PW: Role of basophils, mast cells and vasoamines in hypersensitivity reactions with a delayed time course. *Prog Allergy* 23:199, 1977
3. Austen KF: Biological implications of the structural and functional characteristics of the chemical mediators of immediate-type hypersensitivity. *Harvey Lect* 73:93, 1979
4. Beaven MA: Histamine. *New Engl J Med* 294:30, 1976
5. Becker KE, Ishizaka T, Metzger H, Ishizaka K, Grimley PM: Surface IgE on human basophils during histamine release. *J Exp Med* 138:395, 1973
6. Belcon MC, Collins SM, Castelli MF, Qizibash AH: Gastrointestinal hemorrhage in mastocytosis. *CMA Journal* 122:311, 1980
7. Benditt EP, Wong RL, Arase M, Roeper E: 5-Hydroxytryptamine in mast cells. *Proc Soc Exp Biol Med* 90:303, 1955
8. Bloom F: Spontaneous solitary and multiple mast cell tumors (Mastocytoma) in dogs. *AMA Arch Pathol* 33:661, 1942
9. Bloom G, Larrson B, Aberg B: Canine mastocytoma. *Zentr Venterinaermed* 5:443, 1958
10. Brinkman GL: The mast cell in normal human bronchus and

lung. *J Ultrastruct Res* 23:115, 1968

11. Campbel EW, Hector D, Gossain V: Heparin activity in systemic mastocytosis. *Ann Int Med* 90:940, 1979
12. Caulfield JP, Lewis RA, Hein A, Austen KF: Secretion in dissociated human pulmonary mast cells. Evidence for solubilization of granule contents before discharge. *J Cell Biol* 85:299, 1980
13. Cawley EP, Hoch-Ligeti C: Association of tissue mast cells and skin tumors. *Arch Derm* 83:146, 1961
14. Chi EY, Lagunoff D, Koehler JK: Freeze-fracture study of mast cell secretion. *Proc Natl Acad Sci USA* 78:2823, 1976
15. Chi EY, Henderson WR, Klebanoff SJ: Phospholipase A$_2$-induced rat mast cell secretion; Role of arachidonic acid metabolites. *Lab Invest* 47:579, 1982
16. Clark RA, Klebanoff SJ, Einstein AB, Fefer A: Peroxidase-H$_2$O$_2$-halide system: cytotoxic effect on mammalian tumor cells. *Blood* 45:161, 1975
17. Clark RAF, Gallin J, Kaplan AP: The selective eosinophil chemotactic activity of histamine. *J Exp Med* 142:1462 1975
18. Cohen HF, Raisbeck MJ, Baer RL: Acquired (adult) urticaria pigmentosa. Disappearance after removal of intestinal carcinoma. *Dermatologia* 121:386, 1960
19. Combs JW, Purnell DM: Functional characteristics of mast cells associated with rat mammary tumors induced by 7, 12 dimethylbenz{α}anthracene. *J Natl Cancer Inst* 50:1003, 1973
20. Cutz E, Chan W, Track NS, Goth A, Said SI: Release of vasoactive intestinal peptide in mast cells by histamine liberators. *Nature* 275:661, 1978
21. Demis DJ: The mastocytosis syndrome: clinical and biological studies. *Ann Int Med* 59:194, 1963
22. Demis DJ, Walton MD, Higdon RS: Histaminuria in urticaria pigmentosa and the mastocytosis syndrome. *Arch Derm* 83:127, 1961
23. Dolovich J, Punthakee ND, MacMillan AB, Osbaldeston GJ: Systemic mastocytosis: control of lifelong diarrhea by ingested disodium cromoglycate. *Can Med Assoc J* 111:684, 1974
24. Dunn TB, Potter M: A transplantable mast cell neoplasm in the mouse. *J Natl Cancer Inst* 18:587, 1957
25. Efrati P, Klajman A, Spitz H: Mast cell leukemia? -malignant mastocytosis with leukemia-like manifestations. *Blood* 12:869, 1957
26. Ellis JM: Urticaria pigmentosa: Report of a case with autopsy. *Arch Path* 48:426, 1949
27. Ende N, Cherniss N: Splenic mastocytosis. *Blood* 13:631, 1958
28. Enerback L, Olsson Y, Sourander P: Mast cells in normal and sectioned peripheral nerve. *Z Zellforsch Mikrosk Anat* 60:596, 1965
29. Feldman EJ, Isenberg JI: Effects of metiamide on gastric acid hypersecretion, steatorrhea and bone marrow function in a patient with systemic mastocytosis. *New Engl J Med* 295:1178, 1976
30. Friedman BI, Will JJ, Freiman DG, Braunstein H: Tissue mast cell leukemia. *Blood* 13:70, 1958
31. Fromer JL, Jaffe N: Urticaria pigmentosa and acute lymphoblastic leukemia. *Arch Dermatol* 107:283, 1973
32. Furth J, Hagen P, Hirsch EI: Transplantable mastocytoma in the mouse containing histamine, heparin and 5-hydroxytryptamine. *Proc Soc Exptl Biol Med* 95:824, 1957
33. Ginsburg H, Lagunoff D: The *in vitro* differentiation of mast cells. Culture of cells from immunized mouse lymph nodes and thoracic duct lymph on fibroblast monolayers. *J Cell Biol* 75:685, 1967
34. Ginsburg H, Sachs L: Formation of pure suspensions of mast cells in tissue culture by differentiation of lymphoid cells from the mouse thymus. *J Natl Cancer Inst* 31:1, 1963
35. Graham RM, Graham JB: Mast cells and cancer of the cervix. *Surg Gyn Ob* 123:3, 1966
36. Gross P: Urticaria pigmentosa (solitary lesion). *Arch Derm Symph* 29:451, 1934
37. Havard CWH, Scott RB: Urticaria pigmentosa with visceral and skeletal lesions. *Quar J Med* 28:459, 1959
38. Henderson WR, Kaliner M: Immunologic and non-immunologic generatin of superoxide from mast cells and basophils. *J. Clin Invest* 61:187, 1978
39. Henderson WR, Kaliner M: Mast cell peroxidase: location, secretion and SRS-A inactivation. *J Immunol* 122:1322, 1979
40. Henderson WR, Chi EY, Klebanoff SJ: Eosinophil peroxidase-induced mast cell secretion. *J Exp Med* 152:265, 1980
41. Henderson WR, Chi EY, Jong EC, Klebanoff SJ: Mast cell-mediated tumor-cell cytotoxicity. Role of the peroxidase system. *J Exp Med* 153:520, 1981
42. Hills E, Dunstan CR, Evans RA: Bone metabolism in systemic mastocytosis. *J Bone Joint Surgery* 63-A:665, 1981.
43. Hirschowitz BI, Groarke JF: Effect of cimetidine on gastric hypersecretion and diarrhea in systemic mastocytosis. *Ann Int Med* 90:769, 1979
44. Horner HH: Macromolecular heparin from rat skin. Isolation, characterization and depolymerizations with ascorbate. *J Biol Chem* 246:231, 1971
45. Ishizaka T, Adachi T, Chang T-H, Ishizaka K: Development of mast cells *in vitro* II. Biologic function of cultured mast cells. *J Immunol* 118:211, 1977
46. Johnson AR, Moran NC: Selective release of histamine from rat mast cells by compound 48/80 and antigen. *Am J Physiol* 216:453, 1969
47. Johnson AR, Hugli TE, Muller-Eberhard HJ: Release of histamine from rat mast cells by the complement peptides C$_{3a}$ and C$_{5a}$. *Immunology* 28:1067, 1975
48. Kaliner M, Sigler R, Summers R, Shelhamer J: Effects of infused histamine: analysis of the effects of H-1 and H-2 histamine receptor antagonists on cardiovascular and pulmonary responses. *J Allergy Clin Immunol* 68:365, 1981
49. Keller R, Hess MW, Riley FJ: Mast cells in the skin of normal, hairless and athymic mice. *Experientia* 32:171, 1976
50. Kitamura Y, Shimada M, Go S, Matsuda H, Hatanaka K, Seki M: Distribution of mast cell precursors in hematopoietic and lymphopoietic tissues of mice. *J Exp Med* 150:482, 1979
51. Kitamura Y, Yokoyama M, Matsuda H, Ohno T: Spleen colony forming cell as a common precursor for tissue mast cells. *Nature* 291:159, 1981
52. Lagunoff D: Structural aspects of histamine binding: the mast cell granule. In: Mechanisms of Release of Biogenic Amines, p. 79. von Euler US, Rosell S and Uvnas B, eds. Pergamon Press, Oxford. 1966
53. Lagunoff D: Contributions of electron microscopy to the study of mast cells. *J Invest Derm* 58:296, 1972
54. MacGlashan DW Jr, Schleimer RP, Peters SP, Schulman ES, Adams GK III, Newball HH, Lichtenstein LM: Generation of leukotrienes by purified human lung mast cells. *J Clin Invest* 70:747, 1982
55. Majno G, Gilmore V, Leventhal M: On the mechanism of vascular leakage caused by histamine-type mediators. *Circ Res* 21:833, 1967
56. Metcalfe DD, Klehanoff SJ, Henderson WR: Oxidative degradation of rat mast cell haparin proteoglycan. *Fed Proc* 43:1806, 1984
57. Metzger H, Bach MK: The receptor for IgE on mast cells and basophils: studies on IgE binding and on the structure of the receptor. In: Immediate Hypersensitivity - Modern Concepts and Developments, p. 561. Bach MK, Ed. Marcel Dekker, New York. 1978
58. Mikhail GR, Miller-Milinska A: Mast cell population in human skin. *J Invest Dermatol* 43:279, 1964
59. Morishima T: 5-Hydroxy tryptamine (serotonin) and 5-hydroxytryptophan in mast cells in human mastocytosis. *Tohoku J Exp Med* 102:121, 1970
60. Nettleship E: Rare forms of urticaria. *Brit Med J* 2:323, 1869
61. Norris HT, Zamcheck N, Gottlieb L: The presence and distri-

bution of mast cells in the human gastrointestinal tract at autopsy. *Gastroenterology* 44:448, 1963

62. Oates JA, Marsh E, Sjoerdsma A: Studies on histamine in human urine using a fluorometric method of assay. *Clin Chim Acta* 7:488, 1962

63. Ouwendijk RJT, Zijlstra FJ, Wilson JHP, Bonta IL, Vincent JE, Stolz E: Raised plasma levels of thromboxane B_2 in systemic mastocytosis. *Eur J Clin Invest* 13:227, 1983

64. Parker F, Odland GF: The mastocytosis syndrome. Chapter 87, In: Dermatology in General Medicine, Fitzpatrick TK, Eisen AZ and Wolff K et al. (Eds), McGraw-Hill, New York, 1979

65. Razin E, Mencia-Huerta, J-M, Stevens RL, Lewis RA, Liv F-T, Corey EJ, Austen KF: IgE-mediated release of leukotriene C_4, chrondroitin sulfate E proteoglycan, B-hexosaminadase, and histamine from cultured bone marrow-derived mouse mast cells. *J Exp Med* 157:189, 1983

66. Riley JF, West GB: Mast cells and histamine in normal and pathological tissues. *J Physiol* 119:44, 1953

67. Roberts LJ, Lewis RA, Oates JA, Austen KF: Prostaglandin, thromboxane and 12-hydroxy-5,8,10,14-eicosatetraenoic acid production by ionophore-stimulated rat serosal mast cells. *Biochim Biophys Acta* 575:185, 1979

68. Roberts LJ II, Sweetman BJ, Lewis RA, Austen KF, Oates JA: Increased production of prostaglandin D_2 in patients with systemic mastocytosis. *New Eng J Med* 303:1400, 1980

69. Rothwell TLW, Dineen JK: Cellular reactions in guinea pigs following primary and challenge infection with *Trichostrongylus colubriformis* with special reference to the roles played by eosinophils and basophils in the rejection of the parasite. *Immunol* 22:733, 1972

70. Sagher F, Even-Paz Z: Mastocytosis and the Mast Cell. Year Book Medical Publishers, Inc., Chicago. 1967

71. Lucaya J, Perez-Candela V, Aso C, Calvo J: Mastocytosis with skeletal and gastrointestinal involvement in infancy. Two case reports and a review of the literature. *Radiology* 131:363, 1979

72. Sher A: Complement-dependent adherence of mast cells to schistosomula. *Nature* 263:334, 1976

73. Schultz HF, Code CF, Brunsting LA: Blood histamine and basophil-eosinophil counts in skin diseases. *Arch Derm* 80:44, 1959

74. Soter NA, Austen KF, Wasserman SI: Oral disodium cromoglycate in the treatment of systemic mastocytosis. *New Engl J Med* 301:465, 1979

75. Szweda JA, Abraham JP, Fine G, Nixon RK, Rupe CE: Systemic mast cell disease. A review and report of three cases. *Am J Med* 32:227, 1962

76. Uvnas B: Chemistry and storage function of mast cell granules. *J Invest Dermatol* 71:76, 1978

77. van Kammen E: Generalized mastocytosis. *Acta Haemat* 52:129, 1974

78. Weiler JM, Yurt RW, Fearon DT, Austen KF: Modulation of the formation of the amplification convertase of complement C_3b, Bb by native and commercial heparin. *J Exp Med* 147:409, 1978

79. Wesley Fr, Vinik AI, O'Dorisio TM, Glaser B, Fink A: A new syndrome of symptomatic cutaneous mastocytosis producing vasoactive intestinal polypeptide. *Gastroenterology* 82:963, 1982

80. Yurt RW, Leid RW, Austen KF, Silbert JE: Native heparin from rat peritoneal mast cells. *J Biol Chem* 252:518, 1977

81. Yurt RW, Leid RW, Spragy J, Austen KF: Immunologic release of heparin from purified rat peritoneal mast cells. *J Immunol* 118:1201, 1977

82. Zachariae H: Histamine: Spectrofluorometric studies on normal and diseased skin. Munksgaard, Copenhagen, 1965

83. Zeiger RS, Colten HR: Histaminase release from human eosinophils. *J Immunol* 118:540, 1977

84. Zeiger RS, Twarog FJ, Colten HR: Histaminase release from human granulocytes. *J Exp Med* 144:1049, 1976

HISTIOCYTIC TUMORS: IMMUNOLOGIC CLASSIFICATION

SHAW WATANABE

HETEROGENEITY OF HISTIOCYTES

The term "histiocytes" was first proposed by Kiyono (53) and Aschoff (3). They distinguished myeloid cells, lymphoid cells and histiocytes in terms of phagocytosis of *in vivo* administered lithium carmine. Histiocytes with active phagocytic ability are now considered to be derived from bone marrow monocytes as described later, but their fetal development still needs experimental elucidation. Fetal differentiation of histiocytes from fetal mesenchymal cells in the yolk sac was studied by Kiyono, and he observed that histioid cells showed transition between primitive endothelial cells and mononuclear lymphoid cells. This very early stage of hematopoiesis has not yet been studied by modern immunological methods, therefore the possibility that these primitive histioid cells could migrate to the whole body and stay there as facultative histiocytes should be reexamined, because phagocytic cells play an important role for organogenesis during fetal development, and usually these cells appear earlier than the complete development of myeloid cells and early hepatic hematogenesis mainly produces erythrocytes (105).

After Aschoff proposed the concept of the reticuloendothelial system (RES) in 1924 by categorizing cells with strong phagocytic ability, the origin of histiocytes was considered to be reticulum cells which were considered to be pluripotent stem cells of hematolymphoid cells, resembling the concept of primitive mesenchymal cells proposed by Maximow in 1924 (68). The condition of proliferation of reticulum cells and their derivatives was called reticuloen-

dotheliosis or reticulosis, and the neoplastic proliferation was termed reticulum cell sarcoma (80). The terminology for proliferative disorders of histiocytes would not be comprehensible without this historical background (Table 1).

On the other hand, the term "macrophage", which was first proposed by Metschnikoff (70), who distinguished two kinds of phagocytic cells, microphage and macrophage, has been widely used mainly in the field of immunology. Studies on experimentally collected macrophages clarified their origin, turnover, population size, etc. (17, 23, 97), and blood monocytes are now candidates for the role of precursor cells of these macrophages, and a cell line from monoblasts in the bone marrow to macrophages in the tissue via monocytes in the bloodstream is called the mononuclear phagocytic system or monocyte-macrophage system (MPS) (95, 100).

They have common characters, as listed in Table 2 (35, 36, 38, 42, 60, 67, 83, 87, 111), but several differences are also recognized. The macrophages are usually distinguished by the site where they are, i.e., peritoneal macrophages, alveolar macrophages, splenic macrophages, Kupffer cells and tissue macrophages (histiocytes). Their function seems to vary slightly according to site. For example, splenic macrophages show strong erythrophagocytosis but peritoneal macrophages do not, alveolar macrophages phagocytize many sphingolipid (myeline figures), Kupffer cells have many worm-like structures on their surface, etc.

Recent work on macrophage heterogeneity has revealed several problems in terms of different phenotypes of macrophage populations, whether they correspond to different maturation stages in a single cell lineage, or multiple lineages

Table 1. Changes in terminology used in regard to histiocytic proliferative disorders and their probable cell origin.

Old terms	Present disease entity	Phenotype
Leukemic reticuloendotheliosis	Hairy cell leukemia	? B/mono
	Monocytic leukemia	monocyte
Aleukemic reticuloendotheliosis	Letterer–Siwe disease	T-zone histiocyte
Reticulosis		
	Eosinophilic granuloma	T-zone histiocyte
Malignant reticulosis	Histiocytic medullary reticulosis	
	(Robb-Smith)	T-zone histiocyte
	Malignant histiocytosis	
	(Rappaport)	various
	(Isaacson)	tissue macrophage
	Histiocytic sarcoma	various
Reticulosarcoma	T-malignant lymphoma	T-lymphocyte
	B-malignant lymphoma	B-lymphocyte

K.W. Brunson (ed) Local invasion and spread of cancer.

Table 2. Macrophage heterogeneity.

| | ϕ | Immunohistochemical reactivity | | | | | |
		OKM1	NCA	Lys	S100	T6	Others
Monoblast	−	+ +	+	+	−	−	
Monocyte	+ +	+ +	+ +	+ +	−	−	$Ia^{+/-}$, Fc receptor, C3 receptor
Tissue macrophages							
Splenic (red pulp)	+ +	+	+	+ +	−	−	Erythrophagocytosis
Peritoneal	+ +	+ / −	+	+ +	−	−	
Alveolar	+ +	+ / −	+	+ +	−	−	Anthracosis, Myelin-like inclusion
Kupffer	+	+ / −	+	+	−	−	Worm-like structure
Specific histiocytes							
(T-zone histiocytes)							
Interdigitating cells in lymph node, spleen, thymus	−	−	−	−	+	+ +	ATPase +
Langerhans cells	−	−	−	−	+	+ +	Birbeck granules

ϕ: phagocytosis; Lys: lysozyme.

with a different differentiation pathway (4, 96, 97). Many problems have been proposed from the basis of human oncology, for example, cells in malignant histiocytosis do not always have markers of MPS (69, 108).

We found that special kind of histiocytes, such as Langerhans cells in the epidermis, interdigitating cells in the lymph nodes, spleen and thymic medulla were stained with anti-S100 protein antibody, but not with anti-lysozyme or anti-NCA antibodies which are the common markers of MPS (Fig. 1) (14, 22, 32, 72, 93, 105, 106, 108). They also have T6 antigen on their surface, which is considered to be specific for immature thymic T-lymphocytes (Fig. 2) (29, 77, 107). These histiocytes are first recognized in fetal life by immunohistochemical methods in the thymic medulla at the end of the third month of gestation and they spread to the peripheral lymphoid organs in accordance with the homing of T-lymphocytes (105). They seem to be independent of MPS, which show different distribution in the liver, red pulp of the spleen and other connective tissues. We termed them T-zone histiocytes because of their intimate relationship with T-lymphocytes and their preferred location in T cell dependent areas in normal lymphoid tissues. As the term "Langerhans cells" is defined by the presence of Birbeck granules confirmed by an electron microscopy (11), a term

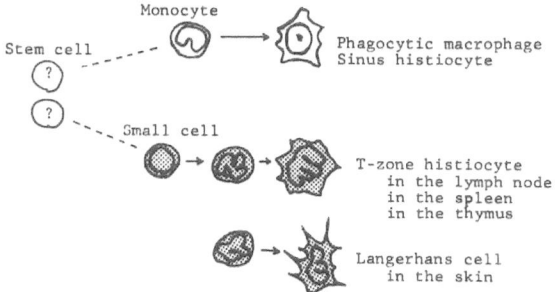

Figure 1. A hypothesis of dual histiocytic cell lines. Upper cell line is characterized by the phenotype of $100^- lysozyme^{-+}NCA^+$, while the other $S100^+ lysozyme^- NCA^-$.

"T-zone histiocytes" is convenient to summarize cells, which are called by different names including their precursors.

Furthermore, many histiocytoma cells in the connective tissues do not fit the definition of cells in MPS (30, 52). In such occasion, the presence of facultative histiocytes in the mesenchymal cells is preferable. Hairy cell leukemia, which usually shows both immunoglobulin production and phagocytic ability (18), suggests the presence of phagocytic cells derived from B-lymphocytes. Actually, pre-B lymphoma cells are transformed to typical macrophages by 5-azacytidine treatment in *in vitro* experiment (12).

As described above, a multiple lineage hypothesis of histiocytes seems to more easily explain the nature of neoplastic histiocytes and facilitates the categorization of these disorders (Table 3).

HISTIOCYTOSIS X

The neoplastic conditions of histiocytes are not well understood (7, 21, 33, 51, 108). The borderline between the neoplasm and hyperplasia is often obscure. Histologic findings of malignancy are not necessarily related to prognosis. One such example is histiocytosis X, which includes Letterer–Siwe disease, Hand–Schuller–Christian disease and eosinophilic granuloma of the bone (62, 63).

Letterer–Siwe disease (59, 89) is characterized by cutaneous infiltration of histiocytes (Fig. 3). Infiltrating cells are often unicellular, and mitotic figures are sometimes frequent, but chromosome analysis usually reveal normal diploid histogram. The presence of Birbeck granules in these cells has suggested their relationship to Langerhans cells in the epidermis (16, 74, 86). Visceral organs, such as spleen, liver, bone marrow, lymph nodes, thymus are also involved and pulmonary infiltration often becomes a cause of death (88, 89).

When the skin lesion becomes chronic, it makes granulomatous lesions often aggregating around the skin appendages and dermal vessels (2). Eosinophils, lymphocytes or macrophages are occasionally associated with the lesion. Xanthoma cells and multinuclear giant cells are often inter-

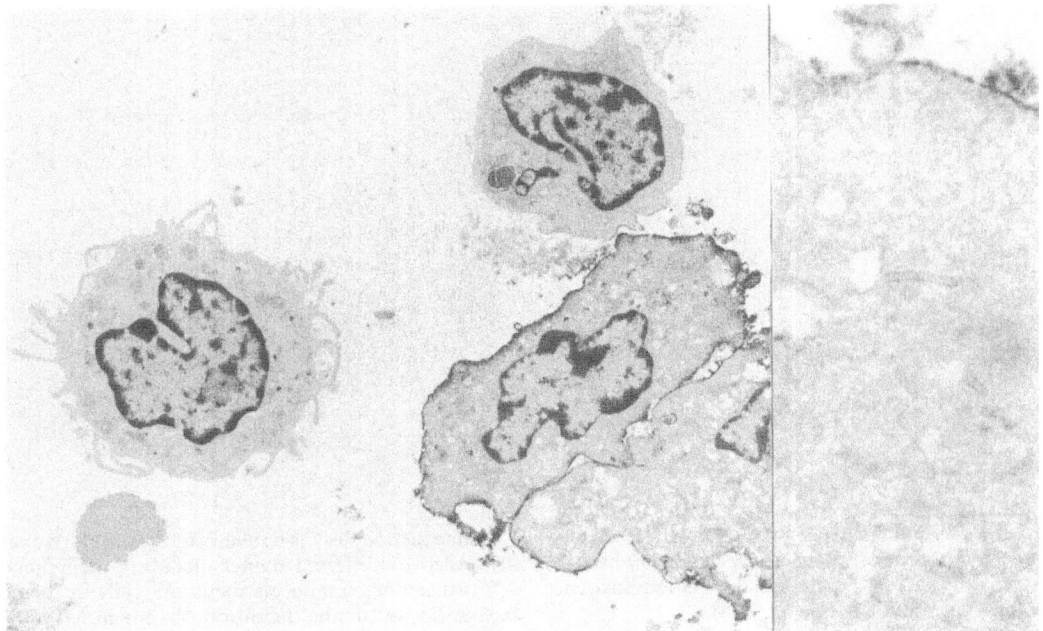

Figure 2. T6⁺ T-zone histiocytes and macrophages in the alveolar space. Birbeck granules are present in the cytoplasm of T-zone histiocytes. Immunohistochemical stain with OKT6 monoclonal antibody. × 6,000 (× 30,000 inset).

mingled, but Touton type giant cells, which are common in xanthoma disseminatum, are not present in the lesion.

Multifocal eosinophilic granuloma (Hand–Schuller–Christian disease) is characterized by more solid infiltration of histiocytes in the skull, vertebrae, ribs or other flat bones, internal ears, skin and rarely in visceral organs (Fig. 4). When the hypophysis is involved, the classical triad of diabetes insipidus, exophthalmos and bone defects appears (112). Transition and/or overlapping of clinical manifestation are often present between the Letterer–Siwe disease and multifocal eosinophilic granuloma. These findings suggest the same origin of cells in Letterer–Siwe disease and multifocal eosinophilic granuloma.

Solitary eosinophilic granuloma usually develops in long

bones in older people, although the infiltrating cells show the same character as the former two. These three diseases have been summarized under the term "histiocytosis X", but there have been recent proposals to divide them, because of their different clinical manifestation and prognosis (33, 54, 64, 76).

Cell suspensions from the lesion of histiocytosis X usually contain both T6-positive and T6-negative histiocytes. T6+ cells take the form of dendritic cells, and stained with anti-S100 protein antibody, and T6−cells appear as S100 − typical macrophages after short term culture (Fig. 5). Presence of Fc receptors is considered to relate to erythrophagocytic ability (57, 75).

Proliferating cells in most cases show characteristics of

Table 3. Relationship between various histiocytic proliferation and neoplasms by cell lineage.

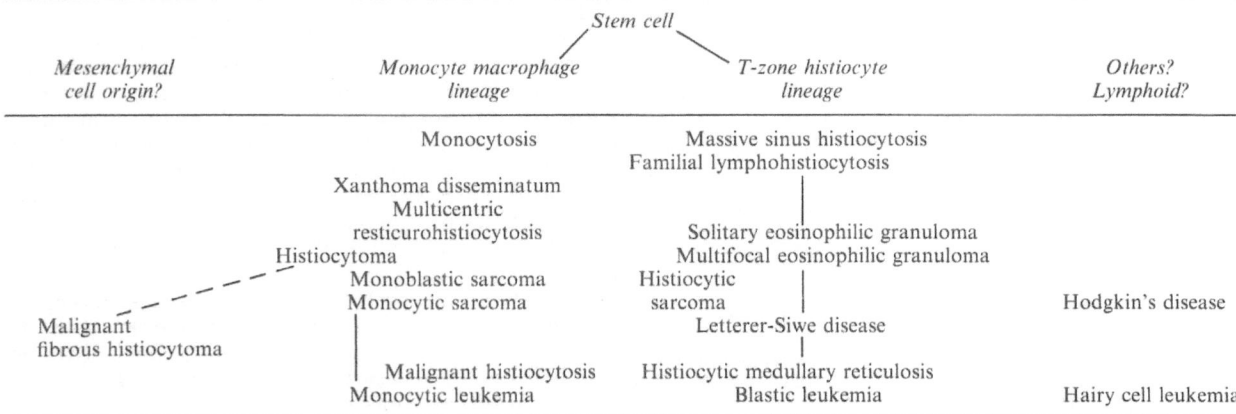

Mesenchymal cell origin?	Monocyte macrophage lineage	*Stem cell*	T-zone histiocyte lineage	Others? Lymphoid?
	Monocytosis		Massive sinus histiocytosis	
			Familial lymphohistiocytosis	
	Xanthoma disseminatum			
	Multicentric			
	resticurohistiocytosis		Solitary eosinophilic granuloma	
Histiocytoma			Multifocal eosinophilic granuloma	
	Monoblastic sarcoma		Histiocytic	
	Monocytic sarcoma		sarcoma	Hodgkin's disease
Malignant fibrous histiocytoma			Letterer-Siwe disease	
	Malignant histiocytosis		Histiocytic medullary reticulosis	
	Monocytic leukemia		Blastic leukemia	Hairy cell leukemia

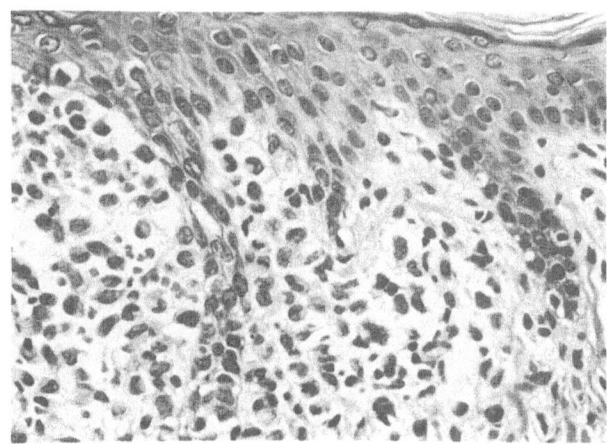

Figure 3. Skin lesion of Letterer–Siwe disease. Diffuse monomorphic infiltration of histiocytes is noted. Mitotic figures are frequent. H&E, × 400.

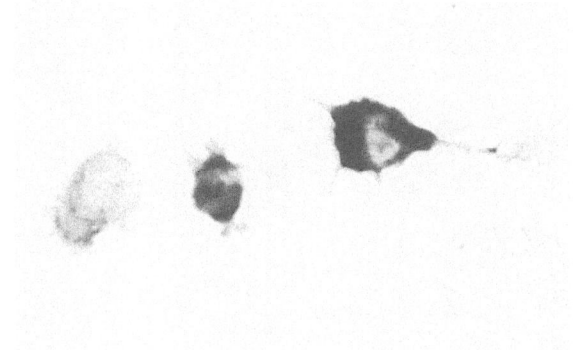

Figure 5. Cell suspension of multifocal eosinophilic granuloma. Dendritic cells stain with anti-S100 protein antibody, while typical macrophage does not. PAP-immunostain with anti-S100 protein antibody. × 400.

T-zone histiocytes, but a few cases (probably less than one-tenth) of multifocal eosinophilic granuloma reveal a MPS character. These cases show a better prognosis, even though they have diabetes insipidus. In this regard, both diseases should be distinguished, although their clinical manifestation is similar.

The causative agent of histiocytosis X has not been known. Infection at birth during the passage of the baby is considered by the fact of highly preferential site of the lesion in the skull. However, this hypothesis could not explain the racial difference of occurrence of histiocytosis X. So, the study on the distribution of histiocytes in late fetal life may be necessary to know the possibility of congenital abnormal overgrowth like self-heating neuroblastoma in the baby.

Eosinophilic granulomas of the lymph node, lung, stomach or in soft tissue (Kimura's disease) are often considered to be disorders related to histiocytosis X, but these conditions usually occur in adults and seem to be more reactive in nature. So they have to be treated under the separate entity from histiocytosis X (6, 8, 9, 41, 71, 101, 108).

MALIGNANT PROLIFERATION OF HISTIOCYTES

Malignant histiocytosis

Immunologic marker studies on histiocytic tumors reveals their heterogeneity. Rappaport (78) discards the term "reticulosis" and distinguishes (1) the reactive histiocytic proliferation that occurs in response to known infectious agents or as the result of metabolic disturbances, (2) the systemic proliferation of neoplastic, morphologically malignant histiocytes and their precursors (malignant histiocytosis), and (3) the systemic proliferation of differentiated histiocytes that are characteristic of Letterer–Siwe disease and Hand–Schuller–Christian disease. After his report, malignant histiocytosis has become a popular term, but this disease entity includes the rather broad proliferative

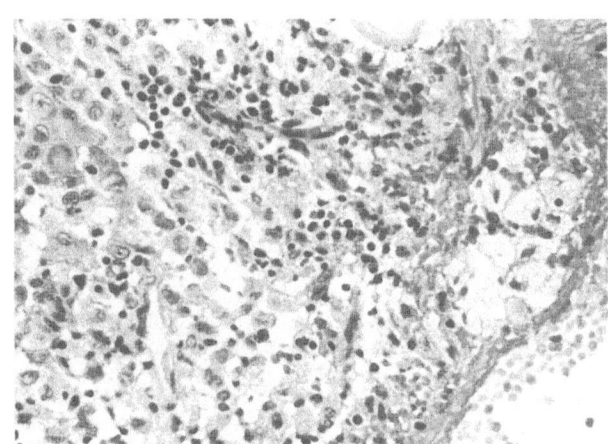

Figure 4. Granulomatous lesion in bone marrow with multifocal eosinophilic granuloma. In addition to the histiocytic aggregates, xanthoma cells are noted in the right of picture. H&E, × 400.

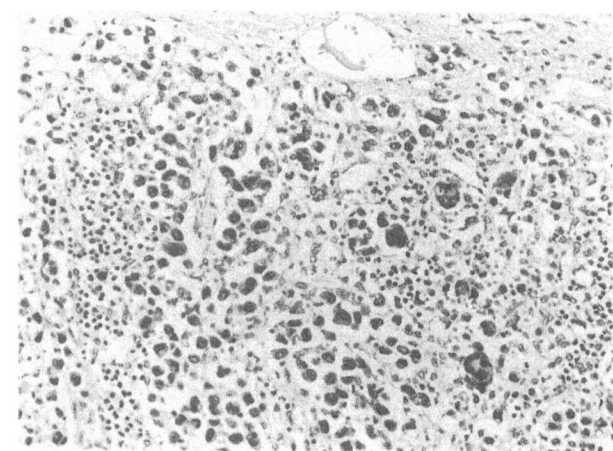

Figure 6. Histiocytic medullary reticulosis. Atypical histiocytes infiltrate in the lymphatic sinuses of the lymph node. Phagocytosis of large neoplastic cells is noted. H&E, × 200.

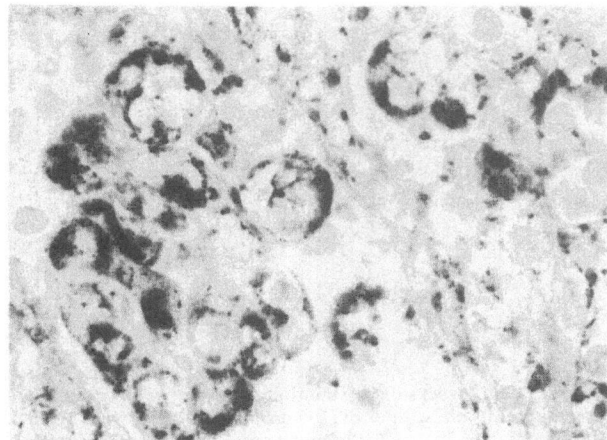

Figure 7. Histiocytic medullary reticulosis. Erythrophagocytic histiocytes in the spleen reveal strong activity of 5'nucleotidase. Enzyme histochemistry. × 800.

stage of histiocytes with neoplastic features, in contrast to that of histiocytic medullary reticulosis (HMR) which seems to be a more distinct clinicopathological entity (81, 85). It is unfortunate that Rappaport used the term "histiocytic lymphoma" instead of reticulum cell sarcoma, because it becomes apparent that the so-called reticulum cell sarcoma is a lymphocyte neoplasm, except for very rare instances. Although there has been some confusion in this regard, solid proliferation of histiocytes should be dealt with within a concept of histiocytic tumors, unrelated to the lymphomas (92). According to the nosology of neoplasms, solid proliferation of histiocytes may be called histiocytic sarcoma, and diffuse infiltrative neoplasms may be called malignant histiocytosis.

Malignant histiocytosis of the Robb-Smith type is characterized by rapidly progressive anemia or pancytopenia due to erythrophagocytosis by proliferating histiocytes in the spleen, liver, bone marrow and lymph nodes (Fig. 6) (15, 24, 102). They show infiltrative growth, but destructive growth is also present in the portal area of the liver and/or lymphatic sinus of the lymph nodes. Most histiocytes show marked erythrophagia, but immature ones (prohistiocyte) without phagocytosis are often observed intermingled. They usually have round nuclei, different from the indented or twisted nuclei of histiocytosis X.

Neoplastic cells show strong activity of lysosomal enzyme, nucleotidase and ATPase (Fig. 7). They are stained with anti-S100 protein antibody and OKT6 monoclonal antibody, except for about one-tenth of the cases of our series, which show MPS character (69, 106). The difference between the two has not been clarified, but the oncogenic stimuli on the different lineages of histiocytes may provoke proliferation of different kind of cell clone.

HMR-like disorders are reported with viral or toxoplasma infection (19, 47, 61, 65, 79). They are distinguished from neoplastic growth by a more mature appearance of the histiocytes and less involvement of hepatosplenomegaly.

HMR is sometimes followed by T-lymphoblastic leukemia or blastic leukemia develops in the terminal stage (20,

37, 48, 84, 90, 91, 106). The presence of T-lymphoma suggests an intimate relationship between T-lymphocytes and phagocytic cells (45, 46). These phenomena may indicate an intimate relationship between the neoplastic cells and T-lymphocyte differentiation.

Familial lymphohistiocytosis or erythrophagocytic reticulohistiocytosis is considered related to HMR (10, 27, 31). Familial lymphohistiocytosis is an autosomal recessive disease characterized by fever, pancytopenia or lymphocytosis, and hepatosplenomegaly (43, 73). Farquhar *et al.* (27) considered this condition to be an infantile form of adult HMR. Two of our autopsy cases revealed proliferation of histiocytes in the spleen, liver, lymph nodes, bone marrow, ovaries, and pleura. The thymus was remarkably atrophic or hypoplastic and only the reticular framework was present. In this regard, it does not appear to have relationship to Letterer–Siwe disease, which usually shows a thymic mass due to infiltration of histiocytes, but is more closely related to HMR. The relationship between the familial lymphohistiocytosis, systemic Letterer–Siwe disease, infantile HMR and immunodeficient states should be examined as well as etiologic work (19). Increased triglycerids and normal cholesterol level, which may be caused by altered metabolism of histiocytes and seems to be indirectly related to the cause of disease, are reported in some patients (34, 56).

Malignant histiocytosis of the intestinal type, as reported by Isaacson *et al.* (39, 40) was characterized by the proliferation of histiocytes in the intestinal wall with resultant malabsorption syndrome (Figs. 8ab). The neoplastic cells contain lysozyme, α-1 anti-trypsin and α-1 anti-chemotrypsin, but not stained with anti-S100 protein antibody (103). Characteristic clinicopathological findings may form a distinct disease entity in histiocytic tumors.

Histiocytic sarcoma

The definition of histiocytic sarcoma has not been generally established and the acceptance or rejection of this concept is still under debate (92, 99). Occasional tumor formation in histiocytosis X, HMR, and monocytic leukemia is present. However, they are neoplasms primarily showing diffuse infiltrative growth patterns, so they are excluded from histiocytic sarcoma (1, 24, 66, 94, 104, 108, 110). Cases with terminal dissemination or leukemic change may be included as well as the relationship between the lymphoblastic lymphoma and its leukemic change.

Four tumorous conditions might be separable; i.e., monoblastic or monocytic sarcoma, histiocytic sarcoma of tissue macrophage or relevant cells, histiocytic sarcoma of T-zone histiocytes (interdigitating reticulum cell sarcoma as reported by Feltkamp *et al.*, in 1981 (28)), and morphologically histiocytic sarcoma of so far undetermined origin.

The first group usually occurs in young children as Lennert (58) reported, under the term histiocytic sarcoma, as blastic cell proliferation with lysozyme activity. They take a blastic form in childhood and a more mature form with a moderate amount of pale cytoplasm and medium-sized nuclei with some indentation in adults. These cases usually show high leukemic tendency. Bone marrow examination did not reveal proliferation of monocytic cells in the early stage or throughout the course, so these cases should be

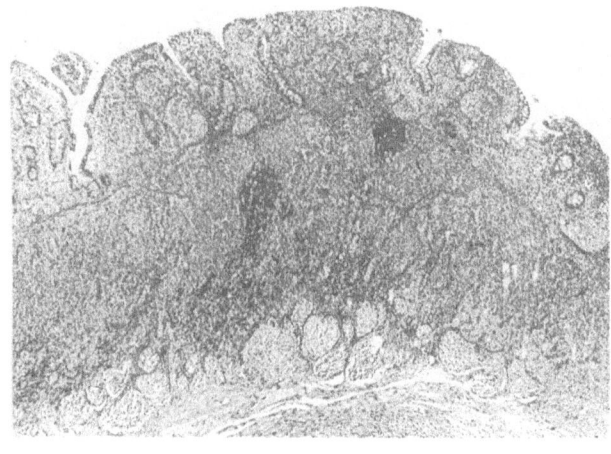

(a)

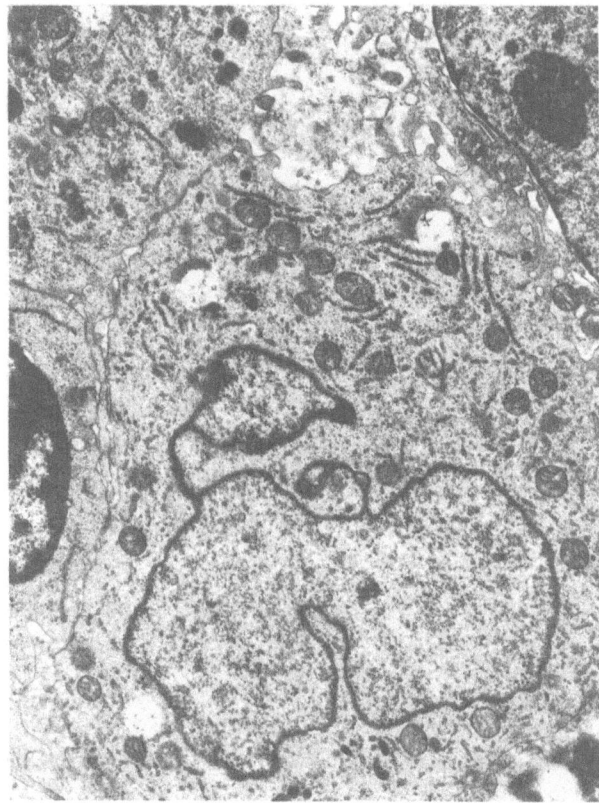

(b)

Figure 8. Malignant histiocytosis of the intestinal type. (a) Diffuse infiltration of histiocytes in the intestinal mucosa and emboli of histiocytes in the lymphatics is prominent. (b) Ultrastructurally neoplastic histiocytes have rich organelles, such as lysosomes, small mitochondria, short rough endoplasmic reticula, etc. (a) H&E, × 40, (b) × 10,000.

distinguished from monocytic leukemia originating in the bone marrow (50).

Neoplastic cells in the second group appeared to be more mature forms of tissue macrophages with abundant cytoplasm (Fig. 9) (25, 42). Tumorous growth of the third group is also rare, and we experienced only 4 cases. Tumor formation with monomorphic composition and atypical mitoses suggest their sarcomatous character (Fig. 10), (28, 108). Both the latter two groups show local growth, do not become leukemic, and are well controlled by irradiation and/ or combined chemotherapy, regardless of their malignant histologic features.

Assumptions that Reed-Sternberg cells of Hodgkin's diseases may derive from interdigitating cells of the lymph nodes may require consideration for inclusion in this category (26, 44). Van der Valk *et al.* (98) reported the presence of dendritic reticulum cell sarcoma of the lymph node, but their tumors seem to be composed of heterogeneous groups as described above.

The fourth group is morphologically histiocytic but lacks any detectable markers on paraffin section. They are often soft tissue tumors. In malignant fibrous histiocytoma cases, monomorphic proliferation of histiocytic cells are occasionally found (30, 109). Neoplastic cells usually stain for α-1 anti-chymotrypsin but lysozyme staining is exceptional.

Other more reliable markers of histiocytes are also negative. As their origin seemed to be different from MPS or T-zone histiocyte system, although some authors consider them tissue macrophages on the basis of the presence of α1-anti-chemotrypsin.

OTHER HISTIOCYTIC TUMORS OR HYPERPLASTIC REACTION OF HISTIOCYTES

There are many tumors considerably related to histiocytes in the field of dermatology (13). Among them histiocytes in xanthoma disseminatum and multicentric reticulohistiocytosis seems to belong to MPS by their immunohistochemical staining pattern (5). Secondary xanthoma to hyperlipidemia, such as xanthoma tuberosum, is also composed of cells of MPS.

Rather systemic proliferation of histiocytes is observed in massive sinus histiocytosis with lymphadenopathy (49, 55, 82). Cervical lymph node enlargement associated with fever, mild anemia, neutrophilia and hyperglobulinemia are usual clinical manifestations. Lymph node biopsy reveals marked infiltrates of histiocytes not only in the sinuses but also in paracortical area, as in the dermatopathic lymphadenopathy (Fig. 11). These histiocytes have abundant cytoplasm,

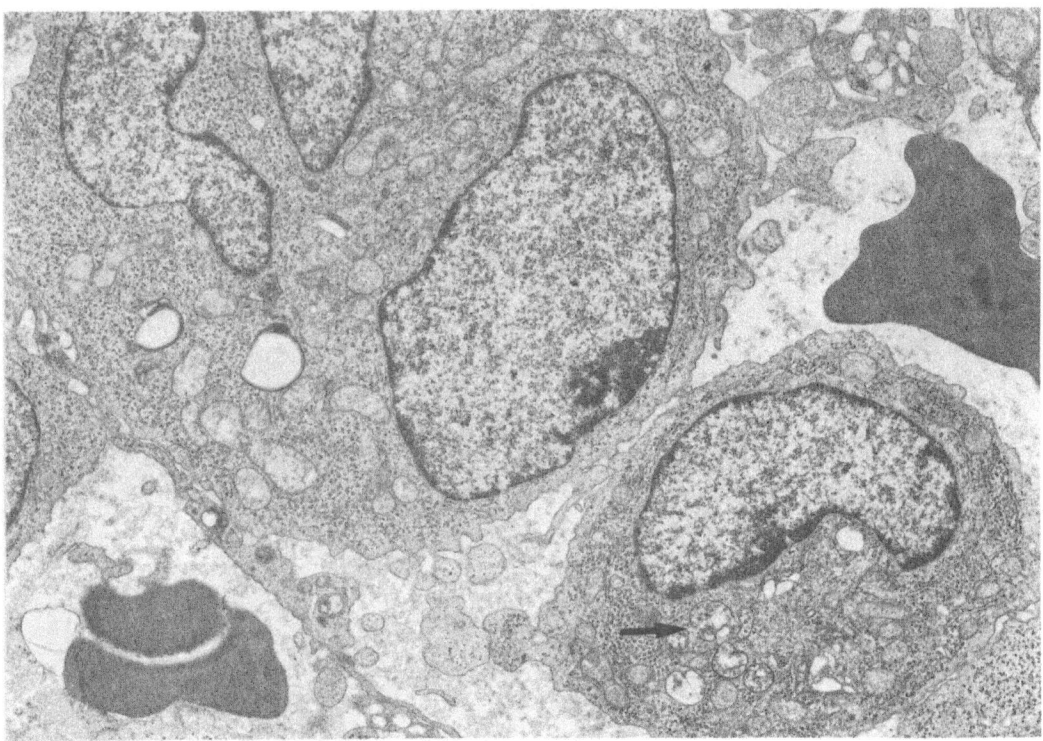

Figure 9. Histiocytic sarcoma of MPS origin. Cytoplasm of neoplastic cells is full of polyribosomes. Occasional phagosomes are noted (arrow). × 5,000.

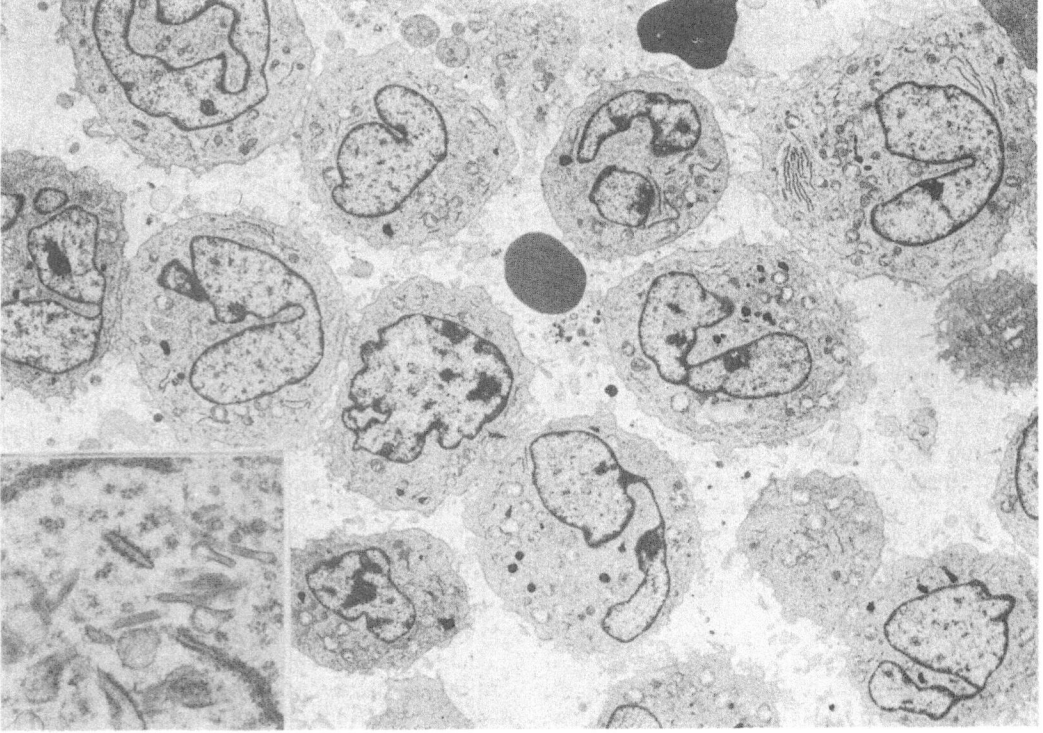

Figure 10. Histiocytic sarcoma of T-zone histiocyte origin. Infiltration of T-zone histiocytes is monomorphic and typical Birbeck granules are found in the cytoplasm (inset). × 2,700 (× 30,000 inset).

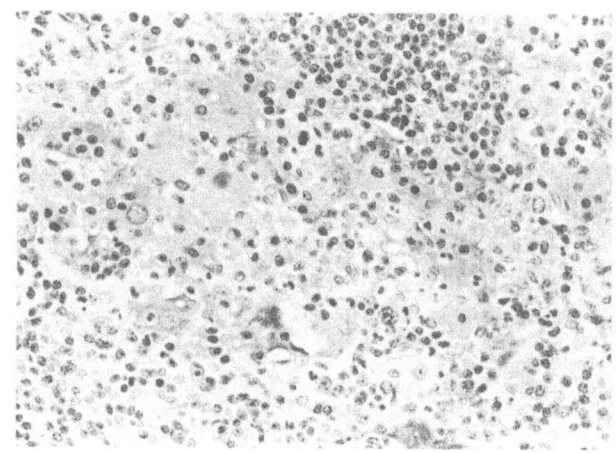

Figure 11. Massive sinus histiocytosis with lymphadenopathy. Infiltrating histiocytes stain with anti-S100 protein antibody, suggesting their T-zone histiocyte origin.

in which many lymphocytes are phagocytized, and small round nuclei. They stain with anti-S100 protein antibody but neither lysozyme nor NCA, so they belong to the T-zone histiocyte system. The possibility of special kind of infection is suspected, but further investigation is necessary.

CONCLUSION

Histiocytes play important roles in host defense mechanism by phagocytosis of foreign materials and antigen presentation for lymphocytes. Histiocytes or macrophages proliferate through these processes, so that proliferation of histiocytes is often hard to classify as reactive or neoplastic.

In experimental animals, histiocytic tumors comparable with humans are not yet known, except for monocytic leukemia. In this regard, it is important to find animal models for histiocytic tumors.

Complex heterogeneity of histiocytic proliferation may be better classified on the basis of a multiple lineage hypothesis by using multiple markers. Further examinations are necessary to know the characterization of cells for their neoplastic nature and condition of neoplastic change.

REFERENCES

1. Abele DC, Augusta GA, Griffin TB: Histiocytic medullary reticulosis. Report of two cases and review of the literature. *Arch Dermatol* 106:319, 1972
2. Altman J, Winkelmann RK: Xanthomatous cutaneous lesions of histiocytosis X. *Arch Dermatol* 87:164, 1963
3. Aschoff L: Das retikuloendotheliale System. *Erg Inn Med* 26:1, 1924
4. Bakker JM, de Witt AW, Daems WT: Haematology and Blood Transfusion 27, Disorders of the Monocyte Macrophage System, edited by Schmalzl F, Hohn D, Schaefer HE, Berlin Heidelberg, New York, Springer-Verlag, pp 79–87, 1981
5. Barrow MV, Holubar K: Multicentric reticulohistiocytosis. A review of 33 patients. *Medicine* 48:287, 1969
6. Basset F, Corrin B, Spencer H, Lacronique J, Roth C, Soler P, Battesti JP, Georges R, Chretien J: Pulmonary histiocytosis X. *Amer Rev Rep Dis* 118:811, 1978
7. Basset F, Nezelof C, Mallet R: Nouvelle mise en evidence par la microscopie electronique, de particules d'allure virale dans une second forme clinique de l'histiocytose X, le granulome eosinophile de l'os. *CR Acad Sci (Paris)* 261:5719, 1965
8. Basset F, Nezelof C, Ferrans VJ: The histiocytoses. In Pathology Annual 1983 Part 2, edited by Sommers SC, Rosen P, New York, Appleton-Century-Croft, 1983
9. Beatty EC Jr: Eosinophilic granuloma of parotid gland and thymus. *Am J Dis Child* 105:507, 1963
10. Berard CW, Cooper RA, Freireich EJ, Rabson AS: Disseminated histiocytosis associated with atypical lymphoid cells (lymphohistiocytosis). *Cancer* 19:1429, 1966
11. Birbeck MS, Breathnach AS, Everall JD: An electron microscopic study of basal melanocytes and high level clear cells (Langerhans cells) in vitiligo. *J Invest Dermatol* 37:51, 1961
12. Boyd AW, Schrader JW: Derivation of macrophage-like lines from the pre-B lymphoma ABLS8.1 using 5-azacytidine. *Nature* 297:691, 1982
13. Burgdorf WHC, Duray P, Rosai J: Immunohistochemical identification of lysozyme in cutaneous lesions of alleged histiocytic nature. *Am J Clin Pathol* 75:162, 1981
14. Burtin P, Quan PC, Savin MC: Nonspecific cross-reacting antigen as a marker for human polymorphs, macrophages, and monocytes. *Nature* 255:714, 1975
15. Byrne GE, Rappaport H: Malignant histiocytosis. Gann Monograph on Cancer Research 15, pp 145-, Tokyo, Tokyo University Press, 1973
16. Cancilla PA, Lahey ME, Carnes WH: Cutaneous lesions of Letterer–Siwe disease. Electron microscopic study. *Cancer* 20:1986, 1967
17. Carr I, Daems WT (eds): The Reticuloendothelial System. I Morphology. New York, London, Plenum Press, 1980
18. Catovsky D, Pettit JE, Galetto J, Okos A, Galton DAG: The B-lymphocyte nature of the hairy cell of leukemic reticuloendotheliosis. *Br J Haematol* 26:29, 1974
19. Cederbaum SD, Niwayama G, Stiehm ER, Neevhout RC, Amman AJ, Berman W Jr: Combined immunodeficiency presenting as the Letterer–Siwe syndrome. *J Pediat* 85:466, 1974
20. Clark BS, Dawson PJ: Histiocytic medullary reticulosis presenting with a leukemic blood picture. *Am J Med* 47:314, 1969
21. Cline MJ, Golde DW: A review and reevaluation of the histiocytic disorders. *Am J Med* 55:49, 1973
22. Cocchia D, Michetti F, Donato R: Immunochemical and immunocytochemical localization of S100 antigen in normal human skin. *Nature* 294:85, 1981
23. Cohn ZA: The activation of mononuclear phagocytes: Fact, fancy and future. *J Immunol* 121:813, 1978
24. Colby TV, Carrington CB, Mark GJ: Pulmonary involvement in malignant histiocytosis; a clinicopathologic spectrum. *Am J Surg Pathol* 5:61, 1981
25. Deura K, Ishii Z, Shimoyama M, Minato K, Matsuda M: A case of "monocytic sarcoma of the peritoneal type" with minimal involvement of the bone marrow, liver, spleen and lymph node. *Rinsho-Ketsueki* 19:372, 1978
26. Diehl V, Kircher HH, Burrichter H et al: Characteristics of Hodgkin derived cell lines. *Cancer Treat Rep* 66:615, 1982
27. Farquhar JW, MacGregor A, Richmond J: Familial hemophagocytic reticulosis. *Br Med J* 2:1561, 1958
28. Feltkamp CA, Van Heerde P, Feltkamp-Vroom TM, Koudstaal J: Malignant tumor arising from interdigitating cells. Light microscopic, ultrastructural, immuno- and enzyme histochemical characteristics. *Virchows Arch A (Pathol Anat)* 393:183, 1981
29. Fithian E, Kung P, Goldstein G, Rubenfeld M, Fenoglio C,

Edelson R: Reactivity of Langerhans cells with hybridoma antibody. *Proc Natl Acad Sci USA* 78:2541, 1981

30. Fu Y, Gabbiani G, Kaye GI, Lattes R: Malignant soft tissue tumors of probable histiocytic origin (malignant fibrous histiocytoma); general considerations and electron microscopic and tissue culture studies. *Cancer* 35:176, 1975

31. Goodall HB, Guthrie W, Buist NR: Familial hemophagocytic reticulosis. *Scot Med J* 10:425, 1965

32. Greenberger JS, Campos-Neto A, Parkman R, Moloney WC, Karpas A, Schlossman SF, Rosenthal DS: Immunologic detection of intracellular and cell-surface lysozyme with human and experimental leukemic leukocytes. *Clin Immunol Immunopathol* 8:318, 1977

33. Groopman JE, Golde DE: The histiocytic disorders: A pathophysiologic analysis. *Ann Intern Med* 94:95, 1981

34. Hagberg B, Hultquist G, Svennerholm L, Voss H: Malignant hyperlipemia in infancy. *Am J Dis Child* 107:267, 1964

35. Hayashi M, Nakajima Y, Fishman WH: The cytologic demonstration of β-glucoronidase employing naphthol AS-BI glucuronide and hexazonium pararosanilin, a preliminary report. *J Histochem Cytochem* 12:293, 1964

36. Huber H, Polley MH, Linscott WD, Fudenberg JJ, Muller-Eberhard HJ: Human monocytes: distinct receptor sites for the third component of complement and for immunoglobulin G. *Science* 162:1281, 1968

37. Imamura M, Sakamoto S, Hanazono H: Malignant histiocytosis: A case of generalized histiocytosis with infiltration of Langerhans granule-containing histiocytes. *Cancer* 28:467, 1971

38. Isaacson P, Jones DB, Millward-Sandler GH, Judd MA, Payne S: Alpha-1-antitrypsin in human macrophages. *J Clin Pathol* 34:982, 1981

39. Isaacson P, Wright DH: Malignant histiocytosis of the intestine. Its relationship to malabsorption and ulcerative jejunitis. *Human Pathol* 9:661, 1978

40. Isaacson P, Wright DH: Coeliac disease and malignant histiocytosis of the intestine (MHI). *Recent Adv Clin Oncol* 1:233, 1982

41. Ishikawa E, Tanaka H, Kakimoto S, Takasaki S, Kirino Y, Sakata A, Suzuki M: A pathologic study on eosinophilic lymphfolliculoid granuloma (Kimura's disease). *Acta Pathol Jpn* 31:767, 1981

42. Jaffe ES, Braylan RC, Nanba K, Frank MM, Berard CW: Functional markers: A new perspective on malignant lymphomas. *Cancer Treat Rep* 61:953, 1977

43. Janka GE, Belohradsky BH, Daumling S et al: Familial lymphohistiocytosis. In: Haematology and Blood Transfusion 27, Disorders of the Monocyte Macrophage System, edited by Schmalzl F, Huhn D, Schaefer HE, Berlin, Heidelberg, New York, Springer-Verlag, pp 245–253, 1981

44. Kadin ME: Possible origin of the Reed-Sternberg cell from an interdigitating cell. *Cancer Treat Rep* 66:601, 1982

45. Kadin ME: T gamma cells: A missing link between malignant histiocytosis and T-cell leukemia lymphoma? *Hum Pathol* 12:771, 1981a

46. Kadin ME, Kamoun M, Lamberg J: Erythrophagocytic Tγ lymphoma. A clinicopathologic entity resembling malignant histiocytosis. *New Engl J Med* 304:648, 1981b

47. Kalderon AE: Histiocytic medullary reticulosis associated with cytomegalic inclusion disease. *Cancer* 27:659, 1971

48. Karcher DS, Head DR, Mullins JD: Malignant histiocytosis occurring in patients with acute lymphocytic leukemia. *Cancer* 41:1967, 1978

49. Karpas A, Arno J, Cawley J: Sinus histiocytosis with massive lymphadenopathy – properties of cultured histiocytes. *Eur J Cancer* 9:729, 1973

50. Kass L, Schnitzer B: Monocytes, Monocytosis and Monocytic leukemia. Springfield, Illinois, Charles C Thomas, 1973

51. Kaufman A, Bukbery PR, Werlin S, Young IS: Multifocal eosinophilic granuloma ("Hand–Schuller–Christian disease"). Report illustrating H–S–C chronicity and diagnostic challenge. *Am J Med* 60:541, 1976

52. Kauffman SL, Stout AP: Histiocytic tumors (fibrous xanthoma and histiocytoma) in children. *Cancer* 14:469, 1961

53. Kiyono K: Die vitale Karminspeicherung. Jena, G. Fischer, 1914

54. Lahey ME: Histiocytosis X – an analysis of prognostic factor. *J Pediatr* 87:184, 1975

55. Lampert F, Lennert K: Sinus histiocytosis with massive lymphadenopathy. Fifteen new cases. *Cancer* 37:783, 1976

56. Landrieu P, Choulot JJ: Reticulose hemophagocytaire avec hypertriglyceridemie. *Arch Fr Pediatr* 33:497, 1976

57. Leikin S, Puruganan G, Frankel A, Steerman R, Chandra R: Immunologic parameters in histiocytosis X. *Cancer* 32:796, 1973

58. Lennert K: Malignant lymphomas other than Hodgkin's disease. In: Handbuch der Speziellen Pathologischen Anatomie und Histologie. Berlin, Springer-Verlag, 1978

59. Letterer E: Aleukämische Retikulose. *Frank Z Pathol* 30:377, 1924

60. Li CY, Yam LT, Crosby WH: Histochemical characterization of cellular and structural elements of the human spleen. *J Histochem Cytochem* 20:1049, 1972

61. Liao KT, Rosai J, Daneshbod K: Malignant histiocytosis with cutaneous involvement and eosinophilia. *Am J Clin Pathol* 57:438, 1972

62. Lichtenstein L: Histiocytosis X (eosinophilic granuloma of bone, Letterer–Siwe disease, and Schuller–Christian disease). *J Bone Joint Surg* 46A:76, 1964

63. Lichtenstein L, Jaffe HL: Eosinophilic granuloma of bone with report of a case. *Am J Pathol* 16:595, 1940

64. Lieberman PH, Jones CR, Dargeon HWK, Begg CF: A reappraisal of eosinophilic granuloma of bone, Hand–Schuller–Christian syndrome, and Letterer–Siwe syndrome. *Medicine* 48:375, 1969

65. Manoharan A, Catovsky D: Histiocytic medullary reticulosis, revisited. In: Haematology and Blood Transfusion 27. Disorders of the Monocyte Macrophage System, edited by Schmalzl F, Huhn D, Schaefer HE, Berlin, Heidelberg, New York, Springer-Verlag p 205, 1981

66. Marshall AH: Histiocytic medullary reticulosis. *J Pathol Bacteriol* 71:61, 1956

67. Mason DY, Taylor CR: The distribution of muramidase (lysozyme) in human tissues. *J Clin Pathol* 28:124, 1975

68. Maximow AA: Relation of blood cells to connective tissues and endothelium. *Physiol Rev* 4:533, 1924

69. Mendelsohn G, Eggleston JC, Mann RB: Relationship of lysozyme (muramidase) to histiocytic differentiation in malignant histiocytosis: an immunohistochemical study. *Cancer* 45:273, 1980

70. Metchnikoff E: Lecons sur la pathologie comparée de l'inflammation, edited by Masson G, Libraire de L'Academie de Médicine, 1892

71. Motoi M, Helbron D, Kaiserling E, Lennert K: Eosinophilic granuloma of lymph nodes – a variant of histiocytosis X. *Histopathol* 4:585, 1980

72. Nakajima T, Watanabe S, Shimosato Y, Ishihara K, Isobe T: Immunoelectron microscopic demonstration of S100 protein in epidermal Langerhans cells. *Biomed Res* 3:226, 1982

73. Nelson P, Santamaria A, Olson RL, Nayak NC: Generalized lymphohistiocytic infiltration. A familial disease not previously described and different from Letterer–Siwe disease and Chediak–Higashi syndrome. *Pediatrics* 27:931, 1961

74. Nezelof C, Basset F, Rousseau MF: Histiocytosis X. Histogenetic arguments for a Langerhans cell origin. *Biomedicine* 18:365, 1973

75. Nezelof C, Diebold N, Rousseau-Merck MF: Ig surface receptors and erythrophagocytic activity of histiocytosis X

cells *in vitro. J Pathol* 122:105, 1977

76. Otani S: A discussion on eosinophilic granuloma of bone, Letterer–Siwe disease, and Schuller–Christian disease. *J Mount Sinai Hosp* 24:1079, 1957
77. Poppema S, Bhan AK, Reinherz EL, McCluskey RT, Schlossman SF: Distribution of "T"-cell subsets in human lymph nodes. *J Exp Med* 153:30, 1981
78. Rappaport H: Histiocytosis. In: Tumours of the Hematopoietic System. Armed Forces Institute of Pathology Fascicle 8, Washington, DC, pp 48–91, 1966
79. Risdal RJ, McKenna RW, Besbit ME, Krivit WK, Balfour HH Jr, Simmons RL, Brunning RD: Virus-associated hemophagocytic syndrome. A benign histiocytic proliferation distinct from malignant histiocytosis. *Cancer* 44:993, 1979
80. Robb-Smith AHT: Reticulosis and reticulosarcoma: A histologic classification. *J Pathol Bacteriol* 47:457, 1938
81. Robb-Smith AHT, Taylor CR: In Lymph Node Biopsy, London, Miller Heyden, pp 127–135, 1981
82. Rosai J, Dorfman RF: Sinus histiocytosis with massive lymphadenopathy: a pseudolymphomatous benign disorder. Analysis of 34 cases. *Cancer* 30:1174, 1972
83. Rowden G: Expression of Ia antigen on Langerhans cells in mice, guinea pigs, and man. *J Invest Dermatol* 75:22, 1980
84. Schreiner DP: Acute lymphocytic leukemia terminating as histiocytic medullary reticulosis. *JAMA* 231:838, 1975
85. Scott RB, Robb-Smith AHT: Histiocytic medullary reticulosis. *Lancet* 2:194, 1939
86. Shamato M: Langerhans cell granule in Letterer–Siwe disease. An electron microscopic study. *Cancer* 26:1102, 1970
87. Shnitka TK, Seligman AM: Role of esteractic inhibition on localization of esterase and the simultaneous cytochemical demonstration of inhibitor sensitive or resistant enzyme species. *J Histochem Cytochem* 9:504, 1961
88. Sims DG: Histiocytosis X. Follow-up of 43 cases. *Arch Dis Child* 52:433, 1977
89. Siwe SA: Die Retikuloendotheliose – ein neues Krankeitsbild unter den Hepatosplenomegalien. *Z Kinderheilk* 55:212, 1933
90. Skarin AT, Karb K, Reynolds ES: Acute lymphoblastic leukemia terminating as histiocytic medullary reticulosis. *Arch Pathol* 93:256, 1972
91. Starkie CM, Kenny MW, Mann JR, Cameron AH, Hill FGH: Histiocytic medullary reticulosis following acute lymphoblastic leukemia. *Cancer* 47:537, 1981
92. Symposium on "histiocytic" or large cell lymphoma. In Malignant Lymphomas, A Pathology Annual Monograph, edited by Sommers SC, Rosen P, New York, Appleton-Century-Croft, 109–168, 1983
93. Takahashi K, Yamaguchi H, Ishizeki et al.: Immunohistochemical and immunoelectron microscopic localization of S100 protein in the interdigitating reticulum cells of the lymph node. *Virchows Arch (Cell Pathol)* 37:125, 1981
94. Taunton OD, Yeshurun D, Jarratt M: Progressive nodular histiocytoma. *Arch Dermatol* 114:1505, 1982
95. Thomas ED, Ramberg RE, Sale GE, Sparkes RS, Golde DW: Direct evidence for a bone marrow origin of the alveolar macrophage in man. *Science* 192:1016, 1976
96. Thorbecke GJ, Silberberg-Sinakin I, Flotte TJ: Langerhans cells as macrophages in skin and lymphoid organs. *J Invest Dermatol* 75:32, 1980
97. Unaue ER (ed): The regulatory role of macrophages in antigenic stimulation. *Adv Immunol* 31:1, 1981
98. Van der Valk P, Ruiter DJ, Den Ottolander GJ, TeVelde J, Spaander PJ, Meijer CJ: Dendritic reticulum cell sarcoma? Four cases of a lymphoma probably derived from dendritic reticulum cells of the follicular compartment. *Histopathology* 6:269, 1982
99. Van der Valk P, TeVelde J, Jansen J, Ruiter DJ, Spaander PJ, Cornelisse CJ, Meijer CJ: Malignant lymphoma or true histiocytic sarcoma. A morphological, ultrastructural, immunological, cytochemical, and clinical study of 10 cases. *Virchows Arch A (Pathol Anat)* 391:249, 1981
100. Van Furth R: Macrophage activity and clinical immunology. Origin and kinetics of mononuclear phagocytes. *Ann NY Acad Sci* 278:161, 1976
101. Vazquerz JJ, Ayestaran JR: Eosinophilic granuloma of the stomach similar to that of bone. *Virchows Arch (Pathol Anat)* 366:107, 1975
102. Warnke RA, Kim H, Dorfman RF: Malignant histiocytosis (histiocytic medullary reticulosis). I. Clinicopathologic study of 29 cases. *Cancer* 35:215, 1975
103. Watanabe S, Hirota T, Shimosato Y, Ito A, Zeze F, Hojo K: Unusual histiocytic tumor of the small intestine. *Human Pathol* 11:289, 1980
104. Watanabe S, Mikata A, Toyama K, Kitamura K, Minato K: Sarcomatous variant of malignant histiocytosis. A case report and review of the literature. *Acta Pathol Jpn* 28:963, 1978
105. Watanabe S, Nakajima T, Shimosato Y, Shimamura K, Sakuma H: T-zone histiocytes with S100 protein: Distribution and development in human fetuses. *Acta Pathol Jpn* 33:15, 1983
106. Watanabe S, Nakajima T, Shimosato Y, Shimizu K: Malignant histiocytes and Letterer–Siwe disease. Neoplasms of T-zone histiocytes with S100 protein. *Cancer* 51:1412, 1983
107. Watanabe S, Sato Y, Kodama T, Shimosato Y: Immunohistochemical study on immune reaction of human lung cancer. *Cancer Res*, 43(12 ptl) 5883, 1983
108. Watanabe S, Shimosato Y, Nakajima T: Proliferative disorders of histiocytes. *Pathol Ann Monograph*, edited by Sommers SC, Rosen P, New York, Appleton-Century-Croft, pp 65–108, 1983
109. Weiss SW, Enzinger FM: Malignant fibrous histiocytoma. An analysis of 200 cases. *Cancer* 41:2250, 1978
110. Wolfson WL, Gossett T, Pagani J: Systemic giant cell histiocytosis. Report of a case and review of the adult form of Letterer–Siwe disease. *Cancer* 38:2529, 1976
111. Yam LT, Li CY, Crosby WH: Cytochemical identification of monocytes and granulocytes. *Am J Clin Pathol* 55:283, 1971
112. Zinkham WH: Multifocal eosinophilic granuloma: Natural history, etiology, and management. *Am J Med* 60:457, 1976

UPDATED REFERENCES

1. Furukawa T, Watanabe S, Kodama T, et al.: T-zone histiocytes in adenocarcinoma of the lung in relation to postoperative prognosis. *Cancer* 56:2651–2656, 1985
2. Ishii E, Watanabe S: Biochemistry and biology of the Langerhans cell. *Hematolgoy/Oncology Clinics of North America.* 1:99–118, 1987
3. Roholl PJ, Kleyne J, Prins ME, et al.: Immunologic marker analysis of normal and malignant histiocytes. A comparative study of monoclonal antibodies for diagnostic purposes. *Am J Clin Pathol* 89: 187–94, 1988
4. Sheibani K, Burke JS, Swartz WG, et al.: Monocytoid B-cell lymphoma. Clinicopathologic study of 21 cases of a unique type of low-grade lymphoma. *Cancer* 62:1531, 1988
5. van der Valk P, Meijer CJ: The histology of reactive lymph nodes. *Am J Surg Pathol* 11:866–82, 1987

14

EOSINOPHILIC GRANULOMA

WILLIAM R. HENDERSON and EMIL Y. CHI

STRUCTURE AND FUNCTION OF EOSINOPHILS

Closely associated with mast cells in areas of allergic reactions are eosinophils. Mast cell secretory products may attract eosinophils at inflammatory sites of mast cell activation. Histamine (6) and the lipoxygenase product of arachidonic acid, leukotriene B_4 (12, 32) are examples of mast cell derived factors which are potent chemoattractants for eosinophils.

Production of eosinophils in the bone marrow is T lymphocyte dependent (4). After release from the marrow, eosinophilic leukocytes egress from the blood and pass primarily into epithelial tissues (skin, respiratory and gastrointestinal tracts and uterus) where they may reside for several days.

DEGRANULATION

When eosinophils are stimulated by soluble or particulate stimuli (such as opsonized zymosan) there is an increase in oxygen consumption (respiratory burst) with production of superoxide anion and hydrogen peroxide (2, 27).

Activation of eosinophils also induces characteristic secretory changes. Eosinophils have large cytoplasmic granules which contain a crystalloid body in most species (Figs. 1 and 2). The crystalloid body which contains major basic protein (14) is surrounded by a peroxidase-containing granule matrix (Fig. 3) (3).

Eosinophils obtained from patients with eosinophilia differ ultrastructurally from cells obtained from normal individuals. Cells from eosinophilic patients often appear vacuolated when viewed by light microscopy (38) because of intragranular vacuoles seen by transmission electron microscopy (Fig. 1b). Eosinophils from patients with the hypereosinophilic syndrome (HES) contain fewer and smaller granules than normal cells. Some HES patients' cells contain large cytoplasmic structures similar to Charcot-Leyden crystals (Fig. 1b).

Phagocytes of particles by eosinophils (Fig. 4) leads to the release of peroxidase and other granule constituents into a phagocytic vacuole (8) and also extracellularly (1). Bacteria are killed as a consequence of the peroxidase oxidative

system activated by eosinophils during phagocytosis. The degranulation process of calcium ionophore A23187-stimulated horse and human eosinophils (21, 22) differs from that induced by phagocytosis and is similar to that observed in mast cells (Fig. 5). Eosinophil degranulation is characterized by fusion of granules, with loss of granule density and the formation of large intracellular vacuoles which communicate with the cell exterior through surface pores. Intact granule matrices are not observed within these cytoplasmic vacuoles suggesting that the granule material dissolves completely and is secreted (Fig. 5b).

CYTOTOXIC ACTIVITY

Elevated levels of eosinophils are found both circulating and in the tissues of patients with a variety of tumors (4). Eosinophilia is found in Hodgkin's disease, mycosis fungoides, Sézary syndrome, acute lymphoblastic leukemia and in some carcinomas (mucin secreting carcinomas of epithelial origin). *In vitro* studies have shown that activated eosinophils can kill mammalian tumor cells with cytotoxicity mediated by the peroxidase oxidative system (25). Mast cells and eosinophils may interact to form mast cell granule-eosinophil peroxidase complexes (see chapter on systemic mastocytosis) in areas of inflammation around tumors to play a role in the host defense against malignancies (20). Eosinophils are also found in increased numbers in various parasitic infestations. Eosinophils accumulate in areas of tissue invasion by helminthic parasites and bind to the surface of parasite targets in the presence of antibody and/or complement *in vitro* (Fig. 6). Eosinophils also cause morphologic damage and death to helminthic larvae (e.g. *Trichinella spiralis*, *Schistosoma mansoni*). Eosinophilia is found clinically in helminthic parasite infections where there is tissue invasion by helminths such as in schistosomiasis, filariasis, trichinosis and strongyloidiasis.

LEUKOTRIENE FORMATION

Allergic asthma is thought to result from IgE-mediated mast cell degranulation with release of chemical mediators of hypersensitivity and eosinophils are a prominent cellular constituent of immediate hypersensitivity reactions. Eosinophilia is commonly seen in patients with bronchial asthma (4), where a rise in circulating eosinophils has been associated with a deterioration of pulmonary function and an

Supported in part by National Institutes of Health grant AI17758. William R. Henderson is the recipient of Allergic Diseases Academic Award AI00487 from the National Institutes of Allergy and Infectious Diseases.

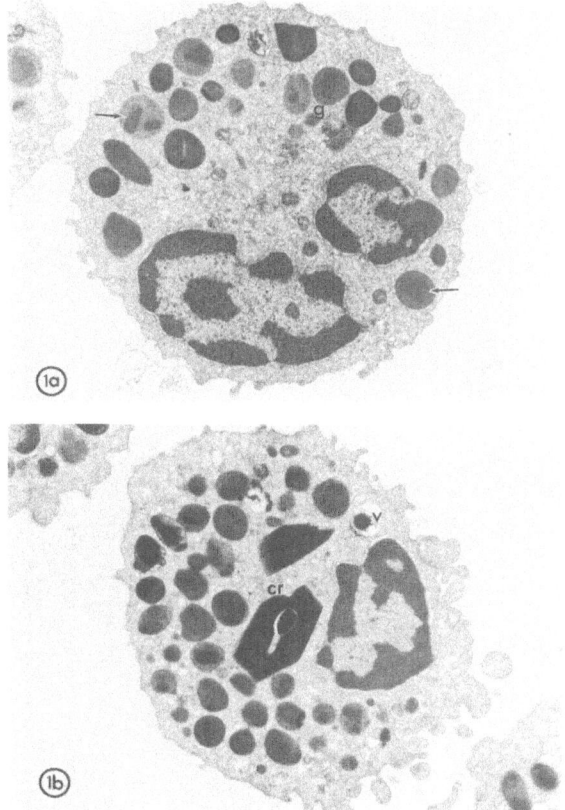

Figure 1. Human circulating eosinophils. Transmission electron microscopy of eosinophils obtained from the peripheral blood of a normal individual (a; × 16,000) and a patient with the hypereosinophilic syndrome (HES) (b; × 14,000). The normal cell seen in (a) shows the characteristic large, oval to round, membrane bound cytoplasmic granules (g) with central crystalloid cores (arrows). Eosinophils have the usual array of cytoplasmic organelles, including mitochondria and Golgi vesicles and have the typical multilobed nucleus of polymorphonuclear leukocytes. In contrast, HES eosinophils, as seen in (b), often have large crystalloid (cr) cytoplasmic structures similar to Charcot-Leyden crystals. Vacuolated granules (v) are also often noted in HES cells.

increase in clinical symptoms (24). Eosinophils may play an important role in asthma by their formation of sulfidopeptide leukotrienes C_4 and D_4 (19, 23) which are the slow reacting substance (SRS) of anaphylaxis that have potent bronchoconstrictive activity. Leukotriene SRS activity may be modulated by peroxidase and/or hydroxyl radical mediated inactivation of leukotrienes by eosinophils as well as other phagocytes (17–19).

HYPEREOSINOPHILIC DISORDERS

Other diseases, not previously mentioned, that are characterized by hypereosinophilia include immunodeficiency disorders (hyper-IgE syndrome, Wiscott-Aldrich syndrome and selective IgA deficiency), connective tissue disorders (Churg-Strauss syndrome of systemic necrotizing vasculitis,

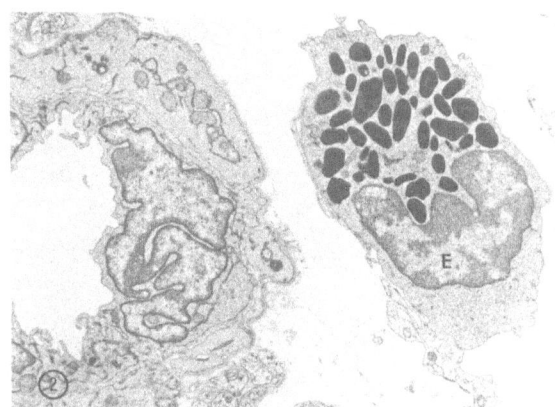

Figure 2. Tissue eosinophil. Submucosal eosinophil (E) present in the ileum of a guinea pig and examined by transmission electron microscopy (× 10,600). This eosinophil which has migrated to the tissues has an elongated, spreading shape in contrast to the round (spherical) shape of the circulating normal eosinophil seen in Fig. 1a. The guinea pig eosinophil granules are primarily oval in shape and contain prominent crystalloid core material.

eosinophilic fasciitis), skin diseases (dermatitis herpetiformis, atopic dermatitis, pemphigus and drug reactions) and pulmonary disorders (bronchopulmonary aspergillosis, eosinophilic pneumonia and Löffler's syndrome) (4). Tissue injury may result when high levels of circulating eosinophils persist for extended periods of time, as seen in the hypereosinophilic syndrome (HES). In this idiopathic disorder, patients have 1500 eosinophils/mm³ for a period of greater than 6 months without discernible cause but with evidence of organ system dysfunction (hepatosplenomegaly, cardiac and neurological involvement) related to the high levels of eosinophils (5, 11). Endocardial damage is particularly characteristic of the HES patients with resulting endomyocardial fibrosis leading to cardiomyopathy and congestive

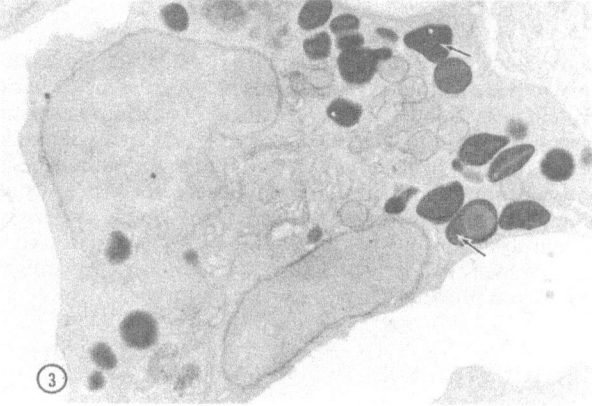

Figure 3. Eosinophil granule peroxidase. An eosinophil present in the peripheral lung tissue of a rabbit was examined for peroxidase activity by diaminobenzidine cytochemistry (× 22,000). The section was not counterstained with either lead or uranyl acetate. Eosinophil peroxidase is noted as the electron-dense material (arrows) in the matrix of the cytoplasmic granules. The crystalloid core of these granules does not react for peroxidase activity.

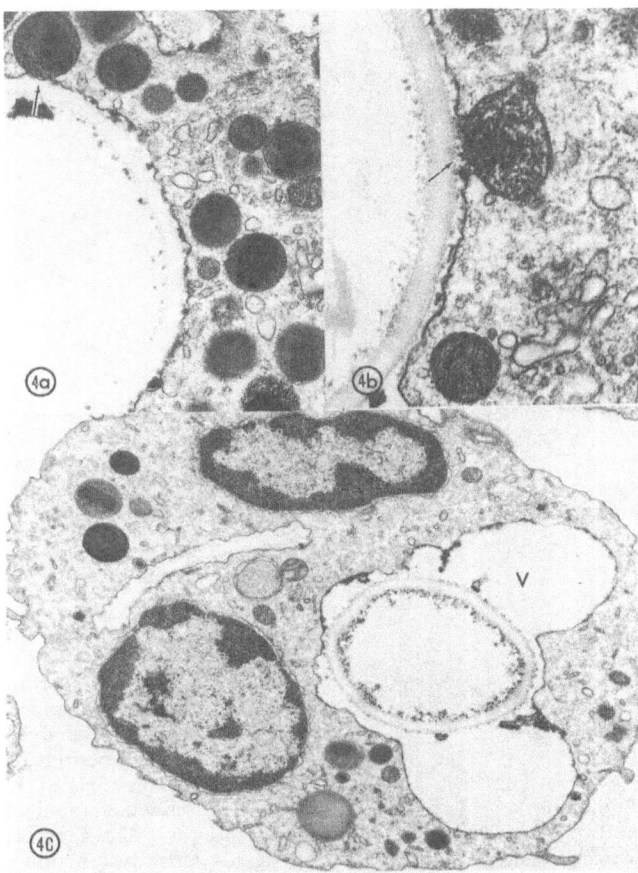

Figure 4. Eosinophil phagocytosis of zymosan particles. Human eosinophils were incubated with zymosan particles (1 mg/ml) in buffer at 37°C for 5 min (a; × 40,000, b; × 52,500) or 20 min (c; × 21,000). In (a), there is fusion (arrow) of the perigranular membrane on the surface of the ingested zymosan particle. In (b), granule contents (arrow) are discharged onto the surface of the zymosan particle as seen by the decrease in electron density of the granule which has fused with the phagolysosome. In (c), a zymosan particle is seen within a large phagocytic vacuole (v). These vacuoles contain peroxidase-positive material by diaminobenzidine cytochemistry (not shown).

heart failure (10, 11). Tissue damage is thought to be secondary to release of toxic granule enzymes such as major basic protein, eosinophil cationic protein and peroxidase enzyme systems. Other chemical mediators released by eosinophils such as the leukotrienes may be involved in the pathogenesis of tissue injury. Therapy of HES patients consists initially of prednisone in individuals with evidence of progressive organ system dysfunction with the addition of a cytotoxic agent such as hydroxyurea if prednisone alone does not control the disease process (11, 36).

HISTIOCYTOSIS X

Eosinophilic granuloma

Histiocytosis X constitutes a triad of clinical conditions: eosinophilic granuloma, Hand–Schuller–Christian disease and Letterer–Siwe disease, in which there is a proliferation of histiocytes and eosinophils. The most limited form of this syndrome, eosinophilic granuloma, is characterized by an

eosinophilic infiltration of a granuloma in bone (29, 35). It presents most commonly in children as swelling or pain of a solitary bone although multiple bones may also be involved (31). Multifocal eosinophilic granuloma can involve many other organ sites including the lungs (30), gastrointestinal tract and lymph nodes (15). Solitary pulmonary lesions can occur without skeletal or visceral involvement (9). The etiology of eosinophilic granuloma is unknown, and cultures of affected tissues have failed to identify an infectious agent.

Eosinophilic granuloma characteristically involves the metaphyseal and/or diaphyseal regions of long bones whereas in osteomyelitis there is typically epiphyseal involvement (31). Eosinophilic granuloma appears as osteolytic lesions radiologically secondary to destruction of the bony trabeculae by the cellular proliferation (31).

Histologically, variable numbers of eosinophils and histiocytes are found in the granuloma; plasma cells, neutrophils and lymphocytes may also be noted. Hemorrhagic necrosis of blood vessels can occur in the granuloma. The infiltrating histiocytes are often multinucleated and may be Langerhans' cells (33). The bone marrow derived Langer-

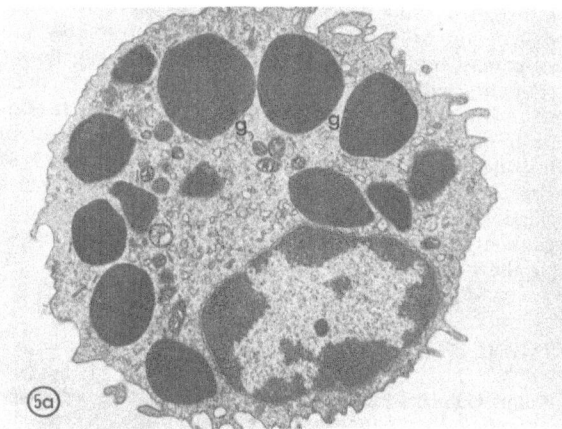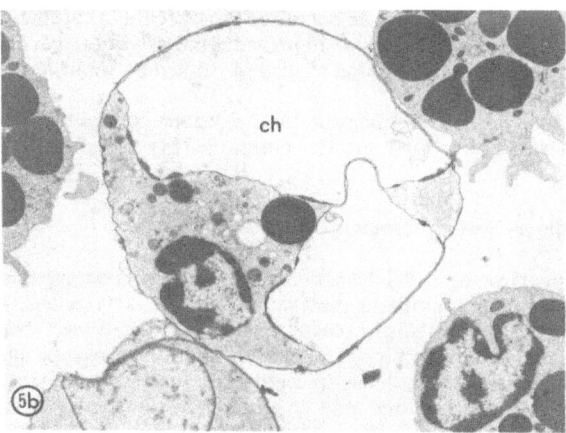

Figure 5. Eosinophil degranulation. Horse eosinophils were incubated in buffer alone (a; × 10,000) or with 10 µg/ml concentration of the calcium ionophore A23187 (b; × 9,000) for 15 min at 37°C. As seen in (a), horse eosinophils have very large cytoplasmic granules (g) of uniform electron density. No central crystalloid core material is seen in contrast to human eosinophil granules shown in Fig. 1a. In (b), eosinophil degranulation is characterized by the formation of large intracytoplasmic channels (ch) into which granule contents are released. These channels communicate with the extracellular environment through surface pores (not shown) for extracellular release of granule contents.

hans' cells which are similar to macrophages in their functional properties, are specifically identified by the presence of T6 surface antigens. Mouse monoclonal antihuman T6 antigen IgG has been used to detect Langerhans' cells by immunofluorescent techniques in biopsy material of an eosinophilic granuloma involving a vertebral body (13). Histiocytic cells containing the distinctive Birbeck granules characteristic of Langerhans' cells have also been noted in lesions from a patient with multifocal eosinophilic granuloma (26).

An experimental model of pulmonary eosinophilic granuloma has been developed in rabbits (16). Endobronchial injection of mycobacterial constituents were found to induce pulmonary granulomas without eosinophilic infiltration.

Addition of long chain fatty acids, in particular arachidonic acid, to the instillation produced a prominent eosinophilic infiltration. Eosinophils were noted to infiltrate the lesions by migration through arteriolar walls. The infiltration was inhibited by aspirin treatment of the animals suggesting involvement of a cyclooxygenase product of arachidonic acid as mediating this influx of eosinophils; PGE_2 was the most potent prostaglandin examined in inducing infiltration (16). How eosinophils are attracted to the sites of these granulomas in man is unknown as is whether eosinophils are directly involved in the pathogenesis of these lesions. Eosinophil production of leukotrienes could be expected to increase vascular permeability in granulomas and release of granule enzyme products such as major basic protein and

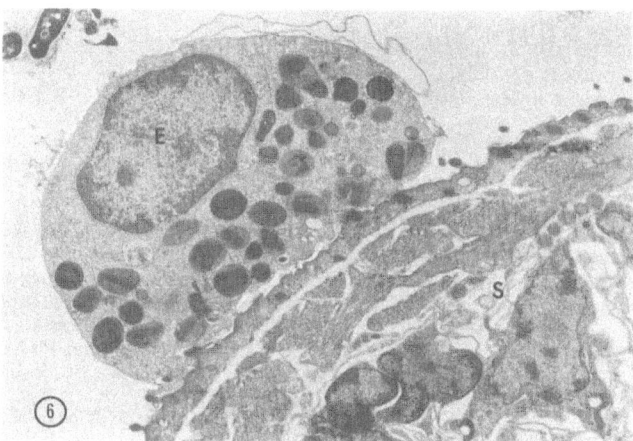

Figure 6. Eosinophil-helminth interaction. Normal human eosinophils were incubated with schistosomula of *Schistosoma mansoni* in buffer containing fresh normal human serum and heated human immune (antischistosomular) serum for 1 min and examined by transmission electron microscopy (× 12,000). Adherence of the eosinophil (E) to the tegumental surface of the schistosomula (S) is seen. Degranulation of the eosinophil with release of granule contents such as peroxidase on the surface of the helminth occurs as a consequence of this interaction (not shown).

peroxidase could induce significant extracellular cytotoxicity. Lipids released from damaged tissues would then be phagocytosed by the macrophage-histiocytes found at the granuloma site.

Unifocal eosinophilic granuloma lesions commonly heal either spontaneously or after curettage (31).

Letterer–Siwe syndrome

Approximately 10% of patients with eosinophilic granuloma develop multifocal disease (31). In the acute disseminated form of this disease termed Letterer–Siwe, there occurs an infiltration of moderately well differentiated histiocytes in the skin, liver, spleen, lymph nodes and bones (7, 28, 37). These lesions may be similiar histologically to the well differentiated form of reticulum cell sarcoma and have variable numbers of infiltrating eosinophils. This acute form occurs usually in children less than 2 years of age and is often complicated by a bleeding diathesis and infections. Letterer–Siwe disease has occurred in identical twins and is associated with an increased incidence of mental retardation and associated congenital developmental anomalies (15). This syndrome has a progressive and frequently fatal course.

Hand–Schuller–Christian syndrome

Surviving Letterer–Siwe patients may develop the chronic disseminated form of Histiocytosis X termed Hand–Schuller–Christian disease (Hand, 1921; 7). This chronic phase may also occur as a consequence of a unifocal eosinophilic granuloma without development of the acute disseminated phase. These patients are most commonly children under four years of age and often present with otitis media. Other characteristic features of this disease are large destructive bony lesions (involvement of the calvarium, sinuses, mastoid bones and mandible), hypopituitarism, exophthalmous and skin involvement. Lymphadenopathy and hepatosplenomegaly may also be present. The histiocytes found in Hand–Schuller–Christian disease sometimes have a foamy appearance and eosinophils are not a prominent participant in the inflammatory process (7). Usually this is a chronic disease with a fatal outcome in less than 15% of patients (7).

TREATMENT OF HISTIOCYTOSIS X

The treatment results of 127 patients with Histiocytosis X (multifocal eosinophilic granuloma, Letterer–Siwe disease and Hand–Schuller–Christian disease) seen at the Children's Cancer Research Foundation and Children's Hospital Medical Center in Boston from 1941 to 1975 have recently been reported (15). Patients older than 2 years at the time of diagnosis had a much better prognosis than younger patients (85% survival at 10 years compared to 42% by acturial analysis). Patients were staged for extent of disease involvement; those patients with disseminated disease and greater than 6 cm of palpable splenomegaly all died despite various combination chemotherapeutic regimens. Individuals with less extensive disease involvement had a much

better prognosis and were typically responsive to single cytotoxic agents or local radiation to prevent fractures and control pain of bone lesions or to reverse diabetes insipidus (15). Patients with less extensive disease also have been treated with thymic humoral factor (34). Of particular concern in the treatment of Histiocytosis X is that 5 patients in the Boston series who had received radiation therapy and cytotoxic drug therapy developed secondary malignancies (anaplastic thyroid carcinoma, acute undifferentiated leukemia, acute myelogenous leukemia, hepatocellular carcinoma and papillary-follicular thyroid carcinoma).

REFERENCES

1. Archer GT, Hirsch JG: Motion picture studies on degranulation of horse eosinophils during phagocytosis. *J Exp Med* 118:287, 1963
2. Baehner RL, Johnston RB Jr: Metabolic and bactericidal activities of human eosinophils. *Br J Haematol* 20:277, 1971
3. Bainton DF, Farquhar MG: Segregation and packaging of granule enzymes in eosinophilic leukocytes. *J Cell Biol* 45:54, 1970
4. Beeson P, Bass DA: In: The Eosinophil. Major Problems in Internal Medicine Series. WB Saunders Co., Philadelphia. Vol. 14, 1977
5. Chusid MJ, Dale DC, West BC, Wolff SM: The hypereosinophilic syndrome: analysis of fourteen cases with review of the literature. *Medicine* 54:1, 1975
6. Clark RAF, Gallin JI, Kaplan AP: The selective eosinophil chemotactic activity of histamine. *J Exp Med* 142:1462, 1975
7. Cline MJ, Golde DW: A review and reevaluation of the histiocytic disorders. *Amer J Med* 55:49, 1973
8. Cotran RS, Litt M: The entry of granule-associated peroxidase into the phagocytic vacuole of eosinophils. *J Exp Med* 129:1291, 1969
9. Cruthirds TP, Johnson HR: Solitary primary eosinophilic granuloma. *JAMA* 196:195, 1966
10. Davies JNP: Endocardial fibrosis in Africans. *East Afr Med J* 25:10, 1948
11. Fauci AS, Harley JB, Roberts WC, Ferrans VJ, Gralnick HR, Bjornson BH: The idiopathic hypereosinophilic syndrome. Clinical, pathophysiologic syndrome. *Ann Int Med* 97:79, 1982
12. Ford-Hutchinson AW, Bray MA, Doig MV, Shipley ME, Smith MJH: Leukotriene B, a potent chemokinetic and aggregating substance released from polymorphonuclear leukocytes. *Nature* 286:264, 1980
13. Fox JL, Berman B: T6-antigen-bearing cells in eosinophilic granuloma of bone. *JAMA* 249:3071, 1983
14. Gleich GJ, Loegering DA, Maldonado JE: Identification of a major basic protein. *J Exp Med* 137:1459, 1973
15. Greenberger JS, Crocker AC, Vawter G, Jaffe N, Cassady JR: Results of treatment of 127 patients with systemic histiocytosis (Letterer–Siwe syndrome, Schuller–Christian syndrome and multiple eosinophilic granulomal). *Medicine* 60:311, 1981
16. Hamamoto Y, Kinoshita K, Hashimoto K, Matsushita T, Kogishi K, Yasuhira K: Experimental production of pulmonary granulomas. IV. Eosinophilic granuloma. *Br J Exp Path* 64:177, 1983
17. Henderson WR, Klebanoff SJ: Leukotriene B_4, C_4, D_4 and E_4 inactivation by hydroxyl radicals. *Biochem Biophys Res Commun* 110:266, 1983a
18. Henderson WR, Klebanoff SJ: Leukotriene production and inactivation by normal, chronic granulomatous disease and myeloperoxidase-deficient neutrophils. *J Biol Chem* 258:13522, 1983b

19. Henderson WR, Jörg A, Klebanoff SJ: Eosinophil peroxidase-mediated inactivation of leukotrienes B$_4$, C$_4$ and D$_4$. *J Immunol* 128:2609, 1982

20. Henderson WR, Chi EY, Jong EC, Klebanoff SJ: Mast Cell mediated tumor cell cytotoxicity: role of the peroxidase system. *J Exp Med* 153:520, 1981

21. Henderson WR, Chi EY, Jörg A, Klebanoff SJ: Horse eosinophil degranulation induced by the ionophore A23187. Ultrastructure and role of phospholipase A$_2$. *Am J Path* 111:341, 1983

22. Henderson WR, Harley JB, Fauci AS, Chi EY: Hypereosinophilic syndrome human eosinophil degranulation induced by soluble and particulate stimuli. *Dr J Haematol* 69: 13, 1988

23. Henderson WR, Harley JB, Fauci AS: Arachidonic acid metabolism in normal and hypereosinophilic syndrome human eosinophils: generation of leukotrienes B$_4$, C$_4$, D$_4$ and 15-lipoxygenase products. *Immunology* 51: 679, 1984

24. Horn BR, Robin ED, Theodore J, Van Kessel A: Total eosinophil counts in the management of bronchial asthma. *N Engl J Med* 292:1152, 1975

25. Jong EC, Klebanoff SJ: Eosinophil-mediated mammalian tumor cell cytotoxicity: role of the peroxidase system. *J Immunol* 124:1949, 1980

26. Kato T, Matsuda M, Ando H, Sasaki H: A case of multifocal proliferations of histiocytic cells containing Langerhans' cell granules. *Amer J Clin Pathol* 76:480, 1981

27. Klebanoff SJ, Durack DT, Rosen H, Clark RA: Functional studies of human peritoneal eosinophils. *Infect Immun* 17:167, 1977

28. Letterer E: Aleukämische Reticulose (Ein Beitrag zu den proliferativen Erkrankungen des Retikuloendothelialapparates). *Frankfurt Z Path* 30:377, 1924

29. Lichtenstein L, Jaffe HL: Eosinophilic granuloma of bone. *Amer J Path* 16:595, 1940

30. Mazzitello WF: Eosinophilic granuloma of the lungs. *New Engl J Med* 250:804, 1954

31. Mirra JM: Bone tumors: Diagnosis and Treatment. Philadelphia, JB Lippincott Co, pp 376–391, 1980

32. Nagy L, Lee TH, Goetzl EJ, Pickett WC, Kay AB: Complement receptor enhancement and chemotaxis of human neutrophils and eosinophils by leukotrienes and other lipoxygenase products. *Clin Exp Immunol* 47:541, 1982

33. Nezelof C, Basset F, Rousseau MF: Histiocytosis-X: Histogenetic arguments for a Langerhans' cell origin. *Biomedicine* 18:365, 1973

34. Osband M, Lipton J, Lavin P, Levey R, Vawter G, Greenberger JS, McCaffrey RP, Parkman R: Histiocytosis-X: Demonstration of abnormal immunity, T-cell histamine H$_2$ receptor-deficiency and successful treatment with thymic extract. *N Engl J Med* 304:146, 1981

35. Otani S, Ehrlich JC: Solitary granuloma of bone simulating primary neoplasm. *Amer J Path* 16:479, 1940

36. Parillo JE, Fauci AS, Wolff SM: Therapy of hypereosinophilic syndrome. *Ann Int Med* 89:167, 1978

37. Siwe SA: Die Retikuloendotheliose–ein neues Krankheisbild unter den Hepatosplenomegalien. *Z Kinderheilk* 55:212, 1933

38. Tai P-C, Spry CJF: The mechanism which produce vacuolated and degranulated eosinophils. *Br J Haematol* 49:219, 1981

15

MALIGNANT LYMPHOMAS: IMMUNOLOGIC ASPECTS

SHAW WATANABE

Histologic classification of malignant lymphomas has been dramatically influenced by the application of immunological techniques for the characterization of neoplastic cells (1, 3, 12, 22, 23, 40, 41, 45, 61). Large neoplastic cells were interpreted as reticulum cells or histiocytes on the basis of histologic examinations several years ago, but these cells are now considered to be transformed lymphocytes by cell culture study and other cytologic experiments.

Lymphocytes with ability to produce immunoglobulins (Ig) are designated as B-lymphocytes and cells spontaneously forming rosettes with sheep erythrocytes (E+) are designated as T-lymphocytes (8). Recently developed monoclonal antibodies further characterize more detailed phenotypes of lymphocytes in various stages of differentiation and maturation in both reactive and neoplastic state (12, 30, 53).

B-CELL LYMPHOMAS

Rapidly accumulating data suggest that the neoplastic cells preserve their surface markers and immunologic functions in close relation to the differentiation and maturation of normal lymphoid cells (25, 62). Normal differentiation stages of B-lymphocytes and their markers can be represented schematically as in Fig. 1.

The preservation of Ig synthesis and receptors of neoplastic cells has been considered to resemble their parent cells which had become malignant at a certain stage of maturation. The representative neoplasms of B-lymphocytes are considered to be Burkitt's tumor, follicular lymphoma, large cell lymphoma or immunoblastic sarcoma and plasmacytoma. Leukemic forms of B-cells are acute lymphoblastic leukemia in childhood, chronic lymphocytic leukemia in the elderly and lymphosarcoma cell leukemia, which usually develops from follicular lymphoma composed of smaller cell type (medium-sized cell type).

This section describes recent lymphoma studies.

Burkitt's lymphoma

Since the Epstein-Barr virus (EBV) was isolated from Burkitt's lymphoma in 1964, this tumor has been considered to be the first human tumor caused by tumor-virus infection. However, later etiologic work failed to certify the direct relationship between EBV infection and tumorigenicity. Viral infection is considered to be the initiation of the tumor. Other promoting activities, such as malaria infection, are held to be necessary to cause actual tumors (29). However, lymphoblastoid cell lines obtained by infection of EBV B95-8 in normal lymphocytes can yield tumors in nude mice and some showed metastasis (59) (Fig. 2).

Burkitt's tumor is composed of monomorphic cells, medium to large in size, with relatively regular nuclear size and limited atypism (Fig. 3). Their nuclear chromatin is fine, and they are often called undifferentiated cells. The African Burkitt's tumor is frequent in the maxillary and mandibulary bones, but the non-African Burkitt's tumor occurs in

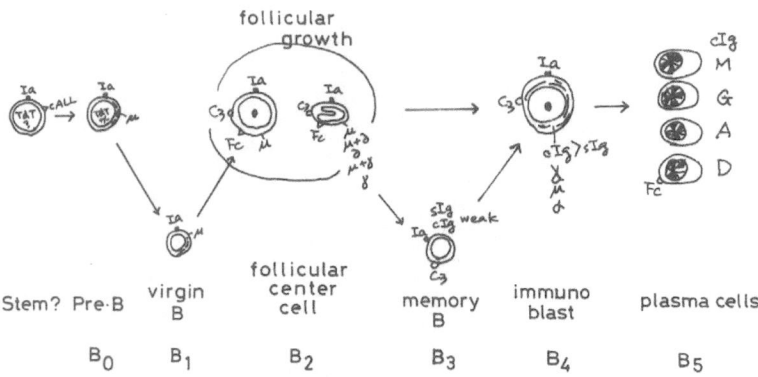

Figure 1. B-cell differentiation and maturation in relation to their surface markers and other functions. Follicular center cells, immunoblasts (progenitor cells of plasma cells) and plasma cells proliferate in the tissues, mainly in the peripheral lymphoid organ. Neoplastic change of other cells is usually represented as leukemia.

K.W. Brunson (ed) Local invasion and spread of cancer.
© 1989, Kluwer Academic Publishers, Dordrecht.

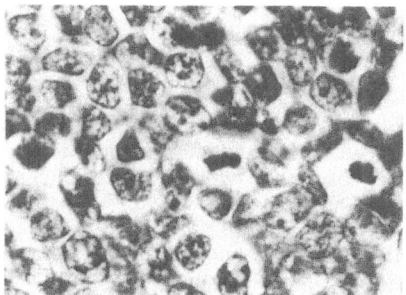

Figure 2. Tumor of lymphoblastoid cells transformed by EBV B95-8 strain in nude mice. H&E, × 800.

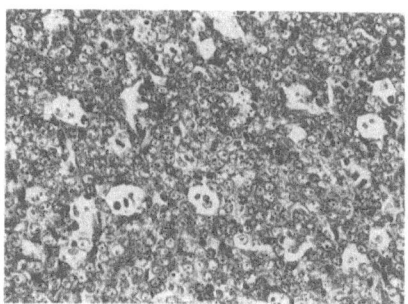

Figure 3. Burkitt's lymphoma of the ovary. Uniform proliferation of large cells with round nuclei and starry-sky arrangement of histiocytes are noted. H&E, × 330.

intestine, ovaries or other intraabdominal organs. High EBV titer is not necessarily found in these cases.

Most cases have μ-sIg and are considered to correspond pre-B or virgin B cells. Neoplastic cells rarely showed follicular growth in metastatic lesion.

Chromosome analysis reveals a very high frequency of translocation between chromosomes number 8 and 14, t(8;14)(q24;q32) (4, 9, 20, 38, 49). The band of 8q24 has been considered to be identical with c-*myc* viral oncogene. Other chromosome translocation, such as t(2;8)(q12;q24) or t(8;22)(q24;q11), are also reported, but 8q24 is concerned in all these cases. Lymphoma cells with t(2;8) express k chain, and those with t(8;22) express λ-chains. In this regard, Burkitt's tumor may in the future be more firmly defined by chromosome analysis.

Follicular lymphoma

Nodular (follicular) growth is considered to represent one of the definite histologically recognized stages of B-cell differentiation and/or maturation (54, 62). The cultured cell line of follicular lymphoma, as well as other lymphoblastoid cell lines with B-cell nature, shows ball-like growth (57). The reason for follicular growth has been obscure, but a high frequency of both Fc and C3 receptors compared to those of diffuse lymphomas of B-cell origin was reported.

Dominancy of μ chain, double production of $\mu + \gamma$ chain, and frequent expression of sIg rather than cIg coincide with the intrafollicular maturation of B-lymphocytes.

Neoplastic cells of follicular lymphomas have characteristic features, and Lukes divided them into cleaved and noncleaved cells (23). It is well known that follicular lymphoma changes its histology according to the progression of the disease (35). One of these is the diffuse change due to destructive and rapid growth of large cells resulting in the fusion of neoplastic follicles. Diffuse change can also be caused by infiltrative spread of lymphoma cells with a strong leukemic tendency. The cells in the latter type of change are composed of medium-sized cells with cleaved nuclei. This leukemic stage is usually called lymphosarcoma cell leukemia. Direct maturation toward plasma cells may also occur after the cells go out from the neoplastic follicles, as evidenced by the monoclonality of both cIg of plasma cells and sIg of neoplastic follicular center cells. This indicates maturation ability of follicular lymphoma cells toward the end stage of differentiation as seen in chronic myelogenous leukemia cells.

Distribution pattern of Igs and receptors in Ig-positive diffuse lymphoma of the medium-sized cell type may suggest the relation of B-cells with follicular growth. Loss of Fc receptors may correlate to the loss of nodular growth. Chromosome translocation t(14;18)(q32;q31) is frequent in follicular lymphoma (4, 33).

B-large cell lymphoma and immunoblastic sarcoma

B-large cell lymphoma is divided to follicular center cell type and immunoblastic type (56). The neoplastic cells have vesicular nuclei with prominent large nucleoli (Fig. 4). Lukes uses the term immunoblast for a wide range of transformed lymphocytes, but others use it for a narrow range corresponding to the committed stem cells toward plasma cells (plasmablast). Most sIg positive large cell lymphomas were also stained for cIg. SIg negative but cIg positive cells indicate cytoplasmic maturation toward plasma cells, and their feature are usually consistent with immunoblastic sarcoma.

About one-fourth of non-T-large cell lymphoma seems to lose the ability of Ig synthesis, but some cases begin to produce Ig by heterotransplantation into nude mice, or other methods of induction for differentiation. They usually have C3 receptors more often than Ig negative cases, and express Ia (HLA-Dr) antigen on their surface.

Chromosome abnormality varies, such as t(1;14)(p23; q23), t(8;14)(q22;q32), t(10;14)(q24;q32), t(11;14)(q13;q32),

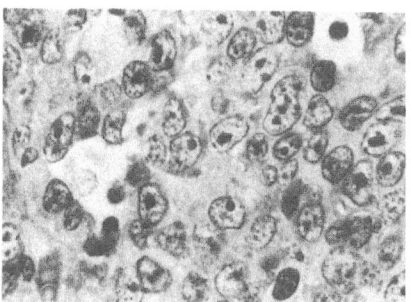

Figure 4. B-large cell lymphoma. Vesicular nuclei with conspicuous nucleoli and moderate amount of cytoplasm are noted. Some nuclei are elongated, suggesting similarity with large cleaved cells in the germinal center. H&E, × 600.

t(14;14)(q24;q32), or t(18;14)(q21;q32). High frequency of del(6)(q21) is reported (4). Chromosome band 8q22 is known as c-*mos* oncogene. It needs further analysis whether different expression of c-*myc* or c-*mos* yields Burkitt's tumor or large cell lymphoma, when they show the same t(8;14) translocation. Other abnormality is also present, and when the Ig producing genes (chromosome No. 14; heavy chain, No. 2 k light chain, No. 22; λ light chain) are involved, the Ig production of neoplastic cells seems to be influenced.

Plasmacytoma

Multiple myeloma was formerly considered as a separate entity from malignant lymphomas, because of different clinical manifestation and different histology from malignant lymphoma. Since the maturation way of B-lymphocytes to plasma cells has been clarified, multiple myeloma and extraosseous plasmacytoma are now accepted as lymphoid neoplasms.

Recent analysis indicates that neoplastic change may occur in the lymphocyte stage, because peripheral blood lymphocytes have the same idiotype as that of myeloma cells in some patients. The preferential occurrence of myeloma in bone has not been clarified and selective homing of neoplastic lymphocytes to the bone marrow is considered possible. Alternatively direct maturation toward plasma cells from committed B-lymphoid stem cells could happen in bone marrow (2).

T-CELL LYMPHOMAS

Three maturation stages of T-lymphocytes are differentiated as pre-T (T0), thymic T (T1) and peripheral T (T2) lymphocytes (Fig. 5ab). T-lymphocytes mature from progenitor cells in the thymus. Intrathymic differentiation of pre-T-lymphocytes is well studied by using monoclonal antibodies (34). Thymic T-lymphocytes have T6, T4 and T8 surface antigens, and they lose T6 antigen with maturation, and differentiate toward helper/inducer T-lymphocytes (T4+) or suppressor/cytotoxic T-lymphocytes (T8+) (28, 34, 46). Thymic T-lymphocytes show terminal deoxynucleotidyl transferase (TdT) activity, which is lost in peripheral T-lymphocytes (65). Peripheral T-lymphocytes respond to various kinds of lectins, such as phytohemagglutinin (PHA) and concanavalin A (ConA), and transform to large cells. Various kinds of interferons are secreted during these reactions (37).

Neoplastic T-lymphocytes usually preserve their surface markers and/or any other characteristics, showing their degree of differentiation and maturation (60, 61). Acute lymphoblastic leukemia, and diffuse lymphoblastic lymphoma belong to the T0/T1 stage. There are various neoplastic states of peripheral T-lymphocytes, and recent research has deepened our knowledge, especially in relation to retrovirus infection. This section deals with diffuse lymphoblastic lymphoma, adult T-cell leukemia, mycosis fungoides, and other types of peripheral T-cell lymphomas.

Diffuse lymphoblastic lymphoma (DLB)

This type of lymphoma has a strong leukemic tendency and is considered to be identical to acute lymphoblastic leukemia except for the precedence of tumorous growth before leukemic involvement (31, 44, 58). DLB is the most common lymphoma in childhood, but rarely occurs in adults. Neoplastic cells are more uniform in childhood cases (L1 by FAB classification) compared to those in adults (L2 by FAB classification). Childhood cases usually have a thymic mass (Fig. 6), and neoplastic cells do not express Ia-like antigen in such cases unlike the Ia-positive pre-T or nonT–nonB DLB (51, 62). Most of these cells have TdT activity and dexamethasone receptors, but certain number of cases do not show TdT activity, which are considered to represent a stage of maturation toward peripheral T-lymphocytes. A

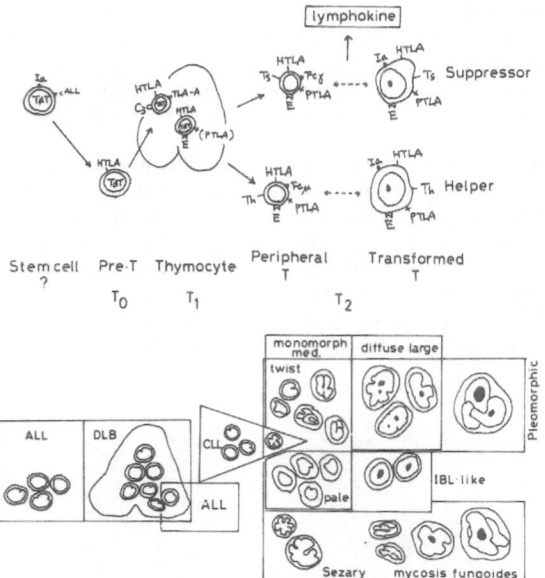

Figure 5. (a) T-cell differentiation and maturation in relation to functional markers. Peripheral T-cells are divided into suppressor/cytotoxic and helper/inducer. HTLA; human T-lymphocyte antigen, TLA-A; thymic leukemia associated antigen, PTLA; peripheral T-lymphocyte antigen, Ts; suppressor/cytotoxic T cell antigen, Th; helper/inducer T cell antigen. (b) Neoplastic counterparts of T-lymphocytes. Marked pleomorphism is one of characteristics of peripheral T cell lymphoma, and histologic subclassification is arbitrary.

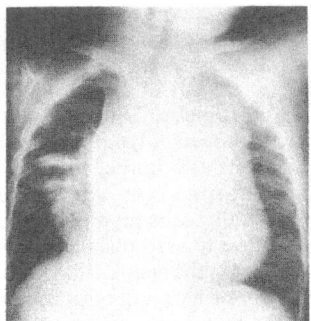

Figure 6. Mediastinal mass in a child with diffuse lymphoblastic lymphoma.

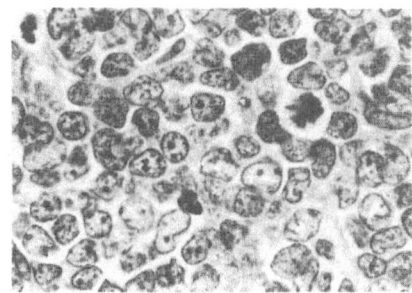

Figure 7. Diffuse lymphoblastic lymphoma (T1). Neoplastic cells have round or convoluted nuclei with stippled chromatin and thin nuclear membrane. Mitotic figures are frequent. H&E, × 800.

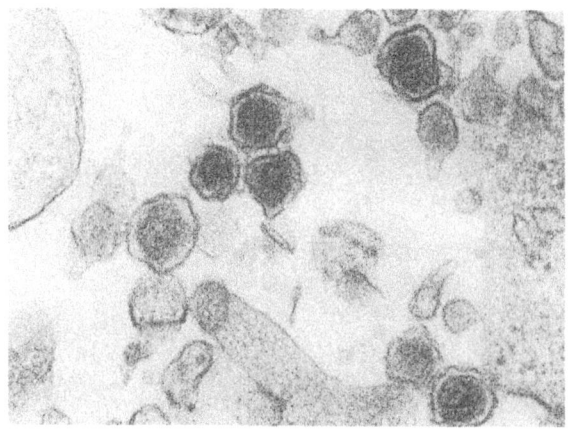

Figure 8. C-type viral particles of ATL cells. × 40,000.

certain number of cell lines have been established, and some showed phenotypic change for maturation by induction with phorbol esters and other substances. DLB reveals a diffuse monomorphic proliferation of cells with frequent mitotic figures (Fig. 7). The nuclei have small nucleoli and fine chromatin aggregates bordered by a thin nuclear membrane. Nuclear contour is often indented giving a raisin-like appearance (convoluted nuclei) in the paraffin embedded section. The amount of cytoplasm is scanty, often containing PAS-positive granules and acid phosphatase and/or β-glucuronidase positive dots. These reaction products coincide with the clustered dense body by an electron microscopy (61).

The prognosis is poor, especially when the neoplastic cells show T cell character. Cells with chromosome numbers in the hyperdiploid range may indicate better reaction to combined chemotherapy (21, 52).

Adult T-cell leukemia (ATL) and pleomorphic T-cell lymphoma

ATL/pleomorphic T-cell lymphoma shows a geographic accumulation in the Southern part of Japan and in the Caribbean. The patients have a natural antibody against special kind of retrovirus, which has been termed ATL virus in Japan and HTLV type 1 in U.S.A. (14, 36). The number of normal healthy carriers of ATLV in Japan is estimated to be one million, and one or two hundred ATL cases occur annually, so that the ATLV infection and ATL seemed to be etiologically related. Actually, ATLV is able to transform normal T-lymphocytes, just as EBV B95-8 transforms B-lymphocytes (27). Type C viral particles are observed by short-term culture of neoplastic cells with BUDR or TCGF (15) (Fig. 8).

ATL is characterized by the irregular leukemic cells in both size and shape, especially with lobulated nuclei (Fig. 9). Lymph node biopsy usually reveals pleomorphic composition of cells, including giant cells (13, 47, 61, 62, 64) (Fig. 10ab). Immunologic markers of neoplastic cells show T4$^+$ helper/inducer T-cell phenotype, but their function on Ig production of PWM stimulated B-lymphocytes is suppression. The neoplastic cells also express core antigen of ATLV, which are detected by monoclonal antibodies Gin2 and Gin14 (14, 15, 42).

Chromosome analysis of ATL usually reveals a broad range of chromosome abnormality from pseudodiploid range to tetraploid range. In pseudodiploid range 14q$^+$ and 6q$^-$ chromosomes are reported to be the most frequent abnormality (26).

The clinical features of ATL are characteristic, such as high white blood cell counts, frequent skin lesions, hepatosplenomegaly, lymphadenopathy, and a rapidly fatal terminal course, usually by opportunistic infection (7, 41, 48, 68). Hypercalcemia is a noticeable laboratory finding.

Several variants of the clinical course are known in addition to the typical acute form of ATL. One is a chronic form, which begins T-CLL or T-small cell type lymphoma with survival of 5 to 10 years until final crisis, and another is a smouldering type, which usually begins with skin lesions in the form of erythema, papules or nodules for several years and then flares up to typical acute ATL (42, 69). Cases show a small percent atypical cells with lobulated nuclei in the peripheral blood.

Some cases of ATL evince the same clinical and laboratory manifestation as those of Sezary's syndrome, which is characterized by generalized exfoliative erythroderma and leukemic involvement by atypical cells with cerebriform nuclei. In this regard, all peripheral T-cell neoplasms should be reevaluated in relation to the retrovirus infection.

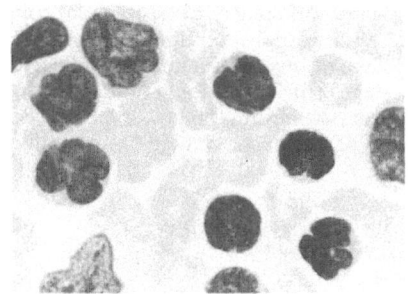

Figure 9. Peripheral blood smear of ATL. The variety of size and shape and the irregularly lobulated nuclei are characteristic. May-Giemsa. × 800.

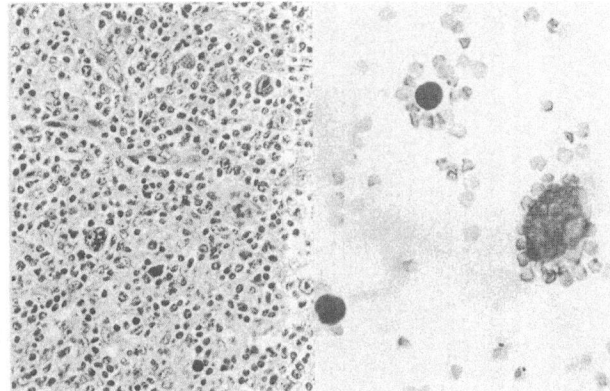

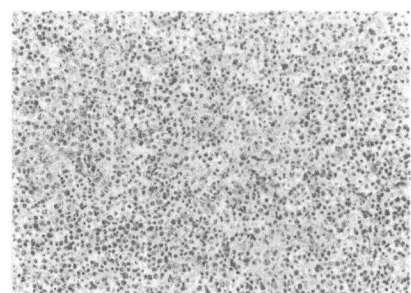

Figure 11. Peripheral T-cell lymphoma. Foci of pale cells with clear cytoplasms and irregularity of nuclear size and shape are noted, but are less than in the case of pleomorphic T-cell lymphoma. H&E, × 330.

Figure 10. T-diffuse lymphoma, pleomorphic type. (a) Pleomorphic composition of cells from small to large giant cells is characteristic. Giant cells often mimic Reed-Sternberg cells but irregularity of small lymphocytes in the background is a point of differential diagnosis. H&E, × 330. (b) E-rosetted cells in the suspension of pleomorphic T-cell lymphoma. May-Giemsa, × 660.

Mycosis fungoides and cutaneous T-cell lymphomas

Mycosis fungoides is a chronic skin lesion which is caused by the infiltration of T-lymphocytes with both helper phenotype and helper action on Ig production of B-lymphocytes (5, 6, 39). Increase of IgA or other immunoglobulins is often observed in mycosis fungoides. Typical mycosis fungoides cases with Pautrier's microabscess are composed of relatively regular small to medium-sized cells. These cases are ATLA-negative. ATLA positive cases should be excluded from mycosis fungoides, because they usually show terminal aggravation, regardless of their benign appearance due to a long course. In addition to the difference of cellular composition, e.g., skin manifestation of ATL is more pleomorphic compared to mycosis fungoides, skin lesions of ATLA-positive patients contained numerous T8[+] suppressor T-lymphocytes, which is scant in ATLA-negative mycosis fungoides (67).

Patients with mycosis fungoides have a high frequency of antecedent allergies, fungal and viral skin infections, sun sensitivity and employment in the manufacture of chemicals and drugs. The long duration of such types of stimulation is considered to provoke neoplastic change of T-lymphocytes under the influence of epidermal Langerhans cells. Actually the number of Langerhans cells and their precursors is high in the early stage of mycosis fungoides, and decreases in the later tumor stage (16). Three stages of the disease are widely accepted, i.e., erythematous, plaque and tumor stage. However, the point of neoplastic change has been unequivocally demonstrated.

Peripheral T-cell lymphoma

Peripheral T-cell lymphoma is usually composed of pleomorphic or mixed cells from small to large transformed cells (Fig. 5b). Some cases are composed of monomorphic cells, but the variety of size and shape is usually present compared

to the B-cell lymphomas. Foci of cells with rich clear pale cytoplasm are often present (Fig. 11). These features suggest their peripheral T-cell nature (32, 55, 61). Peripheral T-cell tumors often reveal many biological abnormalities, such as eosinophilia, hypercalcemia, polyclonal hypergammaglobulinemia, accumulation of histiocytes, vascular proliferation, increase of reticulin fiber, etc. These findings may be induced by biological substances, such as lymphokines, secreted from the neoplastic T-cells. Modified histologic findings, which clearly indicate their histologic characteristics, permit classification of lymphomas in different subtypes, such as IBL-like T-cell lymphoma, T-zone lymphoma and so-called Lennert lymphoma (18, 19, 43, 63).

The prognosis of these cases is not significantly different, therefore histologic subclassification of peripheral T-cell lymphoma seems to be meaningless. Rather, functional classification into helper T-cell lymphoma or suppressor T-cell lymphoma may be more valuable to indicate the nature of neoplastic cells (64).

PRELYMPHOMATOUS LESIONS

Several diseases are considered to be prelymphomatous lesions. These include immunoblastic lymphadenopathy, lymphomatoid granulomatosis of the lung and lymphomatoid papulosis of the skin, etc. Borderline lesions are also present, such as in Hashimoto's thyroiditis, orbital lymphoma, celiac disease prior to intestinal lymphoma, reactive lymphoid hyperplasia of the stomach, etc. Other conditions, such as transplantation of organs and Sjögren's syndrome, show higher incidence of lymphoma in these patients.

Although active proliferation of lymphocytes against antigenic stimulation is a physiological phenomenon (66), neoplastic clones may occur among these proliferating lymphocytes. Frequent B-cell lymphomas in the gastrointestinal tract and frequent T-cell lymphomas in the skin and respiratory tract suggest the possibility that the influence of different uptake of antigenic or carcinogenic substances determines the neoplastic change among populations of reacting lymphocytes. It has been unclear whether a single cell becomes neoplastic to make a neoplastic clone or a certain number of cells becomes neoplastic and makes a single neoplastic clone.

It is not difficult to recognize neoplastic growth from

hyperplastic lymphoid reaction in extranodal sites. However, the borderline between the two is often unclear. Emergence of foci composed of monomorphic cells in hyperplastic areas in aged people and infiltration of these cells into the surrounding connective tissues suggests neoplastic change even though reactive follicles remain in some areas.

Proliferation of B-lymphocytes with borderline malignancy is also observed in the systemic type of Castleman's disease or some cases of benign monoclonal gammopathy. In these diseases, functional abnormalities of T-lymphocytes are often found, so that the interaction of T-lymphocytes should be considered.

Secondary leukemia or lymphoma after chemotherapy and/or irradiation for the first cancer is another problem.

Immunoblastic lymphadenopathy

Immunoblastic lymphadenopathy (IBL) or angioimmunoblastic lymphadenopathy (AILD) are thought to be abnormal immune states (11, 24). Clinical manifestations are general malaise, systemic lymphadenopathy and splenomegaly. Polyclonal hypergammaglobulinemia is one of characteristic laboratory findings. This disease is considered to be a hyperimmune state of B-lymphocytes, which may be produced by impaired suppressor T-cell function on B-lymphocytes. Occurrence of true B-cell lymphoma, usually taking a form of immunoblastic sarcoma, is rarely reported.

T-cell lymphomas often cause a hypergammaglobulinemia, and its typical form is IBL-like T-cell lymphoma or peripheral T-cell lymphoma with hypergammaglobulinemia (41, 63). Unlike mycosis fungoides, neoplastic cells have a phenotype of suppressor/cytotoxic T-lymphocytes ($T3^+ T8^+$). This special type of T-cell lymphoma is considered to be treated under the diagnosis of IBL or AILD.

Lymphomatoid granulomatosis of the lung

Lymphomatoid granulomatosis of the lung shows patchy infiltration of lymphoid and/or lymphoplasmacytoid cells in the perivascular region of the lung parenchyma, showing features of vasculitis or granulomatous inflammation. The disease is usually discovered by chest X-ray in adults but the lesion also occurs in the skin, kidney or central nervous system. A certain number of cases develop overt lymphoma after 5 to 10 years, and most cases show T-cell nature (10).

Lymphomatoid papulosis is also considered to be a reactive lesion, but some develop cutaneous T-cell lymphoma. The differentiation of the smouldering type of lymphoma from these prelymphomatous conditions is sometimes very difficult (61).

COMPARISON WITH EXPERIMENTAL MODELS

Lymphomas and leukemias have been thoroughly studied in mice, rats, guinea pigs and cats. Lymphomas in dogs and cows are also well known. Some of these tumors are related to retrovirus infection.

However, the lymphoma models in experimental animals are rather limited, because of the lack of histologic variety

(17). The common lymphoma-leukemias are T-cell lymphoma-leukemia with mediastinal (thymic) involvement, B-immunoblastic sarcoma and plasmacytoma. Follicular growth is occasionally observed in the spleen, but the follicularity is not as well demarcated as in human. Peripheral T-cell lymphoma is considered to be very rare, or non-existent.

Immunologic characterization of neoplastic cells lugs behind that of human materials, but recent knowledge on viral oncogenes needs further development of lymphoma-leukemia research in experimental animals.

REFERENCES

1. Aisenberg AC, Wilkes BM, Long JC, Harris NL: Cell surface phenotype in lymphoproliferative disease. *Am J Med* 68:206, 1980
2. Azar HA, Potter M: Multiple Myeloma and Related Disorders. Vol 1, Chapters 1 and 2. Hagerstown, Harper & Row Pub Inc, 1973
3. Berard CW, Jaffe ES, Braylan RC, Mann RB, Nanba K: Immunologic aspects and pathology of the malignant lymphomas. *Cancer* 42:911, 1978
4. Bloomfield CD, Authur DC, Frizzera G, Levine EG, Peterson BA, Gajl-Peczalska KJ: Nonrandom chromosome abnormalities in lymphoma. *Cancer Res* 43:2975, 1983
5. Broder S, Bunn P Jr: Cutaneous T-cell lymphoma. *Seminars Oncol* 7:310, 1980
6. Broder S, Edelson R, Lutzner MA: The Sezary syndrome. A malignant proliferation of helper T cells. *J Clin Invest* 58:1297, 1976
7. Bunn PA Jr, Schechter GP, Jaffe E, Blayney D, Young RC, Matthews MJ, Blattner W, Broder S, Robert-Guroff M, Gallo RC: Clinical course of retrovirus-associated adult T-cell lymphoma in the United States. *New Eng J Med* 309:257, 1983
8. Chess L, Schlossman SF: Human lymphocyte subpopulations. In: *Adv Immunol* Vol 25 pp 213–241, edited by Kinkel HG, Dixon FJ, New York–San Francisco–London, Academic Press, 1977
9. Dalla-Favera R, Bregni M, Erikson J, Patterson D, Gallo RC, Croce CM: Human c-*myc* onc gene is located on the region of chromosome 8 that is translocated in Burkitt's lymphoma cells. *Proc Natl Acad Sci* 79:7824, 1982
10. Fauci AS, Haynes BF, Costa J, Katz P, Walff SM: Lymphomatoid granulomatosis: Prospective clinical and therapeutic experiences over 10 years. *N Eng J Med* 306:68, 1982
11. Frizzera G, Moran EM, Rappaport H: Angioimmunoblastic lymphadenopathy. Diagnosis and clinical course. *Am J Med* 59:803, 1975
12. Habeshaw JA, Bailey D, Stansfeld AG, Greaves MF: The cellular content of non-Hodgkin's lymphomas: A comprehensive analysis using monoclonal antibodies and other surface marker techniques. *Br J Cancer* 47:327, 1983
13. Hanaoka M, Sasaki M, Matsumoto H et al.: Adult T-cell leukemia – histological classification and characteristics. *Acta Pathol Jpn* 29:723, 1979
14. Hinuma Y, Komoda H, Chosa T, Kondo T, Kohakura M, Takenaka T, Kikuchi M, Ishimaru M, Yunoki K, Sato I, Matsuo R, Takiuchi Y, Uchino H, Hanaoka M: Antibodies to adult T-cell leukemia-virus associated antigen (ATLA) in sera from patients with ATL and controls in Japan. A nation-wide sero-epidemiologic study. *Int J Cancer* 29:631, 1982
15. Hoshino H, Esumi H, Miwa M, Shimoyama M, Minato K, Tobinai M, Hirose S, Watanabe S, Inada N, Kinoshita K, Kamihira S, Ichimaru M, Sugimura T: Establishment and characterization of new cell lines derived from patients with

adult T cell leukemia. *Proc Natl Acad Sci USA* 80:6061, 1983

16. Igisu K, Watanabe S: Langerhans cells and their precursors stained antiS100 antibody in mycosis fungoides. *Jpn J Clin Oncol* 13:693, 1983

17. Kaiser H (Ed): Neoplasms comparative pathology of growth in animals, plants, and man. Williams & Wilkins, London, 1981

18. Kim H, Nathwani BN, Rappaport H: So-called "Lennert's lymphoma": Is it a clinicopathologic entity? *Cancer* 45:1379, 1980

19. Lennert K: T-zone lymphoma. In: *Malignant lymphomas other than Hodgkin's disease*. pp 196–209, New York–Heidelberg–Berlin, Springer Publisher, 1978

20. Lenoir GM, Preud'homme JL, Bernheim A, Berger R: Correlation between immunoglobulin light chain expression and variant translocation in Burkitt's lymphoma. *Nature (Lond)* 298:474, 1982

21. Levine AM, Shackney SE, Cunningham RE, Smith CA, Schuette WS, Teitelbaum AH, Nichols PW, Stolinsky DC, Lukes RJ: Therapeutic response and survival in B and T-cell lymphomas in relation to tumor cell aneuploidy and proliferative state. *Proc Am Assoc Cancer Res* 22:520, 1981

22. Lukes RJ, Collins RD: Lukes–Collins classification and its significance. *Cancer Treat Rep* 61:971, 1977

23. Lukes RJ, Parker JW, Taylor CR, Tindle BH, Cramer AD, Lincoln TL: Immunologic approach to non-Hodgkin's lymphomas and related leukemias. Analysis of the results of multiparameter studies of 425 cases. *Seminar Hematol* 15:322, 1978

24. Lukes RJ, Tindle BH: Immunoblastic lymphadenopathy. A hyperimmune entity resembling Hodgkin's disease. *N Engl J Med* 292:1, 1975

25. Melchers F: B-lymphocyte development and growth regulation. In: *Differentiation of normal and neoplastic hematopoietic cells*, pp 485–503, edited by Clarkson B et al, Cold Spring Harbor, Cold Spring Harbor Laboratory, 1978

26. Miyamoto K, Sato J, Kitajima K, Togawa A, Suemaru S, Sanada H, Tanaka T: Adult T-cell leukemia: chromosome analysis of 15 cases. *Cancer* 52:471, 1983

27. Miyoshi I, Kubonishi I, Yoshimoto S, Akagi T, Ohtsuki Y, Shiraishi Y, Nagata K, Hinuma T: Type C virus particles in a cord T-cell line derived by co-cultivating normal human cord leukocytes and human leukemic T-cells. *Nature (London)* 294:770, 1981

28. Moretta L, Webb SR, Grossi CE et al.: Functional analysis of two human T-cell subpopulations: help and suppression of B-cell responses by T-cells bearing receptors for IgM or IgG. *J Exp Med* 146:184, 1977

29. Moss DJ, Burrows SR, Castelino DJ, Kane RG, Pope JH, Rickinson AB, Alpers MP, Heywood PF: A comparison of Epstein-Barr virus-specific T-cell immunity in malaria-endemic and nonendemic regions of Papua new guinea. *Int J Cancer* 31:727, 1983

30. Nadler LM, Stashenko P, Hardy R, Schlossman SF: A monoclonal antibody defining a lymphoma-associated antigen in man. *J Immunol* 125:570, 1980

31. Nathwani BN, Kim H, Rappaport H: Malignant lymphoma, lymphoblastic. *Cancer* 38:964, 1976

32. Palutke M, Tabaczka P, Weise RW et al.: T-cell lymphomas of large cell type. A variety of malignant lymphomas: "histiocytic" and mixed lymphocytic-"histiocytic". *Cancer* 46:87, 1980

33. Reeves BR, Pickup VL: The chromosome changes in non-Burkitt lymphomas. *Hum Genet* 53:349, 1980

34. Reinherz EL, Kung PC, Goldstein G, Levey H, Schlossman SF: Discrete stages of human intrathymic differentiation: Analysis of normal thymocytes and leukemic lymphoblasts of T-cell lineage. *Proc Natl Acad Sci USA* 77:1588, 1980

35. Risdall R, Hoppe RT, Warnke R: Non-Hodgkin's lymphoma.

A study of the evolution of the disease based upon 92 autopsied cases. *Cancer* 44:529, 1979

36. Robert-Guroff M, Nakao Y, Notake K, Ito Y, Sliski A, Gallo RC: Natural antibodies to human retrovirus HTLV in a cluster of Japanese patients with adult T cell leukemia. *Science* 215:975, 1982

37. Rocklin RE, MacDermott RP, Chess L et al.: Studies on mediator production by highly purified human T and B lymphocytes. *J Exp Med* 140:1303, 1974

38. Rowley JD: Human oncogene locations and chromosome aberrations. *Nature (Lond)* 301:290, 1983

39. Schein PS, Macdonald JS, Edelson R: Cutaneous T-cell lymphoma. *Cancer* 38:1859, 1976

40. Seligmann M: B-cell and T-cell markers in lymphoid proliferations. *N Engl J Med* 290:753, 1974

41. Shimoyama M, Minato K, Kitahara T, Watanabe S: Comparisons of clinical, morphologic and immunologic characteristics of adult T-cell leukemia/lymphoma and cutaneous T-cell lymphoma. *Jpn J Clin Oncol* 9:357, 1979

42. Shimoyama M, Minato K, Tobinai M, Nagai T, Setoya T, Takenaka T, Ishihara K, Watanabe S, Miwa M, Kinoshita M, Okabe S, Fukushima N, Inada N: Atypical adult T-cell leukemia-lymphoma: Diverse clinical manifestations of adult T-cell leukemia-lymphoma. *Jpn J Clin Oncol* 13 (Suppl 2):165, 1983

43. Shimoyama M, Minato K, Watanabe S: Immunoblastic lymphadenopathy-like T cell lymphoma. *Jpn J Clin Oncol* 9:347, 1979

44. Silverstone AE, Rosenberg N, Baltimore D, Sato VL, Scheid MP, Boyse EA: Correlating terminal deoxynucleotidyl transferase and cell-surface markers in the pathway of lymphocyte ontogeny. In: *Differentiation of normal and neoplastic hematopoietic cells* pp 433–453, edited by Clarkson B et al, Cold Spring Harbor, Cold Spring Harbor Laboratory, 1978

45. Stein RS, Cousar J, Flexner JM, Collins RD: Correlations between immunologic markers and histopathologic classifications: Clinical implications. *Seminars Oncol* 7:244, 1980

46. Stutman O: Intrathymic and extrathymic T-cell maturation. *Immunol Rev* 42:138, 1978

47. Suchi T, Tajima K, Nanba K, Watanabe S, Mikata A, Mori S, Kikuchi M: Some problems on the histopathological diagnosis of non-Hodgkin's malignant lymphoma – A proposal of a new type. *Acta Path Jpn* 29:755, 1979

48. T- and B-lymphoma Study Group: Statistical analysis of immunologic, clinical and histopathologic data of lymphoid malignancies in Japan. *Jpn J Clin Oncol* 11:15, 1981

49. Taub R, Kirsch I, Morton C, Lenoir G, Swan D, Tronick S, Leder P: Translocation of the c-*myc* gene into the immunoglobulin heavy chain locus in human Burkitt's lymphoma and murine plasmacytoma cells. *Proc Natl Acad Sci USA* 79:7837, 1982

50. Taylor CR: Immunohistologic studies of lymphomas: new methodology yields new information and poses new problems. *J Histochem Cytochem* 27:1180, 1979

51. Thiel E, Rodt H, Huhn D, Netzel B, Grosse-Wilde H, Ganeshaguru K, Thielfelder S: Multimarker classification of acute lymphoblastic leukemia: Evidence for further T subgroups and evaluation of their clinical significance. *Blood* 56:759, 1980

52. Third International Workshop on Chromosomes in Leukemia: Clinical significance of chromosomal abnormalities in acute lymphoblastic leukemia. *Cancer Genet Cytogenet* 4:111, 1981

53. Tobinai K, Hirose H, Yamada K, Minato K, Shimoyama M: Cellular origin of human lymphoid malignancies based on immunologic analysis of membrane differentiation antigens. *Jpn J Clin Oncol* 12:73, 1982

54. Tolksdorf G, Stein H, Lennert K: Morphological and immunological definition of a malignant lymphoma derived from germinal center cells with cleaved nuclei. *Br J Cancer* 41:168, 1980

55. Waldron JA, Leech JH, Glick AD, Flexner JM, Collins RD: Malignant lymphoma of peripheral T lymphocyte origin. *Cancer* 40:1604, 1977
56. Warnke R, Miller R, Grogan T, Pederson M, Dilley J, Levy R: Immunologic phenotype in 30 patients with diffuse large cell lymphoma. *N Engl J Med* 303:293, 1980
57. Watanabe S, Kuroki M, Sato Y, Shimosato Y, Hasegawa T: The establishment of a cell line (NH-AR) from a human nodular lymphoma and a comparison with lymphoblastoid cell line. *Cancer* 46:2438, 1980
58. Watanabe S, Shimosato Y, Kuroki M, Kitahara T: Leukemic distribution of a human acute lymphocytic leukemia cell line (Ichikawa strain) in nude mice conditioned with whole body irradiation. *Cancer Res* 38:3494, 1978
59. Watanabe S, Shimosato Y, Kuroki M, Hirohashi S, Okada H, Suzuki S, Tsutsumi Y: Tumorigenicity of Epstein–Barr virus-transformed human lymphocytes in conditioned nude mice. Proc 3rd Intn'l Workshop on Nude Mice. Ed: Norman D Hunt pp 481–492, NY, Gustav Fischer New York Inc, 1982
60. Watanabe S, Shimosato Y, Nakajima T, Shimoyama M, Minato K: T cell malignancies: Subclassification and interrelationship. *Jpn J Clin Oncol* 9:423, 1979
61. Watanabe S, Shimosato Y, Shimoyama M: Leukemia and lymphoma of T-lymphocytes. In: *Pathology Annual*, Vol 16, pp 155–205, edited by Sommers SC, New York, Appleton-Century Crofts, 1981
62. Watanabe S, Shimosato Y, Shimoyama M, Minato K: Studies with multiple markers on malignant lymphomas and lymphoid leukemias. *Cancer* 50:2372, 1982
63. Watanabe S, Shimosato Y, Shomoyama M, Minato K, Suzuki M, Abe M, Nagatani T: Adult T-cell lymphoma with hypergammaglobulinemia. *Cancer* 46:2472, 1980
64. Watanabe S, Shimoyama M: T-cell lymphomas in relation to subpopulation of T-lymphocytes. In: *Gann Monograph on Cancer Res*, Vol 28, pp 107–120, Tokyo, Tokyo University Press, 1982
65. Watanabe S, Tsutsumi Y, Shimosato Y, Shimoyama M: Terminal deoxynucleotidyl transferase activity in leukemia and lymphoma, with special reference to adult T-cell related neoplasms. *Acta Haemat Jpn* 48:139, 1980
66. Watanabe S, Watanabe K, Ohishi T, Kageyama K: The development of extranodal lymphoid follicles in experimental bronchopneumonia. *Acta Pathol Jpn* 29:533, 1979
67. Watanabe S: Pathology of peripheral T-cell lymphomas and leukemias. *Haematol Oncol* 4:45, 1986
68. Uchiyama T, Yodoi J, Sagawa K, Takatsuki K, Uchino H: Adult T-cell leukemia: Clinical and hematologic features of 16 cases. *Blood* 50:481, 1977
69. Yamaguchi K, Nishimura H, Kawano F, Kohrogi H, Jono M, Miyamoto Y, Takatsuki K: A proposal for smouldering adult T-cell leukemia – Diversity in clinical pictures of adult T-cell leukemia. *Jpn J Clin Oncol* 13 (Suppl 2):189, 1983

POSTSCRIPT

In August 1987, International Colloquium on Lymphoid Malignancy was held in Kyoto. Recent development of immunological and molecular biological methods on lymphoma research contributed much to the classical clinicopathological diagnosis with more profound understanding about the nature of lymphoid malignancy, so that it was timely to summarize the present situation and to find the future direction. Four items were discussed; adult T-cell leukemia, angioimmunoblastic lymphadenopathy, monoclonal growth detected by DNA rearrangement and/or chromosome analysis, and geographic pathology of lymphoid malignancy.

Immunohistochemical methods using various monoclonal antibodies clarified the varying aspects of T-cell lymphomas (2–4, 15). HTLV-I related lymphomas and leukemia were categorized by the expression of CD_4 and IL-2 receptor in addition to the proviral DNA in the neoplastic cells (5, 9). HTLV-I infection was also found to be related to the tropical spastic paresis or HTLV-I associated myelopathy (HAM) (8). Ki-1 lymphoma, which contains peculiar large anaplastic cells with probable T-cell origin, was still in debate about its independency (1, 16). In this regard, histologic classification of T-cell lymphomas needs further basic research, although several proposals have been present (10).

Neoplastic nature of angioommunoblastic lymphadenopathy or immunoblastic lymphadenopathy became more clear by chromosome study and T-c-beta gene rearrangement (11, 14). Early stage of T-cell lymphomas, so far considered to be atypical hyperplasia or dysplasia, was detected by these methods.

Geographic pathology yielded many breakthrough in lymphoma research; Burkitt tumor, adult T-cell leukemia, and recently HIV-related lymphomas (12). Several leukemogenic viruses are known to cause other diseases. Studies on immigrants should be important from etiologic standpoint (6). Mathematical models may be available to suggest the etiologic events (7, 13).

POSTSCRIPT REFERENCES

1. Agnarsson BA et al.: Ki-1 positive large cell lymphoma. A morphologic and immunologic study of 19 cases. *Am J Surg Pathol* 12:264, 1988
2. Bunn PA Jr: Diagnostic factors in intermediate and high-grade lymphomas: pathologic, immunologic, and clinical. *J Clin Oncol* 6:1073, 1988
3. Coiffier B et al.: T-cell lymphomas: immunologic, histologic, clinical, and therapeutic analysis of 63 cases. *J Clin Oncol* 6:1584, 1986
4. Foon FA et al.: Immunologic classification of lymphoma and lyphoid leukemia. *Blood Rev* 1:77, 1987
5. Griesser H et al.: Rearrangement of the beta-chain of the T-cell antigen receptor and immunoglobulin genes in lymphoproliferative disorders. *J Clin Invest* 78:1179, 1986
6. Lippman SM et al.: Clonal ambiguity of human immuno-deficiency virus-associated lymphomas. Similarity to post-transplant lymphomas. *Arch Pathol Lab Med* 112:128, 1988
7. Okamoto T et al.: Multi-step carcinogenesis model for adult T-cell leukemia. *Jpn J Cancer Res* (in press)
8. Osame M et al.: HTLV-I associated myelopathy, a new clinical entity. *Lancet i:* 1031, 1986
9. Seiki M et al.: Human adult T-cell leukemia virus: complete nucleotide sequence of the provirus genome integrated in leukemic cell DNA. *Proc Natnl Acad Sci* USA 80:3618, 1988
10. Suchi T et al.: Histopathology and immunohistochemistry of peripheral T cell lymphomas: a proposal for their classification. *J Clin Pathol* 40:995, 1987
11. Tobinai K et al.: Clinicopathologic, immunophgenotypic, and immunogenotypic analyses of immunoblastic lymphadenopathy-like T-cell lymphoma. *Blood* 72:1000–1006, 1988
12. Tsugane S et al.: Infectious states of human T-lymphotropic virus type 1 and hepatitis B virus among Japanese immigrants in the republic of Bolivia. *Am J Epidem* (in press)
13. Watanabe S et al.: Cumulative incidence rates for Hodgkin's disease and other hematologic malignancies, with special reference to age-related carcinogenesis. *Jpn J Cancer Res* 77:743, 1986
14. Watanable S et al.: Immunoblastic lymphadenopathy, angioimmunoblastic lymphadenopathy, and IBL-like T-cell lymphoma. A spectrum of T-cell neoplasia. *Cancer* 58:2222, 1986
15. Watanabe S et al.: Peripheral T-cell lymphoma. CANCER Metast Rev (in press)
16. Weiss LM et al.: Large-cell hematolymphoid neoplasms of uncertain lineage. *Hum Pathol* 19:967, 1988

16

DORMANCY AND LOCAL RECURRENCE OF NEOPLASMS

F.E. WHEELOCK and T. OKAYASU

Recurrent tumors may appear locally or at distant sites to which cells of the primary tumor have metastasized. Generally, recurrent tumors can be classified as early (less than two years after primary therapy), intermediate, and late (more than five years after primary therapy). Many factors, such as the biological characteristics of the tumor and the physiologic condition of the host, influence the time of appearance and the site of tumor recurrence.

Recurrent tumors which appear at the end of a clinical remission are by definition regrowths of tumor cells which survived treatment of the primary tumor and persisted throughout the clinical remission. Tumor cells that persist in a clinically normal host for a prolonged period of time are said to be in a tumor dormant state (see Chapter 3/Volume IV).

Recurrent tumors must be distinguished from second primary tumors that arise during the clinical remission. This distinction can be made either by demonstrating a parent:progeny relationship between the primary amd second tumors using karyotypic, biochemical, or immunologic markers, or by obtaining clinical evidence that the second tumor is a recurrent tumor. Currently karyotyping of tumor cells is, the most definitive procedure and also the most difficult. Performance of karyotype comparisons between the primary and second tumor must be part of a prospective study and therefore requires either the immediate processing of the primary tumor or freezing its cells for future analysis. Examples of convincing clinical evidence for tumor recurrence, as opposed to second primary tumors, are second cancers of the breast which are histologically identical to the primary cancer and which develop in the scar tissue of a mastectomy performed for the primary cancer 20–30 years earlier (see Chapters 17/Volume IV, 8/Volume VI). Another example is a malignant melanoma which grows out in the liver years after surgical removal of a primary uveal melanoma (see Chapter 16/Volume VIII).

Histologic identity between a primary and a second tumor by itself is insufficient evidence to classify a second tumor as recurrent. This is because a second tumor which results from a second neoplastic transformation event in the same population of cells in which the primary transformation event occurred and initiated by the same oncogenic agent, would be expected to be histologically identical to the primary tumor. Thus, more rigorous specific comparisons must be performed to prove a parent:progeny relationship.

Recurrent tumors develop as a result of the failure of treatment to kill all cells of a primary tumor as also in residual cells of acute leukemias (1). The ability of a subpopulation of the primary tumor to survive treatment and persist in a tumor dormant state is usually a consequence of both the heterogeneity of the primary tumor cell population and the inherent resistance of the surviving tumor cell subpopulation to the therapeutic modality (see Chapters 8/Volume I, 7/Volume III, 1/Volume IV). Heterogeneity results from the genetic instability of tumor cells and is one of the major obstacles to cancer cure. Major effort must be made to identify tumor cells that persist in patients during clinical remissions and to devise therapeutic regimens to destroy them before they form recurrent tumors.

REFERENCE

1. Loewenberg B, Hagenbeek A (eds): Minimal Residual Disease in Acute Leukemia. Martinus Nijhoff Publishers, Boston–The Hague–Dordrecht–Lancaster, 1984

LOCAL RECURRENCE

H.E. KAISER

LOCAL RECURRENCE, A TYPE OF NEOPLASTIC SPREADING, MADE POSSIBLE BY THERAPY

Neoplastic progression in man is, in general, modified from its normal course by therapy. Cases are known where no treatment took place of humans afflicted with neoplastic disease. (See Chapter 8/Volume VI).

The usual ways of neoplastic spreading are either by closed spreading, known as intrusion, or by distant spreading, known as metastasis. The primary tumor exhibits some inhibition toward metastatic spreading. The positive aspect of tumor growth is found in tumor regression which can affect primary as well as secondary tumors. (See Chapters 4–8, Volume IV.)

In an untreated organism, the primary tumor will grow continuously, perhaps turning necrotic in its center. Depending on the type of tumor it will persistently seed metastatic cells. During operative treatment of a primary tumor in man the whole tumor may be exterminated but in more advanced cases remnants of the tumor tissue remain in the patient's body. To control these, preoperative, interoperative and postoperative radiation and chemotherapy are the usual methods employed. Radiation or chemotherapy are often carcinogenic themselves; they may stimulate weakened cells of the already diseased organism to become malignant in turn. The parent tissue of the primary tumor may be more sensitive than surrounding healthy tissues. Local recurrence is found in man, laboratory and domestic animals. Either the cell rests remaining from the primary tumor or new cells made malignant by therapy are the source of local recurrence of a neoplasm.

LOCAL RECURRENCE AS AN INDICATION OF WEAKENED INTERACTION BETWEEN HOST AND TUMOR AND LOCAL INVOLVEMENT OF THE HOST

After an operation the body of the patient is no longer under the influence of the metabolic burden of the primary tumor. But the interaction of the removed primary neoplasm and the host is still felt. At this time the body's metabolism can be considered the same as during the time when the primary tumor was still present. With the redevelopment of malignancy in form of local recurrence the metabolic condition in the patient turns around. The cells of the locally recurring tumor gain influence first on the local area and then on the whole body of the host. This is due to the humoral, hor-

monal or other toxic products of the locally recurring tumor. It will be different in various types of tumors (see Chapters 11–14, Volume VIII).

COMPARABILITY, EXTENDING FROM MAN TO LABORATORY ANIMALS TO DOMESTIC ANIMALS AND THROUGH ALL ORGANS OF THE BODY, AT LEAST OF THE MAMMALIAN ORGANISM

As stated elsewhere, the human body is the one whose histology of neoplasms is best known because we have the largest amount of data available to us. Naturally most cases of local recurrence are known from man because man is the species undergoing the greatest number of surgeries. Other species which follow in this regard are the laboratory mouse, the rat, the hamster, the dog and the cat. More or less occasional cases have been seen in other laboratory and domestic animals.

CLINICAL IMPORTANCE

Neoplasms are known either with a high metastatic potential or a very low one. Similarly, we find neoplasms with a very high potential of recurrence (Table 1), such as basal cell carcinoma, and those with a very low local recurrence. For many neoplasms, a radical operation is the therapy of choice. This should not be done for neoplasms with high local recurrence because they occur again and again. Such neoplastic diseases may continue over decades and several operations over larger time intervals may be required. Other neoplasms reoccur generally over a time interval of one year postoperatively and are followed during the next years by metastatic dissemination. Table 2 shows selected cases of locally recurring and metastasizing neoplasms.

SCIENTIFIC IMPORTANCE

As we have already said, neoplasms with a high potential of local recurrence and those with high metastatic dissemination are known. Both are not equally distributed through the spectrum of tissues in the mammalian body. This is not by chance, but is tied in with the host-tumor interrelationship in the specific area where the process of local recurrence takes place. To learn the reasons why some of the parental

Table 1. High potential of local recurrence.

Tissue	Tumor	Patient(s)	Treatment	Remarks	References
2	Basal cell skin cancer	Adult female/male	Laser irradiation		(50)
4	Rectal neoplasms	Middle aged male	Pericutaneous aspiration biopsy	New method for demonstrating perineal recurrence after abdominoperineal extirpations	(18)
2	Tumor of the hand, forearms	Aged male	Below elbow amputation	Tumor recurred following excision and irradiation	(66)
2/4	Cervical cancer	539 patients	Restricted hysterectomy in 91%	5-yr. survival rate 97.6%; 50/9 recurrences might have been avoided by better follow-up: curative treatment in 7/9	(37)
3/4	Uterine carcinoma	Female	Computed tomography	Use of CT in diagnosis compared with other imaging techniques	(52, 53)
4	Colorectal neoplasms		Chordotomy, percutaneous	Investigation of drug therapies for pain soothing	(63)
4	Rectal and colonic neoplasms		Computed tomography	Use for detecting recurrences following surgery	(60)
4	Esophageal neoplasms	35 patients		Factors responsible for relapse following radical treatment; tumor stage, area of location, degree of local expansion	(9)
4	Esophageal neoplasms		Reoperation		(83)
4	Stomach neoplasms	47 adults	Gastrectomy	Resection yielded significantly lower mean and median survival than other procedures	(38)
4	Rectal neoplasms	11 patients	Secondary amputation	Lymphatic metastasis	(1)
4	Colorectal neoplasms		Secondary surgery	Patients under postoperative care were diagnosed one-third better; resection in twice as many	(56)
4	Rectal neoplasms	Aged adults		Use of clinico-endoscopic diagnosis	(31)
4	Rectal/sigmoid neoplasms			Frequency and pattern of recurrence and malignant transformation following electrocoagulation	(57)
4	Colonic neoplasms	Aged m + f 100	Secondary laparotomy	Incidence of recurrence 37.4%; of these 33% resected curatively	(42)
4	Stomach neoplasm			Frequency of recurrence in (a) rapidly growing penetrating type, (b) slowly growing superficial type	(26)
4	Sigmoid/colon neoplasms	57 patients	Extirpation	19/57 local recurrences; question of extirpation vs. resection dependent on distance of tumor from anus	(80)
4	Rectal cancer		Second resection	Curative second operation possible only if recurrence caused by techniques used in primary operation	(15)
5	Tracheal cancer		Tracheostomy, radiotherapy	Of 340 laryngectomy, 20 stomal recurrences	(2)
5	Tracheal tumor		Manubriectomy	Reconstruction using a musculocutaneous flap	(21)
8	Bladder neoplasms	27 m + f middle age		18-yr. follow-up to study TCC incidence of upper tract. No tumors in upper collecting system detected	(43)
8	Bladder neoplasm			Thomsen-Friedenreich antigen detected by specific antibody; possible marker for recurrence	(46)
8	Bladder neoplasms	5 patients	Ureteral and bilateral resections	Electrocoagulation and resection of superficial tumors leads to iatrogenic refluxes	(55)
8	Bladder neoplasm			Analysis of a study on prophylactic superficial bladder neoplasms	(74)
8	Bladder neoplasm		Methotrexate dry therapy	Clinical trials of this therapy are evaluated	(22)
8	Bladder neoplasm		Adjuvant therapy	Doxorubicin hydrochloride, ethoglucid, and TUR-alone are evaluated	(33)

Table 1. Continued.

Tissue	Tumor	Patient(s)	Treatment	Remarks	References
8	Bladder neoplasms	184 patients	Chemotherapy	92 primary, 92 recurrent tumors; thiotepa adriamycin, or cis-platinum following surgery; no significant differences	(36)
8	Bladder neoplasms	129 patients	Transabdominal ultrasonic scanning	Results composed with cytoscopy; size of tumor of significance	(59)
8	Bladder cancer, non-invasive	24 patients, middle ages	Intravesical ethoglucid	New tumors in 60–80% after termination of treatment	(34)
8	Bladder neoplasms and genital cancer	5 males, advanced and middle age 2 women	Salvage cystectomy	Fairly safe procedure even in elderly patients	(45)
10	Breast cancer	400 patients	Estrogen with progesterone receptor	Used for prediction of short-term relapse	(47)
10	Breast ca 231 primary, 85 metastatic	232 middle age or aged females		Indices of body weight are relatively weak, but real, prognostic factors	(17)
10	Breast cancer	175 females		Investigation of disease-free interval and estrogen-receptor activity showed that it affects prognosis only for the short term	(54)
10	Breast ca*	Females	Computed tomography	Assessment of postoperative recurrences mediastinal metastases	(60)
10	Breast	Female	Lumpectomy	Pathology with reference to recurrence and multicentricity	(19)
19	Spinal paraganglioma	Male, middle age	Angiography	First report, similarity w/paragangliomas of craniocervical region	(69)
19	Adrenal cortical ca	18 adults, m + f	CT following adrenalectomy		(67)
21	Ovarian neoplasms	47 females		Cellular immunity indices were found adversely affected in primary patients as a result of surgery and chemotherapy; they returned to normal during remission but were badly deranged in relapsing patients	(79)
21	Ovarian tumor	Middle age female	CT	Excellent imaging modality for evaluation	(3)
21	Ovary	Female		Lipid-bound serum sialic acids in complex diagnosis	(8)
32	Head and neck mediastinal neoplasms	177 patients	Radiation therapy	Complete remission after radiotherapy; local relapse can be exposed to repeated radiation w/good results	(32)
36	Melanoma, skin	161 patients		Secondary tumors in zone of postoperative scar or transplanted skin flap; lesions pathogenetically different	(4)
47	Neuroblastoma	Infant female	Radionuclide imaging	Detection for diagnosis	(81)
48(?)	Astrocytoma, brain neoplasms	17 patients	Chemotherapy (AZQ)	Recurrence after chemo- and/or radiotherapy; regression in 4/17	(14)
	Basal cell ca	Middle age m + f		Recurrence followed cryosurgery	(65)

Explanations of code numbers for tissues: 2 = stratified squamous epithelium; 3 = simple cuboidal epithelium; 4 = simple columnar epithelium; 5 = pseudostratified columnar epithelium; 8 = transitional epithelium; 10 = mammary glands; 11 = salivary glands; 16 = pituitary glands; 19 = adrenal cortex and medulla; 20 = testis; 21 = ovary; 32 = reticular connective tissue; 36 = melanogenic system; 41 = bone; 43 = smooth musculature; 47 = neurons of the central nervous system; 48 = neurons of the peripheral nervous system; 52 = central glia.
*ca = cancer or carcinoma.

tissues of the primary tumor exhibit a high local recurrence and others do not will help scientists and physicians to understand the process of local recurrence and to treat patients afflicted with it.

MALIGNANT POTENTIAL OF TISSUES AND INTRASPECIFIC TUMOR TYPES, REFLECTED IN LOCAL RECURRENCE

The tissues of the human body, just as those of other species, have a varying malignant potential reflected in intraspecies tumor types and their local recurrence. Prognostic factors for 1,015 women with recurrent breast cancer showed that the site of initial recurrence is an important indicator of survival time, followed by estrogen receptor status and conditions of lymph nodes. Estrogen-negative tumors recur more often in viscera and soft tissue sites and estrogen-positive ones more often in bone (11). The recurrence of superficial bladder tumors, which have this characteristic either in the same stage or deeply invading, can be predicted by certain risk factors and altered by treatment (77). A retinoblastoma with orbital recurrence presented with contrast enhancement of the subarachnoidal space in CT (51).

INTRASPECIES SPECTRUM OF LOCAL RECURRENCE OF HUMAN NEOPLASMS BASED ON A COMPARISON OF TISSUES

Tissues vary according to their potential towards local recurrence but, in addition, there are other factors which influence local recurrence, such as the radiosensitivity of the neoplastic cells of the recurrent tumor. Important is the location. Locally recurring neoplasms in the skull cavity are extremely dangerous. To date, no clear picture of the behavior of local recurrence exists; many more aspects will come to light in the near future.

TISSUES WITH HIGH NEOPLASTIC POTENTIAL OF LOCAL RECURRENCE

High neoplastic potential of local recurrence depends not only on the cell types involved but also on the interaction of the environment with the particular tissue, as can be observed in the simple columnar epithelium of the intestinal tract and other structures. It also depends on the extension of the tissue in the body and, therefore, the weight and space of this particular tissue. We may consider simple columnar epithelium in relation to chordal tissue in the human body. A selection of tissues with high potentials for neoplastic recurrence is given in the appropriate tables.

TISSUES WITH NO OR LOW NEOPLASTIC POTENTIAL OF LOCAL RECURRENCE

As the material investigated indicates, there are tissues in the human body which have a low potential recurrence. These are either partial tissues with a restricted distribution or those, like striated musculature, with a wide distribution but a low neoplastic potential in general. The tables of this section show selected tissue types with low potential of local recurrence.

THE ACTION OF TISSUE SUBTYPES

Mankind once was divided into races, but became more and more intermingled by marriage, a process which resulted in the nearly total disappearance of pure races and the development of geographic human types. These various people, exhibit differences in the tumor potential of the same tissues in their body, but tissues in various positions of the body of racial or typical similar configuration also exhibit a difference in tumor potential.

CASE REPORTS: THE BASIC FOUNDATION

This largest section of the chapter offers a review of case material characterized by local recurrences and arranged by the main tissue types. To avoid any distortion of the cases, the abstracted material has been shortened but left in its individual way of presentation.

THE INFLUENCE OF THE PRIMARY TUMOR TREATMENT ON LOCAL RECURRENCE

Treatment of the primary tumor has basic influence on the later development of local recurrence. Follow-up of postsurgery adenoid cystic carcinoma of the breast requires physical examinations to detect local recurrence (72). Cardiac myxoma, the most common primary intracardiac tumor histologically benign, may behave malignant, and shows also unusual manifestations (40). Patients with IB cervical carcinoma had an incidence of 11.3% recurrence (17.4% in patients with adenocarcinoma or adenosquamous carcinoma, and 9.2% in those with pure squamous tumors); 35% of cases showed central pelvic location, 39% pelvic side-wall location, and 20.6% distant recurrence. Distant recurrence was more common after postoperative radiotherapy of the pelvis for positive nodes or surgical margins (7).

TISSUE EVALUATION OF MULTIPLE PRIMARY NEOPLASMS, THERAPY-INDUCED NEOPLASMS, LOCAL RECURRENCE, AND METASTASIS

Multiple primary neoplasms can develop from the same tissue type as, for example, from colon epithelium or they can develop from different primary tissues (Chapter 6/Volume III). Therapy-induced neoplasms (see Chapters 14, 15, 21, 22/Volume VI) develop occasionally in the same tissue of the primary tumor but at different locations. The majority is produced in tissues other than the primary tumor. Local recurrence, as the name implies, is characterized by the appearance in the same tissue of the primary tumor. Metastases, although generally heterogenous, show the characteristics of the tissue of the primary tumor. As for disseminated leukemias, one type may change to another at the end stage. This is possible because of development from a mesenchymatic stem cell.

Table 2. Locally recurring and metastasizing neoplasms

Tissue	Tumor	Patient(s)	Treatment	Remarks	References
2	Skin neoplasms		Mohs surgery	Review of the technique used for primary non-melanoma skin tumors not treated successfully by conventional methods	(73)
4	Malignant mixed Mullerian tumors of uterus	180 females	Surgery	No difference in recurrence between homologous, heterologous, or undifferentiated sarcomatous elements. Locoregional recurrence rate was 17%	(70)
4	Colonic/rectal neoplasms			Study to determine cost of serial monitoring of carcinoembryonic antigen (CEA) to provide early indication of recurrence	(62)
4	Combined anus neoplasms	5 aged m + f	Synchronous chemo/radiotherapy	Suggested alternative to abdominoperineal resection; probability of cure at least equal to resection; patients retain normal anal function	(75)
4	Colorectal neoplasms	Middle age m + f	CEA-initiated laparotomy	Hepatic and pulmonary resection for metastatic disease accepted. About 20% of patients w/recurrence can be cured by local reresection	(5)
4	Rectal adenoca		Adjuvant pelvic radiation	Risk of pelvic recurrence can be reduced to 15% or less	(13)
4	Gastric adenoca			Use of endoscopy for early diagnosis	(16)
5	Juvenile laryngeal papillomas	627 patients	Suction diathermy (also: laser beams ultrasound)	Recurrence-free rate of 55% of more than 3 yrs. in children, 72.2% in adults	(85)
8	Superificial bladder ca*		Intravesical chemotherapy	Agents appear to lower recurrence rate and extend disease-free interval	(76)
8	Bladder ca		Intervesical adriamycin	Preliminary results indicate significant reduction in recurrence rate; treatment well tolerated	(48)
8	Bladder ca		Platinum coordination compounds	Review provides basis for selection of optimum regime	(68)
10	Gynecologic tumors	Females	Radiotherapy and hyperthermia	Rates of remission for local recurrences: breast ca: 80%, cervical ca 50–80%. Side effects of radiotherapy are not enhanced by hypothermia	(24)
10	Adenoid ca of breast	11 new cases, aged females	Surgery	Slow progression, local recurrence is inadequately resected, absence of lymph node metastases	(49)
10	Breast neoplasm			Progesterone receptor as important prognostic factor; more important than estrogen receptor for predicting time to recurrence	(10)
10	Breast ca		Adjuvant chemotherapy, postoperative	Among node-negative patients those w/a relatively high recurrence rate should be given adjuvant chemotherapy	(27)
10	Tumor breast ca		Chemotherapy	Bibliographic review	(64)
11	Primary malignant tumors of salivary gland			52 yr. review; this tumor comprises 30% of salivary gland neoplasms; long duration, repeated local recurrence, occasional metastases to regional lymph nodes, frequent metastases to lungs	(25)
16	Prolactin adenomas	963 patients	Transsphenoidal surgery or bromocriptine	First mode of treatment if serum prolactin levels below 100 mg/ml, second mode if above; heavy ion radiation may eventually be most effective treatment	(84)

Table 2. Continued.

Tissue	Tumor	Patient(s)	Treatment	Remarks	References
20	Primary mediastinal seminoma	3 new cases 129 reviewed white males	Radiotherapy	Testicular atrophy in only 7 patients; spread by distant metastases	(6)
32	Primary lymphoma central nervous system	12 middle age, m + f	Radiotherapy	CTU most successful diagnostic tool for initial detection and follow-up; recurrence noted from/to 33 months after diagnosis	(41)
41	Extraskeletal osteosarcoma	Female child	Surgery	Appeared in an ectopic hamartomatous thymus	(78)
43	Leiomyosarcoma of gastro-intestinal tract			About $\frac{1}{3}$ developed metastases, of which 90% were intra-abdominal (primarily liver) peritoneal seeding and local recurrence or extension	(35)
52	Pleomorphic xanthoastrocytoma	Male, 32 yr. old	Surgery	Relatively rapid fatal outcome 21 months following diagnosis; presence at autopsy of extensive recurrent tumor w/features of a malignant astrocytoma	(82)

Explanations of code numbers for tissues: 2 = stratified squamous epithelium; 3 = simple cuboidal epithelium; 4 = simple columnar epithelium; 5 = pseudostratified columnar epithelium; 8 = transitional epithelium; 10 = mammary glands; 11 = salivary glands; 16 = pituitary glands; 19 = adrenal cortex and medulla; 20 = testis; 21 = ovary; 32 = reticular connective tissue; 36 = melanogenic system; 41 = bone; 43 = smooth musculature; 47 = neurons of the central nervous system; 48 = neurons of the peripheral nervous system; 52 = central glia.
*ca = cancer or carcinoma.

SUMMARY AND CONCLUSIONS

Local recurrence of neoplasms in the human body has never before been compared on the basis of tissues involving an extensive a collection of materials, as in this chapter. The following conclusions are presented:

1. Local recurrence is a therapy-produced phenomenon, a failure of neoplastic progression.
2. Certain tumors of specific tissues are more prone to local recurrence than others.
3. Local recurrence occurs during tumor dissemination; generally one or two years after surgery.
4. Local recurrence generally precedes metastasis.
5. Local recurrence can be as devastating as metastasis.
6. Local recurrence may require several operations for the same tumor in the same patient several decades.
7. Local recurrence often occurs together with tumor metastasis in the same patient.
8. The frame of comparison is restricted to man, laboratory animals, domestic animals, and a few zoo animals.

REFERENCES

1. Adloff M, Arnaud JP: Secondary amputation of the rectum for neoplastic recurrence after rectal resection. Personal experience in 11 cases. *Chirurgie* 111(2):1985
2. Amatsu M, Makino K, Kinishi M: Stomal recurrence – etiologic factors and prevention. *Auris Nasus Larynx* 12(2):103, 1985
3. Amendola MA: The role of CT in the evaluation of ovarian malignancy. *CRC Crit Rev Diagn Imaging* 24(4):329, 1985
4. Anisimov VV: Meaning of the concept "local recurrence" following surgical treatment of malignant melanoma of the skin. *Vopr Onkol* 31(1):32, 1985
5. August DA, Ottow RT, Sugarbaker PH: Clinical perspective of human colorectal cancer metastasis. *Cancer Metastasis Rev* 3(4):303, 1984
6. Aygun C, Slawson RG, Bajaj K, Salazar OM: Primary mediastinal seminoma. *Urology* 23(2):109, 1984
7. Bassalyk LS, Novikov AM, Makhova EE, Kozachenko VP: Lipid-bound serum sialic acids in the complex diagnosis of recurrences of cancer of the ovary. *Vestn Akad Med Nauk SSSR* (9):67, 1985
8. Burke TW, Hoskins WJ, Heller PB et al.: Clinical patterns of tumor recurrence after radical hysterectomy in stage IB cervical carcinoma. *Obstet Gynecol* 69(3 Pt 1):382, 1987
9. Cholokashvili LD: Factors affecting the occurrence of cancer relapses in the intrathoracic portion of the esophagus after radical treatment. *Vopr Onkol* 31(7):39, 1985
10. Clark GM, McGuire WL: Progesterone receptors and human breast cancer. *Breast Cancer Res Treat* 3(2):157, 1983
11. Clark GM, Sledge GW Jr, Osborne CK, McGuire WL: Survival from first recurrence: relative importance of prognostic factors in 1,015 breast cancer patients. *J Clin Oncol* 5(1):55, 1987
12. Cooper RG: Adjuvant chemotherapy and the practicing oncologist. *Surg Clin North Am* 64(6):1173, 1984
13. Cummings BJ: Adjuvant radiation therapy for rectal adenocarcinoma. *Dis Colon Rectum* 27(12):826, 1984
14. Decker DA, Al Sarraf M, Kresge C, Austin D, Wilner HI: Phase II study of aziridinylbenzoquinone (AZQ: NSC-182986) in the treatment of malignant gliomas recurrent after radiation. Preliminary report. *J Neurooncol* 3(1):19, 1985
15. Dommes M, Thiede A, Hamelmann H: Locoregional recurrence following the operative treatment of rectal cancer. Basic principles of prevention and therapy. *Zentralbl Chir* 110(2–3):159, 1985
16. Douglass HO Jr, Nava HR: Gastric adenocarcinoma – management of the primary disease. *Semin Oncol* 12(1):32, 1985
17. Eberlein T, Simon R, Fisher S, Lippman ME: Height, weight, and risk of breast cancer relapse. *Breast Cancer Res Treat* 5(1):81, 1985

18. Eros A, Ritter L, Bajtai A: Percutaneous aspiration biopsy in perineal recurrences after abdominoperineal extirpations. *Acta Chir Hung* 26(3):145, 1985
19. Fisher ER: The pathology of lumpectomy with particular reference to local breast recurrence and multicentricity. *Verh Dtsch Ges Pathol* 69:51, 1985
20. Flamm J, Grof F: Prophylactic use of topical adriamycin after transurethral resection of transitional cell bladder tumours. *Int Urol Nephrol* 17(2):143, 1985
21. Gehanno P, Andreassian B, Guedon C, Veber F et al.: Surgery of pericannular recurrence and extensive tumors of the trachea. *Ann Otolaryngol Chir Cervicofac* 102(2):105, 1985
22. Hall RR: Methotrexate for superficial bladder cancer. *Prog Clin Biol Res* 185B:143, 1985
23. Henry C, Mahieu PH, Pringot J, Detry R: Contribution of the barium enema to the diagnosis of postoperative recurrence of malignant tumors of the rectum and sigmoid colon. *J Belge Radiol* 68(4):263, 1985
24. Herbst M: Palliative radiotherapy with and without hyperthermia in gynaecology. *Geburtshilfe Fraunheilkd* 43(8):520, 1983
25. Hunter RM, Davis BW, Gray GF Jr, Rosenfeld L: Primary malignant tumors of salivary gland origin. A 52-year review. *Am Surg* 49(2):82, 1983
26. Inokuchi K: Early gastric cancer viewed from its growth patterns. *Surg Annu* 18:111, 1986
27. Jungi WF: Adjuvant chemotherapy in breast cancer: status in 1984. *Wien Klin Wochenschr* 96(13):486, 1984
28. Kaiser HE (ed.): *Neoplasms – Comparative Pathology of Growth in Animals, Plants, and Man.* Baltimore: Williams & Wilkins, 1981
29. Kazeev KN, Chachibaia VA: Recurrent chromaffinoma. *Vestn Akad Med Nauk SSSR* (11):52, 1985
30. Kindermann G, Genz T: A comparison between the results of simple mastectomy and tumorectomy for breast cancer: the problem of local recurrence. *Arch Gynecol* 237(2):67, 1985
31. Knysh VI, Poddubnyi BK, Ozhiganov EL, Veselov VV, Mamedov EA: Clinicoendoscopic diagnosis of recurrences of cancer of the rectum. *Sov Med* (8):119, 1985
32. Kruglova GV, Pendkharkar DIa: Clinical picture and treatment of recurrent lymphosarcomas after radiotherapy. *Ter Arkh* 57(5):110, 1985
33. Kurth KH, Debruyne FJ, Senge T, Carpentier PJ, Riedl H et al.: Adjuvant chemotherapy of superficial transitional cell carcinoma: an E.O.R.T.C. randomized trial comparing doxorubicin hydrochloride, ethoglucid and TUR-alone. *Prog Clin Biol Res* 185B:135, 1985
34. Larson A, Fritjofsson A: Intravesical ethoglucid (Epodyl) for treatment of noninvasive bladder cancer (Stage 1a). *Ups J Med Sci* 90(2):127, 1985
35. Lee YT: Leiomyosarcoma of the gastro-intestinal tract: general pattern of metastasis and recurrence. *Cancer Treat Rev* 10(2):91, 1983
36. Llopis B, Gallego J, Mompo JA et al.: Thiotepa versus adriamycin versus *cis*-platinum in the intravesical prophylaxis of superficial bladder tumors. *Eur Urol* 11(2):73, 1985
37. Lotze W, Richter P: Recurrence following staged treatment of cervical cancer in stage Ia. *Zentralbl Gynakol* 107(7):411, 1985
38. Mäkelä J, Kairaluoma MI: Rationale of reoperation for gastric malignancies. *Ann Chir Gynaecol* 74(2):77, 1985
39. Marguth F, Deckler R: Recurrent pituitary adenomas. *Neurosurg Rev* 8(3–4):221, 1985
40. Markel ML, Waller BF, Armstrong WF: Cardiac myxoma. *Medicine (Baltimore)* 66(2):114, 1987
41. Mendenhall NP, Thar TL, Agee OF et al.: Primary lymphoma of the central nervous system. Computerized tomography scan characteristics and treatment results for 12 cases. *Cancer* 52(11):1993, 1983
42. Mentges B, Stahlschmidt M, Brückner R: The problem of recurrence in colonic cancer. *Langenbecks Arch Chir* 367(1):51, 1985
43. Mukamel E, Nissenkorn I, Glanz I, Vilcovsky E et al.: Upper tract tumours in patients with vesico-ureteral reflux and recurrent bladder tumours. *Eur Urol* 11(1)1:6, 1985
44. Newman AN, Colman M, Jayich SA: Verrucous carcinoma of the frontal sinus: a case report and review of the literature. *J Surg Oncol* 24(4):298, 1985
45. Norlen BJ, Malmström PU: Salvage cystectomy for bladder and gynaecologic cancer after irradiation failure. *Ups J Med Sci* 90(2):133, 1985
46. Ohoka H, Shinomiya H, Yokoyama M, Ochi K et al.: Thomsen-Friedenreich antigen in bladder tumors as detected by specific antibody: a possible marker of recurrence. *Urol Res* 13(2):47, 1985
47. Pascual MR, Macias A, Moreno L, Lage A: Factors associated with prognosis in human breast cancer. V. The simultaneous use of estrogen and progesterone receptor measurements for prediction of short-term relapse. *Neoplasms* 32(2):247, 1985
48. Pavone-Macaluso M, Ingargiola GB et al.: Treatment of bladder cancer with intravesical instillation of adriamycin. *Prog Clin Biol Res* 162B:181, 1984
49. Peters GN, Wolff M: Adenoid cystic carcinoma of the breast. Report of 11 new cases: review of the literature and discussion of biological behavior. *Cancer* 52(4):680, 1983
50. Pletnev SD, Artamonov NV, Fomin NS, Karpenko OM: Treatment of recurrent basal-cell skin cancer with laser irradiation. *Sov Med* (4):92, 1985
51. Poppe P, Appel B, Gysellinck J: Pathological contrast enhancement of the subarachnoidal space in CT of a retinoblastoma case with orbital recurrence. *J Belge Radiol* 67(5):329, 1984
52. Räber G, Pötzschke B: Use of computed tomography in the diagnosis of uterine carcinoma recurrence – comparison with other imaging technics. *Radiol Diag (Berl)* 26(3):325, 1985
53. Räber G, Pötzschke B: Computer tomography in the diagnosis of space-occupying gynecologic processes. 3. Use of computer tomography in the diagnosis of recurrence of uterine cancers. *Zentralbl Gynakol* 107(3):146, 1985a
54. Raemaekers JM, Beex LV, Koenders AJ et al.: Disease-free interval and estrogen receptor activity in tumor tissue of patients with primary breast cancer: analysis after long-term follow-up. *Breast Cancer Res Treat* 6(2):123, 1985
55. Rampal M, Coulange C, Lacoste J et al.: Is iatrogenic vesicorenal reflux a negligible factor in the evolution of recurrent superficial tumors of the bladder. *Ann Urol (Paris)* 19(2):132, 1985
56. Rampf W, Bittner R, Wiborg A, Beger HG: Early detection and chances for healing in recurrences of colorectal cancers. *Langenbecks Arch Chir* 366:480, 1985
57. Rivkin VL, Khakhanova MV, Egorov IuN: Recurrences of adenomas of the large intestine. *Vopr Onkol* 31(12):49, 1985
58. Rodriguez J, Point D, Esteve M, Brugere J: Total glossectomy without laryngectomy for recurrence after initial irradiation (2 year follow-up). *Ann Otolaryngol Chir Cervicofac* 102(6):421, 1985
59. Rosenkilde Olsen P, Jörgensen PM, Roed-Petersen K et al.: Control for recurrences of urinary bladder tumours by transabdominal ultrasonic scanning. *Scand J Urol Nephrol* 19(2):105, 1985
60. Rotte KH: Computer tomography in the diagnosis of recurrence of rectal and colonic cancer. *Zentralbl Chir* 110(2–3):89, 1985
61. Rotte KH, Hüttner J, Kriedemann E, Welker K: Value of computed tomography for the assessment of postoperative breast cancer recurrences and mediastinal metastases as a basis for irradiation planning. *Radiobiol Radiother (Berl)* 26(6):731, 1985

62. Sandler RS, Freund DA, Herbst CA Jr, Sandler DP: Cost effectiveness of postoperative carcinoembryonic antigen monitoring in colorectal cancer. *Cancer* 53(1):193, 1984

63. Schilling K: Pain therapy in the recurrence of colorectal cancer. *Zentralbl Chir* 110(2–3):177, 1985

64. Scolozzi R, Boccafogli A, Tocchetto M et al.: Prognostic factors and response to chemotherapy in breast cancer, bibliographic review. *Minerva Med* 74(18):1021, 1983

65. Sebastian G, Scholz A: Recurrence following cryosurgical basalioma therapy. *Dermatol Monatsschr* 171(1):38, 1985

66. Sennwald G, Segmüller G, Stanisic M, Wiederkehr P: Tumor of the hand, free flap and irradiation. Anatomo-pathologic study apropos of 1 case. *Ann Chir Main* 4(4):328, 1985

67. Shirkhoda A: Computed tomography after adrenalectomy in adrenal cortical carcinoma. *Urol Radiol* 7(3):132, 1985

68. Sidorik EP, Burlaka AP, Sirdorik OA, Korchevaia LM: Prospects for using platinum coordination compounds possessing antitumor activity. *Eksp Onkol* 6(6):6, 1984

69. Solymosi L, Ferbert A: A case of spinal paraganglioma. *Neuroradiology* 27(3):217, 1985

70. Spanos WJ Jr, Wharton JT, Gomez L et al.: Malignant mixed Müllerian tumors of the uterus. *Cancer* 53(2):311, 1984

71. Staab HJ, Brümmendorf T, Anderer FA et al.: Differentiation of disease recurrence in various primary malignancies using CEA slope analysis. *Tumour Biol* 6(2):157, 1985

72. Sumpio BE, Jennings TA, Merino MJ, Sullivan PD: Adenoid cystic carcinoma of the breast. Data from the Connecticut Tumor Registry and a review of the literature. *Ann Surg* 205(3):295, 1987

73. Swanson NA: Mohs surgery. Technique, indications, applications, and the future. *Arch Dermatol* 119(9):761, 1983

74. Sylvester R: The analysis of results in prophylactic superficial bladder cancer studies. *Prog Clin Biol Res* 1858:3, 1985

75. Tiver KW, Langlands AO: Synchronous chemotherapy and radiotherapy for carcinoma of the anal canal – an alternative to abdominoperineal resection. *Aust NZ J Surg* 54(2):101, 1984

76. Torti FM, Lum BL: The biology and treatment of superficial bladder cancer. *J Clin Oncol* 2(5):505, 1984

77. Torti FM, Lum BL: Superficial bladder cancer. Risk of recurrence and potential role for interferon therapy. *Cancer* 59(3 Suppl):613, 1987

78. Valderrama E, Kahn LB, Wind E: Extraskeletal osteosarcoma arising in an ectopic hamartomatous thymus. Report of a case and review of the literature. *Cancer* 51(6):11, 1983

79. Vinokurov VL, Nikolaeva LIa: Cellular immunity indices of ovarian cancer patients. *Vopr Onkol* 32(1):60, 1986

80. von Gottberg C, Kroczek H: Comparative studies of local recurrence following sphincter preserving anterior rectal resection and primary rectal excision 1980–1983. *Zentralbl Chir* 110(2–3):172, 1985

81. Voute PA, Hoefnagel CA, Marcuse HR, de Kraker J: Detection of neuroblastoma with 131I-meta-iodobenzylguanidine. *Prog Clin Biol Res* 175:389, 1985

82. Weldon-Linne CM, Victor TA, Groothuis DR, Vick NA: Pleomorphic xanthoastrocytoma. Ultrastructural and immunohistochemical study of a case with a rapidly fatal outcome following surgery. *Cancer* 52(11):2055, 1983

83. Wilson RE: Reoperation for gastro-esophageal cancer. *Ann Chir Gynaecol* 74(2):49, 1985

84. Wollesen F, Bendsen BB: Effect rates of different modalities for treatment of prolactin adenomas. *Am J Med* 78(1):114, 1985

85. Wolters B, Eichhorn T, Kleinsasser O: Critical review of the therapy of juvenile laryngeal papillomas. *Laryngol Rhinol Otol (Stuttg)* 63(8):396, 1984

18

EFFUSIONS

RUDOLF C. ULIRSCH and DENA M. GOMEZ

Effusions may develop in any of the serous membrane-lined body cavities. The peritoneal, pleural, and pericardial spaces are the principal mesothelial-lined body cavities that cause clinical diagnostic problems. All three major body cavities share the characteristic that they are normally more accurately described as potential spaces. When fluid of any type develops in this "potential space", it separates the layers of the body cavity. Excessive accumulation of fluid may result in compromise of normal organ functions. In this respect, the heart is particularly subject to the effects of fluid accumulation in the pericardial sac. Compromise of ventricular filling in diastole may result in cardiac tamponade and rapid death. In the pleural cavities, fluid accumulation will lead to respiratory compromise by preventing normal lung expansion. Fluid accumulation is perhaps best tolerated in the peritoneal cavity, but eventually this also results in discomfort, respiratory compromise, and difficulty with mobility.

Clinically, early recognition of the presence of disease is an important consideration. When far advanced, the presence of an effusion will be easily recognized. Specialized laboratory studies are required for a more timely definitive evaluation. These studies include radiographic studies as a first modality (143).

False diagnostic signs may be generated by benign anatomical anomalies. Cardiac levorotation with medial rotation of the right coronary artery has been reported to cause confusion with a thickened pericardial stripe on chest radiographs (70).

More sensitive techniques have been developed which allow a prompt identification and even formation of a differential diagnosis before the development of the severe complications already described. Ultrasonography may be helpful, particularly in identifying an early pericardial effusion.

Early effusions have been detected by prenatal ultrasonic diagnosis. A case of pleural and pericardial effusion diagnosed by this modality has been reported (76).

CAT scanning may be helpful in defining pleural-based diseases and small effusions (167, 198). Magnetic resonance imaging (MRI) has also been applied to the identification of pericardial effusions with some success (177).

It is important to distinguish true fluid accumulation in the body cavities from other space-occupying lesions. A mediastino-abdominal lipomatosis without obesity, consisting of fatty tissue causing "pseudo-ascitic" abdominal enlargement has been described. Insulin-dependent diabetes mellitus, and type IV hyperlipidemia are associated with this syndrome (51).

Metastatic carcinoma can surround the heart and result in a picture simulating pericardial effusion, without the presence of fluid in the pericardial space (86).

"Pseudo-ascites" may also be seen with massive ovarian cysts. Elevated serum and "ascitic" amylase levels may be seen in this setting (66). Steroid therapy may be associated with pseudoeffusion of the pericardium, again due to lipomatosis (120). Malignant neoplasms primary to the omentum are quite rare, but may result in clinical findings that mimic hemorrhagic ascites. A primary omental leiomyosarcoma causing hemorrhagic pseudoascites has been described (47).

CLASSIFICATION OF EFFUSIONS

Much clinical interest is focused on effusions. Even small effusions may represent the harbinger of a progressive stage of neoplastic transformation: metastatic disease. The presence of an effusion, in and of itself, should not be considered evidence for progression of disease. An effusion may result from many causes, both benign and malignant. Proper evaluation of an effusion requires assessment of the clinical situation and fluid sampling, if possible. Frequently, the withdrawal of excess fluid has a beneficial clinical effect, even if only for a brief period. The fluid obtained may be subjected to many diverse types of analyses. However, the classical initial evaluation of an effusion demands that an attempt be made to classify it either as a transudate or an exudate (Table 1) (157). This approach may be somewhat simplified and has been applied primarily to pleural effusions, but it serves a useful purpose. Transudates tend to be caused by any of several benign conditions, whereas exudates tend to be associated with actual neoplastic progression into the site sampled. Some causes of transudates and exudates are listed (Table 2) (12, 85, 133). These broad categories of types of effusions should be used as a general guide only. The studies used to define these groups relate only to second-

The views expressed herein are those of the authors, and should not be construed as official.

The authors wish to express their appreciation to Dr. Eileen B. King, Chief, Cytopathology, UCSF, for sharing her wealth of case material for use in preparation of this chapter.

The authors also express their thanks to David Geller for preparing the manuscript.

Table 1. Criteria for effusion classification.

	Transudate	Exudate
Appearance	Clear, pale yellow	Cloudy
Cells	Few	Abundant
Specific gravity	< 1.015	> 1.015
Glucose	High	Low (40 mg/dl < serum)
Total protein	< 2 g/dl	> 2 g/dl
Fibrin content	Low	High
White blood cell count	< 1,000/µl	> 1,000/µl
Red blood cell count	–	> 10,000/µl
pH (correlates with glucose)	–	> 7.4
LDH	–	Elevated

ary phenomena, not to the actual presence or absence of neoplastic cells. Therefore, they should not be used as the sole basis of definitive therapy or prognosis.

Classification of effusions can be simplified for practical clinical purposes. Early studies indicated a correlation of malignancy and elevated lactic dehydrogenase (201). Exudates may be differentiated from transudates on the basis of ratios of protein and LDH in the pleural fluid and serum. An exudate is identified when one of the following is present: (a) pleural fluid protein elevation to exceed 0.5 times the serum level, (b) pleural fluid LDH elevation to exceed 0.6 times the serum level, or (c) pleural fluid LDH elevation to exceed 0.66 times the upper reference level for serum LDH (103). Such criteria are meaningful only if they show correlation with the clinical state of the patient, rather than an arbitrary grouping of effusion types. One study of 318 patients has shown that application of these criteria allows for the identification of a transudate group which may not require further diagnostic testing for their effusions (133). A group of 83 patients with transudates identified by Peterman showed two missed malignant effusions, but more significantly, they reported 7 "false-positive" results on transudates, and these were subjected to further laboratory tests. This apparently included one false-positive finding of malignancy. This was a case of

Table 2. Causes of effusions (in approximate order of frequency within group).

Transudaates
1. Congestive heart failure
2. Systemic hypoproteinemia
3. Cirrhosis of liver
4. Chronic renal failure
5. Pneumonia
6. Neoplasm
7. Autoimmune disease

Exudates
1. Infections (especially pneumonia and tuberculosis)
2. Neoplasms (especially carcinoma of lung, breast, ovary, and lymphoma/leukemia)
3. Congestive heart failure
4. Trauma (including thoracotomy)
5. Pancreatitis
6. Autoimmune diseases
7. Pulmonary embolism
8. Chronic renal failure
9. Myocardial infarction (Dressler's syndrome)

Table 3. Effusions/serous membrane disease: useful diagnostic techniques.

I. *Biopsy*
  A. "Blind"
  B. Thorascopy directed

II. *Fluid aspiration*
  A. *Physico-chemical analysis*
    1. Red blood cell count
    2. White blood cell count
    3. Specific gravity
    4. Lactate dehydrogenase (LDH), including isoenzymes
    5. pH (primarily for pleural fluid)
    6. Total protein
  B. *Immunologic studies*
    1. Flow cytometry
    2. Immunoperoxidase, e.g., terminal deoxynucleotidyl transferase (TdT)
  C. *Microbiologic studies*
    1. Gram stain
    2. Aerobic culture
    3. Anaerobic culture
    4. Mycobacterial culture
    5. Fungal culture
  D. *Chromosomal studies*
    1. Cytogenetics
    2. DNA content

lymphoma which subsequently was tested for T- and B-cell markers, which did not support this diagnosis. An alternate interpretation of these data might be that separation of effusions into transudate and exudate categories is not always reliable, and that confirmatory tests should be performed on some cytologic specimens which appear to contain malignant cells.

In another study of diagnoses of 584 specimens from 472 consecutive patients, the author reports that there were no false positive diagnoses of malignancy (80). Further studies are required for accurate and precise diagnostic classification. The various techniques available, including modern research methods, are described (Table 3).

MECHANISMS OF EFFUSION ACCUMULATION

Effusions result from an imbalance of capillary fluid dynamics, as described by E.H. Starling. Such disturbances may have their roots in many specific disease processes. In general, systemic abnormalities result in formation of transudates. Transudates are essentially ultrafiltrates of plasma that form in the presence of intact vascular and capillary walls. Exudates form when there is a localized breakdown of the structural integrity of the vascular system (133, 187). These are general priniciples that usually apply to actual clinical problems.

Increased capillary pressure may occur due to an elevation of hydrostatic pressure. Congestive heart failure and its associated increase in venous pressure transmitted to the capillaries is a prototypical example of this mechanism. Rarely, similar mechanisms may affect the right heart circulation. Massive pulmonary thromboembolism has resulted in acute right heart failure and an associated 700-cc transudative pericardial effusion (176). Portomesenteric venous occlusion may occur secondary to intraabdominal neoplasm, or hepatic cirrhosis. This event is associated with rapidly increasing ascites, and variceal hemorrhage (200).

A decrease in serum proteins results in a decline in intravascular colloid osmotic pressure. If this decline is extreme, it may result in sufficient disturbance of the balance of fluid forces to result in accumulation of an effusion.

Obstruction of lymphatic channels may result in increased pressures within the potential spaces of the serous-lined body cavities. Obstruction may result from multiple causes, including (a) metastatic carcinoma with "mass effect" on large lymphatic channels, such as the thoracic duct; (b) lymphangiectatic spread of carcinoma; (c) filariasis and other parasitic diseases; (d) trauma or operations disturbing the normal lymphatic channels.

Alterations in fluid and electrolyte balance in patients with hypothyroidism seem to have a relationship to the development of pericardial effusions. Interestingly, a recent study has shown some, albeit weak, correlation between human atrial natriuretic peptide (hANP) levels and the amount of pericardial effusion present (196).

Finally, effusions may develop because of an increase in capillary permeability. This increase may be due to a breakdown of normal tissues by neoplasm, or by intense inflammatory infiltrates. Even more interesting is the isolation of a "vascular permeability factor" from guinea pigs, hamsters, and mice. Tumor cells from these animals have been found to produce a distinct 34,000 to 42,000-dalton protein which rapidly increases vascular permeability and results in ascitic fluid accumulation (162). The possible relevance of this mechanism to human disease is unknown at this time.

Experimental studies have been undertaken to define the mechanism of spread of neoplastic cells within serosal-lined body cavities. Mouse ascitic hepatoma cells did not attach to intact mesothelium-lined surfaces. However, these neoplastic cells did attach to peritoneum from which the mesothelial lining cells had been removed (150).

Other experimental studies on mechanisms of ascites development in mice with cancer cells injected into the peritoneum have been performed. Cancer cells in these studies established subperitoneal colonies associated with local capillary rupture (165).

Ascitic fluid from women with advanced ovarian carcinomas was found to contain a factor, or factors, that inhibit T-lymphocyte mitogenesis. Macrophages isolated from the ascitic fluid of these patients have been shown to be a source of these factors. It has been suggested that this results in a localized immunosuppression, which could result in enhanced metastasis within the peritoneal cavity (163).

THE USE OF BIOPSY

Biopsies may be performed, especially on pleural-based lesions. Such biopsies are usually undertaken closed ("blind"). Diagnostic yield of blind needle biopsies has been studied by multiple investigators, and some have compared biopsies to results obtained by the use of cytologic examination. Use of biopsy alone gives the lowest sensitivity for detection of malignant disease. Pleural malignant disease was found on biopsy in 43% (142) and 51.6% (199) of cases of demonstrated malignancy, when considered alone. Most

investigators have shown some improved sensitivity of the biopsy technique through multiple biopsies. A 2% increase in sensitivity was seen on second biopsy in one study (199). Multiple biopsies (up to 10) with an Abrams needle through a single entry site increased biopsy sensitivity to 72% in one series (121). Almost all of the 33 patients examined by Mungall showed no malignancy on some of the biopsies obtained.

Sensitivity of cytologic examination alone has been found to be superior to biopsy alone in the evaluation of pleural-based malignancy. Sensitivity of cytologic examination has been reported in the range of 57.6% (142) to 89.4% (106) by various authors. Use of cytologic examination alone yields some cases of false negative results, which are detected by biopsy examination. In different series, 7.1% of 281 patients (142), and 10.9% of 181 patients (199) with malignant disease were missed when biopsy examination was excluded. It is for this reason that a combined approach is most prudent (136, 199).

Recently, direct visualization of the pleural surfaces by thoracoscopy has been developed. The use of direct visualization of the serous membrane surfaces generates excellent sensitivity with the biopsy technique, resulting in diagnostic findings in 119/127 patients studied (93.7%) in one series (195).

Neoplasms primary to the serosal surfaces are quite uncommon. In addition to mesotheliomas (discussed elsewhere), several other disorders may primarily involve the lining surfaces of the body cavities. Hemangiomatosis has been described as a rare cause of hemorrhagic pleural effusion in the neonate (74). However, malignant vascular lesions arising in serous membranes can also occur. Angiosarcomas may arise in any of the major body cavity linings, including peritoneum, pleura, and pericardium (Fig. 1). A cystic lymphangiosarcoma showing progression throughout the peritoneum and right pleural cavity in a manner similar to the usual mode of spread of mesothelioma has been described (113). Hemangiomyosarcoma arising in the pleura has been reported (22).

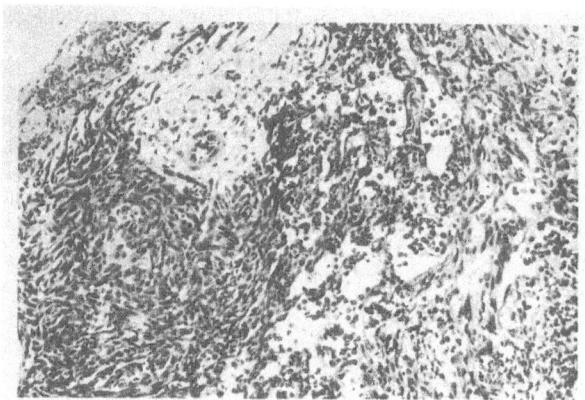

Figure 1. Angiosarcoma of pericardium in a 50-year-old male with pleuritic chest pain and hemopericardium. An infiltrative vascular lesion composed of cytologically malignant cells is evident. A prominent spindle cell component is present (left side of field) (Hematoxylin and eosin stain, 100 ×).

Lymphangioleiomyomatosis is a rare disease of women in their reproductive years, which results from proliferation of smooth muscle around lymphatic channels in the lung, chest, and abdomen (27). The smooth muscle proliferation tends to become extensive, with infiltration of pulmonary alveolar walls, pleural surfaces, and lymph nodes (36). Repeated spontaneous pneumothoraces are frequently seen. As a consequence of extensive muscle proliferation, lymphatic channels tend to become obstructed and rupture. This results in the frequent development of chylous pleural effusions in these patients, which are best identified by the analysis of triglyceride levels. Gross examination is not always reliable, but triglyceride levels above 110 mg/dl are very suggestive of the presence of a chylous effusion (175). This should be differentiated from the "milky" effusion seen in some patients with tuberculosis. These effusions are high in cholesterol, but not truly chylous in nature (14). Lymphangioleiomyomatosis tends to recur and progress despite operation, chemotherapy, and radiotherapy. Disease arising in, or progressing to, peritoneal involvement may also cause intractable chylous ascites. Peritoneo-venous drainage has been applied as a palliative measure in this situation (46). A unique approach of dietary fat restriction has met with success in one case of chylous ascites due to lymphangioleiomyomatosis (25).

Very rarely, chylopericardium can be seen as a primary disease process. Such a case has been reported to be successfully treated with ligation of the thoracic duct at the level of the diaphragm (192).

Non-neoplastic, reactive processes may occasionally simulate malignant or benign neoplasms of the serosal surfaces. Foreign body reactions to talc from surgical gloves are well known to be associated with proliferative foreign body responses within body sites previously operated upon. This can cause considerable diagnostic difficulty in the separation of metastatic carcinoma from benign reaction, especially upon frozen section examination. Administration of talc injected by intravenous drug users may cause systemic granulomatous disease simulating sarcoidosis (56). Cornstarch, an alternate surgical glove powder, may also produce a granulomatous response when deposited on serosal surfaces. Rarely, caseating granulomas simulating tuberculosis may be formed (128).

A variety of processes can be seen to primarily affect the serosal surfaces. Occasionally, the laboratory examination of an effusion provides only a clue to the correct, specific diagnosis without demonstration of actual malignant cells. However, the presence of footprints of cancer is not sufficient evidence to establish a diagnosis of cancer. Serosal biopsy may be helpful in the setting of non-exfoliative neoplasms.

CYTOLOGY

Specimen collection

Morphologic cytologic examination constitutes a significant and frequently definitive technique for examining effusions (21, 108, 191). It has the advantage of bathing any localized lesion which may be present on the pleural, peritoneal, or pericardial surfaces. Any shedding neoplastic cells are then likely to be captured and only need to be concentrated by any of a variety of techniques.

Effusions frequently have the capacity to clot. Anticoagulation should be performed promptly after receipt of the specimen, if it has not already been done at the time of specimen aspiration. This is accomplished with 1% heparin in saline, with up to 2 ml/liter of fluid. Any fibrin strands already present in the specimen should be removed with the use of an applicator stick (197).

Fluids may be collected and stored under refrigeration for several days. Alternatively, the specimen can be mixed with equal parts of 50% ethanol (or methanol), and then refrigerated. Smears may be rapidly fixed with an alcohol fixative (85). The specimen must then be concentrated by any of several techniques. Filter or cytocentrifuge preparations may be prepared directly for low volume specimens. Otherwise, the specimen is first spun down to concentrate the cellular elements and the supernatant is discarded. Such concentration techniques permit the examination of large numbers of cells in a short time, despite an initially dilute specimen.

Another approach to examination of high volume pleural fluid samples for malignant cells using Percoll density gradient centrifugation has been described (123). The technique involves discontinuous density gradient centrifugation under physiologic conditions. Malignant cells are not only separated, but actually enriched in the 1.050 g/ml density layer.

Preparation of smears for morphologic examination from bloody effusions can be a significant technical problem. Such specimens adhere poorly to glass slides. In addition, the large numbers of red blood cells can obscure important cytologic details of rare nucleated cells. A technique of centrifugation in capillary tubes to produce a "buffy coat" preparation has recently been described (204). This technique concentrates the desired nucleated cells, and has the advantage that it does not require specialized laboratory equipment for implementation.

Benign effusions

Numerous causes of benign effusions exist (26). Congestive heart failure is a common etiology of such benign, usually transudative, effusions. Some other specific causes of benign effusions deserve special mention because of their special nature and potential for causing confusion with malignant disease.

Meig's syndrome is defined as the presence of ascites and hydrothorax with benign fibrous lesions of the ovary. Variations of this pattern have been described in which other lesions, including stroma ovarii, involve the ovary. Such variations are designated pseudo-Meig's syndrome (117).

Rarely, ascites may develop in association with endometriosis involving the abdominal cavity (Fig. 2). Hormonal therapy has been used to control this condition (68, 79, 125). The existence of effusions associated with benign neoplasms, and other non-neoplastic diseases emphasizes the critical nature of actual examination of an abnormal collection of fluid. Reliance cannot be placed solely on the clinical presentation.

Rarely, patients with severe kidney disease requiring

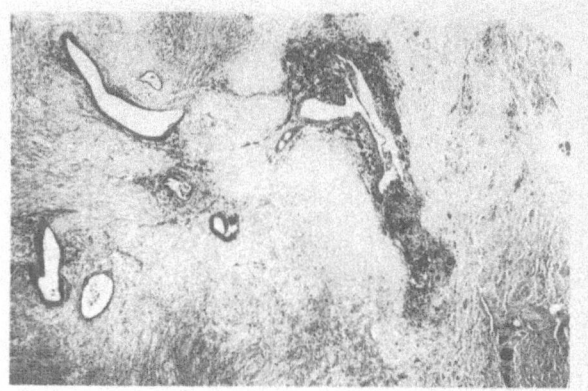

Figure 2. Endometriosis of the pelvic peritoneum. The glands of endometriosis have simple columnar, cytologically bland epithelium and associated endometrial stromal cells. This lesion should not be confused with metastatic adenocarcinoma (Hematoxylin and eosin stain, 25 ×).

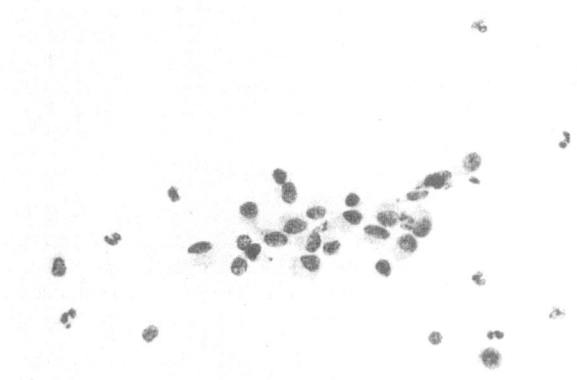

Figure 3. Benign mesothelial cells in peritoneal fluid. Cuboidal cells with uniform nuclei with central located chromocenter or nucleolus. Cytoplasm is pale with distinct cell borders (Papanicolaou stain, 250 ×).

dialysis, develop severe ascites. The mechanism of this atypical reaction is unclear and multiple treatment modalities including peritoneal dialysis, and peritoneovenous shunt placement have been used in such patients (13, 71).

Occasional pleural fluids may show pronounced eosinophilia. Koss has suggested a 10% level of eosinophils to qualify as an eosinophilic pleural effusion. These effusions may be associated with diverse etiologies, including drug reaction, allergic reaction, chest trauma, autoimmune disease, tuberculosis, and rarely cancer. Other cases are idiopathic in nature. Synchronous peripheral blood eosinophilia is rarely observed. Eosinophilic pleural effusions share the characteristic that they almost always eventually resolve spontaneously (88). Eosinophilic infiltrates are also quite commonly observed in pleural biopsies. Pleural eosinophilia has been observed in association with spontaneous pneumothorax. This lesion is distinct from eosinophilic granuloma, and has been designated reactive eosinophilic pleuritis (5). This process represents a distinctive form of inflammatory response rather than a specific disease entity.

Pleural effusions may be seen in association with autoimmune diseases, particularly systemic lupus erythematosus (SLE). These effusions are usually late manifestations of disease, but may represent the initial presentation on rare occasions. In rare cases, intractable pleural effusions may become a serious treatment problem (50).

Fluids from SLE are characterized as exudates with high leukocyte counts, and are composed predominantly of lymphocytes and neutrophils. Plasmacytoid lymphocytes may be seen (145). On occasion, lupus erythematosus (LE) cells may be seen in effusions. These cells consist of neutrophils engulfing a round, distinct, and homogeneous nuclear mass (84, 131, 132, 145).

Mesothelial cells and their reactive counterparts are frequently encountered in cytologic examination of all types of effusions. These lining cells show a wide spectrum of appearances. Mesothelial cells are found singly, in small clusters, or in rosette-like formations (Fig. 3). The nuclei are small, round to oval, and centrally located. Cytoplasmic features are highly variable, with clear, finely vacuolated to dark

basophilic appearance. Reactive changes in mesothelial cells are quite common and pose a frequent differential diagnostic problem for the cytopathologist (Fig. 4) (180). Reactive mesothelial cells may become enlarged, show cytoplasmic inclusions such as vacuoles and pigment, become multinucleated, and show prominent nucleoli and chromocenters. Differentiation from primary mesothelioma of the serosal surfaces, or metastatic adenocarcinoma is sometimes quite difficult, but nonetheless essential.

Atypical reactive changes may occur in mesothelial cells in various circumstances. These changes include proliferation of mesothelial cells, and enlargement of cells. Pseudoglandular clusters may be observed. Abnormal chromatin patterns and prominent nucleoli may also be seen. These atypical features are found in a large number of nonneoplastic processes (Table 4). Such changes are known to occur in ascitic fluid with cirrhosis. Congestive heart failure, pulmonary infarction, uremia, bronchopneumonia and its

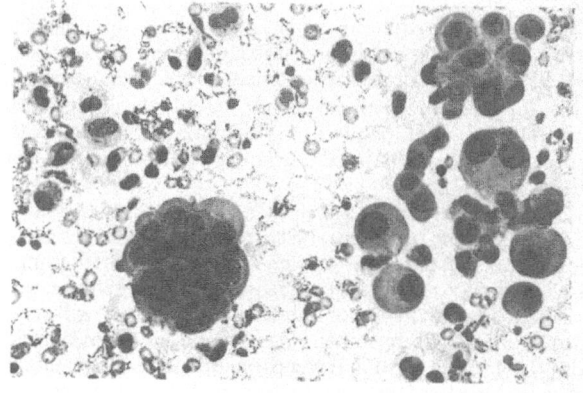

Figure 4. Reactive mesothelial cells. Clusters of enlarged cells with well-defined cell borders and uniform nuclei with nucleoli. Note the apparent increase in size with air-dried preparation (Giemsa stain, 250 ×).

Table 4. Reactive mesothelial cells. Associated disorders.

1. Liver disease, especially cirrhosis
2. Necrosis or infarction
3. Autoimmune disease (e.g., SLE)
4. Radiation
5. Any chronic irritation

complications, and tuberculosis have all been associated with the production of occasionally difficult to interpret reactive mesothelial processes. Pancreatitis has recently been added to the list of lesions that lead to atypical reactive processes which cause false positive malignant diagnoses (95).

MALIGNANT NEOPLASMS

Different anatomical areas of the body are preferentially affected by metastases from specific organ sites. Pleural involvement and generation of effusions is seen most commonly from breast carcinoma (24%), lung (19%), and lymphoreticular neoplasms (16%). In the peritoneal cavity, the most commonly observed primary neoplasms are as follows: ovarian carcinoma (32%), breast carcinoma (13%), and lymphoreticular neoplasms (7%) (160).

Mesothelioma

The lining cells of the body cavities (mesothelium) can give rise to localized or diffuse primary tumors. Localized lesions, usually of papillary or adenomatoid configuration (see adenomatoid tumor, below) are generally benign. Diffuse malignant mesothelioma is an aggressive infiltrative neoplasm which involves large areas of lining surfaces.

Asbestos exposure as an etiologic factor in the development of diffuse malignant mesothelioma is well established (99). Crocidolite, amosite, and chrysotile, in decreasing order, are the fibers most strongly implicated in the subsequent development of mesothelioma (11). Lung involvement with other primary lung carcinomas (33) and lymphoid and plasma cell malignancies (82) also follow exposure to asbestos. However, ferruginous bodies have been found in a large percentage of lungs without significant parenchymal disease (34). An increased risk for lung cancer has been associated with shipyard employment during World War II (17). The possibility of an epidemic of mesothelioma in the late 20th century appears real since the latency period ranges from 20–25 years (38).

One postulated mechanism of malignant transformation secondary to the presence of asbestos exposure draws analogies to the subcutaneous foreign-body sarcomas in animals after introduction of plastic, glass, and metal (38).

The predominant site of involvement is the pleural cavity, with over 70% of mesotheliomas originating from this site. About 25% are found in the peritoneum, with the remaining mesotheliomas arising pleural/peritoneal, within the pericardium, or from the tunica vaginalis (114).

Clinical symptoms and signs are related to the location of the tumor and a characteristic, locally infiltrative growth pattern. A gradual onset of dyspnea and chest pain is noted

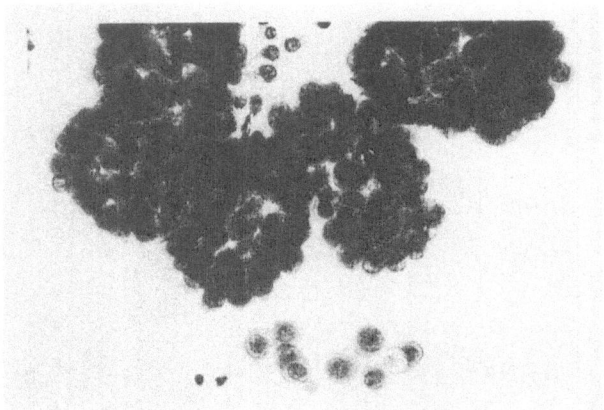

Figure 5. Malignant mesothelioma in pleural fluid specimen. Papillary cell clusters with ill-defined borders are seen. Nuclei are large and hyperchromatic with distinct nucleoli (Papanicolaou stain, 400 ×).

with pleural-based mesotheliomas, with pleural effusions and later encasement of the lung parenchyma. Nonspecific abdominal discomfort and ascites may precede the diagnosis of peritoneal mesotheliomas. Involvement of the gastrointestional tract by the tumor may lead to obstruction. Similarly, the heart may become encased by mesothelioma of the pericardium.

Exfoliative cytology is that of cellular smears generally containing groups of cells ranging from small clusters to large papillary configurations, as well as single cells. The clusters may have smooth, discreet outlines, but the majority have an irregular periphery (Fig. 5). Individual cells are larger than benign mesothelial cells and some may be gigantic. Cytoplasm stains densely, and can take on a variety of colors with Papanicolaou stain. Nuclei may be large, have irregular contours, hyperchromatic and coarse chromatin, and prominent nucleoli (126). The cytology of effusions in the presence of malignant mesothelioma can appear deceptively benign, with only slightly enlarged cells showing minimal nuclear abnormalities. Recently, pleural fluids from three cases of diffuse malignant mesothelioma demonstrated foamy macrophage-like cells, some lacking the nuclear features of malignancy (174).

Three histologic patterns of diffuse malignant mesothelioma are recognized: epithelial, sarcomatous, and biphasic (Fig. 6), with the predominant form being epithelial (50–75%) (114). The epithelial component is often papillary in configuration. Cells vary from well differentiated to anaplastic. Malignant mesotheliomas are strongly positive with anticytokeratin antibody, and may also stain for vimentin, particularly if fixed in alcohol (5/5) vs. formalin (10/30) (33). The special stain most widely used to confirm mesothelioma is Alcian blue. Alcian blue positive material, which disappears when pretreated with hyaluronidase, is strongly suggestive of mesothelial cell origin.

Diffuse malignant mesothelioma must be differentiated from a metastatic or locally invasive adenocarcinoma. This is difficult when the tumor is poorly differentiated; however, demonstration of intracytoplasmic mucin with PAS pretreated with diastase, or mucicarmine stains confirms an

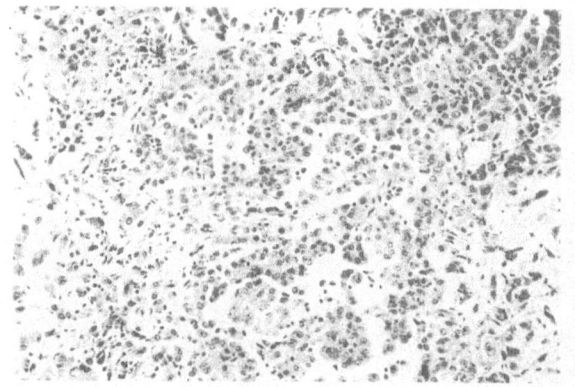

Figure 6. Malignant mesothelioma involving peritoneal wall in a 55-year-old male. A biphasic pattern is evident, with papillary mesothelial and spindle cell components (extreme lower right) (Hematoxylin and eosin stain, 100×).

adenocarcinoma. The use of CEA staining, also is helpful for the diagnosis of adenocarcinoma (119).

Diffuse malignant mesothelioma should also be differentiated from mesothelial hyperplasia, fibrosis, and other carcinomas and sarcomas. The benign mesothelioma, or adenomatoid tumor, is easily distinguished by its classic location along the genital tract and bland cytologic appearance (Fig. 7).

Adenocarcinoma

Metastatic adenocarcinomas comprise the largest group of malignant neoplasms showing progression to body cavity involvement (21, 23, 80). Adenocarcinomas arise from multiple different organs, and generally show a predilection for spread to body cavities closest to the primary site. Pronounced differences in patterns of metastasis exist between

male and female patients, as might be expected from the differences in distribution of primary malignancies. Pleural effusions with adenocarcinoma, in order of frequency in male patients, arise in (1) lung, (2) gastrointestinal tract, and (3) genitourinary tract. In female patients, the likely primary sites to be explored for adenocarcinoma are (1) breast, (2) female genital tract, (3) lung, (4) gastrointestinal tract, and occasionally (5) urinary tract (80). In the female patient with malignant ascites, ovarian carcinoma is the most common primary site.

Many disease processes cause reactive mesothelial changes which can simulate adenocarcinoma. In addition, adenocarcinoma is the most commonly observed histologic pattern of metastatic neoplasm in effusions. These observations suggest that precise criteria must be applied for the accurate separation of benign from malignant processes. False positive diagnoses may subject patients to unnecessary treatment, or result in failure to give appropriate treatment for what is actually localized disease not yet showing body cavity involvement. Fortunately, most authors report that positive results of malignancy based on cytologic examination have a very high predictive value for true malignancy. Some authors report no false positive diagnoses over the period studied (88, 80). Excellent results such as these demand strict adherence to diagnostic criteria by experienced observers.

Mesothelial cells tend to form cell aggregates, but do not form true glandular clusters. These aggregates of mesothelial cells tend to show a spectrum of sizes and shapes which merge with recognizable mesothelial cells. Clusters should be small and infrequent. If very prominent, a diagnosis of primary mesothelioma should be considered. Adenocarcinoma forms larger cell groups. Careful examination for glandular lumens should be undertaken. Adenocarcinoma groups are so large as to extend above and below the usual

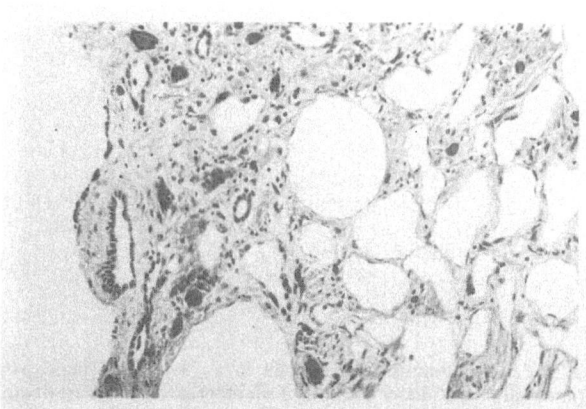

Figure 7. Adenomatoid tumor (benign mesothelioma) of Fallopian tube. Multiple tubular spaces lined by a single layer of flattened cells. Peritoneal mesothelial lining is to the left (Hematoxylin and eosin stain, 100×).

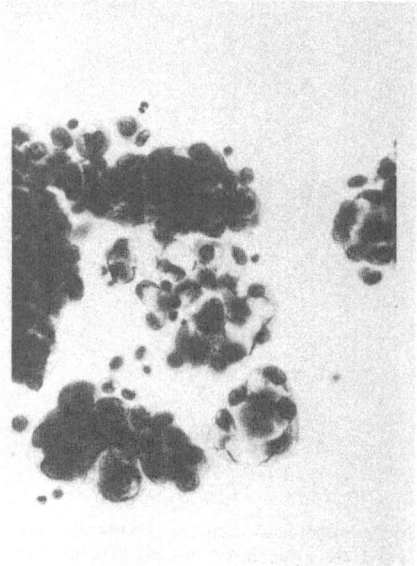

Figure 8. Ovarian carcinoma in ascitic fluid. Three-dimensional papillary structures composed of cytologically malignant cells (Papanicolaou stain, 250×).

plane of focus (188). This results in the presence of so-called "three dimensional" clusters (Fig. 8).

General cytologic criteria of malignancy should also be applied. Increased nuclear-cytoplasmic (N:C) ratio, and absolute increase in nuclear size is observed in malignancy. Nucleoli may be prominent and multiple. Mitotic figures may be present in frequent numbers. Very helpful is the presence of abnormal mitotic figures, such as tripolar or tetrapolar forms. All these criteria are helpful in the distinction of reactive mesothelial cells and adenocarcinoma, but none of them should be considered absolute (Figs. 9 and 10).

Special stains may occasionally be helpful in the differential diagnosis of reactive mesothelial cells, mesothelioma, and metastatic carcinoma. The periodic-acid-Schiff (PAS) stain for neutral mucopolysaccharides is expected to be negative in mesotheliomas (158). Early studies suggested use of nonspecific esterase staining to recognize malignant cells (6) (see discussion of mesothelioma and immunochemical methods).

Carcinomas of the lung may occasionally present with pleural or pericardial effusions. Rarely, peripheral lung carcinoma may disseminate via subpleural lymphatics. This pattern of carcinoma has been described as pseudomesotheliomatous, based on its pattern of spread. Such a pattern of carcinoma, with pleural effusion negative for malignancy on repeated examination, has been reported (158).

Cases of lung cancer presenting with pericardial effusion have been reported. Repeated examination of pericardial effusion fluid, pericardial biopsy, or a search for a primary neoplasm may be required in the presence of an exudative pericardial effusion. The importance of arriving at a correct

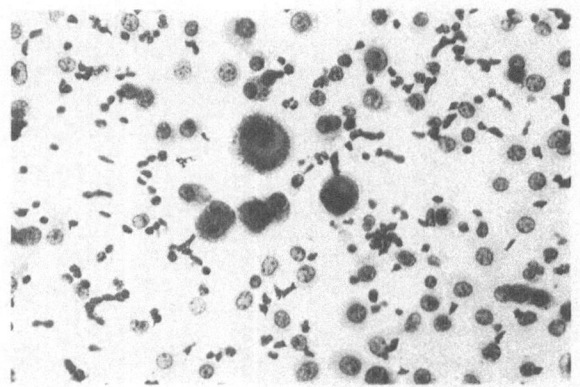

Figure 10. Breast carcinoma in pleural fluid of a 51-year-old woman. Larger cells with prominent nucleoli are suggestive of adenocarcinoma. Background histiocytes are prominent (Papanicolaou stain, 250 ×).

diagnosis is underscored by reported cases of death due to cardiac tamponade in pericardial effusions due to lung carcinoma (29, 40).

Careful examination of pleural surfaces in patients with breast cancer has shown visceral pleural involvement much more frequently (59%) as compared to parietal pleural metastasis (15%). Combinations of visceral and parietal pleural metastases were not observed (58).

Renal cell carcinoma may involve serous body cavities. Metastases to thoracic structures, especially mediastinal lymph nodes, may occur more frequently than previously appreciated. A recent study found evidence for such metastases in 37% of patients with renal cell carcinoma at the time of initial diagnosis (96).

Pseudomyxoma peritonei is a type of carcinomatosis in which a neoplasm producing abundant mucin is dissemi-

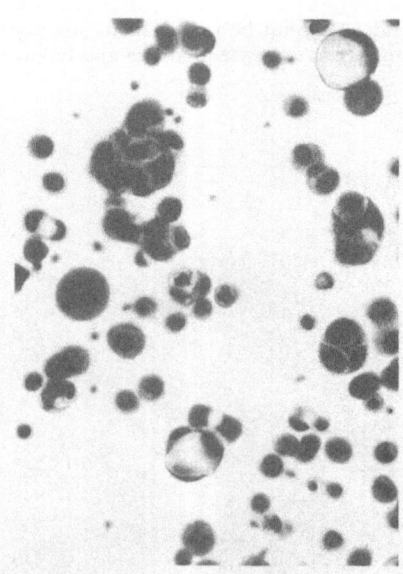

Figure 9. Metastatic adenocarcinoma involving pericardial fluid in a 51-year-old male. Aggregates of cells with nuclear molding are present. Marked nuclear enlargement, pleomorphism, and hyperchromasia are seen. Nucleoli are present, but difficult to appreciate in this specimen. Many cells contain abundant cytoplasmic mucin, which compresses and distort the nuclei off to one side (Papanicolaou stain, 250 ×).

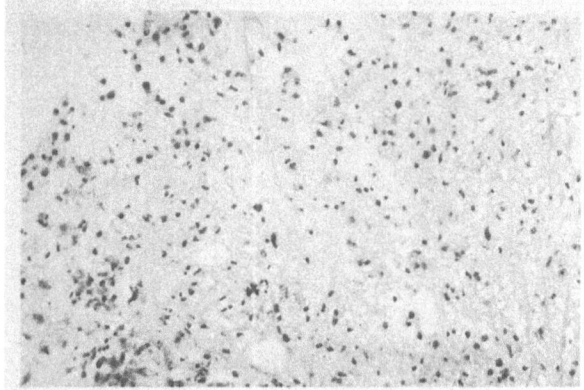

Figure 11. Pseudomyxoma peritonii in a 33-year-old male with abdominal cavity dissemination of chondrosarcomatous elements from a testicular seminoma/teratocarcinoma. Abundant mucinous material filled the abdomen. Some structures reminiscent of lacunae of cartilage are evident in the right-hand side of the field (Hematoxylin and eosin, 100 ×; case material from San Francisco General Hospital).

nated throughout the peritoneal cavity. Benign adenomas of the ovary and appendix may rupture and lead to accumulation of mucin, but this condition resolves spontaneously. The diagnostic label "pseudomyxoma peritonei" should not be applied to this process (148). True pseudomyxoma peritonei shows malignant cells in the mucinous fluid, is highly refractory to therapy, and is most often associated with malignant ovarian neoplasms (37, 135, 154). An unusual variant of this syndrome was recently observed. Exploratory laparotomy of a patient with metastatic teratocarcinoma revealed an abdomen filled with viscid gelatinous material. Microscopic examination revealed extensive embedded malignant chondrosarcoma cells (Fig. 11).

Lymphoma/leukemia

Large numbers of small, round, "mature" lymphocytes may be seen in effusions that are due to a variety of inflammatory processes, including particularly tuberculosis (159), viral infections, and sarcoidosis (124). This may present a difficult problem in differential diagnosis from malignant lymphoma, especially of the small lymphocytic type (well differentiated lymphocytic of Rappaport), and other low-grade lymphomas (202). The clinical setting in some cases may provide helpful clues in arriving at a correct diagnosis. Heavy chromatin clumping ("cellules grumelees") is said to be present in chronic lymphocytic leukemia and not benign reactive lymphocytes, but this feature is dependent on the cytopreparatory techniques employed (161).

It should be noted that, although lymphocytosis in pleural effusions is classically associated with tuberculosis, only 62% of a recent series of 26 cases had greater than 50% lymphocytes on their initial examination of pleural fluid (52).

In one large series of 472 patients with malignant pleural effusions, the lymphoma/leukemia group constituted the second most common group, and made up 15% of all malignancies studied (80). In another series of 101 patients with pleural, peritoneal, or pericardial effusions found to contain malignant cells, lymphoma also made up the second most common malignancy at 22% (21). One group found only 72 of 8700 effusions to contain non-Hodgkin's lymphoma, but they emphasized the difficulty of differential diagnosis (202). Thus, the proper interpretation of hematopoietic elements, including lymphoid cells, is a common and important problem in the study of effusions.

The first line of examination of an effusion is morphologic examination. Recent studies have emphasized the importance of modern approaches to classification of malignant lymphomas in the study of lymphoid malignancies seen in effusions (77). The Lukes–Collins classification of lymphomas relates these neoplasms to morphologic stages in the normal mitogen-stimulated transformation of lymphocytes (109). This system has the advantage of not only relating more closely to actual normal biological processes than traditional classification systems, but it also uses a more cytologically descriptive terminology. Some examples illustrate the difference in approach. Well differentiated lymphocytic lymphoma is referred to as small lymphocytic lymphoma, and poorly differentiated lymphocytic is essenti-

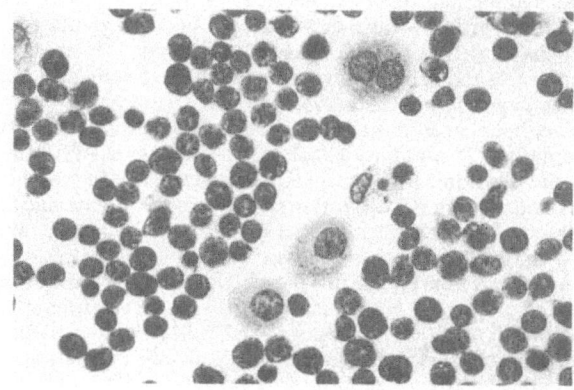

Figure 12. Pleural tap from a 9-year-old boy revealing numerous uniform, small, non-cleaved, malignant lymphocytes with multiple prominent nucleoli. Interspersed are histiocytes with abundant, pale cytoplasm. This pattern is characteristic of Burkitt's lymphoma (Papanicolaou stain, 400 ×).

ally equivalent to small cleaved lymphoma in the Lukes–Collins nomenclature.

Cytologic examination may be very useful in determining the extent of disease, particularly in high grade lymphomas (30). These high grade lesions show a pattern of single detached cells without formation of clusters (115). Individual cells show variable quantities of cytoplasm and round nuclei. Nucleoli and chromocenters may be quite prominent (Fig. 12).

Immunoblastic sarcoma is a large cell lymphoma which shows the presence of particularly prominent nucleoli. Occasional to frequent mitotic figures may be observed. These characteristic and distinctive cytologic features are recognizable in numerous body fluids, including sputum, pleural fluid, cerebrospinal fluid, and urine (30).

Granulocytic sarcoma (chloroma) may present with mediastinal or pleural involvement (91, 94, 138, 203). These patients may present with, or develop, pleural effusions in association with these tumorous, leukemic infiltrates. All major body cavities, including pleural, pericardial, and peritoneal cavities, have been reported to be involved by granulocytic sarcoma. Such lesions may be seen in association with acute leukemia, or blast crisis of chronic granulocytic leukemia. Identification of azurophilic granules in cells, or the presence of eosinophilic myelocytes may be a clue to the diagnosis of granulocytic leukemia. The identity of a suspicious lesion can usually be confirmed by the use of the naphthyl AS-D chloroacetate esterase (Leder) stain, or other specific esterase stains.

Myelomonocytic leukemia may cause ascites due to peritoneal involvement. Direct ascitic fluid examination is necessary in this situation (168). A recent report has also described an association with serous effusions in four patients and monocytic leukemia. These effusions resolved with systemic chemotherapy (118).

Rarely, cases of multiple myeloma have been reported to present with pleural effusions and ascites (28, 53, 151). A case of non-Hodgkin's lymphoma presenting with malignant pericardial effusion has been reported (3). Non-Hodgkin's lymphomas may occasionally produce atypical and unusual types of effusions. A case of hemorrhagic ascites associated with primary splenic "histiocytic" lymphoma emphasizes the need for a specific diagnosis before deciding the therapeutic approach (67).

Chylopericardium has been described in association with lymphoma (7), and lymphangioma of the thymus (43). Pericardial effusion has been seen in association with lymphoblastic leukemia (72). Pyothorax may occur in association with non-Hodgkin's lymphoma (75). Lymphoma may take on a mass appearance in pleural involvement (164).

Advanced non-Hodgkin's lymphoma massively involving the bone marrow has been described in association with peritoneal myeloid metaplasia (182). Such findings may cause difficulty in interpretation without full evaluation of the clinical setting. Cerebrospinal fluid contamination with normal bone marrow elements has been described (90). This, similarly, may cause diagnostic difficulty, and may lead to possible inappropriate treatment if the cells examined are not specifically recognized as normal cellular elements in an atypical context.

Mycosis fungoides (cerebriform lymphoma) may involve the lung and can be detected by cytologic examination of sputum in such cases. Two characteristic cell types are observed: (a) large cells with hyperchromatic nuclei, and (b) small cells. Both cell types are characterized by hyperconvoluted (cerebriform) nuclei, and scant, poorly-defined cytoplasm. In four cases with pulmonary involvement by mycosis fungoides, none showed pleural effusions (149).

Extension of Hodgkin's disease to the body cavities may occur late in the course of this disease. Rarely, characteristic Reed-Sternberg cells may be seen in effusions (190). Radiation therapy for Hodgkin's disease or other disorders may result in late complications and development of effusions (185).

Recently, examples of massive ascites associated with systemic mast cell disease have been described (19, 147).

Squamous cell carcinoma

Primary lung carcinomas are a frequent primary site for malignant neoplasms with progression to serious body cavity involvement. In the male, lung is the most frequent primary site associated with malignant pleural effusion, by a factor of over 2:1 as compared to the next most frequent group, lymphoma/leukemia (80).

Within the lung, squamous cell carcinoma is the most common form of malignancy, and usually pursues a highly aggressive and lethal course for the patient. These observations would suggest that squamous cell carcinoma should be encountered very frequently in the examination of serous body fluids, and particularly in pleural effusions. However, most large series of effusions document a relatively small number of identifiable squamous cell carcinomas.

In a series of 584 pleural pleural fluid specimens from 472 patients, squamous cell carcinoma was recognized in 5.0% of specimens (80). A series of 101 patients with pleural, peritoneal, or pericardial effusions showed only a 1% prevalence of squamous cell carcinoma (21). Another series of 108 patients with confirmed malignant pleural, pericar-

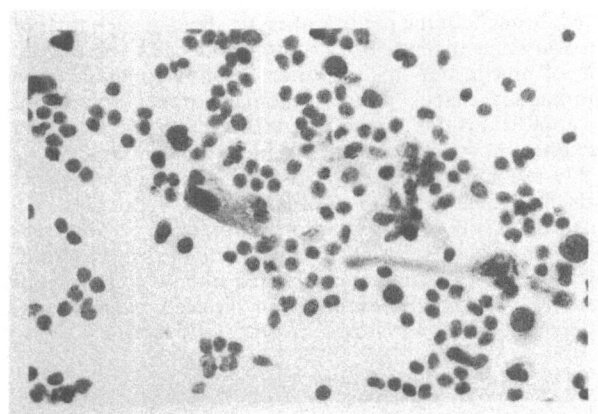

Figure 13. Malignant squamous cells in a unilateral pleural effusion of a 62-year-old woman with lung carcinoma. A tadpole form is seen, with keratohyalin granules in the tail. Background shows an admixture of acute and chronic inflammatory cells (Papanicolaou stain, 250 ×).

dial, or peritoneal effusions showed 5.6% of patients to have squamous cell carcinoma (24).

Some of the observed variability may be due to differing patterns of practice and geographic variability. As a general principle, the exact sites of involvement considered by various studies must also be taken into account. A study confined to pleural effusions can be expected to show a higher frequency of squamous cell carcinoma, or other lung primaries, than one considering all effusions. Despite these considerations, there is a disproportionately small number of squamous cell carcinomas which progress to body cavity metastasis. The tumor biology responsible for this phenomenon is not known.

Squamous cell carcinoma in effusions may be keratinizing or nonkeratinizing. Keratinizing carcinomas may have deep eosinophilic cytoplasmic hue, but this finding is quite variable and unreliable in effusions. Architectural features are not reliable in effusions, since these may be absent or poorly shown. Obvious keratin production is quite unusual, but helpful when present (Fig. 13). The presence of large numbers of even very well-differentiated squamous cells is suspicious for the presence of malignancy, even in the absence of clearly defined nuclear atypia (88).

Other malignant neoplasms

Small cell ("oat cell") carcinoma of lung may occasionally be found in effusions. These cells are small only in comparison to other neoplastic cells arising in the lung. These highly malignant neoplasms are referred to as having a "lymphocyte-like" appearance with a high nuclear to cytoplasmic ratio, and a round to oval nucleus. Spindled neoplastic cells may also be observed occasionally. Small cell carcinoma tends to form small clusters and chains. Such tendency to cluster is characteristically absent from lymphoid malignancies, and serves as an important differential diagnostic criterion (153). Although not considered characteristic of this neoplasm, psammoma bodies have been de-

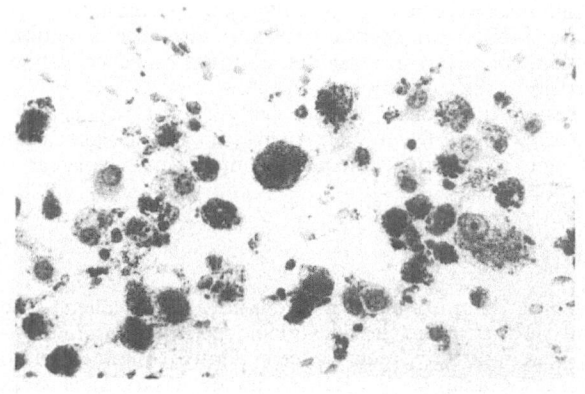

Figure 14. Malignant pleural effusion showing large cells with big nuclei, prominent nucleoli, and abundant intracytoplasmic granular melanin pigment typical of malignant melanoma (Papanicolaou stain, 250 ×).

scribed in an effusion due to metastatic small cell carcinoma with pleural surface metastasis (9).

Malignant melanoma may present with an effusion and cause considerable diagnostic difficulty. Prominent nucleoli are characteristic, and melanin pigment may frequently be observed (Fig. 14). Amelanotic cases occur and may be more difficult to identify specifically (83).

Sarcomas may involve the body cavities and show frequent spindled and pleomorphic cells. The nature of the primary neoplasm determines the precise characteristics of the metastasis, as would be expected. Fibrosarcomas show no giant cells, but many other sarcomas, including liposarcoma, rhabdomyosarcoma, malignant fibrous histiocytoma, and osteosarcoma show the presence of pleomorphic giant cells when they metastasize to body cavities (124).

AIDS

The acquired immune deficiency syndrome (AIDS) occasionally results in the development of various types of effusions because of the large number of opportunistic infections to which these patients are subject. Tuberculous pericardial effusion has been reported (42). Pleural effusion due to pleural cryptococosis has been reported in association with AIDS.

NEW APPROACHES TO THE EVALUATION OF EFFUSIONS

The existence of a residual, difficult-to-classify group of effusions after the application of traditional tests, including cytologic examination, has stimulated a search for additional new approaches to the separation of benign and malignant fluids.

Immunochemical methods

Immunohistochemical techniques, particularly immuno-

peroxidase, have gained constantly increasing importance in surgical pathology. Many modifications and variations of the technique, each with special characteristics, have been applied to the study of antigens present in biopsy specimens (55). A particular strength of this method of immunologic study of tissues is that it permits direct visualization of the cells, showing the presence of a given antigen (marker). Thus, a small suspect population of cells can be selected from a vast background, and individually examined with certainty of their identity. The use of immunoperoxidase in cytologic material was explored and found to be applicable to most specimen types, with the exception of filter preparations, which give a high degree of background staining (122).

Immunocytologic examination has recently been applied as an aid to the evaluation of hematologic diseases extending to body cavities. Application of the avidin-biotin-immunoperoxidase technique has been used to prove the presence of lymphoid malignancy in a pleural effusion also infected with *Mycobacterium tuberculosis* (10). Antibodies to the B-cell markers, α, γ, and μ heavy chains, and light chains, and T-cell markers Leu-1, Leu-2a, and Leu-3a have been found to be useful in identifying low grade lymphomas. Low grade lymphomas are particularly difficult to identify on morphologic grounds alone, but are usually identifiable by their monoclonal B-cell marking with these antibodies. Reactive processes are characterized by a mixture of helper and suppressor cells (111). Cases of lymphoblastic lymphoma (convoluted lymphoma in the Lukes–Collins classification) and lymphoblastic leukemia are characterized by terminal deoxynucleotidyl transferase (TdT) positivity, which has been found to be a useful marker in detection of these neoplasms in effusions (18, 111). Pan-hematopoietic markers, which can be extremely helpful in the differential diagnosis of lymphoid malignancy from carcinoma, have been described (8). Additional markers for hematologic malignancy, such as CALLA (common acute lymphoblastic leukemia antigen), continue to be explored, and have been found to be useful in diagnosis of malignant effusions (78). Several studies have shown excellent correlation of intracellular carcinoembryonic antigen (CEA) positivity with malignancy, particularly adenocarcinoma (97, 193). These results are especially significant since reactive mesothelial cells and mesothelioma are negative or only weakly positive. This provides a practical differential stain for the frequent problem of differential diagnosis of metastatic adenocarcinoma from mesothelial abnormalities (130).

Studies of malignant cells in effusions have also found the identification of epithelial membrane antigen (EMA) to be useful in the identification of carcinoma, and in the differential from mesothelial cells. A variant of the immunocytochemical approach using immuno-alkaline phosphatase has been used in such studies (35, 184).

Immunofluorescent identification of specific components of the intracellular matrix has been shown to be useful in identification of carcinoma cells. Mouse monoclonal antibodies (RGE53) directed against keratin from HeLa cells have been shown to be sensitive for epithelial malignant cells, including various adenocarcinomas, squamous cell carcinoma, and mesothelioma. Mesenchymal cells, including lymphomas, melanomas, and sarcomas do not react with this antibody (144). A new monoclonal antibody, designated B72.3, derived from human breast carcinoma, has been shown to be highly sensitive for the presence of adenocarcinoma primary to breast, ovary, and lung. This antibody is also highly specific, with essentially no reaction to mesothelial cells, or to a number of other neoplasms (81, 179).

New monoclonal antibodies, designated Ca2 and Ca3, have been found to be positive in malignant mesotheliomas and carcinomas in a pattern complementary to reaction with CEA (20). Staining with Ca2 and Ca3 antibody is negative in oat cell (small cell) carcinoma of lung. An oat-cell specific antibody (534F-8) has been developed which can identify this neoplasm also (205). Monoclonal antibodies to antigens found in breast (MBr1) and ovarian (MOv2) carcinomas have been used to detect malignancy in patient specimens interpreted as negative by morphologic studies alone (116).

Tumor markers may also be helpful in the analysis of cerebrospinal fluids. Examination of cytocentrifuge preparations can be quite helpful in the examination of patients with acute lymphoblastic leukemia (87). Application of immunoperoxidase, or immunofluorescent stains for TdT to such preparations, further enhances the detection of small numbers of leukemic cells in cerebrospinal fluid.

Therapy for central nervous system neoplasms can be monitored, and recurrence detected, by searching for such markers as polyamines, α-fetoprotein (AFP), and the beta subunit of human chorionic gonadotrophin (HCG) (49).

Immunochemical methods now represent an extremely powerful tool for the study of all types of effusions. Further refinement of techniques and development of additional antibodies can be expected to make this approach an indispensable tool for the study of effusions (157).

Flow cytometry

The technique of flow cytometry fundamentally consists of measurement of absorbance and scatter of light beamed at individual cells. A cell suspension is pumped through a narrow aperture in a precisely shaped flow cell. This presents one cell at a time to the light source in very rapid succession. It is readily apparent that passage of each cell through the aperture generates much information. At a minimum, forward angle (proportional to cell size) and right angle (proportional to cytoplasmic complexity) scatter intensities are measured. Capture of these data requires a high-speed digital computer since cells flow past the light source at up to 10,000 cells/second (157). The computer can then be applied to provide totals, statistical analyses, and graphical presentation of the data it has captured.

Stains for DNA may be applied to samples to be studied. This provides information regarding nuclear DNA content of the cells examined. Aneuploidy found in this manner has been shown to correlate with the presence of malignancy (54, 59). Variable results have been reported, with some authors finding large numbers of false negative results (69).

The technique of flow cytometry is advanced still further with the addition of a fluorescent-labeled antibody to the test sample. Numerous antibodies have been used in this manner. Application of a new monoclonal antibody, Ca1, to the study of pleural and peritoneal effusions has been found to be quite sensitive and specific for the diagnosis of malignancy. Seventeen malignant effusions were studied by this method, and all except an endometrial carcinoma and two

lymphomas were positive (39). Panels of specific antibodies, perhaps tailored to specific body sites or clinical situations could theoretically increase the sensitivity and specificity of this aid in the evaluation of effusions.

Technical problems in the analysis of DNA patterns generated by flow cytometry make diagnostic application difficult. In addition, adequate sampling of neoplasms is essential (155).

Morphometrics

Quantitative morphologic methods have been applied to the analysis of visual images of cytologic specimens. An interesting and innovative new concept allows computer based interactive analysis of cytologic images (110). Such techniques promise to allow the real time combination of human judgment and direction, with the power for exact quantitative analysis provided by a computer. This will prove to be an interesting research, and perhaps diagnostic tool.

Biochemical analysis

Quantitative analysis of various substances found in effusions has been studied as an aid in the detection of malignant and other lesions. Carcinoembryonic antigen (CEA), present in markedly elevated concentrations by radioimmunoassay, has been found to be highly predictive for the presence of malignancy (105, 112, 189).

The protein β_2-microglobulin correlates with the presence of lymphoma, but it is not completely specific. Ceruloplasmin, α_2-macroglobulin, orosomucoid, lysozyme, and hexosamidase levels are of no diagnostic value in the identification of malignant effusions (189).

Biochemical analysis of ascitic fluid from patients with malignant neoplasms has shown the presence of several glycolipids not normally found in serum. These substances, including lactoneotetraosylceramide, could have application as tumor markers (181).

Cytogenetics

Chromosome analysis has been adopted by some investigators. It should be noted that this can be accomplished on a practical, more basic level by examination of neoplasms in female patients for multiple sex chromatin (Barr) bodies. The presence of two or more Barr bodies is indicative of hyperdiploidy, and this finding correlates with malignancy (88). Formal chromosome studies have shown high sensitivity for diagnosis of carcinoma in effusions. In one study, 79% of malignant tumors were identified when cytogenetic studies were used alone (64). The technique has been modified to allow culture of effusion cells in order to enhance sensitivity, and maintain viability of cells pending results of other studies. However, some difficulty with false positive results has been encountered (194).

Electron microscopy

Electron microscopy has been applied to the study of cells in effusions (157). Mucin vacuoles, intracellular lumens, and luminal tight junctions are characteristic of adenocarcinoma. These findings were absent from mesothelial cells similarly examined. Mesothelial cells were found to have characteristic long, slender, "bushy" microvilli, and numerous pinocytotic vesicles (15). Ultrastructural examination has been proposed as an adjunct to conventional studies for the differentiation of reactive mesothelial cells and carcinoma (48, 134).

Miscellaneous

The presence of blood in an effusion has sometimes been assumed to correlate with malignancy. In fact, this is a nonspecific finding (23). An indirect immunoperoxidase technique has been developed to study A, B, and H blood group antigens on the surfaces of cells in effusion fluids. Malignant cells failed to stain by this method, while various other cell types did (170). Interpretation of a lack of staining by such a technique might be expected to be difficult.

Fibronectin concentration was found to be highly sensitive and specific in separating malignant from benign ascitic fluids in one more recent study. It has been suggested that this parameter would be particularly valuable if used on conjunction with other measurements designed to screen out effusions due to infectious agents or pancreatitis (156).

An ammonia tolerance test has been designed as a "screening test" to differentiate between benign and malignant ascites. The test consists of rectal administration of ammonia, and subsequent arterial sampling at 15 and 30 minutes. Plasma ammonia concentrations in the patients with benign ascites due to cirrhosis have been observed to be significantly different from those patients with malignant ascites (57).

Examination of pleural fluid and serum by protein electrophoresis and quantitative immunoglobulins was undertaken in one recent study. An elevated ratio of pleural to serum immunoglobulin level was found to correlate with malignancy. Pleural to serum IgG ratio greater than 0.6 was found to have a sensitivity of 69% and specificity of 74% (44).

Examination for pH has been advocated in the evaluation of pleural effusions (62, 73, 101, 102, 103, 104, 139). Pleural fluid pH and glucose concentration have been shown to fall rapidly in an experimental model of empyema (152). An interrelationship for glucose and pH levels, possibly dependent on pleural fluid leukocyte metabolism has been proposed (140, 141, 152). Pleural fluid may be used to study patients with parapneumonic effusions in order to predict which patients will require chest drainage. Despite widely overlapping results, patients with very low (< 7.00) pH values have been found to have more frequent complications requiring early thoracostomy (101).

TREATMENT OF EFFUSIONS

Malignant disease with progression to peritoneal involvement and consequent development of intractable accumulation of ascitic fluid is an ominous clinical occurrence. Most patients in this clinical situation have a very short life span

with survival of less than 8 weeks expected in most cases (146). Specific therapy requires clinical assessment of the expected survival of the patient. Breast and ovarian carcinomas frequently show an indolent course despite widespread dissemination of disease. Thus, the exact type of neoplasm, its extent of dissemination, and unknown host resistance factors all play key roles in determining the rapidity of the patient's demise. These factors must be carefully weighed in the selection of appropriate means of therapeutic intervention.

Some patients with severe neoplastic ascites require control of fluid accumulation for palliative purposes. In this clinical situation, drainage of ascitic fluid and venous reinfusion has been performed. A more definitive variant of this procedure involves placement of a peritoneo-venous shunt. This approach is frequently successful in the control of ascites (65). Dissemination of the malignant neoplasm is enhanced by such a procedure. In some circumstances, placement of an in-line filter to remove cellular material from drained fluid has been advocated in order to reduce the dissemination of neoplasm (186). A frequent problem with the peritoneo-venous shunt is obstruction and consequent failure of drainage (172, 173). This problem appears to be less frequent with the Denver shunt as opposed to the LeVeen shunt (129).

Another approach to drainage of malignant ascitic fluid is through the use of a peritoneo-cystic shunt (178). This procedure was well tolerated, but achieved only minimal flow rates. It was speculated that this was due to an insufficient pressure gradient between the peritoneal cavity and the urinary bladder. Modifications to allow manual or automatic increase in the pressure gradient generated in this system could potentially improve its effectiveness. Other innovative approaches to the drainage of ascitic fluid include drainage into the subcutaneous tissues of the thigh (63).

Management of malignant ascites includes not only various shunting procedures as described, but also attempts to eradicate neoplastic cells in the local area where they cause complicating fluid accumulations. Approaches such as these must still be considered palliative since they do not attack the primary site of disease, or even other sites of dissemination. Such treatments include intracavitary radiotherapy, intracavitary chemotherapy, radioactive colloids, and immunotherapeutic approaches (98). One group applied Adriamycin, and Adriamycin Nocardia rubra cell wall skeleton as an immunopotentiator. This combination resulted in a 73.4% response rate (61).

Rare cases of extracardiac malignancy may present as acute pericardial effusion. Most commonly, the primary site for such neoplasms is lung. Patients receiving pericardiectomy, with or without ancillary therapy, survived longer than patients treated by radiation, chemotherapy, or drainage alone (60).

As might be anticipated, the placement of shunts in body cavities in order to drain persistently accumulating fluids is associated with significant complications. One obvious consideration is the theoretical propensy of such a procedure to disseminate neoplastic cells involving the body cavities still further. Although this problem has not been studied extensively, it does not appear to be a clinical problem in this group of patients with already widely disseminated disease. One author (173) reported postmortem lung examination of

12 patients who had undergone peritoneovenous shunts in the management of malignant ascites. There was a wide spectrum of findings ranging from absence of neoplastic cells, to developing metastases. Tumor embolization was suspected in two of eight patients in one group treated for malignant ascites (107). The incidence of tumor emboli in another autopsy study was approximately 5% (31).

In some circumstances, the effects of mechanical transport of fluid in contact with neoplastic cells can be quite significant clinically. Metastatic spread of an optic glioma through a ventriculo-peritoneal shunt resulting in accumulation of malignant ascites has been reported (186). Such an occurrence is particularly important since extra-cranial metastases from a low-grade glioma would not be expected. Other cases of intractable CSF ascites have been reported in association with the placement of ventriculo-peritoneal shunts (1, 2).

Complications other than the further dissemination of malignant disease may become major clinical problems in the placement of peritoneovenous shunts. Removal of substantial amounts of ascitic fluid preoperatively may decrease the acute adverse occurrences of fluid overload, disseminated intravascular coagulation, and fever (107). Rarely, complications from placement of the peritoneovenous shunt are devastating and may cause fatal pulmonary embolization (171). Mild prolongation in clotting studies are commonly observed following peritoneovenous shunt placement (92). These patients also show thrombocytopenia, in a pattern of low grade disseminated intravascular coagulation (DIC). Patients generally tolerate this complication fairly well (183). Other complications include pulmonary edema, fever (without organisms demonstrable by culture), and pneumonia (183).

Patients with malignant ascites seem to have a lower incidence of spontaneous bacterial peritonitis than patients with ascites due to cirrhosis of the liver. In one series of 101 patients with demonstrated malignant ascites, no definite cases of spontaneous bacterial peritonitis were observed. Three patients developed positive ascitic cultures for what were thought to be other specific reasons. This compares with an expected incidence of spontaneous bacterial peritonitis of 8% in patients with cirrhotic ascites. These authors suggest that liver disease must be present for the development of spontaneous bacterial peritonitis (93).

These are some approaches to the palliative treatment of neoplasms that show progression to neoplastic involvement of the serosal surfaces. Appropriate application of these modalities can aid and improve the quality of life for those with advanced neoplastic disease.

PROGNOSIS OF EFFUSIONS

There is a tendency to regard all malignant effusions as an indication of far advanced, and therefore hopeless, disease (16). This may not always be a correct interpretation. For example, in pleural effusions associated with metastatic breast carcinoma, patients in one study experienced a median survival of 48 months. As always, the entire clinical situation should be taken into account. Patients with other distant metastases and pleural effusions have a significantly worse prognosis, with median survival of 12 months (137).

It is interesting to note that a high incidence of ipsilateral effusions occurs in patients with breast cancer without distant metastases. Thus, in this circumstance, serosal surface and body cavity involvement may represent a local extension type of phenomenon rather than a true metastatic process (137). In another series of 660 patients with breast cancer, 79 were found to have pleural or extrapleural metastases. Ten patients with solitary thoracic metastases also showed a prolonged median survival of 42 months (89).

Involvement of the peritoneal cavity, as opposed to pleural surfaces, by breast carcinoma represents advanced spread of disease and has been found to carry an ominous prognosis with a median survival of 47 days (4). In addition, the presence of liver involvement carries a much worse prognosis, with less than one-third the median survival seen without such involvement, despite serosal metastases.

Prognosis of ovarian neoplasms is related to cytologic evidence of peritoneal involvement by malignant cells. Serous and endometrioid carcinomas more commonly involve the peritoneal surfaces. Spread of these neoplasms to the serosal surfaces carries a worse prognosis, and this may be related to the clinical and pathologic staging of these neoplasms (207). In another study, ascites in patients with malignant epithelial ovarian tumors had an effect on survival only in Stage III patients who had minimal or no neoplasm after resection of their primary lesion (116).

In a series of 22 patients with malignant disease and intractable ascites treated by peritoneovenous shunts, survival was significantly related to the results of cytologic examination of the peritoneal fluid. Patients with a positive cytologic examination had a median survival of 26 days, as compared to 140 days for those with negative examinations (31).

Patients with hepatocellular carcinoma and cirrhosis of the liver frequently experience ascites. In one series, only 14% of 59 patients with this lesion showed malignant cells in cytologic examination (208). Despite this low yield of positive cytologic examinations, 96% of hepatocellular carcinoma patients with ascites go on to die of their disease without improvement. In comparison, patients with cirrhosis, without malignant disease, very frequently improve after an episode of ascites (208).

The presence of a bloody ascitic fluid in a patient with cirrhosis is an ominous finding. Over one-third of 32 patients in one series had hepatocellular carcinoma. All patients required surgical exploration, and had a worse prognosis than patients with clear fluid only (45).

Resection of the primary site of neoplasm correlates with a slightly improved prognosis in patients with malignant effusions. In general, pleural effusions show a better prognosis than peritoneal effusions. Numbers of neoplastic cells and associated mononuclear inflammatory cells show no correlation with prognosis in malignant effusions (206).

It is critical to establish that an effusion in a patient is actually due to neoplastic involvement of the body cavity in question. In one study, only two patients with malignant pericardial effusions had prolonged survival, as opposed to 11/13 patients with benign effusions (169). Therefore, the decision to treat or not to treat the patient with an effusion should not be based on clinical evaluation alone. To do so risks failure to identify patients who have not yet developed serous membrane involvement and have effusions due to benign disease (false positives). These patients may suffer the adverse effects of unneeded therapy. On the other hand, the sensitive and specific techniques previously described are needed to confirm the presence of neoplastic cells when they have progressed to involve the body cavities. These patients can then receive appropriate medical and surgical therapy to improve the quality and length of their lives.

REFERENCES

1. Adegbite AB, Khan M: Role of protein content in CSF ascites following ventriculoperitoneal shunting. Case Report. *J Neurosurg* 57:423, 1982
2. Agha FP, Amendola MA, Shirazi KK et al.: Unusual abdominal complications of ventriculo-peritoneal shunts. *Radiology* 146:323, 1983
3. Almagro UA, Remeniuk E: Non-Hodgkin's lymphoma presenting as a malignant pericardial effusion and cardiac tamponade. *Hum Pathol* 16:315, 1985
4. Appelqvist P, Silvo J, Salmela L, Kostiainen S: On the treatment and prognosis of malignant ascites: Is the survival time determined when the abdominal paracentesis is needed? *J Surg Oncol* 20:238, 1982
5. Askin FB, McCann BG, Kuhn C: Reactive eosinophilic pleuritis: A lesion to be distinguished from pulmonary eosinophilic granuloma. *Arch Pathol Lab Med* 101:187, 1977
6. Bakalos D, Constantakis N, Tsicricas TH: Recognition of malignant cells in pleural and peritoneal effusions. *Acta Cytol* 18:118, 1974
7. Barton JC, Durant JR: Isolated chylopericardium associated with lymphoma. *South Med J* 73:1551, 1980
8. Battifora H, Trowbridge IS: A monoclonal antibody useful for the differential diagnosis between malignant lymphoma and non-hematopoietic neoplasms. *Cancer* 51:816, 1983
9. Bauer TW, Erozan YS: Psammoma bodies in small cell carcinoma of the lung: A case report. *Acta Cytol* 26:327, 1982
10. Bauman MD, Borowitz MJ, Johnston WW: Immunocytologic evaluation of lymphoid aspirates and effusions (Abstract). *Acta Cytol* 28:628, 1984
11. Becklake MR: Exposure to asbestos and human disease (editorial). *N Engl J Med* 306:1480, 1982
12. Bell RC, Andrews CP: Pleural effusions: Meeting the diagnostic challenge. *Geriatrics* 40:101, 1985
13. Bennett RR, Moore J Jr: Dialysis-induced ascites treated with peritoneal dialysis. *South Med J* 80:379, 1987
14. Bessone LN, Ferguson TB, Burford TH: Chylothorax. *Ann Thorac Surg* 12:527, 1971
15. Bewtra C, Greer KP: Ultrastructural studies of cells in body cavity effusions. *Acta Cytol* 29:226, 1985
16. Biran S, Brufman G, Klein E, Hochman A: The management of pericardial effusion in cancer patients. *Chest* 71:182, 1977
17. Blot WJ, Harrington JM, Toledo A et al.: Lung cancer after employment in shipyards during World War II. *N Engl J Med* 299:620, 1978
18. Bollum FJ: Terminal deoxynucleotidyl transferase as a hematopoietic cell marker. *Blood* 54:1203, 1979
19. Bonnet P, Smadja C, Szekely AM et al.: Intractable ascites in systemic mastocytosis treated by portal diversion. *Dig Dis Sci* 32:209, 1987
20. Bramwell ME, Ghosh AK, Smith WD et al.: Ca2 and Ca3: New monoclonal antibodies evaluated as tumor markers in serous effusions. *Cancer* 56:105, 1985
21. Britt DA, Schumann GB: Frequency of malignant body cavity effusion cytology (Abstract). *Acta Cytol* 28:637, 1984
22. Britt K, Kaneko M, Chuang MT: Hemangioleiomyosarcoma of the pleura: A case report and review of the literature. *Mt Sinai J Med (NY)* 50:64, 1983
23. Broghamer WL Jr, Richardson ME, Faurest SE: Malignancy-associated serosanguinous pleural effusions. *Acta Cytol* 28:46, 1984
24. Buhaug J, Rone R, Ramzy I: Presentation of squamous-cell carcinoma in effusions (Abstract). *Acta Cytol* 27:567, 1983
25. Calabrese PR, Frank HD, Taubin HL: Lymphangiomyomatosis with chylous ascites: Treatment with dietary fat restriction and medium chain triglycerides. *Cancer* 40:895, 1977
26. Cardoza PL: A critical evaluation of 3000 cytologic analyses of pleural fluid, ascitic fluid, and pericardial fluid. *Acta Cytol* 10:455, 1966
27. Carrington CB, Cugell DW, Gaensler EA et al.: Lymphangioleiomyomatosis: Physiologic-pathologic-radiologic correlations. *Am Rev Respir Dis* 116:977, 1977
28. Chee YC, Chea A: IgA myeloma with primary pleural involvement. *Eur J Respir Dis* 65:136, 1984
29. Chen KT: Extracardiac malignancy presenting with cardiac tamponade. *J Surg Oncol* 23:167, 1983
30. Cheson BD, Johnston JL, delJunco G, Kjeldsberg CR: Cytologic evidence for disseminated immunoblastic lymphoma. *Am J Clin Pathol* 75:621, 1981
31. Cheung DK, Raaf JH: Selection of patients with malignant ascites for a peritoneovenous shunt. *Cancer* 50:1204, 1982
32. Churg A: Immunohistochemical staining for vimentin and keratin in malignant mesothelioma. *Am J Surg Pathol* 9:360, 1985
33. Churg A: Lung cancer cell type and asbestos exposure. *JAMA* 253:2984, 1985
34. Churg A, Warnock ML, Green N: Analysis of the cores of ferruginous (asbestos) bodies from the general population II. True asbestos bodies and pseudoasbestos bodies. *Lab Invest* 40:31, 1979
35. Coleman DV, To A, Dearnaley DP, Ormerod MG: An immunocytochemical approach to the cytodiagnosis of malignancy in serous effusions (Abstract). *Acta Cytol* 25:716, 1981
36. Corrin B, Liebow AA, Friedman PJ: Pulmonary Lymphangiomyomatosis: A review. *Am J Pathol* 79:347, 1975
37. Courant C, Brun G: [Mucoid peritonitis. Apropos of 2 case reports. Review of the literature]. *Rev Fr Gynecol Obstet* 79:641, 1984
38. Craighead JE, Mossman BT: The pathogenesis of asbestos-associated diseases. *N Eng J Med* 306:1446, 1982
39. Czerniak B, Papenhausen PR, Herz F, Koss LG: Flow cytometric identification of cancer cells in effusions with Ca1 monoclonal antibody. *Cancer* 55:2783, 1985
40. Danova M, Riccardi A, Girino M et al.: Severe pericarditis as a presenting sign of bronchogenic carcinoma. *Tumori* 71:81, 1985
41. Das DK, Gupta SK, Ayyagari S et al.: Pleural effusions in non-Hodgkin's lymphoma. A cytomorphologic, cytochemical and immunologic study. *Acta Cytol (Baltimore)* 31:119, 1987
42. D'Cruz IA, Sengupta EE, Abrahams C et al.: Cardiac involvement, including tuberculous pericardial effusion, complicating acquired immune deficiency syndrome. *Am Heart J* 112:1100, 1986
43. deHaan HP, Kolff J, Buis B: Isolated chylopericardium due to lymphangiomatous dysplasia of the thymus. *Eur Heart J* 5:846, 1984
44. Desai SD, Sackett DL: Ratios of pleural fluid to serum immunoglobulins in malignant pleural effusions. *Cancer* 52:2151, 1983
45. Desitter L, Rector WG: The significance of bloody ascites in patients with cirrhosis. *Am J Gastroenterol* 79:136, 1984
46. Dienemann H, Witte J, Szabo L: [Chylaskos in lymphangioleiomyomatosis. Peritoneo-venous drainage with Denver shunt]. *Dtsch Med Wochenschr* 7:920, 1985
47. Dixon AY, Reed JS, Dow N, Lee SH: Primary omental

leiomyosarcoma masquerading as hemorrhagic ascites. *Hum Pathol* 15:233, 1984

48. Duane GB, Sanchez CA, Sugahara R et al.: Mesothelial cell transformation: Morphologic classification and biologic implications deduced from light and transmission electron microscopic investigation (Abstract). *Acta Cytol* 28:658, 1984

49. Edwards MSB, Davis RL, Laurent JP: Tumor markers and cytologic features of cerebrospinal fluid. *Cancer* 56:1773, 1985

50. Elborn JS, Conn P, Roberts SD: Refractory massive pleural effusion in systemic lupus erythematosus treated by pleurectomy. *Ann Rheum Dis* 46:77, 1987

51. Enzi G, Digito M, Marin R et al.: Mediastino-abdominal lipomatosis: Deep accumulation of fat mimicking a respiratory disease and ascites. Clinical aspects and metabolic studies *in vitro*. *Q J Med* 53:453, 1984

52. Epstein DM, Kline LR, Albedla SM, Miller WT: Tuberculous pleural effusions. *Chest* 91:106, 1987

53. Estrov Z, Berrebi A, Hazani E, Resnitzky P: Pleural effusion and ascites as presenting signs of IgA myeloma. *Haematologica (Pavia)* 68:104, 1983

54. Evans DA, Thornthwaite JT, Ng ABP, Sugarbaker EV: DNA flow cytometry of pleural effusions: Comparison with pathology for the diagnosis of malignancy (Abstract). *Acta Cytol* 25:707, 1981

55. Falini B, Taylor C: New developments in immunoperoxidase techniques and their application. *Arch Pathol Lab Med* 107:105, 1983

56. Farber HW, Fairman RP, Glauser FL: Talc granulomatosis: Laboratory findings similar to sarcoidosis. *Am Rev Respir Dis* 125:258, 1982

57. Felding C, Christensen RF, Lindhal F: Ammonia tolerance test used to differentiate between ascites of cirrhotic and malignant genesis. *Scand J Gastroenterol* 19:365, 1984

58. Fentiman IS, Rubens RD, Hayward JL: The pattern of metastatic disease in patients with pleural effusions secondary to breast cancer. *Br J Surg* 69:193, 1982

59. Flint A, Lovett EJ, Stoolman LM et al.: Flow cytometric analysis of DNA in diagnostic cytology. *Am J Clin Pathol* 84:278, 1985

60. Fraser RS, Viloria JB, Wang NS: Cardiac tamponade as a presentation of extracardiac malignancy. *Cancer* 45:1697, 1980

61. Fukuoka M, Takada M, Tamai S et al.: [Local application of anti-cancer drugs for the treatment of malignant pleural and pericardial effusion]. *Gan To Kagaku Ryoho* 11:1543, 1984

62. Funahashi A, Sarkar TK, Kory RC: Measurements of respiratory gases and pH of pleural fluid. *Am Rev Respir Dis* 108:1266, 1973

63. Gagushin VA: [Method of treating ascites by draining into the subcutaneous compartment of the thigh]. *Vestn Khir* 132:122, 1984

64. Gallareto M, Ghiazza GF, DeGiogis L, Gabutto U: [Chromosome analysis performed in 176 cases of pleural effusions of various types]. *Arch Sci Med (Torino)* 139:193, 1982

65. Gough IR: Control of malignant ascites by peritoneovenous shunting. *Cancer* 54:2226, 1984

66. Grobe JL, Kozarek RA, Sanowski RA, Earnest DL: "Pseudo-ascites" associated with giant ovarian cysts and elevated cystic fluid amylase. *Am J Gastroenterol* 78:421, 1983

67. Hacker JF III, Richter JE, Pyatt RS, Fink MP: Hemorrhagic ascites: An unusual presentation of primary splenic lymphoma. *Gastroenterology* 83:470, 1982

68. Halme J, Chafe W, Currie JL: Endometriosis with massive ascites. *Obstet Gynecol* 65:591, 1985

69. Hedley DW, Philips J, Rugg CA, Taylor IW: Measurement of cellular DNA content as an adjunct to diagnostic cytology in malignant effusions. *Eur J Cancer Clin Oncol* 20:749, 1984

70. Hirji MK, Johnson MA, Hennig RC: Cardiac levorotation:

A cause of false-positive epicardial fat pad sign. *Radiology* 161:659, 1986

71. Hobar PC, Turner WW Jr, Vaentine RJ: Successful use of the Denver peritoneovenous shunt in patients with nephrogenic ascites. *Surgery* 101:161, 1987

72. Horikoshi T, Hiyoshi Y, Ota M et al.: A child with acute lymphoblastic leukemia complicated by pericardial effusion. *Nippon Ketsueki Gakkai Zasshi* 49:900, 1986

73. Houston MC: Pleural effusion: Diagnostic value of measurements of PO_2, PCO_2, and pH. *South Med J* 74:585, 1981

74. Hurvitz CH, Greenberg SH, Song CH, Gans SL: Hemangiomatosis of the pleura with hemorrhage and disseminated intravascular coagulation. *J Pediatr Surg* 17:73, 1982

75. Iuchi K, Sawamura K, Mori T et al.: [A case of non-Hodgkin's lymphoma with pyothorax]. *Nippon Kyobu Shikkan Gakkai Zasshi* 22:1165, 1984

76. Jaffe R, Di Segni E, Altaras M et al.: Ultrasonic real-time diagnosis of transitory fetal pleural and pericardial effusion. *Diagn Imag Clin Med* 55:373, 1986

77. James LP: Cytopathology of lymphoid lesions in serous effusions (abstr). *Acta Cytol* 25:715, 1981

78. Janckila AJ, Yam LT, Li CY: Immunocytochemical diagnosis of acute leukemia with pleural involvement. *Acta Cytol* 29:67, 1985

79. Jenks JE, Artman LE, Hoskins WJ, Miremadi AK: Endometriosis with ascites. *Obstet Gynecol* 63(Suppl 3):75S, 1984

80. Johnston WW: The malignant pleural effusion: A review of cytopathologic diagnoses of 584 specimens from 472 consecutive patients. *Cancer* 56:905, 1985

81. Johnston WW, Szpak CA, Lottich SC et al.: Use of a monoclonal antibody (B72.3) as an immunocytochemical adjunct to diagnosis of adenocarcinoma in human effusions. *Cancer Res* 45:1894, 1985

82. Kagan E, Jacobson RJ: Lymphoid and plasma cell malignancies: Asbestos-related disorders of long latency. *Am J Clin Pathol* 80:14, 1983

83. Kapila K, Chopra P, Verma K: Cytologic diagnosis of amelanotic melanoma (Letter to the editor). *Acta Cytol* 29:498, 1985

84. Keshgegian AA: Lupus erythematosus cells in pleural fluid (Letter to the editor). *Am J Clin Pathol* 69:570, 1978

85. Kjeldsberg CR, Knight JA: Body fluids: Laboratory examination of cerebrospinal, synovial, and serous fluids: A textbook atlas. pp 28–47. Chicago: American Society of Clinical Pathologists, 1982

86. Klein AL, Baird MG, Walley V: Tumor encasement of the heart simulating pericardial effusion. *Can J Cardiol* 2:341, 1986

87. Komp DM, Cox BJ: Cytocentrifugation in the management of central nervous system leukemia. *J Pediatr* 81:992, 1972

88. Koss LG: Diagnostic Cytology and its Histopathologic Bases, 3rd Ed, pp 878–970. Philadelphia: JB Lippincott Co., 1979

89. Kreisman H, Wolkove N, Finkelstein HS et al.: Breast cancer and thoracic metastases: Review of 119 patients. *Thorax* 38:175, 1983

90. Kruskall MS, Carter SR, Ritz LP: Contamination of cerebrospinal fluid by vertebral bone-marrow cells during lumbar puncture. *N Engl J Med* 308:697, 1983

91. Kubonishi I, Ohtsuki Y, Ken-Ichi M et al.: Granulocytic sarcoma presenting as a mediastinal tumor: Report of a case and cytological and cytochemical studies of tumor cells *in vivo* and *in vitro*. *Am J Clin Pathol* 82:730, 1984

92. Kudsk K, Fabian TC, Minton JP: Leveen shunts in patients with intractable malignant ascites. *J Surg Oncol* 13:61, 1980

93. Kurtz RC, Bronzo RL: Does spontaneous bacterial peritonitis occur in malignant ascites? *Am J Gastroenterol* 77:146, 1982

94. Kusaka H, Itabashi K, Suzuki J et al.: [A case of granulocytic

sarcoma with near tetraploidy and pleural and pericardial effusions as initial manifestations]. *Nippon Naika Gakkai Zasshi* 73:1170, 1984

95. Kutty CPK, Remeniuk E, Varkey B: Malignant-appearing cells in pleural effusion due to pancreatitis: Case report and literature review. *Acta Cytol* 25:412, 1981

96. Kutty CPK, Varkey B: Incidence and distribution of intrathoracic metastases from renal cell carcinoma. *Arch Intern Med* 144:273, 1984

97. Kyrkou KA, Iatridis SG, Athanassiadou PP et al.: Detection of benign or malignant origin of ascites with combined indirect immunoperoxidase assays of carcinoembryonic antigen and lysozyme. *Acta Cytol* 29:57, 1985

98. Lacy JH, Wieman TJ, Shively EH: Management of malignant ascites. *Surg Gynecol Obstet* 159:397, 1984

99. Levine RJ (ed): Asbestos: An Information Resource. DHEW Publication No. (NIH) 79-1681. National Cancer Institute, Bethesda, 1978

100. Light RW, Erozan YS, Ball WC: Cells in pleural fluid: Their value in differential diagnosis. *Arch Intern Med* 132:854, 1973

101. Light RW, Girard WM, Jenkinson SG, George RB: Parapneumonic effusions. *Am J Med* 69:507, 1980

102. Light RW, MacGregor MI, Ball WC, Luchsinger PC: Diagnostic significance of pleural fluid pH and PCO_2. *Chest* 64:591, 1973

103. Light RW, MacGregor MI, Luchsinger PC et al.: Pleural effusions: The diagnostic separation of transudates and exudates. *Ann Intern Med* 77:507, 1972

104. Light RW, Moller DJ, George RB: Low pleural fluid pH in parapneumonic effusion (Letter to editor). *Chest* 68:273, 1975

105. Lirzin P, Zeitoun P, Vandromme L, Salas H: [Carcinoembryonic antigen in ascites and pleural effusions]. *Gastroenterol Clin Biol* 8:222, 1984

106. Liss HP: Cope needle biopsy. *South Med J* 77:837, 1984

107. Lokich J, Reinhold R, Silverman M, Tullis J: Complications of peritoneovenous shunt for malignant ascites. *Cancer Treat Rep* 64:305, 1980

108. López JM, Delgado JL, Tovar E, González AG: Massive pericardial effusion produced by extracardiac malignant neoplasms. *Arch Intern Med* 143:1815, 1983

109. Lukes RJ, Collins RD: New approaches to the classification of the lymphomata. *Br J Cancer* 31:1, 1975

110. Marchevsky AM, Hauptman E, Gil J, Watson C: Computerized interactive morphometry as an aid in the diagnosis of pleural effusions. *Acta Cytol (Baltimore)* 31:131, 1987

111. Martin SE, Zhang H, Magyarosy E et al.: Immunologic methods in cytology. Definitive diagnosis of non-Hodgkin's lymphomas using immunologic markers for T- and B-cells. *Am J Clin Pathol* 82:666, 1984

112. Martinez-Vea A, Gatell JM, Segura F et al.: Diagnostic value of tumoral markers in serous effusions: Carcinoembryonic antigen, alpha$_1$-acid glycoprotein, alpha-fetoprotein, phosphohexose isomerase, and beta-2-microglobulin. *Cancer* 50:1783, 1982

113. McCaughey WTE, Dardick I, Barr JR: Angiosarcoma of serous membranes. *Arch Pathol Lab Med* 107:304, 1983

114. McCaughey WTE, Kannerstein M, Churg J: Tumors and pseudotumors of the serous membranes: Atlas of Tumor Pathology, 2nd series, Fascicle 20. Washington DC: Armed Forces Institute of Pathology, 1985

115. Melamed MR: The cytological presentation of malignant lymphomas and related diseases in effusions. *Cancer* 16:413, 1963

116. Ménard S, Rilke F, Torre GD et al.: Sensitivity enhancement of the cytologic detection of cancer cells in effusions by monoclonal antibodies. *Am J Clin Pathol* 83:571, 1985

117. Morell ND, Frost D, Ziel HK: Pseudo Meigs syndrome. A case report. *J Reprod Med* 25:88, 1980

118. Mufti GJ, Oscier DG, Hamblin TJ et al.: Serous effusions in monocytic leukaemias. *Br J Haematol* 58:547, 1984

119. Mukai K: Malignant mesothelioma and CEA staining (Letter to the editor). *Am J Surg Pathol* 9:159, 1985

120. Mulrow CD, Corey GR: Pericardial pseudoeffusion due to steroid-induced lipomatosis. *NC Med J* 46:179, 1985

121. Mungall IP, Cowen PN, Cooke NT et al.: Multiple pleural biopsy with the Abrams needle. *Thorax* 35:600, 1980

122. Nadji M: The potential value of immunoperoxidase techniques in diagnostic cytology. *Acta Cytol* 24:442, 1980

123. Nagasawa T, Nagasawa S: Enrichment of malignant cells from pleural effusions by Percoll density gradients. *Acta Cytol* 27:119, 1983

124. Naib ZM: Exfoliative Cytopathology, 3rd edn, pp 349–380. Boston: Little, Brown and Co, 1985

125. Naraynsingh V, Raju GC, Ratan P, Wong J: Massive ascites due to omental endometriosis. *Postgrad Med J* 61:539, 1985

126. Naylor B: The exfoliative cytology of diffuse malignant mesothelioma. *J Pathol Bact* 86:293, 1963

127. Newman TG, Soni, A, Acaron S, Huang CT: Pleural cryptococcosis in the acquired immune deficiency syndrome. *Chest* 91:459, 1987

128. Nissim F, Ashkenazy M, Borenstein R, Czernobilsky B: Tuberculoid cornstarch granulomas with caseous necrosis: A diagnostic challenge. *Arch Pathol Lab Med* 105:86, 1981

129. Oosterlee J: Peritoneovenous shunting for ascites in cancer patients. *Br J Surg* 67:663, 1980

130. Orell SR, Dowling KD: Oncofetal antigens as tumor markers in the cytologic diagnosis of effusions. *Acta Cytol* 27:625, 1983

131. Osamura RY, Shioya S, Handa K et al.: Lupus erythematosus cells in pleural fluid: Cytologic diagnosis in two patients. *Acta Cytol* 21:215, 1977

132. Pandyna MH, Agus B, Grady RF: *In vivo* LE phenomenon in pleural fluid. *Arthritis Rheum* 19:962, 1976

133. Peterman TA, Speicher CE: Evaluating pleural effusions: A two-stage laboratory approach. *JAMA* 252:1051, 1984

134. Pinio MM: Electron microscopy of effusions (Abstract). *Acta Cytol* 27:554, 1983

135. Piver MS, Lele SB, Patsner B: Pseudomyxoma peritonei: Possible prevention of mucinous ascites by peritoneal lavage. *Obstet Gynecol* 64:95S, 1984

136. Poe RH, Israel RH, Utell MJ et al.: Sensitivity, specificity, and predictive values of closed pleural biopsy. *Arch Intern Med* 144:325, 1984

137. Poe RH, Qazi R, Israel RH et al.: Survival of patients with pleural involvement by breast carcinoma. *Am J Clin Oncol* 6:523, 1983

138. Pomeranz SJ, Hawkins HH, Towbin R et al.: Granulocytic sarcoma (Chloroma): CT manifestations. *Radiology* 155:167, 1985

139. Potts DE, Levin DC, Sahn SA: Pleural fluid pH in parapneumonic effusions. *Chest* 70:328, 1976

140. Potts DE, Taryle DA, Sahn SA: The glucose-pH relationship in parapneumonic effusions. *Arch Intern Med* 138:1378, 1978

141. Potts DE, Willcox MA, Good JT et al.: The acidosis of low-glucose pleural effusions. *Am Rev Respir Dis* 117:665, 1978

142. Prakash UBS, Reiman HM: Comparison of needle biopsy with cytologic analysis for the evaluation of pleural effusion: Analysis of 414 cases. *Mayo Clin Proc* 60:158, 1985

143. Pugatch RD, Spirn PW: Radiology of the pleura. *Clin Chest Med* 6:17, 1985

144. Ramaekers F, Haag D, Jap P, Vooijs PG: Immunochemical demonstration of keratin and vimentin in cytologic aspirates. *Acta Cytol* 28:385, 1984

145. Reda MG, Baigelman W: Pleural effusions in systemic lupus erythematosus. *Acta Cytol* 24:553, 1980

146. Reinhold RB, Lokich JJ, Tomashefski J, Costello P: Man-

agement of malignant ascites with peritoneovenous shunting. *Am J Surg* 145:455, 1983

147. Reisberg IR, Oyakawa S: Mastocytosis with malabsorption, myelofibrosis, and massive ascites. *Am J Gastroenterol* 82:54, 1987

148. Rosai J: Ackerman's Surgical Pathology, pp 494, 1487. The C.V. Mosby Co., St. Louis, 1981

149. Rosen SE, Vonderheid EC, Koprowska I: Mycosis fungoides with pulmonary involvement: Cytopathologic findings. *Acta Cytol* 28:51, 1984

150. Rovensky YA, Gvichiya AS, Vasiliev JM: SEM study of the attachment of mouse ascitic hepatoma cells to various substrata. *Scan Electron Microsc* 3:71, 1980

151. Safa AM, Van Orstrand HS: Pleural effusion due to myeloma. *Chest* 64:246, 1973

152. Sahn SA, Taryle DA, Good JT: Experimental empyema: Time course and pathogenesis of pleural fluid acidosis and low pleural fluid glucose. *Am Rev Respir Dis* 120:355, 1979

153. Salhadin A, Nasiell M, Nasiell K et al.: The unique cytologic picture of oat cell carcinoma in effusions. *Acta Cytol* 20:298, 1976

154. Sandenbergh HA, Woodruff JD: Histogenesis of pseudomyxoma peritonei. Review of 9 cases. *Obstet Gynecol* 49:339, 1977

155. Schneller J, Eppich E, Greenbaum E et al.: Flow cytometry and feulgen cytophotometry in evaluation of effusions. *Cancer* 59:1307, 1987

156. Schölmerich J, Volk BA, Köttgen E et al.: Fibronectin concentration in ascites differentiates between malignant and nonmalignant ascites. *Gastroenterology* 87:1160, 1984

157. Schumann GB et al (ed): Clinics in Laboratory Medicine: Symposium on Body Fluid Analysis, pp 193–315; 389–403. Philadelphia: WB Saunders, Co, 1985

158. Scully RE (ed): Case records of the Massachusetts General Hospital: Case 46-1978. *N Engl J Med* 299:1179, 1978

159. Scully RE (ed): Case records of the Massachusetts General Hospital: Case 22-1985. *N Engl J Med* 312:1440, 1985

160. Sears D, Hajdu SI: The cytologic diagnosis of malignant neoplasms in pleural and peritoneal effusions. *Acta Cytol (Baltimore)* 31:85, 1987

161. Seidel TA, Garbes AD: Cellules grumelees: Old terminology revised: The cytologic diagnosis of chronic lymphocytic leukemia and well-differentiated lymphocytic lymphoma in pleural effusions (Abstract). *Acta Cytol* 28:659, 1984

162. Senger DR, Galli SJ, Dvorak AM et al.: Tumor cells secrete a vascular permeability factor that promotes accumulation of ascites fluid. *Science* 219:983, 1983

163. Sheid B, Boyce J: Inhibition of lymphocyte mitogenesis by factor(s) released from macrophages isolated from ascitic fluid of advanced ovarian cancer patients. *Cancer Immunol Immunother* 17:190, 1984

164. Shuman LS, Libshitz HI: Solid pleural manifestations of lymphoma. *AJR* 142:269, 1984

165. Siegler R, Koprowska I: Mechanism of ascites tumor formation. *Cancer Res* 22:1273, 1962

166. Sigurdsson K, Alm P, Gullberg B: Prognostic factors in malignant epithelial ovarian tumors. *Gynecol Oncol* 15:370, 1983

167. Silverman PM, Harell GS, Korobkin M: Computed tomography of the abnormal pericardium. *AJR* 140:1125, 1983

168. Simel DL, Weinberg JB: Leukemic ascites complicating acute myelomonoblastic leukemia. *Arch Pathol Lab Med* 109:365, 1985

169. Skinner DB: Operation for diagnosis and treatment of pericardial effusions. *Surgery* 96:738, 1984

170. Smith NJ, Dziura BR, Gondos B: Use of blood group isoantigens in distinguishing benign and malignant cells in effusions (Abstract). *Acta Cytol* 24:66, 1980

171. Smith RR, Sternberg SS, Paglia MA, Golbey RB: Fatal

172. Souter RG, Tarin D, Kettlewell MG: Peritoneovenous shunts in the management of malignant ascites. *Br J Surg* 70:478, 1983

173. Souter RG, Wells C, Tarin D, Kettlewell MG: Surgical and pathologic complications associated with peritoneovenous shunts in management of malignant ascites. *Cancer* 55:1973, 1985

174. Spriggs AI, Grunze H: An unusual cytologic presentation of mesothelioma in serous effusions. *Acta Cytol* 27:288, 1983

175. Staats BA, Ellefson RD, Budahn LL et al.: The lipoprotein profile of chylous and nonchylous pleural effusions. *Mayo Clin Proc* 55:700, 1980

176. Stang JM, Ruff PD, McEnany MT et al.: Acute massive (pericardial effusive) pulmonary thromboembolism–pulmonary embolectomy revisited. *Clin Cardiol* 6:613, 1983

177. Stark DD, Higgins CB, Lanzer P et al.: Magnetic resonance imaging of the pericardium: Normal and pathologic findings. *Radiology* 150:469, 1984

178. Stehman FB, Ehrlich CE: Peritoneocystic shunt for malignant ascites. *Gynecol Oncol* 18:402, 1984

179. Szpak CA, Johnston WW, Littich SC et al.: Patterns of reactivity of four novel monoclonal antibodies (B72.3, DF3, B1.1, and B6.2) with cells in human malignant and benign effusion. *Acta Cytol* 28:356, 1984

180. Takagi F: Studies on tumor cells in serous effusion. *Am J Clin Pathol* 24:663, 1954

181. Taki T, Kojima S, Seto H et al.: Glycolipid composition of acitic fluids from patients with cancer. *J Biochem (Tokyo)* 96:1257, 1984

182. Tamura K, Kawano K, Ishizaki J et al.: Ascites with peritoneal myeloid metaplasia in a patient with advanced non-Hodgkin's lymphoma. *Jpn J Clin Oncol* 15:25, 1985

183. Tempero MA, Davis RB, Reed E, Edney J: Thrombocytopenia and laboratory evidence of disseminated intravascular coagulation after shunts for ascites in malignant disease. *Cancer* 55:2718, 1985

184. To A, Dearnaley DP, Ormerod MG et al.: Epithelial membrane antigen: Its use in the cytodiagnosis of malignancy in serous effusions. *Am J Clin Pathol* 78:214, 1982

185. Tötterman KJ, Pesonen E, Siltanen P: Radiation-related chronic heart disease. *Chest* 83:875, 1983

186. Trigg ME, Swanson JD, Letellier MA: Metastasis of an optic glioma through a ventriculoperitoneal shunt. *Cancer* 52:599, 1983

187. Turton CW: Pleural effusions. *Br J Hosp Med* 23:239, 244; 246, 1980

188. Vellios F, Griffin J: Examination of body fluids for tumor cells. *Am J Clin Pathol* 24:676, 1954

189. Vladutiu AO, Adler RH, Brason FW: Diagnostic value of biochemical analysis of pleural effusions: Carcinoembryonic antigen and beta$_2$ microglobulin. *Am J Clin Pathol* 71:210, 1979

190. Volpe R, Carbone A: Reed-Sternberg cells in pericardial fluid. *Acta Cytol* 26:61, 1982

191. Von Haam E: Cytology of transudates and exudates. *Monogr Clin Cytol* 5:1, 1977

192. Von Scheidt W, Kandolf R, Denecke H, Erdmann E: [Primary and secondary chylopericardium] *Dtsch Med Wochenschr* 111:1842, 1986

193. Walts AE, Said JW: Specific tumor markers in diagnostic cytology: Immunoperoxidase studies of carcinoembryonic antigen, lysozyme and other tissue antigens in effusions, washes and aspirates. *Acta Cytol* 27:408, 1983

194. Watts KC, Boyo-Ekwueme H, To A, Posnansky M, Coleman DV: Chromosome studies on cells cultured from serous effusions: Use in routine cytologic practice. *Acta Cytol* 27:38, 1983

195. Weissberg D, Kaufmann M: Diagnostic and therapeutic pleuroscopy. Experience with 127 patients. *Chest* 78:732, 1980

196. Weissel M, Punzengruber C, Hartter E et al.: Thyroid hormones and pericardial effusion may influence plasma levels of atrial natriuretic peptide (ANP) in humans. *Klin Wochenschr* 64:93, 1986

197. Wied GL, Koss LG, Reagan JW (eds): Compendium on Diagnostic Cytology, 5th ed, pp 465–486. Chicago: The Tutorials of Cytology, 1983

198. Williford ME, Hidalgo H, Putman CE et al.: Computed tomography of pleural disease. *AJR* 140:909, 1983

199. Winkelmann M, Pfitzer P: Blind pleural biopsy in combination with cytology of pleural effusions. *Acta Cytol* 25:373, 1981

200. Witte CL, Brewer ML, Witte MH, Pond GB: Protean manifestations of pylethrombosis. A review of thirty-four patients. *Ann Surg* 202:191, 1985

201. Wroblewski F, Wroblewski R: Clinical significance of lactic dehydrogenase activity of serous effusions. *Ann Intern Med* 48:813, 1958

202. Wünsch PH, Müller HA: [Cytodiagnosis of malignant non-Hodgkin's lymphomas in effusions]. *Virchows Arch* 36:275, 1981

203. Yam LT: Granulocytic sarcoma with pleural involvement. Identification of neoplastic cells with cytochemistry. *Acta Cytol* 29:63, 1985

204. Yam LT, Jackila AJ: A simple method of preparing smears from bloody effusions for cytodiagnosis. *Acta Cytol* 27:114, 1983

205. Yam LT, Winkler CF: Immunochemical diagnosis of oat-cell carcinoma in pleural effusion. *Acta Cytol* 28:425, 1984

206. Yamada S, Takeda T, Matsumoto K: Prognostic analysis of malignant pleural and peritoneal effusions. *Cancer* 51:136, 1983

207. Yoshimura S, Scully RE, Taft PD, Herrington JB: Peritoneal fluid cytology in patients with ovarian cancer. *Gynecol Oncol* 17:161, 1984

208. Yuasha S, Itoshima T, Nagashima H: Clinical studies of hepatocellular carcinoma with liver cirrhosis and ascites. *Acta Med Okayama* 38:291, 1984

INFECTION IN THE PATIENT WITH CANCER

STEPHEN C. SCHIMPFF

Infection and hemorrhage are the major limiting, life threatening toxicities occurring during the "standard" therapy for patients with leukemia and the intensive treatment of patients with solid tumors. This chapter will therefore review the current approach to the diagnosis, treatment and prevention of infection.

PREVENTION AND TREATMENT OF INFECTIONS IN PATIENTS WITH CANCER

The term "compromised host" indicates an individual at increased risk of developing infection because of dysfunction of basic defense mechanisms (13). Most infections in the compromised host are nosocomial (hospital-associated). The diagnosis of infection in the patient with cancer, a prime example of the compromised host, is challenging but reasonably straight-forward once those factors predisposing to infection are clarified (15). This will allow for early diagnosis and an understanding of the unusual presentations of infection, an empiric approach to early therapy and, of great importance, the development of an effective program for infection prevention.

Predisposing factors

A patient's underlying disease is the most important determinant of the types of infections that may occur, but even in patients with the same underlying tumor diagnosis, infections vary depending on other predisposing factors (18, 2) (Table 1). For example, there are great differences in infections that occur in the adult with acute myelocytic leukemia receiving chemotherapy, the same patient following bone marrow transplantation, or a child with acute lymphocytic leukemia receiving maintenance therapy. The most important conditions predisposing to infection in these patients are granulocytopenia, usually in association with substantial damage to the alimentary canal mucosal membranes and respiratory tract mucociliary function, cellular immune abnormalities, humoral immune deficiencies, obstruction of natural passages, central nervous system dysfunction and various invasive procedures such as intravascular catheters (18).

Cell-mediated immunity

Defects in cell-mediated immunity, such as those found in

patients with Hodgkin's disease or the child with acute leukemia who is receiving long-term maintenance therapy, predispose toward infections with the following organisms: Bacteria – *Listeria monocytogenes*, *Salmonella* spp., *Nocardia asteroides*, *Mycobacteria* (typical and atypical), and *Legionella pneumophilia*; viruses – Varicella-zoster, Cytomegalovirus, and Herpes simplex; yeasts – *Cryptococcus neoformans*, *Histoplasma capsulatum*, and *Coccidioides immitis*; protozoa – *Toxoplasma gondii* and *Pneumocystis carinii*; helminth – *Strongyloides stercoralis* (13, 24).

These infections associated with the acquired immune deficiency syndrome are those of a patient with major deficit in cellular immune function.

Cellular immunity is important in host-versus-graft rejection, and the defenses against viruses, fungi and bacteria which are obligate intracellular pathogens. The medical literature is confusing as to the frequency of infections caused by these organisms. Other than reactivation of tuberculosis and the development of varicella-zoster infection, most of these organisms infrequently cause infection even in the immunocompromised patient. However, it is in this patient population that these infections are most likely to occur, and, should they occur, are most likely to be widespread and life-threatening. These organisms as a group tend to cause four general patterns of infection: pneumonitis, central nervous system infection, alimentary canal infection and skin lesions.

Pneumonitis tends to be caused by *Listeria monocytogenes*, *Mycobacteria*, *Nocardia*, *Legionella pneumophilia*, the three yeasts mentioned above, varicella-zoster virus and Cytomegalovirus, *Pneumocystis carinii*, *Toxoplasma gondii* and *Strongyloides stercoralis*. Therefore, the finding of pneumonitis alone will not be of much diagnostic value, although the specific clinical-epidemiologic setting along with other findings should narrow the possibilities substantially. For example, *Listeria* is likely to be concurrently associated with pleural effusion, septicemia, meningitis, or all three. *M. tuberculosis* is frequently associated with evidence of old scarring in the lung apices and varicella-zoster pneumonitis almost never occurs in the absence of concurrent cutaneous infection.

Central nervous system infections include *Listeria monocytogenes* with a meningoencephalitis, *Nocardia asteroides* causing localized mass lesions, *Cryptococcus neoformans* causing an encephalitis followed by meningitis, *Toxoplasma gondii* causing mass lesions, meningoencephalitis or both, and the varicella-zoster virus causing meningoencephalitis.

Infections along the alimentary canal include Salmonella

K.W. Brunson (ed) Local invasion and spread of cancer.

Table 1. Factors predisposing to infection among patients with cancer.

Granulocytopenia (e.g., acute leukemia)
  Usually with associated damage to body barriers (especially alimentary canal mucosa, respiratory tract ciliary function and integument)
  Common organisms
    Gram-negative bacilli: *Pseudomonas aeruginosa, Klebsiella pneumoniae* and *Escherichia coli*
    Gram-positive cocci: *Staphylococcus aureus, Staphylococcus epidermidis*
    Yeasts: *Candida* spp., *Torulopsis glabrata*
    Fungi: *Aspergillus* spp., *Mucor*
Cellular immune deficiency (e.g., lymphoma)
  Common Organisms:
    Bacteria: *Listeria monocytogenes, Salmonella* spp., *Mycobacterium* spp., *Nocardia asteroides* and *Legionella pneumophilia*
    Viruses: Varicella-zoster, Herpes simplex, Cytomegalovirus
    Fungi: *Cryptococcus neoformans, Histoplasma capsulatum, Coccidioides immitis*
    Protozoa: *Pneumocystis carinii, Toxoplasma gondii*
    Helminth: *Strongyloides stercoralis*
Humoral immune dysfunction (e.g., multiple myeloma)
  Common Organisms: *Streptococcus pneumoniae, Hemophilus influenzae*
Obstruction to natural passages (e.g., solid tumors)
  Common Sites: Respiratory tract, biliary tract, urinary tract
  Common Organisms: Locally colonizing
CNS Dysfunction (e.g., brain tumors)
  Common sites: Pneumonitis and urinary tract infection
  Common organisms: Locally colonizing
Infections associated with medical procedures
  Procedures: Intravascular catheters, urinary catheters and respiratory assist devices
  Common Organisms: Locally colonizing

---

causing an enteritis in patients with pelvic tumors, Cytomegalovirus-induced esophagitis, small bowel inflammation or colitis, Herpes simplex-induced distal esophagitis, or enterocolitis due to infection by *Strongyloides stercoralis*.

These organisms which have a predominance for skin manifestations include varicella-zoster virus-induced chickenpox or "shingles", herpes simplex lesions, usually near the mouth or perineum, and the secondary skin manifestations of many organisms including *Nocardia, Cryptococcus, Histoplasma* or Cytomegalovirus.

The list of organisms which tend to cause infection in the setting of cellular immune deficiency and the fact that many different organisms can be associated with any given clinical picture such as pneumonitis or enteritis, requires that intensive diagnostic procedures be performed promptly so that the correct therapy can be applied. Obviously, the approach to treatment of these infections varies widely depending upon the etiologic agent. Epidemiologic considerations in association with the clinical picture and initial diagnostic clues can assist in designing a rational approach to empiric therapy.

The patient with AIDS has marked immune deficiency due to major reductions in the number and function of T4 lymphocytes. This places the AIDS patient at great risk for infections which the body normally protects itself from with the cellular immune system. The most frequent infection is *P. carinii* pneumonia with cytomegalovirus, Herpes simplex, *Candida* and mycobacteria, especially *M. avium-intracellulare*, also common infectious agents.

Humoral immune deficiency

Patients who have defects in humoral immunity (multiple myeloma, chronic lymphocytic leukemia) tend to have infections for which antibody is the major means of infection prevention, i.e., *Streptococcus pneumoniae, Hemophilus influenzae* and (rarely) *Neisseria meningitidis* (5, 13, 15). Antibody production against *S. pneumoniae* is depressed following bone marrow transplantation and these patients tend to have an increased risk of pneumococcal infection (27). Patients who have had a splenectomy for any cause, including trauma or as a diagnostic procedure (Hodgkin's disease and staging laparotomy) are at an increased risk of infection with these same organisms. Although pneumococcal bacteremia appears to be quite unusual even in the splenectomized patient with Hodgkin's disease, it is important to recall that a very small but real percentage of patients may develop the "overwhelming pneumococcal sepsis syndrome" (1). This has been reported sporadically in adults in whom an overwhelming septicemia without apparent origin of infection leads to the patient's demise in a matter of a day or less. The syndrome mimmicks in many ways the Waterhouse–Friderichsen Syndrome described with meningococcal sepsis and has also been seen occasionally as a result of Hemophilus sepsis. Therefore, patients who have had a splenectomy should be advised that the sudden onset of fever and chills should prompt immediate medical attention and physicians should be aware that immediate hospitalization with institution of intravenous ampicillin (to cover *S. pneumoniae, H. influenzae* and *N. meningitidis*) is appropriate except in those settings where ampicillin-resistant *H. influenzae* are prevalent.

Obstruction to natural passages

Any lesion which partially obstructs a natural passage, such as the bronchus, biliary or urinary tracts, may lead to infections, such as pneumonitis, ascending cholangitis or urinary tract infection. Obstructions are the most common causes of infection in patients with solid tumors or lymphomas. The organisms causing infection will be those colonizing the patient at or near that site so that pneumonitis is likely to be caused by normal mouth flora unless the patient has been on broad spectrum antimicrobials or has been hospitalized for prolonged periods. Ascending cholangitis is likely to be caused by enteric gram-negative bacilli and perhaps anaerobes, and urinary tract infection is also likely to be caused by aerobic gram-negative rods colonizing the colon. Although antimicrobial therapy is important, the critical issue in resolution of these infections is alleviation of the obstruction.

Central nervous system dysfunction

Major abnormalities associated with CNS dysfunction

which lead to infection are diminution or loss of the gag reflex with development of aspiration pneumonitis or impaired micturition with residual urine and secondary urinary tract infection. These are usually very difficult infections to resolve because of persistence of the neurologic deficit. Pneumonia is therefore a common cause or accompaniment of death in patients with primary or metastatic brain tumors.

Infections associated with procedures

Perhaps second only to obstructive phenomena, infectious morbidity and mortality is commonly associated with invasive procedures. In the general hospital population, an indwelling urinary catheter is the most common source of nosocomial infection and this is no exception in the cancer patient. Not only will catheter avoidance dramatically reduce the incidence of urinary tract infection, but it will substantially reduce the incidence of bacteremia. The association of bacteremia and, to a lesser extent, fungemia, with an indwelling intravascular catheter is well known. The relatively simply expedient of utilizing a butterfly-type needle when a venous catheter is not absolutely essential (i.e., most of the time) and of changing catheters every few days when they are in fact indicated will reduce the frequency of these catheter-associated bacteremias. Respiratory assist units are also associated with nosocomial infection because many gram-negative bacilli are capable of living and multiplying in a nebulizer from which they can be forceably blown into the patient's tracheobronchial tree. Proper attention to maintenance of respiratory assist equipment will reduce the frequency of necrotizing pneumonia. One of the most common iatrogenic causes of infection is related to blood and blood product administration, with resultant nonA/nonB hepatitis and, less frequently, infection caused by Cytomegalovirus or Epstein-Barr virus.

Granulocytopenia

Sites and pathogens
There is an inverse and distinct association between the level of absolute circulating granulocyte count and the incidence of infection (3). Most infections in this patient population occur at sites of damaged mucosa, particularly exacerbation of periodontal infections, pharyngitis, esophagitis (distal esophagus), colitis, perianal cellulitis, pneumonitis and sinusitis (20). The infections are caused by organisms colonizing at or near these areas. Hence, perianal lesions are caused principally by gram-negative bacilli. So too are infections at most other locations, and this is apparently due, in part, to the shifts of microbial flora which are a consequence of the underlying disease process. The normal oral flora changes in a few days to an increasing predominance of gram-negative bacilli (7). As a result, pharyngitis, esophagitis, and pneumonitis are frequently caused by gram-negative bacilli.

The organisms that cause the majority of infections are therefore gram-negative bacilli, especially *Escherichia coli*, *Klebsiella pneumoniae* and *Pseudomonas aeruginosa*. *Staphylococcus aureus*, other gram-negative bacilli and less common organisms, such as *Staphylococcus epidermidis* or *Streptococcus faecalis* will cause the majority of the other bacterial infections. Candida and Aspergillus cause most fungal infections. It is of great importance to recognize that these infections are usually not caused by the patient's own normal endogenous flora but rather by colonizing flora which have reached the patient only during hospitalization. Indeed, well over 50% of infections are caused by hospital-acquired microorganisms and these are often organisms which are either more virulent, more resistant to commonly used antibiotics or both.

Diagnosis
The absence of granulocytes and overall diminution in normal inflammatory mechanisms secondary to cytotoxic therapy often makes diagnosis more difficult than in the patient who has a normal inflammatory response (21). In this situation, prompt use of empiric antibiotic therapy will be appropriate for the granulocytopenic patient who develops new fever. The onset of fever in the granulocytopenic patient (less than $1,000/\mu l$) is associated with bacteremia in about 20%, nonbacteremic microbiologically documented infections in about 20%, clinically documented infection (i.e., the site of infection is apparent but a specific infecting organism cannot be defined) in 20%, and a possible infection (i.e., signs and symptoms are suggestive but nevertheless equivocal with regard to the presence of infection) in 20%. About 20% of patients will be found, in retrospect, when all data are available, to have not had an infectious cause for their fever. Thus, at least 60% of these febrile episodes are related to infection and hence empiric antibiotic therapy is appropriate (16).

Empiric therapy
Antibiotic therapy should be instituted immediately on an empiric basis once the appropriate history, physical examination and initial laboratory studies have been completed. These studies should include chest x-ray, urinalysis performed by the physician, collection of two sets of blood cultures (two separate venipunctures), and perhaps a set of "surveillance cultures" from nose, gingiva and rectum. The purpose of the surveillance cultures is to give the physician an idea of the flora currently colonizing the patient so that if a definitive organism is not isolated from the presumed site of infection, the physician may, if necessary, be able to adjust antimicrobial therapy later if indicated by the presence of resistant organisms. These studies can be completed quickly, and antimicrobial therapy should under no circumstances be delayed before the completion of more sophisticated time-consuming evaluations. The antimicrobial regimen chosen should be broad spectrum, bactericidal, and should be given intravenously at full dosage. It is important to emphasize that the design of an empiric antibiotic combination for an individual patient must depend upon an understanding of the epidemiology of infections current at the particular hospital in question. Published guidelines (19) can be an aid in determining an approach but should be modified as appropriate.

The patient with granulocytopenia and new fever should probably be treated with a combination of antibiotics. Recently, a series of new compounds, notably ceftazidime and imipenem, have become available which have exceedingly broad spectrums of activity. Nevertheless, I recommend combination therapy at best for the first few days until culture information is available. It is believed that the benefit of two drugs compared to one drug is primarily related to a synergistic activity of those two active agents (4, 8, 9, 10). Thus, the choice of the two drugs for combination use should be based on known patterns of *in vitro* synergistic activity with the organisms which most commonly invade this patient population. Useful combinations are those which include an extended spectrum penicillin (carbenicillin, ticarcillin, mezlocillin, piperacillin or azlocillin), an extended spectrum cephalosporin (ceftazidime, cefotaxime or cefoperazone) for imipenem plus an aminoglycoside (gentamicin, tobramycin or amikacin).

Once empiric antibiotics have been begun, it is essential that the patient be reexamined on at least a twice daily basis with emphasis on the subtle clinical clues which suggest infection at specific sites. It is of great importance to detect a specific origin of infection so that either appropriate local measures can be applied and so that additional cultures, if necessary, can be examined for antimicrobial susceptibilities. Furthermore, the length of time antibiotics will be continued depends upon whether or not a site of infection is recognized. As a general rule, antibiotics should be continued for approximately two weeks for a patient who has a microbiologically documented infection with a bacteremia or other severe microbiologically documented infection, such as pneumonia or perianal cellulitis. Patients with clinically documented infections should probably be treated for 10–14 days but longer if response to therapy is slow. It is difficult to have exact criteria for therapy of patients with equivocal (possible) infections, but a reasonable rule of thumb is to continue antibiotics for approximately four to five days after the patient becomes a febrile which usually means a total course of eight to ten days. Finally, the patient in whom infection is considered doubtful should have the antibiotics discontinued as promptly as possible to avoid selective pressure toward resistant organisms. Usually this decision can be made in approximately four days because by that time most blood cultures which are ultimately to be positive will have been reported by the laboratory and because twice daily re-examination of the patient should have clarified whether or not a site of infection is present.

There is a small but real subgroup of patients who, after four to five days of therapy, will still be febrile and neutropenic and in whom it is not clear if the patient was or was not infected at the time antibiotics were started (11). Questions in this group often include whether or not antibiotics should be changed or other agents should be added with regard to the possibility of a resistant bacteria, whether or not granulocyte transfusions should be added or whether or not amphotericin B or other antifungal agents should be instituted. No definitive rule of thumb will be appropriate for all patients. Rather, it is most useful to give careful consideration to the background of the specific patient in context with epidemiologic patterns in the specific hospital.

Infection prevention

As with diagnosis and its therapy, infection prevention first requires recognition of the factors which predispose to infection. A specific approach to infection prevention can then be divided into four categories (12, 25): (1) improve the patient's damaged host defense mechanisms wherever possible; (15) reduce the frequency of invasive procedures which will further compromise the patient's ability to defend against microbial invasion; (18) reduce the acquisition of potential pathogens; and (2) reduce the numbers of potential pathogens already colonizing the patient. These are discussed in turn:

Bolster host defenses

Unfortunately, little can be done to improve the patient's own host defense mechanisms other than treating the patient appropriately to induce total remission of the underlying cancer with consequent restitution of normal bone marrow elements. The influenza vaccine may be useful not because influenza is more common in cancer patients but because the infected patient may be more likely to develop a superimposed serious bacterial pneumonia. At this time there are no other useful vaccines and it should be recalled that attenuated live viral vaccines should be avoided, e.g., measles, rubella, mumps, and oral polio. Despite universal testing of blood and blood products, hepatitis B continues to occur occasionally and can be prevented with the genetically engineered hepatitis B vaccine.

Reduce invasive procedures

Butterfly needles should be utilized for peripheral venous access, changed every 48 hours and inserted with proper skin preparation. Urinary catheters should be avoided if at all possible. Even venipunctures, finger sticks, and bone marrow aspirations should be performed with assiduous attention to skin cleansing and should be followed by a few minutes of pressure to hasten clot formation and lessen blood extravasation into tissues thereby reducing microorganism entrance into an ideal growth media.

Reduce organism acquisition

The major routes of acquisition are hands, food, water and air, probably in that order. The most basic infection prevention is handwashing by staff members (23). A fifteen second wash with regular soap under running water is sufficient to remove most transient organisms. Food is another common source of acquired organisms, especially gram-negative bacilli from green leafy vegetables and tomatoes (14). A low microbial content diet can be prepared by any hospital dietary service by simply utilizing only fully cooked foods, pasteurized liquids and foods/beverages certified as "commercially sterile" such as most canned vegetables and meats, sodas, some fruit juices, etc. Salads should be avoided.

Water supplies from city sources have relatively few viable organisms, but faucet aerators may introduce large numbers of water-loving gram-negative bacilli such as *Pseudomonas aeruginosa* or *Serratia marcescens*. A simple approach is either to remove the faucet aerator permanently or be sure that it is removed and cleansed of organic debris on a weekly basis. Finally, air is the source of spores, such as Aspergillus or of particles which carry respiratory viruses, *Staphylococcus aureus* or *M. tuberculosis*. Other than isolation of patients expectorating potential pathogens such as the patient with *S. aureus* pneumonia, there is relatively little that can be done easily about most airborne organisms short of laminar air flow reverse isolation. The laminar air flow room represents the ultimate method for total reverse isolation, the essential aspects of which are a room with a bank of high efficiency particle air (HEPA) filters along one entire wall of the room through which air is pumped by blowers at a uniform velocity forcing it to move in a laminar pattern and exiting at the opposite end of the room (17). The result is essentially sterile air in the room, minimal air turbulence, minimal opportunity for microorganism build-up, and a consistently clean environment. To complete the isolation, sterile water and sterile or low microbial content food along with sterile supplies are utilized, and staff members and visitors must don sterile garments prior to entry and remain downstream from the patient (12).

Suppressing colonizing organisms

Important areas to control in the granulocytopenic patient are the flora of the alimentary canal and skin. Daily bathing and shampooing with an antiseptic solution such as chlorhexidine or povidone-iodine will substantially reduce skin infections. Since most other infections originate from the alimentary canal flora, suppression of the aerobic organisms from mouth to anus will likewise substantially reduce infections. Although oral nonabsorbable antibiotic combinations, such as gentamicin, vancomycin and nystatin have been proven efficacious, there are disadvantages to their use, most notably the acquisition of gentamicin-resistant gramnegative rods and poor patient compliance due to disagreeable taste. An alternative approach is to use oral agents which selectively suppress the aerobic potential pathogens leaving intact the anaerobic flora which in turn will assist in preventing colonization with other newly acquired organisms (i.e., maintain "colonization resistance") (6, 22, 26). Currently, the most commonly used regimen is trimethoprim/sulfamethoxazole (TMP/SMZ) plus nystatin, but, although proven to have reasonable efficacy, this combination has no effect against some important bacteria such as *Pseudomonas aeruginosa* and may have some potential for delaying return of normal numbers of granulocytes. Finally, it is important to observe patients carefully for the acquisition of TMP/SMZ-resistant organisms, occasionally plasmid-mediated with concurrent resistance to drugs, such as ticarcillin, which are used as primary therapeutic agents.

SUMMARY

Infection among patients with cancer is closely associated with the presence of specific predisposing factors especially granulocytopenia, with concurrent damage to normal body barriers, cellular or humoral immune dysfunction, obstruction to natural passages, damage to the central nervous system or iatrogenic procedures. Each setting has a distinctly different set of infections associated with it and hence the approach to diagnosis, therapy and prevention varies from one setting to another.

REFERENCES

1. Bisno AL: Hyposplenism and overwhelming pneumococcal infection: A reappraisal. *Am J Med Sci* 262:101, 1971
2. Bodey GP: Infections in cancer patients. *Cancer Treat Rev* 2:89, 1975
3. Bodey GP, Buckley M, Sathe YS, Freireich EJ: Quantitative relationships between circulating leukocytes and infection in patients with acute leukemia. *Ann Intern Med* 64:328, 1966
4. de Jongh CA, Joshi JH, Newman KA et al: Antibiotic synergism and response in gram-negative bacteremia in granulocytopenic cancer patients. *Am J Med* 80:96, 1986
5. Fahey JL, Scoggins R, Utz JP, Szwed CF: Infection, antibody response and gamma globulin components in multiple myeloma and macroglobulinemia. *Am J Med* 35:698, 1963
6. Gurwith MJ, Brunton JL, Lank BA et al.: A prospective controlled investigation of prophylactic trimethoprim/ sulfamethoxazole in hospitalized granulocytopenic patients. *Am J Med* 66:248, 1979
7. Johanson WG, Pierce AK, Sanford JP: Changing pharyngeal flora of hospitalized patients. Emergence of gram-negative bacilli. *N Engl J Med* 281:1137, 1969
8. Serum bactericidal assay: Technical aspects and clinical correlations. Klastersky J, Schimpff S (Guest Editors) *Europ J Clin Microbiol* 5:57, 1986
9. Klastersky J, Cappel R, Daneau D: Clinical significance of *in vitro* synergism between antibiotics in gram-negative infections. *Antimicrob Ag Chemother* 2:470, 1972
10. Lau WK, Young LS, Black RE et al.: Comparative efficacy and toxicity of amikacin/carbenicillin versus gentamicin/ carbenicillin in leukopenic patients. A randomized prospective trial. *Am J Med* 62:959, 1977
11. Pizzo PA: After empiric therapy: What to do until the granulocyte comes back. *Rev Infect Dis* 9:214, 1987
12. Pizzo PA, Schimpff SC: Strategies for the prevention of infection in the myelosuppressed or immunosuppressed cancer patient. *Cancer Treat Rep* 67:223, 1983
13. Remington JS: The compromised host. *Hosp Prac* 7:59, 1972
14. Remington JS, Schimpff SC: Please don't eat the salads. *N Engl J Med* 304:433, 1981
15. Schimpff SC: Diagnosis of infection in patients with cancer. *Europ J Cancer* 11:29, 1975
16. Schimpff SC: Therapy of infection in patients with granulocytopenia. *Med Clin No Amer* 61:1101, 1977
17. Schimpff SC: Infection prevention in patients with cancer and granulocytopenia. In: *Infections Complicating the Abnormal Host*, edited by Grieco MH, Yorke Medical Books, New York, pp 926–950, 1980
18. Schimpff SC: Infections in the compromised host. In: *Principles and Practices of Infectious Diseases*, edited by Mandell GL, Douglas RG Jr, Bennett JE (3rd edition), Wiley, New York, 1989
19. Schimpff SC: Empiric antibiotic therapy for granulocytopenic cancer patients. *Am J Med* 80:13, 1986
20. Schimpff SC, Young VM, Greene WH et al.: Origin of infection in acute nonlymphocytic leukemia: Significance of hospital acquisition of potential pathogens. *Ann Intern Med* 77:707, 1972
21. Sickles EA, Greene WH, Wiernik PH: Clinical presentation of infection in granulocytopenic patients. *Arch Intern Med* 135:715, 1975
22. Sleijfer DT, Mulder NH, deVries-Hospers HG et al.: Infection prevention in granulocytopenic patients by selective decontamination of the digestive tract. *Europ J Cancer* 16:859, 1980
23. Steere AC, Mallison GF: Handwashing practices for the prevention of nosocomial infections. *Ann Intern Med* 83:683, 1975
24. Wade JC, Schimpff SC: Infections in patients with suppressed cellular immunity. In: *Medical Complications in Cancer Patients*, edited by Klastersky J, Staquet MJ, Raven Press, New York, pp 273–290, 1981
25. Wade JC, Schimpff SC: Epidemiology and prevention of infection in the compromised host. In: *Clinical Approach to Infection in the Compromised Host, 2nd Edition*, edited by Rubin RH, Young LS, Plenum Press, New York, pp. 5–40, 1988
26. Wade JC, Schimpff SC, Hargadon MT et al.: A comparison of trimethoprim-sulfamethoxazole plus nystatin with gentamicin plus nystatin in the prevention of infections in acute leukemia. *N Engl J Med* 304:1057, 1981
27. Winston DJ, Schiffman G, Wang DC et al.: Pneumococcal infections after human bone-marrow transplantation. *Ann Intern Med* 91:835, 1979

20

EFFECTS OF CANCER CHEMOTHERAPY ON GONADAL FUNCTION

RICHARD L. SCHILSKY

During the past 20 years, major strides have been made in the treatment of neoplastic disease with cytotoxic chemotherapy. Progress in understanding tumor cell biology and mechanisms of drug resistance, the introduction of new, effective antineoplastic drugs and technologic advances which allow for more detailed and complete pharmacokinetic studies have all contributed to the successful application of cancer chemotherapy. Many patients with Hodgkin's disease, acute leukemia, non-Hodgkin's lymphoma, testicular carcinoma and other tumors now regularly achieve sustained clinical remissions and cures. Moreover, adjuvant chemotherapy is now commonly employed for treatment of micrometastatic disease in clinically well patients with breast cancer and soft tissue sarcoma and appears to decrease the relapse rate and perhaps prolong survival for some individuals. Thus many more patients currently receive cytotoxic chemotherapy than ever before and, of greater significance, many more individuals are cured of their tumors and survive to experience the potential late adverse effects of such treatment. Among these, infertility and mutagenesis are often of particular concern to cancer survivors who have new hopes and expectations for a return to a normal life style. This chapter will review the effects of cancer chemotherapy on the gonadal function, sexuality and progeny of patients treated for malignant disease.

EFFECTS OF CANCER CHEMOTHERAPY ON GONADAL FUNCTION

Neoplastic disease and its treatment can potentially interfere with any of the cellular, anatomic, physiologic or behavioral processes which comprise normal sexual and reproductive function. The nature of the patient's illness, the extent of necessary surgery or radiation therapy, and the patient's relationship with spouse and family may all play an important role in reestablishing normal sexual interest and function following treatment for cancer. Further, many drugs used in the treatment of malignant disease have profound and often lasting effects on the testis and ovary. Germ cell production and endocrine function may both be altered, with the magnitude of the effect related to the age, pubertal status and menstrual status of the patient as well as to the particular drug, dosage or combination administered.

Chemotherapy effects in men

The normal adult testis is an organ composed of diverse and highly specialized cell types which may vary in their sensitivity to cytotoxic drugs. The exocrine function of the gland, spermatogenesis, proceeds in the seminiferous tubules, while the interstitial cells of Leydig carry on the primary endocrine function of the testis, testosterone production (75).

The seminiferous tubules, which constitute 75% of the testicular mass, are lined by stratified epithelium composed of two cell types: spermatogenic cells and Sertoli cells. The spermatogenic cells are arranged in an orderly fashion; spermatogonia lie directly on the tubular basement membrane, while primary and secondary spermatocytes, spermatids, and maturing spermatozoa progress centrally toward the tubular lumen. Sertoli cells also lie on the basement membrane and serve to regulate the release of mature spermatozoa from the germinal epithelium as well as to maintain the integrity of the blood-testis barrier.

Spermatogenesis is a dynamic and complex process which may be divided into three phases: (1) proliferation of spermatogonia to produce spermatocytes and to renew the germ cell pool; (2) meiotic division of spermatocytes to reduce the chromosome number in the germ cells by half; and (3) maturation of the spermatids to become spermatozoa (19). Cytotoxic drugs could potentially effect this process in a number of ways: (1) a specific cell type within the germinal epithelium might be selectively damaged or destroyed; (2) the proliferative and meiotic phases of spermatogenesis might proceed normally, but sperm maturation might be abnormal, leading to functionally incompetent mature spermatozoa; or (3) chemotherapy might damage Sertoli cells, Leydig cells or other supportive or nutritive constituents of the testis in such a way as to alter the particular microenvironment necessary for normal germ cell production.

Animal models

Drug effects on the testicular germinal epithelium have been investigated using both animal models and clinical assessment. The use of animal models permits a detailed analysis of drug effects on specific stages of spermatogenesis and provides an opportunity to examine the effects of drugs on the chromosomal complement of primitive gametes.

Interpretation of animal studies requires an understanding of the normal histology of the germinal epithelium and of the kinetics of spermatogenesis in the species being studied. In any area of the seminiferous tubule, several generations of germ cells can be identified. These generations are not randomly distributed but occur in fixed cell associations.

219

Thus, spermatids at a particular stage in their development are always associated with the same types of spermatocytes and spermatogonia. These cell associations synchronously evolve in the process of sperm maturation. A complete series of cell associations constitutes a cycle of the germinal epithelium and each cell association may be considered a stage of the cycle. The entire process of spermatogenesis proceeds continuously throughout the tubule and the time elapsed from spermatogonial stem cell mitosis to release of mature spermatozoa is relatively species-specific (30, 51).

Thus, it is possible to estimate the specific site of a drug's effect either by examining the testis histologically or by performing sperm counts or mating studies at some defined interval after drug administration. The morphology of the spermatids can be used to define the stage of the germinal epithelial cycle at the time of biopsy, and the presence or absence of cells expected to occur in association with those spermatids can be noted. Known kinetic parameters can then be used to determine precisely which cell was destroyed by drug administration. For example, examination of mouse testes 11 days following doxorubicin administration reveals an absence of pachytene primary spermatocytes indicating that type A2 (primitive) spermatogonia are most sensitive to injury by this drug (43). A similar analysis following cisplatin administration demonstrates that intermediate spermatogonia are most sensitive to cisplatin and that at high doses (10 mg/kg) even late stage spermatids may be affected suggesting the occurrence of Sertoli cell damage at this dose level (47).

Serial mating studies, whereby animals are mated at varying intervals after drug administration and the onset of infertility is noted, can provide similar, though less precise information. In the rat, an infertile mating occurring six to seven weeks after drug treatment implies that spermatocytes were primarily affected by the drug in question, whereas infertility occurring ten weeks after drug treatment reflects spermatogonial destruction (35, 36). Table 1 summarizes the information obtained from several animal models concerning the effects of antineoplastic drugs on spermatogenesis.

Clinical assessment

Testicular function in patients receiving cancer chemotherapy can be adequately evaluated with a careful physical examination, semen analysis and determination of serum gonadotropin and testosterone levels. Occasionally, testicular biopsy is necessary to complete the evaluation. Since the seminiferous tubules comprise such a large proportion of the testicular mass, damage to the germinal epithelium frequently results in testicular atrophy which is readily detectable on physical examination. Impaired spermatogenesis is also manifest as a decrease in the number and/or motility of sperm present in the ejaculate and, since pituitary gonadotropin secretion is under feedback control by the testis, an increase in serum follicle stimulating hormone (FSH) level (62, 74). Leydig cell dysfunction may also occur and is detected by an increase in serum luteinizing hormone (LH) level and, if uncompensated, a fall in serum testosterone level. Subclinical abnormalities of Leydig cell function may occasionally be demonstrated by administration of LH releasing hormone. An excessive rise in serum LH levels in this

Table 1. Site of toxicity of antineoplastic drugs in the germinal epithelium.

Drug	Cell type affected	Reference
Actinomycin-D	Stem cells, early spermatogonia	(47)
BCNU	Stem cells, intermediate spermatogonia	(47)
Bleomycin	Intermediate spermatogonia	(43)
Busulfan	Type A spermatogonia	(35, 36)
CCNU	Intermediate spermatogonia, spermatocytes	(47)
Cis-Platin	Spermatogonia, spermatocytes, spermatids	(47)
Cytosine arabinoside	Late spermatogonia	(43)
Cyclophosphamide	Late spermatogonia spermatocytes	(43)
Doxorubicin	Stem cells	(43)
Methotrexate	Early spermatogonia	(47)
Mitomycin-C	Stem cells, spermatogonia	(47)
Nitrogen mustard	Intermediate and late spermatogonia	(47)
Procarbazine	Stem cells, early spermatogonia	(47)

provocative test suggests the presence of abnormal Leydig cell function (12, 46, 77, 78). The clinical assessment of a patient with suspected germinal epithelial aplasia is summarized in Table 2.

Drug effects on spermatogenesis

Following cytotoxic chemotherapy, there appear to be common histopathologic changes that occur in the testis, independent of the type of drug employed but related to the total dose administered. The primary testicular lesion caused by all antitumor agents studied thus far is depletion of the germinal epithelium lining the seminiferous tubules (26, 39, 48, 54, 55). Testicular biopsy in most patients reveals complete germinal aplasia with only Sertoli cells left lining the tubular lumens. Occasionally, scattered spermatogonia, spermatocytes or spermatids may be seen or there may be evidence for maturation arrest occurring at the spermatocyte stage. This latter finding appears most often in

Table 2. Evaluation of the patient with germinal aplasia.

	Normal	Germinal aplasia
Testicular size		
Length × width (cm)	5.0 × 3.0	3.7 × 2.3
Volume (cc)	16–30	8–15
Sperm count (10^6/ml)	20–100	0
FSH (mIU/ml)	4–25	25–90
LH (mIU/ml)	4–20	8–25
LH response to LH–RH	Normal	Exaggerated
Testosterone (ng/dl)	250–1200	200–700

patients receiving short courses of chemotherapy with antimetabolites (44).

Alkylating agents, particularly chlorambucil and cyclophosphamide, deplete the testicular germinal epithelium in a dose related fashion. Progressive but reversible oligospermia occurs in men receiving up to 400 mg of chlorambucil, whereas azoospermia and germinal aplasia occur in those patients treated with total doses higher than 400 mg (55). Similarly, decreased sperm counts may be noted in men treated with 50 to 100 mg of cyclophosphamide daily for courses as brief as two months, although azoospermia is infrequent until 6 to 10 g of the drug has been administered (26). Antimetabolites, in conventional doses, appear to have relatively few effects on spermatogenesis although one study of 1981 suggests that high dose methotrexate (250 mg/kg) may produce transient oligospermia in some patients (64). These data suggest the presence of a threshold dose for the development of testicular germinal aplasia for each particular drug. However, prospective studies of testicular function in large numbers of men receiving a variety of antitumor agents will be necessary to provide more reliable information concerning the threshold drug dose above which severe or irreversible testicular injury occurs.

At present, there is little information available concerning the impact on the testis of recently introduced antineoplastic agents. One report has suggested that Adriamycin may be less toxic to the human testis than expected based on animal studies. In the mouse model, a single injection of 35 mg/m² produces azoospermia, yet two patients treated with Adriamycin-containing chemotherapy regimens developed only mild oligospermia (21, 47). Further, a recent study of the effects of cyclophosphamide, Adriamycin and high dose methotrexate on testicular function has revealed only mild reversible testicular injury occurring in the majority of patients under age 40 (64).

While the effects of Adriamycin on the human testis appear to be less severe than suggested by animal models, the converse may be true for cis-platin. Patients with testicular cancer treated with cis-platin based combination chemotherapy uniformly become azoospermic soon after chemotherapy is initiated (24). Though the specific contribution of cisplatin to the gonadal toxicity of this regimen is difficult to discern, the combination of velban, bleomycin and cis-platin is now routinely employed in the treatment of testicular cancer and its effects on testicular function in a patient population likely to be cured of their malignancy deserve particular emphasis.

As might be expected, other combination chemotherapy regimens, particularly those which include alkylating agents, produce germinal aplasia and infertility in the majority of patients. The effects of nitrogen mustard, vincristine, procarbazine and prednisone (MOPP) and a related regimen in which vinblastine replaces vincristine (MVPP) have been most extensively investigated. At least 80% of men receiving these regimens develop azoospermia, germinal aplasia, testicular atrophy and elevated FSH levels (3, 14, 65). Leydig cell dysfunction may also occur more commonly than previously recognized. Though Leydig cells remain morphologically intact following chemotherapy, and basal serum LH levels tend to remain normal, many patients have now been found to have hypersecretion of LH in response to LH releasing hormone, an indication of Leydig cell dysfunc-

tion (12, 77, 78). Some patients develop evidence of more severe Leydig cell dysfunction and are able to maintain normal serum testosterone levels only at the expense of elevated basal serum LH levels and rarely, frank Leydig cell failure may occur and serum testosterone levels are clearly subnormal. These biochemical abnormalities have not, however, been clearly associated with specific clinical changes in sexual desire or function.

Reversibility of chemotherapy effects

Following cytotoxic chemotherapy, the recovery of spermatogenesis is unpredictable for the individual patient but is likely related to the total dose of drug administered, the type of drug and the duration of time off therapy. Complete recovery of spermatogenesis has been reported in three of five previously azoospermic patients after therapy with chlorambucil in doses of 410 to 2600 mg (16). In these patients, sperm counts were found to be normal at 33, 34 and 42 months following completion of chemotherapy. Two additional patients, who received the highest cumulative drug doses, demonstrated a partial return of spermatogenesis at 38 and 58 months after discontinuing treatment. In a similar study, 26 men treated for five to 34 months with 50 to 100 mg of cyclophosphamide daily all became azoospermic within 6 months of starting therapy (9). Serial sperm counts demonstrated a return of spermatogenesis in 12 patients a mean period of 31 months following discontinuation of cyclophosphamide. Those patients demonstrating a recovery of spermatogenesis tended to receive lower initial drug doses. These studies, along with numerous anecdotal reports (5, 32), clearly demonstrate that the germinal epithelium can regenerate and spermatogenesis can resume following single agent chemotherapy.

Patients who receive combination chemotherapy, particularly the MOPP regimen, are likely to develop long-lasting and frequently permanent, infertility. Sherins and DeVita (65) noted azoospermia and testicular germinal aplasia in patients as long as four years after completion of MOPP chemotherapy and Chapman and colleagues (12) observed a return of spermatogenesis in only 4 of 64 men followed for 15 to 51 months from completion of MVPP chemotherapy. Several other recent studies have confirmed these findings and it seems reasonable to conclude that only about 10% of patients receiving MOPP or MVPP will ultimately have a return of spermatogenesis. One study has suggested that the use of procarbazine in these regimens is particularly damaging to the germinal epithelium (56). Thirty-two patients receiving MOPP, CVP or related regimens for lymphoma were studied. Thirty-one of the 32 developed increased serum FSH levels during therapy and, of 15 studied, all had azoospermia. Sixteen patients were evaluated for recovery of testicular function. In 7 of 10 patients treated with CVP, plasma FSH levels returned to normal during 34 months of follow-up. Of four patients studied, 3 had normal sperm counts and the fourth was oligospermic. In contrast, only one of six patients treated with a procarbazine containing regimen demonstrated a fall of serum FSH or rise in sperm count during 52 months of follow-up. Thus, procarbazine, which is severely toxic to the germinal epithelium in adult monkeys (68), appears to play an important role in the development of permanent infertility in patients receiving the MOPP regimen.

In recent years, a number of alternative combination chemotherapy regimens to MOPP have been proposed for treatment of advanced Hodgkin's disease. Among these ABVD (Adriamycin, bleomycin, vinblastine, DTIC) has been touted as being equally efficacious and less toxic than the MOPP regimen. A comparison of the treatment regimens has revealed that azoospermia occurs in 100% of patients treated with MOPP but in only 35% of patients receiving ABVD and that recovery of spermatogenesis occurs rarely in MOPP-treated patients but nearly always in those treated with ABVD (60). This information may play an important role in treatment planning for young men with Hodgkin's disease who are concerned about preservation of fertility during and after treatment.

Similar concerns face patients with testicular cancer about to embark on a course of chemotherapy with velban, bleomycin and cis-platin. As discussed previously, this chemotherapy regimen renders virtually all patients azoospermic within 2 months of beginning treatment. Unlike MOPP however, there appears to be a high degree of reversibility of this testicular dysfunction with the majority of patients showing evidence of resumption of spermatogenesis within 2 years from the discontinuation of treatment (24).

Chemotherapy effects in women

Oogenesis is the process of maturation of the primitive female germ cell to the mature ovum. This process occurs primarily during intrauterine life and involves multiple mitotic divisions to increase the number of germ cells followed by the beginning of the first meiotic division which will eventually reduce the diploid chromosome number to half prior to fertilization. At the time of birth the oocytes are in the long prophase of their first meiotic division and remain in that state until the formation of a mature follicle prior to ovulation (45).

In the postnatal ovary, most of the ongoing cellular growth and replication is related to the growth and development of follicles. Primordial follicles develop during gestation and consist of a primary oocyte surrounded by a layer of mesenchymal cells called granulosa cells. At birth, the ovary may contain 150,000 to 500,000 primordial follicles many of which subsequently become atretic. From childhood to menopause follicular growth occurs as a continuous process with ovulation occurring in a cyclical fashion (53). The granulosa cells surrounding the primary oocyte proliferate, follicular fluid accumulates, and the ovum completes its first meiotic divison to become a secondary oocyte. At this time the follicle is known as a secondary or graafian follicle. The follicle continues to enlarge until the time of ovulation. During the reproductive life of a woman only 300 to 400 oocytes mature and are extruded in the process of ovulation, the remainder undergo some form of atresia. It is likely that this continuing process of follicular growth and maturation is primarily affected by cytotoxic chemotherapy although the specific site(s) of drug-induced ovarian damage have not yet been identified.

Assessment of ovarian function

The evaluation of chemotherapy effects on ovarian function is hampered by the relative inaccessibility of the ovary to biopsy. Unlike the semen analysis, no direct measurement of the female germ cell population is readily available. Further, no reliable animal model has been developed to assess the effects of cytotoxic drugs on ovarian function. Thus, evaluation of the functional status of the ovary must be based primarily on menstrual and reproductive history and on determination of serum hormone levels.

Follicular growth and maturation and estradiol production are under regulatory control of the pituitary and hypothalamus. Pituitary FSH stimulates granulosa cells to replicate and produce estradiol. The midcycle LH surge promotes ovulation and the ruptured follicle becomes the corpus luteum which produces progesterone thereby suppressing further LH secretion (15). Drug-induced ovarian failure interrupts this delicate hormonal balance and results in abnormally low serum levels of estradiol and progesterone, markedly elevated levels of FSH and LH, amenorrhea and symptoms of estrogen deficiency (Fig. 1).

Drug effects on ovarian function

The primary histologic lesion noted in the ovaries of women receiving antineoplastic chemotherapy is ovarian fibrosis and follicle destruction (4, 49, 70). Among the anticancer drugs, alkylating agents have most often been associated with ovarian dysfunction. During the early clinical trials of busulfan, amenorrhea was a common side effect. Several investigators noted the onset of permanent amenorrhea among patients receiving busulfan in doses of 0.5 to 14 mg/day for at least 3 months (29, 42).

The effects of cyclophosphamide on ovarian function were first noted in the rheumatology literature. Early cessation of menses and menopause symptoms developed in 6 of 33 patients treated for rheumatoid arthritis with daily cyclophosphamide for 6 to 40 months (28). Subsequently, several investigators have documented the occurrence of amenorrhea and primary ovarian failure in at least 50% of premenopausal women receiving 40 to 120 mg of cyclophosphamide daily for an average of 18 months (72, 76).

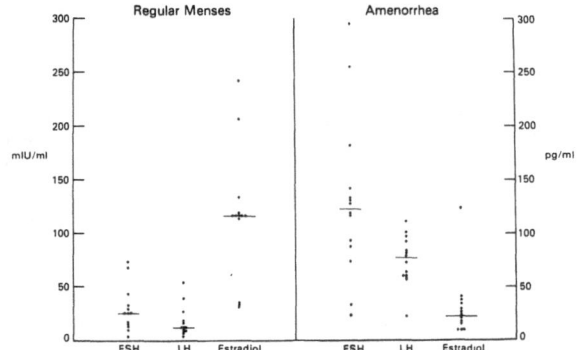

Figure 1. Serum FSH, LH (mIU/ml) and estradiol (pg/ml) levels following combination chemotherapy for Hodgkin's disease. (Reproduced with permission from Schilsky *et al* (61)).

More recent studies of the use of adjuvant chemotherapy for the prevention of recurrence of breast cancer suggest that the onset of amenorrhea and the potential for resumption of menses is related to the age of the patient during chemotherapy and to the total dose administered (23, 58). Amenorrhea has been reported to develop in 17 of 18 women treated with adjuvant cyclophosphamide for 13 to 14 months postoperatively (38). Permanent cessation of menses occurred following a mean total dose of 5.2 gms in all patients 40 years and older. Amenorrhea also developed in 4 of 5 women under 40 years of age but only after a mean cyclophosphamide dose of 9.3 gm was administered. Further, menses subsequently returned in two of these patients within 6 months of discontinuing therapy. A recent prospective study of ovarian function in premenopausal women receiving melphalan alone or in combination with 5-fluorouracil has demonstrated the occurrence of amenorrhea in 22 percent of patients younger than 39 years but in 73 percent of women older than 40 years (27). Clearly then, alkylating agent chemotherapy accelerates the onset of menopause, particularly in the older patient, while younger patients may tolerate higher total drug doses before amenorrhea becomes irreversible. Among the antimetabolites, only high dose methotrexate has been evaluated and appears to have no immediate ovarian toxicity (63).

The risk of ovarian injury following combination chemotherapy is also clearly related to the age of the patient at the time of treatment. Overall, 40–50% of women treated with combination chemotherapy, particularly MOPP or related regimens, become amenorrheic (10, 34, 50). In one study of 1981, follow-up of MOPP-treated patients for a median of nine years following completion of chemotherapy revealed that 46% had developed permanent amenorrhea (61). Further analysis demonstrated that 89% of these women were older than 25 years at the time of treatment (Fig. 2). Moreover, the time of onset of amenorrhea appeared age related in that amenorrhea occurred within one year of discontinuing therapy in all patients age 39 years or older, while in younger patients there was a gradual decrease in frequency of menses occurring over several years post-therapy. Thus, while it is impossible to predict the effect of MOPP chemotherapy on ovarian function for any individual patient, it appears unlikely that those patients treated when younger than age 25 will experience any significant therapy-related ovarian dysfunction during the initial 5 to 10 years following completion of therapy. Continued long term prospective

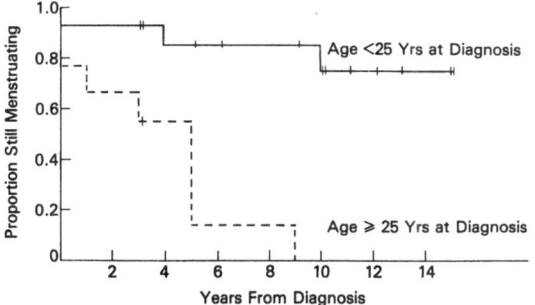

Figure 2. Age-related development of amenorrhea following combination chemotherapy for Hodgkin's disease. (Reproduced with permission form Schilsky *et al* (61)).

follow-up of women such as these is necessary to more accurately determine the degree of risk for premature ovarian failure and early menopause.

Chemotherapy effects in children

Analysis of the effects of cytotoxic chemotherapy on gonadal function in children is particularly complex because of the variables introduced by the continuum of sexual development in this patient population. Thus, the effects of chemotherapy may vary according to when drugs are given and when their effects are evaluated relative to puberty.

Boys
There appear to be differences in the sensitivity of the prepubertal, pubertal and adult testis to alkylating agent chemotherapy. The prepubertal testis, for example, is relatively resistant to moderate doses of alkylating agents. Cyclophosphamide, in cumulative doses up to 20 gm, produces only minor alterations in the testicular histology of prepubertal boys and no abnormalities in serum gonadotropin or testosterone levels. Germinal aplasia has been documented however, at cumulative doses greater than 20 gm (25, 52). Little information is available concerning the effects of other drugs on the immature testis. Cytosine arabinoside in cumulative doses in excess of 1 gm/m^2 has been shown to be damaging to the germinal epithelium (40) yet other commonly used antileukemia drugs, e.g. prednisone, 6-mercaptopurine, methotrexate and vincristine (POMP), appear to cause no adverse effects to testicular function in patients at any pubertal stage (7).

By contrast, chemotherapy administered to pubertal boys may have profound effects on both germ cell production and endocrine function. A study of testicular function in boys treated with MOPP combination chemotherapy for Hodgkin's disease demonstrated the development of gynecomastia in 9 of 13 pubertal patients a mean of 28 months after initiation of treatment (66). These patients were also found to have elevated serum FSH and LH levels and low serum testosterone levels. Testicular biopsy in 6 patients with gynecomastia revealed germinal aplasia. These data suggest that MOPP chemotherapy may be damaging to both Leydig cells and seminiferous epithelium if administered during puberty.

Girls
Little information is available concerning the effects of cytotoxic chemotherapy on ovarian function in children. There appears to be no delay in menarche and no interruption of menses in girls treated with single agent cyclophosphamide (17, 22, 41, 52). One investigator reported normal ovarian histology at postmortem examination of six girls treated with cyclophosphamide for malignancy (2). Other reports, however, have noted absence or inhibition of follicle development following cytotoxic chemotherapy in girls with advanced acute leukemia (31). A careful analysis of ovarian function in girls treated with POMP combination chemotherapy for acute leukemia, however, has demonstrated normal ovarian function in 80% of patients (69). Thus, it would appear that the immature ovary is relatively insensitive to cytotoxic chemotherapy but accurate deter-

mination of drug effects on reproductive potential over time require continued long term follow-up of the survivors of childhood cancer.

COUNSELING PATIENTS

Counseling patients who are about to embark on a course of cancer chemotherapy is often a difficult and perplexing task for physician and patient alike. All too often such discussions deal primarily with the acute and potentially life-threatening toxicities of chemotherapy with little attention given to more delayed side effects such as infertility, hormone deficiency and mutagenesis. Yet, particularly for young patients with curable malignancies, these late toxicities often become increasingly important once chemotherapy has been completed and remission attained. The remainder of this chapter will review three areas of particular importance which should be discussed early in the doctor-patient relationship: semen cryopreservation, hormone replacement therapy and risks of chemotherapy to progeny of treated individuals.

Semen cryopreservation

Pretreatment sperm banking is presently the only potential means of preserving fertility for men who are to receive combination chemotherapy for cancer. Patients must be advised, however, that pretreatment sperm banking does not guarantee a successful pregnancy in future years. Though the technology of freezing, preserving and thawing human sperm has advanced considerably, ultimate conception rates using cryopreserved semen remain only 50–60% due to loss of semen quality following thawing (1, 20, 67). Moreover, recent studies clearly indicate that at least 50% of patients with Hodgkin's disease and testicular cancer may be severely oligospermic or azoospermic prior to initiation of chemotherapy and that only 10–20% of newly diagnosed patients produce semen of sufficient quality to even consider cryopreservation (8, 18, 24, 59, 71). Nevertheless, all patients should be given an opportunity to provide semen for analysis if they wish to consider pretreatment sperm banking. Unfortunately, it now appears that only a small proportion of patients will be candidates for semen cryopreservation and, of these, only about 50% will ultimately produce a successful pregnancy.

Hormone replacement therapy

Women at risk of developing premature ovarian failure due to cytotoxic chemotherapy may also be subject to the physical and emotional disorders that accompany estrogen deficiency. Depressed libido, irritability, sleep disturbances, and poor self-image all occur commonly in women with chemotherapy-related amenorrhea (11). Severe symptoms may, at times, result in alienation of family, friends, children or spouse, not infrequently leading to separation or divorce. Hormone replacement therapy may be of considerable benefit to these patients, frequently producing dramatic relief of hot flashes and irritability. Restoration of normal libido

and renewed self-confidence may be vitally important to allowing patients to resume a normal life-style following completion of cancer chemotherapy.

Other potential benefits of estrogen replacement therapy may be prevention of premature postmenopausal osteoporosis and, in combination with progesterone, protection of the ovary from the damaging effects of cytotoxic drugs (13). However, these uses of hormone replacement therapy must be considered investigational at present.

In male patients, testosterone therapy may benefit those individuals with loss of libido or impotence who have elevated serum LH levels and/or depressed serum testosterone levels. Those patients with psychogenic or neurogenic impotence, however, are not likely to benefit from this therapeutic approach.

Risks to future generations

Successfully treated cancer patients have a host of new concerns about the future and frequently raise questions concerning the risks of spontaneous abortion and the frequency of fetal abnormalities should pregnancy occur. A number of anecdotal reports and small series have appeared which suggest that prior chemotherapy poses no greater risk of spontaneous abortion or fetal abnormality than occurs in the general population (6, 37, 57, 73). One recent study did suggest that women previously treated with both chemotherapy and radiation had a greater chance of pregnancy ending in abortion or with delivery of an abnormal child than did sibling controls (33).

The uncertainty and happenstance that may occur in the collection of these types of retrospective data do not allow, at present, an adequate assessment of the risk of genetic damage to germ cells posed by chemotherapy, nor do they provide any certain guidelines for advice or reassurance for patients concerned with the risks of having abnormal children. Many more careful studies carried over many years will be required before the true risks to subsequent generations are known.

REFERENCES

1. Ansbacher R: Artificial insemination with frozen spermatozoa. *Fertil Steril* 29:375, 1978
2. Arneil GC: Cyclophosphamide and the prepubertal testis. *Lancet* 2:1259, 1972
3. Asbjornsen G, Molne K, Klepp O, Aakvaag A: Testicular function after combination chemotherapy for Hodgin's disease. *Scand J Hematol* 16:66, 1976
4. Belohorsky B, Siracky J, Sandor L, Klauber E: Comments on the development of amenorrhea caused by myleran in cases of chronic myelosis. *Neoplasma* 4:397, 1960
5. Blake DA, Heller RH, Hsu SH, Schecter BZ: Return of fertility in a patient with cyclophosphamide-induced azoospermia. *Johns Hopkins Med J* 139:20, 1976
6. Blatt J, Mulvihill JJ, Ziegler JL, Young RC, Poplack DG: Pregnancy outcome following cancer chemotherapy. *Am J Med* 69:828, 1980
7. Blatt J, Poplack DG, Sherins RJ: Testicular function in boys after chemotherapy for acute lymphoblastic leukemia. *New Engl J Med* 304:1121, 1981
8. Bracken RB, Smith KD: Is serum cryopreservation helpful in

testicular cancer? *Urology* 15:581, 1980

9. Buchanan JD, Fairley KF, Barrie JU: Return of spermatogenesis after stopping cyclophosphamide therapy. *Lancet* 2:156, 1975

10. Chapman RM, Sutcliffe SB, Malpas JS: Cytotoxic-induced ovarian failure in women with Hodgkin's disease. I. Hormone function. *J Amer Med Assoc* 242:1877, 1979

11. Chapman RM, Sutcliffe SB, Malpas JS: Cytotoxic-induced ovarian failure in Hodgkin's disease. II. Effects on sexual function. *J Amer Med Assoc* 242:1882, 1979

12. Chapman RM, Sutcliffe SB, Rees LH, Edwards CRW, Malpas JS: Cyclical combination chemotherapy and gonadal function. *Lancet* 1:285, 1979

13. Chapman RM, Sutcliffe SB: Protection of ovarian function by oral contraceptives in women receiving chemotherapy for Hodgkin's disease. *Blood* 58:849, 1981

14. Chapman RM, Sutcliffe SB, Malpas JS: Male gonadal dysfunction in Hodgkin's disease. *J Amer Med Assoc* 245:1323, 1981

15. Chapman RM: Effect of cytotoxic therapy on sexuality and gonadal function. *Sem in Oncol* 9:84, 1982

16. Cheviakoff J, Calamera JC, Morgenfeld M, Mancini RE: Recovery of spermatogenesis in patients with lymphoma after treatment with chlorambucil. *J Reproduct Fertil* 33:155, 1973

17. Chiu J, Drummond K: Long-term follow-up of cyclophosphamide therapy in frequent relapsing minimal lesion nephrotic syndrome. *J Pediatrics* 84:825, 1974

18. Chlebowski RT, Heber D: Hypogonadism in male patients with metastatic cancer prior to chemotherapy. *Cancer Res* 42:2495, 1982

19. Clermont Y: Kinetics of spermatogenesis in mammals: Seminiferous epithelium cycle and spermatogonial renewal. *Physiol Rev* 52:198, 1972

20. Curie-Cohen M, Luttrel L, Shapiro J: Current practice of artificial insemination by donor in the United States. *New Engl J Med* 300:585, 1979

21. daCunha MF, Meistrich ML, Reid HL, Powell ML: Effect of chemotherapy on human sperm production. *Proc Am Assoc Can Res* 20:100, 1979

22. DeGroot GW, Faiman C, Winter JSD: Cyclophosphamide and the prepubertal gonad: A negative report. *J Pediatrics* 84:123, 1974

23. Dnistrian AM, Schwartz MK, Fracchia AA, Kaufman RJ, Hakes TB, Currie VE: Endocrine consequences of CMF adjuvant therapy in premenopausal and postmenopausal breast cancer patients. *Cancer* 51:803, 1983

24. Drasga RE, Einhorn LH, Williams SD, Patel DN, Stevens EE: Fertility after chemotherapy for testicular cancer. *J Clin Oncol* 1:179, 1983

25. Etteldorf JN, West CD, Pitcock JA, Williams DL: Gonadal function, testicular histology and meiosis following cyclophosphamide therapy in patients with nephrotic syndrome. *J Pediatrics* 88:206, 1976

26. Fairley KF, Barrie JU, Johnson W: Sterility and testicular atrophy related to cyclophosphamide therapy. *Lancet* 1:568, 1972

27. Fisher B, Sherman B, Rockette H, Redmond C, Margolese R, Fisher E: L-phenylalanine mustard in the management of premenopausal patients with primary breast cancer. *Cancer* 44:847, 1979

28. Fosdick WM, Parsons JL, Hill DF: Long-term cyclophosphamide therapy in rheumatoid arthritis. *Arthritis Rheum* 11:151, 1968

29. Galton DAG, Till M, Wiltshaw E: Busulfan: summary of clinical results. *Ann NY Acad Sci* 68:967, 1958

30. Helen CG, Clermont Y: Kinetics of the germinal epithelium in man. *Recent Prog Horm Res* 20:545, 1964

31. Himelstein-Braw R, Peters H, Faber M: Morphological study of the ovaries of leukemic children. *Brit J Cancer* 38:82, 1978

32. Hinkes E, Plotkin D: Reversible drug-induced sterility in a patient with acute leukemia. *J Amer Med Assoc* 233:1490, 1973

33. Holmes GE, Holmes FF: Pregnancy outcome of patients treated for Hodgkin's disease. *Cancer* 41:1317, 1978

34. Horning SJ, Hoppe RT, Kaplan HS, Rosenberg SA: Female reproductive potential after treatment for Hodgkin's disease. *New Engl J Med* 304:1378, 1981

35. Jackson H, Fox BW, Craig AW: Antifertility substances and their assessment in the male rodent. *J Reprod Fertil* 2:447, 1961

36. Jackson H: The effects of alkylating agents on fertility. *Br Med Bull* 20:107, 1964

37. Johnson SA, Goldman JM, Hawkins DF: Pregnancy after chemotherapy for Hodgkin's disease. *Lancet* 2:93, 1979

38. Koyama H, Wada T, Nishizawa Y, Iwanaga T, Aoki T, Terasawa T, Kosaki G, Yamamoto T, Wada A: Cyclophosphamide-induced ovarian failure and its therapeutic significance in patients with breast cancer. *Cancer* 39:1400, 1977

39. Kumar R, Biggart JD, McEvoy J, McGeown MG: Cyclophosphamide and reproductive function. *Lancet* 1:1212, 1972

40. Lendon M, Hann IM, Palmer MK, Shalet SM, Morris-Jones PH: Testicular histology after combination chemotherapy in childhood for acute lymphoblastic leukemia. *Lancet* 2:439, 1978

41. Lentz RD, Bergstein J, Steffes MW, Brown DR, Prem K, Michael AF, Vernier RL: Post-pubertal evaluation of gonadal function following cyclophosphamide therapy before and during puberty. *J Pediatrics* 91:385, 1977

42. Louis J, Limarzi LR, Best WR: Treatment of chronic granulocytic leukemia with Myleran. *Arch Int Med* 97:299, 1956

43. Lu CC, Meistrich ML: Cytotoxic effects of chemotherapeutic drugs on mouse testis cells. *Cancer Res* 39:3575, 1979

44. Maguire LC, Dick FR, Sherman BM: The effects of antileukemia therapy on gonadal histology in adult males. *Cancer* 48:1967, 1981

45. Mayer DL, Odell WD: Physiology of Reproduction. pp 20–27. St. Louis, C. V. Mosby, 1971

46. Mecklenburg RS, Sherins RJ: Gonadotropin response to luteinizing hormone in men with germinal aplasia. *J Clin Endocrinol Metab* 38:1005, 1974

47. Meistrich ML, Finch M, daCunha MF, Hacker U, Au WW: Damaging effects of fourteen chemotherapeutic drugs on mouse testis cells. *Cancer Res* 42:122, 1982

48. Miller DG: Alkylating agents and human spermatogenesis. *J Amer Med Assn* 217:1662, 1971

49. Miller JJ, Williams GF, Leissring JC: Multiple late complications of therapy with cyclophosphamide including ovarian destruction. *Amer J med* 50:530, 1971

50. Morgenfeld MC, Goldberg V, Parisier H, Bugnard SC, Bur GE: Ovarian lesions due to cytostatic agents during the treatment of Hodgkin's disease. *Surg Gynec Obstet* 134:826, 1972

51. Oakberg EF: A description of spermiogenesis in the mouse and its use in analysis of the seminiferous epithelium and germ cell renewal. *Am J Anat* 99:391, 1956

52. Pennisi AJ, Grushkin CM, Lieberman E: Gonadal function in children with nephrosis treated with cyclophosphamide. *Am J Dis Child* 129:315, 1975

53. Peters H, Byskov AG, Himelstein-Braw R, Faber M: Follicular growth: the basic event in the mouse and human ovary. *J Reprod Fertil* 4:559, 1975

54. Qureshi MJA, Goldsmith HJ, Pennington HJ, Cox PE: Cyclophosphamide therapy and sterility. *Lancet* 2:1290, 1972

55. Richter P, Calamera JC, Morgenfeld MC, Kierzenbaum AL, Lavieri JC, Mancini RE: Effect of chlorambucil on spermatogenesis in the human with malignant lymphoma. *Cancer* 25:1026, 1970

56. Roeser HP, Stochs AE, Smith AJ: Testicular damage due to cytotoxic drugs and recovery after cessation of therapy. *Aust*

226   *R.L. Schilsky*

New Zealand J Med 8:250, 1978

57. Ross GT: Congenital anomalies among children born of mothers receiving chemotherapy for gestational trophoblastic neoplasms. *Cancer* 37:1043, 1976

58. Samaan NA, DeAsis DN, Buzdar AU, Blumenschein GR: Pituitary-ovarian function in breast cancer patients on adjuvant chemoimmunotherapy. *Cancer* 41:2084, 1978

59. Sanger WG, Armitage JO, Schmidt MA: Feasibility of semen cryopreservation in patients with malignant disease. *J Am Med Assn* 244:789, 1980

60. Santoro A, Viviani S, Zucali R, Ragni G, Bonfante V, Valagussa P, Banfi A, Bonadonna G: Comparative results and toxicity of MOPP vs ABVD combined with radiotherapy in PS IIB, III Hodgkin's disease. *Proc Am Soc Clin Oncol* 2:223, 1983

61. Schilsky RL, Sherins RJ, Hubbard SM, Wesley MN, Young RC, DeVita VT: Long-term follow-up of ovarian function in women treated with MOPP chemotherapy for Hodgkin's disease. *Amer J Med* 71:552, 1981

62. Schilsky RL, Sherins RJ: Gonadal dysfunction. In: *Cancer: Principles and Practice of Oncology*, edited by DeVita VT, Hellman S, Rosenberg SA, pp 1713–1717, Philadelphia, J.B. Lippincott Co, 1982

63. Shamberger RC, Rosenberg SA, Seipp CA, Sherins RJ: Effects of high dose methotrexate and vincristine on ovarian and testicular functions in patients undergoing postoperative adjuvant treatment of osteosarcoma. *Cancer Treat Rep* 65:739, 1981

64. Shamberger RC, Sherins RJ, Rosenberg SA: The effect of postoperative adjuvant chemotherapy and radiotherapy on testicular function in men undergoing treatment for soft tissue sarcoma. *Cancer* 47:2368, 1981

65. Sherins RJ, DeVita VT: Effects of drug treatment for lymphoma on male reproductive capacity. *Ann Int Med* 79:216, 1973

66. Sherins RJ, Olweny CLM, Ziegler JL: Gynecomastia and gonadal dysfunction in adolescent boys treated with combination chemotherapy for Hodgkin's disease. *New Engl J Med* 299:12, 1978

67. Sherman JK: Synopsis of the use of frozen human semen since 1964: state of the art of human semen banking. *Fertil Steril* 24:397, 1973

68. Sieber SM, Correa P, Dalgard DW, Adamson RH: Carcinogenic and other adverse effects of procarbazine in non-human primates. *Cancer Res* 38:2125, 1978

69. Siris EJ, Leventhal BG, Vaitukaitis JL: Effects of childhood leukemia and chemotherapy on puberty and reproductive function in girls. *New Engl J Med* 294:1143, 1979

70. Sobrinho LG, Levine RA, DeConti RC: Amenorrhea in patients with Hodgkin's disease treated with antineoplastic agents. *Am J Obstet Gynceol* 109:135, 1971

71. Thacil JV, Jewett MAS, Rider WD: The effects of cancer and cancer therapy on male fertility. *J Urology* 126:141, 1981

72. Uldall PR, Kerr DNS, Tacchi D: Sterility and cyclophosphamide. *Lancet* 1:693, 1972

73. VanThiel DH, Ross GT, Lipsett MB: Pregnancies after chemotherapy of trophoblastic neoplasms. *Science* 169:1326, 1970

74. VanThiel DH, Sherins RJ, Myers GH, DeVita VT: Evidence for a specific seminiferous tubular factor affecting follicle-stimulating hormone secretion in men. *J Clin Invest* 51:1009, 1972

75. Walsh PC, Amelar RD: Embryology, anatomy and physiology of the male reproductive system. In: *Male Infertility*, edited by Amelar RD, Dublin L, Walsh PC, pp 3–32, Philadelphia, W.B. Saunders Co, 1977

76. Warne GL, Fairley KF, Hobbs JB, Martin FIR: Cyclophosphamide-induced ovarian failure. *N Engl J Med* 289:1159, 1973

77. Waxman JHX, Terry YA, Wrigley PFM, Malpas JS, Rees LH, Besser GM, Lister TA: Gonadal function in Hodgkin's disease: long-term follow-up of chemotherapy. *British Med J* 285:1612, 1982

78. Whitehead E, Shalet SM, Blackledge G, Todd I, Crowther D, Beardwell CG: The effects of Hodgkin's disease and combination chemotherapy on gonadal function in the adult male. *Cancer* 49:418, 1982

INDEX

Abelson leukemia virus 151
Acid phosphatase 113
Acidic protein 44
Acinous-cell carcinoma 45
Acoustic neuroma 23
   trauma 24
Acquired immune deficiency syndrome (AIDS) 14, 39, 205, 214, 215
Actin-myosin 113
Actinomycin-D 220
Acute granulocytic leukemia (AGL) 122
   leukemia 13, 128, 219
   lymphoblastic leukemia (ALL) 83, 128, 172, 180
   monoblastic leukemia 83
   myelocytic leukemia 214
   non-lymphocytic leukemia (ANLL) 131, 150, 151
Adamantinoma 89
Adenoacanthocarcinosarcoma 45
Adenocarcinoma 112, 201
Adenocystic carcinoma 45
Adenoid cystic carcinoma of the salivary glands 1
Adenolymphoma 45
Adenomas 45
Adenosquamous carcinomas 42
Adipose tissue 33
Adjuvant chemotherapy 219
Adrenal cancer 113
   gland 5, 9, 32, 65
   medulla 20, 49, 50
Adrenocorticotrophic hormone (ACTH) 49
Adriamycin 113, 207, 221
Adult T cell leukemia (ATL) 141, 143, 181
Aganglionosis 54
Aicardi syndrome 43
Alimentary canal mucosal membranes 214
Alkaline phosphatase 113
Alkylating agents 221
Allergic reaction 172, 199
Alpha chain 125, 138
   fetoprotein (AFP) 113, 206
   heavy chain disease 138
   I-antitypsin 113
   lactalbumin 33, 113
   $_2$-macroglobulin 206
Alveolar macrophages 162
Ameloblastoma 63
Ameloblasts 17
Amenorrhea 222
Amine precursor uptake and decarboxylase system (APUD) 20, 49, 71
Ammonia tolerance test 207
Amosite 200
Amphibians 115
Amyloidosis 32

Anaphylatoxins 154
Anaplasia 14
Anaplastic neoplasms 63
Anemia 123, 130, 158, 166
Aneuploidy 206
Angiogenesis 7
Angioimmunoblastic lymphadenopathy (AILD) 183
Angiolipoma 85
Angiosarcoma 197
Animal models of paraganglioma 56
Aniridia 43
Ann Arbor staging classification 131
Anterior hypophysis 54
Antichemotrypsin 166
   S100 protein antibody 164
Antibiotic therapy 216
Antibodies 124, 205
   to desmoplakins 42
   to the keratins 19
   production, site of 126
   to aldolase C 44
   anti-S100 protein 164
Anticoagulant 156
Anticoagulation 198
Antigens, oncofetal 113
Antihistamines 156
Antileukemia drugs 223
Antimetabolites 223
Antithrombin 156
Antoni tissue 22
Aortic paraganglionic tissue 20
Aponeuroses 8
Aponeurosis fasciae 1
Appendix mucocele 31
araC therapy 150
Arachidonic acid 157, 172
Arachidonic acid metabolism 155
Arteries 1
Arthropods 115
Arylsulfatase 155
Asbestos 31
Asbestos exposure 200
Aschoff 162
Ascites 112, 198
   control of 207
Ascitic fluid 197, 207
Aspergillosis 173
Aspiration pneumonitis 216
Asthma 157, 172
Astrocytes 13
Astrocytoma 11
Atopic dermatitis 173
ATPase + 163
Atrial myxoma 101

Auditory 24
Autocrine function 49
Autoimmune disease 199
Autonomic nervous system 49
Avian leukoses 115
Axillary nodes 112
Axolotl 115
5-Azacytidine 163
Azoospermia 221
Azygos vein 2

B and T cell markers 132, 196
B cell chronic lymphocytic leukemia (B cell CLL) 133
    differentiation 125, 178
    genesis 124
    neoplasia of mature cells 138
    symptoms 140, 143
    lymphomas 136, 162, 205
    markers 205
    large cell lymphoma 179
    lymphocyte 122, 162, 178
    lymphoid stem cell 122
    16 melanoma 13, 126
Bacteria 214
Bacterial peritonitis 208
Banding techniques 150
Barr bodies 206
Basal cell adenoma 45
    cancer 14, 20, 63, 64, 67, 187
Basalioma 68
Basement membrane 7, 111
BCNU 220
Benign effusions 198
Beta-1-glycoprotein 43
Beta$_2$-microglobulin 206
Bilateral retinoblastoma 101
Bilharzial carcinoma 5
Biopsy 196, 220
Biopsy technique, sensitivity of the 197
Birbeck granules 163, 175
Birds 115
Bladder 5, 9, 14, 42, 45, 51
    cancer 13, 39, 65, 190
    paragangliomas 51
Blast transformation 128
Blastema 42
Blastic crisis 148, 150
    leukemia 166
Blastoma 73
Bleomycin 220
Blood 123
Blood vessels 1
Blood-testis barrier 219
Bone 11, 13, 33, 112
    defects 164
    marrow (BM) 13, 123, 140, 172, 204
    monocytes 162
    transplantation 125, 154
    metastasis 63
    sarcoma 33
Botryoid sarcoma 43
Bowel 14
Brain 11, 112
    tumors 101, 216
Branchioma 45
Breast 3, 38, 45, 101
    cancer 7, 13, 31, 63, 101, 112, 113, 190, 200, 206, 208, 219, 223
Brenner tumor 63

Bronchus 42
Burkitt's lymphoma 44, 85, 101, 134, 178
Burn scar carcinoma 68
Busulfan 148, 220

C cells 51, 54
    mos viral oncogene 180
    myc oncogene 134
    myc viral oncogene 179
C$_3$ receptor 157, 163
CA-125 113
Calcitonin 49, 51, 113
Calcium, serum 54
Capillary permeability 197
Carcinoembryonic antigen (CEA) 34, 43, 113, 191, 201, 205
Carcinogens 149
Carcinoid cell 76
    syndrome 71
    tumor 3, 31, 51, 54, 71, 95, 102, 112
Carcinoma *in situ* 9, 157
Carcinomas 30
Carcinomatosis 30
Carcinosarcoma of the Fallopian tube 45
Carcinosarcomas 45
Cardiac musculature 13
    myxoma 190
    tamponade 195
    tumor 45, 101
Cardiomyopathy 173
Carney's triad 52
Carotic body 20
Carotid bodies 50
Cartilage 45
    invasion 13
CAT scanning 195
Catecholamines 20, 21, 49
Catheter-associated bacteremias 216
Cattle 34
Cauda equina tumors 51
CCNU 220
Cell colony forming (CFU) assays 123
    lines 111
    nest 49
    origin 162
    surface marker 123
    types 190
    mediated immunity 214
Cellular immune deficiency 215
Cementoblasts 17
Central nervous system (CNS) 13, 15, 33, 44, 50, 53, 101, 127
    dysfunction 215
    infections 214
    lymphomas 127
    tumors 92
Cerebellum 44
Cerebriform lymphoma 204
Cerebrospinal fluid 13, 204
    spaces 1
    direct spread in 8
Ceruloplasmin 206
Cervical cancer 13, 190
    lymph node enlargement 167
Cervix uteri 7, 31, 63, 157
Cestode infection 157
Charcot Leyden crystals 172
Chediak Higashi syndrome 154
Chemoattractants 172
Chemodectoma 13, 20, 76

Chemosensitive paraganglia 55
Chemosensory transduction 50
Chemotherapy 44, 101, 127, 150, 176, 187, 203, 214, 219
  effects in children 223
  in women 222
  effects, reversibility of 221
Childhood cancer 42, 224
Cholangiocarcinoma 75
Cholangitis 215
Cholesteatoma 19
Cholesterol 198
Chondroid syringoma 45
Chondroma 88
Chondrosarcoma 6, 7, 32, 88, 203
Chordal tissue 190
Chordoma 11, 17
Chorionepithelioma 4, 7
Choroid plexus carcinoma 11
Choroidal melanoma 8
Chromatin clumping 203
Chromogranins 49
Chromosomal abnormalities 150
  marker 148
  translocations 56
Chromosome 43, 134
  analysis 206
  translocation 179
Chronic granulocytic leukemia (CGL) 128
  hypoxemia 55
  lymphatic leukemia 32
  lymphocytic leukemia (CLL) 133, 203
  myelocytic leukemia (CML) 148, 150, 151
  pulmonary disease 56, 157, 172
Chrysotile 200
Churg-Strauss syndrome 173
Chylopericardium 198, 204
Chylous effusion 198
Chymotrypsin 155
Ciliary body 43
Cimetidine 156
Circulating antibodies 126
  basophilic leukocyte 154
  cells 101
Circulatory system 7
Cirrhosis 197, 200, 208
Cis-platin 220
Classification of effusions 195
  of lymphoblastic leukemias 129
  of post-thymic T-cell malignancies 141
  of Ann Arbor 131
Clear cell carcinoma 53, 70, 79
  sarcoma 82
Cleaved cells 179
Clonal evolution 149, 150
  overproduction 133
  selection 127
Clonidine 53
Clusters, three dimensional 202
Coelom 30
Coelomic cavity 1, 30
  direct spread of neoplasms in the 8
  fluid 31
Collagenase IV 111
Collision tumor 42, 45, 95
Colon 8, 10, 67, 112
Colonization resistance 218
Colonizing organisms 218
Colony forming units (CFU) 122
Combined types of tumor distribution 8

Comparison, interspecies 62, 115, 187
  intraspecies 62, 115
Complement activation 154
Complete remission (CR) 150
Compromised host 214
Computed tomographic scan (CT) 24, 31, 53
Concanavalin A (ConA) 180
Concepts of spread 111
Condyloma acuminacum 68
Congenital cyanotic heart disease 56
  mesoblastic nephroma 101
Congestive heart failure 196, 198
Connective tissue 8, 33, 111
  disorders 173
  tumors 53
Control of ascites 207
Core antigen of ATLV 181
Counseling patients 224
Cranial nerves 21
Crocidolite 200
Cryopreserved semen 224
Cryptococosis 205
Cutaneous infiltration of histiocytes 163
  T cell lymphoma (CTCL) 141, 182
Cyclic DNA 19
  neutropenia 124
Cyclooxygenase 157
Cyclophosphamide 220
Cylindroma 45
Cystadenoma 45
Cystic fibrosis 56
  lymphangiosarcoma 197
Cystosarcoma phylloides 63, 79
Cytochrome 49
Cytogenetics 206
Cytology 198
Cytomegalovirus 39, 214
Cytosine arabinoside 220
Cytotoxic activity 157
  chemotherapy 219

Dandy-Walker syndrome 43
Darier's sign 157
Deafness 24
Dedifferentiation 42
Degranulation 154, 155, 172, 175
Dense-core granules 49
Denver shunt 207
Deoxycoformycin 129
Dermatitis herpetiformis 173
Dermis 1
Dermoid cysts 11, 30
Desmal epithelium 13, 14, 33
Desmin 18, 32
Desmosomes 46
Dexamethasone receptors 180
Diabetes insipidus 164
  mellitis 195
Differentiation pathways for hematopoietic cells 122
Diffuse lymphoblastic lymphoma (DLB) 180
  lymphomas 138
Diktyoma 42, 43
Diphenhydramine block 156
Direct extension 1
  infiltration 1
  expansion (invasion) via the lymphatic system 1
  spread via the circulatory system 7
  spread in cerebrospinal spaces 8
  of neoplasms in the coelomic cavity 8

spread via nerves 8
spread via veins 7
spread via arteries 7
Dysontogenetic theory 19
Disseminated intravascular coagulation 208
Distant metastases 32
DNA 206
   repair 149
Doege Potter syndrome 32
Dopamine 20, 49
Double minute (DM) chromosomes 44
   positive cells 125
   population 125
Doxorubicin 220
Drug effects on ovarian function 222
   effects on spermatogenesis 220
   reaction 173, 199
   resistance 219
Drug resistance, leukemic cell 150
   therapy 176
   induced ovarian failure 222
Duodenal carcinoids 54
Dysartria 24
Dysphagia 24

Ear disease 19
Ectoderm 30, 42
Effusions 30, 195
   benign 198
   classification 196
   evaluation of 205
   neoplastic 33
   pericardial 202
   prognosis of 208
   treatment of 207
Electrolyte balance 197
Electron microscopic markers 113
   dense cytoplasmic granules 154
Emboli, tumor cell 111
Embolic metastases 13
Embolization of the tumor 101
Embryonal carcinoma 42, 43
   cell lines 43
   of the salivary glands 43
   rhabdomyosarcoma 91
   sarcoma of the liver 101
   tumors 42
Embryonic and mixed tumors 5
   hepatoma 43
   rhabdomyosarcomas 43
   sarcoma 33
Encephalitis 214
Enclavomas 45
Endocrine function 49
Endometrial cancer 13, 87
   carcinosarcomas 45
Endometriosis 198
Endometrium 38, 70
Endothelial tumor 113
Endothelioma 31
Endotoxin 123
Enkephalins 50
Enolase 50
Enteritis 215
Entoderm 30, 42
Environmental factors 55
Enzymatic markers 113
Enzyme 49, 149
Eosinophil chemotactic factor of anaphylaxis (ECF-A) 155
   degranulation 175

Eosinophilia 172, 182, 199
Eosinophilic fasciitis 173
   granuloma 158, 162, 172
   leukocytes 172
   pleural effusion 199
   pneumonia 173
Eosinophils 172
Ependymoma 11, 15
Epidermal cyst 19
Epidermoid carcinoma 18, 45, 69
Epididymis 42
Epidural cord compress 112
Epinephrine 49, 53, 55
Epithelial cavities 1, 8
   membrane antigen (EMA) 205
   surfaces 38
   tumors 30, 42
Epithelioid meningiomas 53
   sarcoma 82
Epstein Barr virus (EBV) 127, 134, 178, 216
Erosion of the major local vessels 17
Erythrocyte 122
Erythroderma 142
   exfoliative 141
Erythroid stem cell 122
Erythroleukemia 122, 130
Erythrophagocytosis 163, 166
Esophageal carcinoma 11
Esophagus 45
Estradiol 113, 222
Estrogen 102
   deficiency 222
   receptor 113, 190
   replacement therapy 224
Ethmoid sinus 13
Eustachian tube compression 19
Evolution of vertebrates 56
Ewing's sarcoma 89
Exfoliative erythroderma 141, 181
Exocrine pancreas 13, 31
Exophthalmos 164
Extracellular matrix of the tumor 111
Extramedullary plasma cell tumors 139
Extravasation of fluid 156
Exudates 196

FAB M_2 152
Facial nerve 24
Fallopian tube 11, 14, 39, 72
   carcinoma of the 45
Familial lymphohistiocytosis 166
   paragangliomas 52
Fasciae 8
Fc receptor 163
   for IgE 154
Fetal differentiation of histiocytes 162
   hepatoblastoma 43
Fever 208
Fibroblasts 17, 39, 111, 154
Fibronectin 207
Fibrosarcoma 6, 18, 33, 87, 101, 205
   of the heart 87
   of the peritoneum 33
Fibrous connective tissue 32
Fibroxanthoma 87
Filaments 49
Filariasis 197
Fishes 115
Floating cells 42
Flow cytometry 196, 206

Fluid aspiration 196
  overload 208
5 Fluorouracil 223
Follicle destruction 222
  stimulating hormone (FSH) 220
Follicular lymphoma 135, 179
Free tumor cells 30
Fungemia 216
Fungi 214

Gag reflex 216
Galactosidase 155
Gall bladder 10, 11, 45
  mixed mesodermal tumor of the 45
Gamma heavy chain disease 127
Gamna Gandy nodules 21
Ganglioglioma 43
Gangliomyoma 44
Ganglioneuroma 33
Gastric cancer 2, 9, 10, 13, 31, 95
  leiomyosarcoma 52
Gastrinoma 76
Gastrointestinal and pancreatic neuroendocrine cells 51
Gene loci 50
Genetic instability 127, 149, 186
  mapping 55
  transmission 21
Genital carcinoma 3
Genitourinary tract neuroendocrine cells 51
Germ cell testis tumors 14
  tumors 46, 65, 79
  cells 219
  layers 42
Germinal tumors 43, 113
Germinoma 14, 79
Giant cell tumor 88
  cells 163
  granules 154
Gingival hypertrophy 131
Glial fibrillary acidic protein 44, 113
  filaments 18
Glioblastoma 11, 15, 93
Glioma 13, 113, 208
Glomus tumors 20
Glucose 6 phosphate dehydrogenase (G6PD) 128, 149
  isoenzymes 56
Glycolipids 206
Glycoprotein 111
Gonadal function 219
Gonadoblastoma 78
Granule associated soluble mediators 156
Granules 172
  Birbeck 163
  electron dense cytoplasmic 154
Granulocyte 122
Granulocytic sarcoma 203
Granulocytopenia 214, 216
Granuloma, eosinophilic 162
Granulosa cell tumor 79

H_2 receptor 156
Hairy cell leukemia 127, 137, 162
Hamartoma 33, 45, 53
Hand Schüller Christian disease 163
  syndrome 176
Hashimoto's thyroiditis 143, 182
Head and neck cancer 2, 17, 113
  paragangliomas 53
Headaches 19, 24

Heart 10
Heavy chain 138
  class switching 135, 139
  enhancer gene 134
Helminthic parasites 172, 214
Helper T cells 142, 143
Hemangioendothelioma 78
Hemangioma 67, 78
  supraglottic 102
Hemangiomatosis 197
Hemangiomyosarcoma 197
Hemangiopericytoma 53, 63, 78, 82
Hematogenic system 30
Hematogenous dissemination 13
Hematologic malignancies 122
Hematopoietic cells, differentiation pathways 122
Hemicerebellectomy 23
Hemorrhage 128
Heparin 154, 156, 198
Hepatic metastases 102
  tumors 3, 101
Hepatoblastoma 42, 43, 75
Hepatocellular carcinoma 65, 208
Hepatoma 33
  mouse ascitic 197
Hepatosplenomegaly 158, 166, 173
Herpes simplex 214
Heterogeneity of tumor cells 43, 186
Heterogeneity of histiocytes 162
Hexosamidase 206
High endothelial post capillary venules (HEV) 125
Hippel Lindau syndrome 54
Hirschsprung's disease 54
Histamine 154, 156, 172
Histidine decarboxylase 156
Histiocytes 182
  fetal differentiation of 162
Histiocytic lymphoma 83
  medullary reticulosis 162
  sarcoma 162, 166
  tumors 162
Histiocytoma 34, 205
Histiocytosis X 163, 174
  treatment of 176
  malignant 162
Hodgkin's disease (HD) 8, 84, 113, 127, 131, 167, 172, 204, 214,
  219, 222
  distribution 132
Homing behavior 140
Hormone deficiency 224
  replacement therapy 224
Hormones 113
Host and tumor, weakened interaction between 187
  defense 217
  tumor interrelationship 187
Host versus graft rejection 214
HTLV type 1 181
Human atrial natriuretic peptide (hANP) 197
  chorionic gonadotrophin (HCG) 113, 206
Humoral immune deficiency 215
Huntingdon's chorea 55
Hydrogen peroxide (H_2O_2) 157
Hydrostatic pressure 196
Hydrothorax 198
Hyper IgE syndrome 173
Hypercalcemia 54, 181
Hypereosinophilic disorders 173
Hypereosinophilic syndrome (HES) 172
Hypergammaglobulinemia 183

Hypergranular promyelocytic leukemia 130
Hyperlipidemia 167, 195
Hyperostosis of the skull 13
Hyperparathyroidism 54
Hypersensitivity reaction, immediate 154
Hyperviscosity 138
Hypopharynx 101
Hypophysis 54, 164
Hypothyroidism 197
Hypoxemia, chronic 55
Hypoxia 123

Iatrogenic spreading by implantation 38
IgA 126, 138, 173
IgD 124, 138
IgG 138
IgM 124
Imidazolylethylamine 156
Immediate hypersensitivity reaction 154, 172
Immune deficiency 214, 215
    dysfunction 143
    system 49, 115
Immunity 39
    cell-mediated 214
Immunoblastic lymphadenopathy (IBL) 183
    sarcoma 138, 179, 203
Immunocytologic examination 205
Immunodeficiency disorders 173
Immunofluorescent identification 205
Immunoglobulins (Ig) 113, 124, 126, 138, 178
    quantitative 207
Immunoperoxidase 196, 205
Immunosuppression 39
Implantation metastases 38
In situ carcinoma 7, 157
Increased capillary pressure 196
Infection 214
    prevention 217
    associated with medical procedures 215
Infertility 222, 224
Inguinal nodes 112
Initiation of the tumor 178
Insects 115
Interdigitating cells of the lymph nodes 167
    reticulum (IR) cells 132
Interferon 33, 137, 180
Interleukin-2 receptor 143
Interspecies comparison 115
Intestinal ganglioneuromatosis 54
Intestines 10
Intra- and extraspecies comparison 62
Intra-adrenal paragangliomas 54
Intracranial hypertension 24
    invasion 21
    tumors 22
Intraspecies comparison 115
    spectrum 190
Intravagal paragangliomas 53
Invasion of tissue spaces 1
    intracranial 21
Invasive adenocarcinoma 201
    procedures 217
Invertebrates 115
Islet cell tumors 54, 76
Isochromosome 17 149
Isoenzymes 50
Isolation, total reverse 217

Jaw tumor 127
Jugularis tumor 21

Kaposi's sarcoma 33, 39, 78
Keratin 18, 32, 43, 113, 204
Keratinocytes 19
Kidney 9, 112
Kiel classification 132
Kimura's disease 165
Kupffer cells 162

L-ornithine decarboxylase 44
Lacrimal gland 45
Lactate dehydrogenase (LDH) 196
Langerhans cells 163
Large cell adenoma 112
Laryngeal cancers 13, 17, 18
Larynx 42, 45, 72
Laser 39
Late complications and effusions 204
Lectins 180
Leiomyoma 14, 95
Leiomyomatosis of the peritoneum 33
Leiomyosarcoma 7, 14, 18, 33, 89
Leptomeningeal metastases 101
Leptomeninges 11
Letterer Siwe disease 162
    syndrome 176
Leukemia 30, 101, 115, 178, 183, 190, 203, 214, 223
    acute 219
    adult T-cell 181
    blastic 166
    chronic lymphocytic 203
    chronic myelocytic 148, 151
    classification of lymphoblastic 129
    hairy cell 127, 137, 162
    lymphoblastic 83, 128, 172, 180, 205
    mast cell 158
    monoblastic 83
    monocytic 162, 203
    myeloblastic 83, 130
    myelocytic 162, 203, 214
    myelomonocytic 203
    nonlymphocytic 131, 150, 151
Leukemia/lymphoma, adult T cell 143
    progression of the myeloid 148
Leukemic cell drug resistance 150
    conversion 140
Leukocytes, eosinophilic 172
Leukoses in amphibians 115
Leukotriene B$_4$ 172
    formation 172
Leukotrienes 155, 157, 173
LeVeen shunt 207
Lewis lung carcinoma 39
Leydig cell dysfunction 220
Life span 95, 207
    of lymphoid cells 125
    threatening toxicities 214
Ligaments 1
Ligation of the thoracic duct 198
Lip 67
Lipomatosis, mediastino-abdominal 195
Liposarcoma 18, 33, 84, 205
    of groin 6
    of the heart 63
Lipoxygenase 157
Listeria 214
Liver 9, 38, 112
Local factors 17
    involvement 187

metastasis 38
  recurrence 17, 180, 186, 187
  recurrence after surgery 17
Loffler's syndrome 173
Long bones 174
Loose connective tissue 154
Lukes Collins classification 132, 203
Lung 9, 13, 38, 45, 101, 112
  cancer 7, 82, 200
  leukostatis 131
  mast cells 157
  metastases 6
  small cell (oat cell) carcinoma of 204
Luschka's gland 20
Luteinizing hormone (LH) 220
Lymph angiosarcoma 78
  node architecture 125
  enlargement 158
  metastasis in mediastinum 2
  nodes 7, 32, 38, 125, 135, 190
  vessels 1
Lymphadenopathy 131, 137, 142, 181, 183
Lymphangioleiomyomatosis 198
Lymphangioma of the thymus 204
Lymphatic channels, obstruction of 197
  system 30, 63, 115
  direct neoplastic expansion (invasion) via the 1
Lymphoblastic leukemia 205
  lymphoma (LL) 63, 140
Lymphocytes 124, 154, 178
Lymphohistiocytosis, familial 166
Lymphoid cells 162
Lymphoma 84, 101, 113, 127, 178, 183, 203, 215
  adult T cell leukemia 143
  B-malignant 162
  cutaneous T cell 141
  diffuse 138
  follicular 135
  nodular 138
  of uncertain cellular origin 131
  peripheral post thymic T cell 142
  pleomorphic T-cell 181
  T-malignant 162
Lymphomatoid granulomatosis of the lung 183
Lymphoproliferative disorders 122
Lymphosarcoma 32, 115, 179
  pulmonary 14
Lysosomal enzyme 166
Lysozyme 166, 206

Macrophage 111, 122, 197
Magnetic resonance imaging (MRI) 195
Maintenance therapy 214
Malignant histiocytosis 162, 165
  lymphoma 127, 178, 203
  potential of tissues 190
Mammals 115
Mammary carcinoma 12
  glands 31, 115
  tumors 65
mAMSA 150
Marfanoid habitus 54
Marker 33, 178
  B and T cell 113, 132
  chromosomal 148
  enzymatic 113
  of MPS 163
  T- and B-cell 196
Marrow fibrosis 151

stem cell precursor 154
  transplantation 214
Mast cell disease 204
  leukemia 158
  neoplasias 86
  secretory products 172
Mast cells 154
  in inflammation 157
Mastocytoma 157
Mastocytosis 154
  classification 157
Maturation arrest 220
Mechanical trapping 101
Mediastinal metastasis 101
  node involvement 131
  tumor 32
Mediastino-abdominal lipomatosis 195
Mediator release 154
Medullary cords (MC) 126
  sinuses (MS) 126
Medulloblastoma 11, 15, 42, 43, 44, 101
Medulloepithelioma 43
Megakaryocyte 122
Meig's syndrome 198
Melanoma 5, 8, 13, 63, 101, 112, 186, 205
  B-16 126
Melphalan 44
Membrane bound granules 154
Memory cell generation 135
Menarche 223
Meningeal melanoma 11
Meninges 13
Meningioma 6, 11, 13, 32
Meningitis 214
Menopause 223
Merkel cell tumor 68
Mesenchymal cells 205
Mesenchyme 33
Mesenteric lymph nodes 132
Mesoderm 30, 42
Mesothelial antigen 113
  cells 30
  lined body cavities 195
Mesothelioma 14, 30, 31, 32, 34, 65, 81, 200
  of the peritoneum 31
Messenger RNA 50
Metachromasia 156
Metachronous paragangliomas 55
Metanephrines 52
Metaphase 150
Metastases to the spine 13
  to thoracic structures 202
  implantation 38
Metastasis 190
  to regional lymph nodes 55
  local 38
Metastatic adenocarcinoma 199
Methotrexate 220
Micrometastatic disease 219
Middle ear 19
Migratory capacity of a cell 111
Mitomycin C 220
  microcapsule therapy 14
Mitotic index 151
Mixed MEN syndromes 54
  mesodermal tumor of the gall bladder 45
  neoplasms 42, 44
  neoplasms of skin 44
  tumor of the Fallopian tube 45

tumor of the vagina 45
   tumor of connective tissue 45
   tumor of the salivary glands tumors 45
   tumor of the thyroid gland 45
Mollusks 115
Monoamines 49
Monoblast 122
Monoclonal antibodies 44, 50, 178, 181, 206
   antibody OKT6 166
   antihuman T6 antigen 175
Monocyte macrophage system (MPS) 162
Monocytic leukemia 130, 162, 203
MOPP 223
Mos oncogene 152
Mouse ascitic hepatoma 197
Mucin 203
   secreting carcinomas 172
   vacuoles 207
Mucociliary function 214
Mucoepidermoid tumors 45, 73
Mucopolysaccharides, neutral 202
Multicentric reticulohistiocytosis 167
Multicystic peritoneal mesothelioma 31
Multifocal eosinophilic granuloma 164
Multiple endocrine neoplasia (MEN) 53, 54, 56
   mucosal neuromas 54
   myeloma (MM) 13, 101, 138, 180, 204
   primary neoplasms 190
Muramidase 113
Mutagenesis 224
Mutation 42, 56, 149
Mycosis fungoides 141, 172, 182, 204
Myelo-monocytic stem cell 122
Myeloblast 122
Myeloblastic leukemia 130, 130
Myelofibrosis 124, 158
Myeloid metaplasia 124
   stem cell 122
Myelomonocytic leukemia 127, 130, 203
Myoglobin 113
Myxoid liposarcoma 17
Myxoma 65, 81, 101
Myxosarcoma 34, 65, 86

Nasopharyngeal carcinoma 2, 11, 72
   liposarcoma 17
Natural barriers against tumor spread 1
   killer cell 122, 124, 132
Necrotizing vasculitis 173
Nematode infection 157
Neoplastic effusion 33
   spontaneous regression 102
Nephrectomy 14
Nephroblastoma 33, 42, 91
Nephroma, congenital mesoblastic 101
Nerve pathways 1
Nerves, direct spread via 8
   vestibular 24
Neural crest 49, 54
   epithelium 22
Neurinoma of the mesenterium 33
Neuroblastoma 5, 8, 15, 33, 42, 44, 92, 165
Neurocristopathies 54
Neuroectoderm 56
Neuroendocrine cells 49, 51
   tumors 49
Neurofibroma 13, 30, 56
Neurofilaments 18, 49
Neuron specific enolase (NSE) 49

Neurotransmitter 50
Neurotransmitting polypeptides 20
Neutral mucopolysaccharides 202
Neutropenia, cyclic 124
Neutrophils 123, 157
Nitrogen mustard 220
Nodular lymphomas 138
Non functional paragangliomas 53
Non Hodgkin's disease 113
   lymphoma 13, 33, 84, 132, 135, 203, 219
NonA/nonB hepatitis 216
Nonkeratinizing carcinomas 204
Norepinephrine 49, 55
Nosocomial 214
Nuclear cytoplasmic (N:C) ratio 202
Nucleotidase 166

Oat cell cancer of the lung 51, 62, 72, 113, 204
   specific antibody 206
Obstruction of lymphatic channels 197
   of the airways 17
   to natural passages 215
Occult primary malignancy (OPM) 111, 112
Odontoblasts 17
OKT6 monoclonal antibody 166
Olfactory tumor 11
Oligodendroglia 22
Oligodendroglioma 11, 95
Oligopeptides 49
Oligospermia 221
Omental leiomyosarcoma 195
Omentum 38
Oncocytoma 13, 45
Oncofetal antigens 113
Oncogene 44, 56, 62, 127, 151
   activation 42
   c-mos viral 180
   sis 151
Oogenesis 222
Opioid peptides (enkephalins) 49
Orchioblastoma 43
Organ capsules 1
   of Zuckerkandl 52, 95
   transplantation 38
   specific collagenase 111
Organism acquisition 217
Orosomucoid 206
Osteoblastoma of the mandible 102
Osteoliposarcoma 85
Osteolytic lesions 174
Osteomyelitis 174
Osteosarcoma 63, 66, 113, 205
   of femur 6
Ovarian cancer 4, 9, 10, 13, 38, 39, 80, 113, 197, 201, 208
   cystadenocarcinomas 31
   fibrosis 222
   function 222
   teratoma 9
Ovary 11, 14, 33, 46, 112
Oxophylic adenoma 45
Oxygen radicals 157

Palatal edema 127
Pancoast syndrome 32
Pancreas 13, 31, 63, 65, 76, 112
Pancreatic cancer 9, 10
   cell tumor 113
   islets 54
Pancreatitis 200, 207

Pancytopenia 137, 166
Papillomatosis 30
Paracrine function 49
Paraganglioma 20, 49, 77
  non-functional 53
Paraganglion of Kohn 20
Parasites, helminthic 172
Parathormone 54
Parathyroid carcinoma 77
  gland 53, 54, 65, 77
Parotid carcinoma 7
Pautrier's microabscess 182
Pemphigius 173
Pericardial carcinomatosis 30
  effusion 196, 202
Pericarditis 33
Pericardium 30
Periosteum 1
Peripheral T (T2) lymphocytes 180
  T cell lymphoma 142, 182
Peritoneal carcinomatosis 9
  cavity 195
  macrophages 162
  mesothelioma 31
  myeloid metaplasia 204
  surface 31
Peritoneo cystic shunt 207
Peritoneo venous shunt 207
Peritoneum 31, 33, 38
Peritonitis 13, 208
Permeability of capillaries 156
Permeation 7
Peroxidase 157
  oxidative system 172
  containing granule matrix 172
Petrous bone 19
Peyers's patches 125
Phagocytosis 162
Pharyngeal carcinoma 2
Pheochromocytoma 51, 54, 77
Philadelphia (Ph^1) chromosome 128, 148, 151
Phospholipase A$_2$ 155
Phytohemagglutinin (PHA) 180
Pineal germinoma 31
  gland 42
Pinealoblastoma 76
Pinealoma 11
Pineoblastoma 43
Pituitary 53
  adenomas 13, 54
  gland 65
  gonadotropin secretion 220
  neoplasms 11
Placenta 43
Placental tumor 113
Plant 17, 42
Plasma cell tumors of bone 139
Plasmacytoma 32, 83, 85, 180
Platelet derived growth factor (PDGF) 151
  function 128
  stem cell 122
Platelets 101, 122
Pleomorphic T-cell lymphoma 181
Pleura 7, 30, 38
Pleural carcinomatosis 9, 30
  cavities 195
  effusions 112, 195, 208
  effusions with adenocarcinoma 201
  eosinophilia 199
  surface 32

Pluripotent stem cell 122
Pneumococcal sepsis syndrome 215
Pneumocystis carinii 214
Pneumonia 208
Pneumonitis 215
Pneumothorax 199
Poikilothermic animals 115
Polyclonal antibodies 50
Polycythemia vera (PV) 128
Polymorphonuclear leukocyte granules 154
Polypeptides, neurotransmitting 20
POMP combination chemotherapy 223
Post-thymic T cell neoplasia 140
Potential of recurrence 187
Pre-neoplastic lesions 55
Pre-T (T0) 180
Predisposing factors 214
Prednisone (MOPP) 174, 221
Pregnancy 102, 224
Preleukemia 151
Prelymphomatous lesions 182
Pressure, hydrostatic 196
  increased capillary 196
Primary and secondary tumors of serosal surfaces 31
  mesothelioma 199
  neoplasms 9, 62
  neoplasms of the coelomic surfaces 30
  tumor treatment 190
Primordium 42
Procarbazine 220
Progesterone 102, 222
Prognosis of effusions 208
Progranulocyte 122
Progression of embryonal neoplasms 42
  mixed neoplasms 42
  the myeloid leukemias 148
Promonocyte 122
Pronormoblast 122
Prostaglandin 155, 175
  biosynthesis 159
  D$_2$ (PGD$_2$) 157
  I$_2$ (PGI$_2$) 157
Prostate 14, 67, 112
  cancer 1, 5, 32, 70, 111, 113
Prostatic nerves 8
Proteases 111
Protein 18, 49, 113, 196
  electrophoresis 207
Proteoglycan macromolecule 156
Proto-oncogene 56
Pruritis 128, 141, 158
Pseudo-ascites 195
Pseudo Meig's syndrome 198
Pseudoeffusion of the pericardium 195
Pseudomyxoma peritonei 31, 86, 203
Pseudopodia 111
Pseudosarcoma 18
Pseudostratified columnar epithelium 14, 32, 64
Puberty 223
Pulmoblastoma 42, 43
Pyothorax 204

Quality of life 208
Quantitative immunoglobulins 207

Radiation 127, 187
Radicals 157
Radiosensitivity 190
Radiotherapy 139, 176
  for Hodgkin 204

Rai staging classification 133
Rappaport classification 132
Rat leukemia basophil (RBL) 155
Reaction processes of the serosal surfaces 198
Receptor, C_3 157
Reciprocal translocation 151
Rectal cancer 2, 8, 112
Red blood cell count 196
Regional direct spread 8
Regression, neoplastic spontaneous 102
Remissions 219
Renal cancer 7, 9, 14, 39, 42, 202
    pelvis 1
    transplantations 39
Repair genes 149
Reproductive function 219
Reticular connective tissue 13, 14, 32, 63
Reticuloendothelial system (RES) 162
Reticulohistiocytosis 83
Reticulosis, histiocytic medullary 162
Reticulum cell sarcoma 176
Retinal infiltration 131
Retinoblastoma 11, 15, 42, 43, 44, 190
    bilateral 101
Retrograde direct spread 1
    invasion 9
Retroperitoneal sarcomas 13
Retrovirus 180, 181
Reversibility of chemotherapy effects 221
Rhabdomyosarcoma 6, 8, 11, 25, 42, 43, 91, 205
Richter's syndrome 133
Risk factors 190
Risks of spontaneous abortion 224
    to future generations 224
Rubra vera 128

S-100 antigen 113
Salivary glands 14, 42, 45
    adenoid cystic carcinoma 1
    embryonal carcinoma of the 43
Salmonella spp 214
Sarcoidosis 198, 203
Sarcoma 5, 30, 89, 95, 115
    lung and pleura 32
    pelvic soft tissues 6
    skull 11
    granulocytic 203
    histiocytic 162
    immunoblastic 138, 203
    subcutaneous foreign-body 200
Scar tissue 186
Schistosoma mansoni 157, 172
Schwann cells 49
Schwannoma 22, 92
Scintigraphy 44
Scrotum 38
Secondary direct spreading 101
    neoplasms 9, 10, 62
    tumors of serosal surfaces, primary and 31
Secretory granules 50, 157
    immunoglobulin 126
Seeding 101
Selective IgA deficiency 173
Semen cryopreservation 224
Seminiferous tubules 219
Seminoma 65, 79
Sensitivity of the biopsy technique 197
Septicemia 215
Serosal carcinomatosis 30

Serotonin 49, 155
Sertoli cell tumor 78
    cells 219
Serum calcium 54
    cell tumors 113
Sessel's pouch 19
Sex chromatin (Barr) bodies 206
    predominance 52
    related neoplasms 95
Sézary syndrome 141, 172, 181
Simple columnar epithelium 8, 14, 31, 64, 190
    cuboidal epithelium 31
    cuboidal/columnar epithelium 8, 14
Sis oncogene 151
Sjøgren's syndrome 143, 182
Skeletal metastases 101
Skeletal muscle 113
Skin 42, 67, 112
    tumors 141
Slow reacting substance of anaphylaxis (SRS-A) 157, 173
Small cell (oat cell) carcinoma of lung 51, 63, 72, 113, 204
    tumor of salivary glands 45
Smooth musculature 14, 33
Soft tissue sarcoma 219
Solitary eosinophilic granuloma 164
Somatostatin 49
Somatostatin-producing tumors 44
Spaces associated with the distribution of fasciae and aponeuroses 1
Species specificity of important tumor types 34
Sperm banking 224
Spermatids 220
Spermatogenesis 219
Spinal cord 11
Spindle cell 18
Spleen 9, 123
Splenectomy 137, 215
Splenic architecture 126
    macrophages 162
    sequestration 137
Splenomegaly 128, 137, 148, 176, 181, 183
Spreading at pericardial surface 33
    by implantation on epithelial surfaces 38
    on the coelomic surface 30
    secondary direct 101
    63
Squamous cell carcinoma 13, 20, 45, 63, 112, 204
    of tongue 2
    of the kidney 7
Staging laparotomy 215
    procedure 131
Stem cell 190
    disorders 128
Sternberg-Reed (SR) cells 127, 132, 204
Steroid hormones 111
    therapy 195
Stomach 10, 45
Storage granules 50
Stratified squamous epithelium 8, 14, 63
Striated musculature 190
Stroma 111
Stromal-gonadal tumor 113
Subcutaneous foreign-body sarcomas 200
Subpopulations 43, 126
Superoxide 157
Suppressor T-cell function 183
Supraclavicular node group 127
Supraglottic hemangioma 102
Surface antigens 123, 180

IgM positive (sIgM⁺) 124
immunoglobulin 133
    marker 125, 135, 143, 178
    markers, T cell 140
    pores 155
Surgery, transtemporal 23
Survival rate, higher 40
Sweat gland 44
Syncytiotrophoblastic 46
Systemic metastasis 55
    granulomatous disease 198
    lupus erythematosus (SLE) 199
    mastocytosis 154
    neoplastic diseases 115

T cell chronic lymphocytic leukemia (T cell CLL) 141
    cell markers 196, 205
    differentiation 180
    helper cells 142, 143
    lymphocytes 122, 154
    lymphoid stem cell 122
    lymphomas 84, 162, 180
    lymphoma, cutaneous 141
    neoplasia of intermediate maturity 140
    peripheral post thymic 142
    surface markers 140
Tartrate resistance acid phosphatase (TRAP) 137
Telangiectatic osteosarcoma 33
Tendons 1
Teratocarcinoma 43
Teratoma 5, 11, 30, 42, 46, 51, 66, 80
    of testis 9, 46
Terminal and deoxynucleotidyl transferase (TdT) 180, 205
Test marker 113
Testicle 112
Testicular adenocarcinoma of infants 42, 43
    biopsy 220
    cancer 219, 224
Testicular neuroblastoma 101
    teratomas 9, 46
Testis 14, 79, 219
Testosterone 113
    production 219
    therapy 224
Therapy, antibiotic 216
Therapy induced neoplasms 190
Thoracic duct 127, 197
    ligation of the 198
Thorascopy 196
Three dimensional clusters 202
Thrombocytopenia 137, 158, 208
Thrombocytosis 128
Thromboembolism, pulmonary 196
Thromboxanes 155, 157, 159
Thymic T (T1) lymphocytes 180
Thymocyte marker 140
Thymoma 86
Thymus 125
Thyrodiditis, Hashimoto's 143
Thyroglobulin 113
Thyroid 4, 13, 76, 113
    cancer 32, 101
    gland 12, 14, 42, 51, 53
Tight junctions 207
Tissue diagnosis 53
    evaluation 190
    grafting 38
    macrophages 162
    spaces 1

subtypes 190
    adipose 33
    aortic paraganglionic 20
    fibrous connective 32
    loose connective 154
    reticular connective 32
    malignant potential of 190
Topographical malignancy 17
Total protein 196
    reverse isolation 217
Toxicities of chemotherapy 224
Toxoplasma gondii 214
    infection 166
Trachea 42
Transitional cell carcinoma 5, 45, 73
    papillary tumors of the bladder 14
    epithelium 8, 14
Translocation 42, 44, 152
    chromosomal 56
Transplantation 38, 39, 182
Transtemporal surgery 23
Transudaates 196
Transverse striated musculature 15
Treatment of effusions 207
    histiocytosis X 176
Trichinella spiralis 172
Triglyceride 198
Trisomy 8 149
Trophoblastic cells 43
    tumor 113
Trophocarcinoma 43
Tuberculosis 198, 199, 214
Tumor biology 204, 219
    cell emboli 13, 111
    embolization 208
    markers 162, 196, 206
    regression 102
    thrombi 3
Type C viral particles 181
    IV collagenase 111
Tyrosine 49
    kinase 56

Ultrasonography 195
Umbilical mass 112
Ureter 1
Ureteral carcinoma 63
Urinary tract infection 215
Urticaria 128
    pigmentosa 157
Uterine carcinoma 3
    mesodermal mixed neoplasm 45
Uveal melanoma 186

Vagal glomus 20
Vanillylmandelic 52
Varicella zoster 214
Vascular lesions 197
    permeability factor 197
    plants 42
    tumor 81
Vasoactive intestinal peptide (VIP) 49, 159
Veins 1
Vertebrates 115
Vestibular dysfunctions 24
    nerves 24
Vibratory capacity 111
Vimentin 18, 32, 44, 200
    filaments 46

Viral infection 178, 203
    oncogene, c-mos 179, 180
    particles, Type C 181
    vaccines 217
Virchow 18
Virus integration site 143
Viruses 214
Von Recklinghausen's neurofibromatosis 22, 54, 93
Vulva 112

Waldenström's macroglobulinemia 138
Waldeyer's ring 127, 132
Walker carcinoma 46
Warthin's tumor 45
Waterhouse Friedrichsen syndrome 215
WDHA syndrome 76
Weakened interaction between host and tumor 187

White blood count 148, 196
Wilms' tumor 5, 42
Wiscott Aldrich syndrome 173

Xanthoma cells 163
    disseminatum 167
    tuberosum 167
Xanthofibrosarcoma 18
Xeroderma pigmentosum 68

Yeasts 214
Yolk sac 123, 162
    carcinoma cell line 43

Zellballen (cell clusters) 21, 49
Zoo animals 192
Zuckerkandl organ 76